Childhood Obesity
Causes, Consequences, and Intervention Approaches

Childhood Obesity
Causes, Consequences, and Intervention Approaches

Edited by
Michael I. Goran

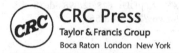

CRC Press
Taylor & Francis Group
Boca Raton London New York

CRC Press is an imprint of the
Taylor & Francis Group, an **informa** business

CRC Press
Taylor & Francis Group
6000 Broken Sound Parkway NW, Suite 300
Boca Raton, FL 33487-2742

First issued in paperback 2021

© 2017 by Taylor & Francis Group, LLC
CRC Press is an imprint of Taylor & Francis Group, an Informa business

No claim to original U.S. Government works

ISBN 13: 978-1-03-209759-6 (pbk)
ISBN 13: 978-1-4987-2065-6 (hbk)

Library of Congress Cataloging-in-Publication Data

Names: Goran, Michael I., editor.
Title: Childhood obesity : causes, consequences, and intervention approaches / editor, Michael I. Goran.
Other titles: Childhood obesity (Goran)
Description: Boca Raton : Taylor & Francis, 2017. | Includes bibliographical references and index.
Identifiers: LCCN 2016014566 | ISBN 9781498720656 (hardcover : alk. paper)
Subjects: | MESH: Pediatric Obesity | Child
Classification: LCC RJ206 | NLM WS 130 | DDC 618.92/398--dc23
LC record available at https://lccn.loc.gov/2016014566

**Visit the Taylor & Francis Web site at
http://www.taylorandfrancis.com**

**and the CRC Press Web site at
http://www.crcpress.com**

Dedication

This book is dedicated to all of my former students and fellows for their dedicated efforts pushing forward the science of childhood obesity and to my family for always being there with love and support.

Contents

SECTION I Epidemiology of Childhood Obesity in Different Populations

SECTION II Nutritional Factors Contributing to Childhood Obesity

SECTION III   Individual and Environmental Factors Contributing to and/or Associated with Childhood Obesity

SECTION IV Behavioral and Metabolic Consequences of Childhood Obesity

SECTION V Treatment and Prevention of Childhood Obesity

SECTION VI Public Health and Policy Based Interventions

Foreword

Childhood obesity is now the most prevalent chronic disease of children and adolescents in the United States. Over 17% of our youth have obesity, and the prevalence is greater among African Americans and Hispanics. Recent data indicate that obesity is declining in 2- to 5-year-old children, and has plateaued in older children and adolescents. Nonetheless, the high prevalence, natural history, and complications of obesity allow no room for complacency. In this context, the comprehensive overview provided by *Childhood Obesity: Causes, Consequences, and Intervention Approaches* is timely, and provides a useful opportunity to assess our progress in the control of the obesity epidemic.

As recently as 40 years ago, childhood obesity was barely recognized. The earliest prevalence data were provided by Stanley Garn, a physical anthropologist at the University of Michigan, writing for an ad hoc committee to review the Ten-State Nutrition Survey conducted between 1968 and 1970. The analyses relied on skinfold thicknesses, and the data were used to provide the first observations on the changes in fatness by age and gender across the life cycle.[1] At about the same time, Gil Forbes at the University of Rochester began to describe changes in body composition associated with obesity. As early as 1963, he noted the increase in fat-free mass[2] and height associated with childhood obesity.[3] Because obesity was not considered a significant problem, few treatment programs existed.

How times have changed. The increase in prevalence since the 1970s has been accompanied by an increase in severity and the recognition that childhood obesity is not a benign cosmetic condition. As with adults, multiple organ systems are affected. Furthermore, the natural history of childhood obesity indicates that it is a significant contributor to the prevalence of obesity in adults and may contribute disproportionately to severe adult obesity. Because few adults with obesity are able to achieve a healthy weight,[4] the prevention and successful treatment of childhood obesity must become a priority.

In many respects, we know more about prevention than we do about treatment. Early efforts by the Centers for Disease Control and Prevention documented the increases in the prevalence of childhood obesity, identified the earliest targets for prevention, and provided funding for state health departments to begin to implement strategies that focused on place-based policy and environmental changes. Schools and early care and education facilities became logical targets, insofar as those were locations where children spent substantial time, consumed substantial quantities of food, and had opportunities for physical activity. Successful changes in the food environment within schools have occurred as a consequence of an agreement between the American Heart Association, the Alliance for a Healthier Generation, and the American Beverage Association to reduce the availability of sugar drinks, as well as the changes in meals and competitive foods in schools mandated by the Healthy Hunger-Free Schools Act. Implementation and retention of physical education and other physical activity programs in schools have been less successful. Similar efforts to change the food and physical activity environments within early care and education facilities have just begun.

Clinical efforts for the treatment of obesity appear more fragmented. The United States Preventive Services Task Force has recommended comprehensive moderate-to-intensive behavioral interventions for weight loss, focused on diet and physical actvitiy.[5] Moderate intensity consists of 26–75 contact hours, and high intensity consists of more than 75 contact hours. However, the practical translation of this treatment to usual pediatric care presents a challenge. Because few insurance plans will reimburse such a program, its scalability is limited. Because few parents and patients can accommodate this time commitment, its efficacy is limited.

In the last 40 years, as our understanding of obesity has expanded, so has our appreciation of its complexity. The microbiome, epigenetics, toxins, obesogens, mobile health strategies, the role of the built environment, and systems thinking all testify to the rapid diversification of knowledge and interest in obesity and its solutions. *Childhood Obesity: Causes, Consequences, and Intervention Approaches* includes this information as well as expanding considerably on what we have learned about treatment and prevention. The challenges that lie ahead are how to integrate this information and whether this knowledge enhances our ability to prevent and treat obesity. In some cases, the issue is no longer about what to do but how to do it effectively.

One of the most important barriers that we must confront and resolve is the pervasive bias and stigma related to obesity. Despite its prevalence, obesity remains one of the most stigmatized conditions in the United States. One of the ways that we all can begin to address bias is to use people-first language. An obese person is an identity. A person with obesity is a person with a disease. Such terminology has political implications. An obese person is more likely to be blamed for his or her condition, whereas a person with obesity may be more likely to be viewed as a person in need of medical care and support.

William H. Dietz
Chair, Redstone Global Center for Prevention and Wellness
George Washington University

REFERENCES

1. Garn SM, Clark DC. Trends in fatness and the origins of obesity: Ad hoc committee to review the Ten-State Nutrition Survey. *Pediatrics* 1976;57:443–56.
2. Forbes GB. Lean body mass and fat in obese children. *Pediatrics* 1964;34:308–14.
3. Forbes GB. Nutrition and growth. *J Pediatr* 1977;91:40–2.
4. Fildes A, Charlton J, Rudisill C, Littlejohns P, Prevost AT, Gulliford MC. Probability of an obese person attaining normal body weight: Cohort study using electronic health records. *Am J Public Health* 2015;105:e1–6.
5. Whitlock EP, O'Connor EA, Williams SB, Beil TL, Lutz KW. Effectiveness of weight management interventions in children: A targeted systematic review for the USPSTF. *Pediatrics* 2010;125:e396–418.

Editor

Michael I. Goran is professor of preventive medicine and pediatrics in the Keck School of Medicine at the University of Southern California in Los Angeles. He is the founding director of the University of Southern California Childhood Obesity Research Center and holds the Dr. Robert C. and Veronica Atkins Endowed Chair in Childhood Obesity and Diabetes. Dr. Goran also serves as codirector of the University of Southern California Diabetes and Obesity Research Institute. Dr. Goran is a native of Glasgow, Scotland, and received his PhD from the University of Manchester, England (1986), prior to postdoctoral training in the United States (1987–1991). He previously served on the Faculty of Medicine at the University of Vermont (1991–94) and the Department of Nutrition Sciences at the University of Alabama at Birmingham (1994–99), prior to joining the University of Southern California in 1999. For the past 30 years, Dr. Goran's research program has focused on the causes and consequences of childhood obesity. His work is focused on understanding the metabolic factors linking obesity to increased disease risk during growth and development and using this information as a basis for developing new behavioral and community approaches for prevention and risk reduction. He is also especially interested in ethnic disparities in obesity and obesity-related diseases, with a special interest in the effects of dietary sugar on obesity and metabolic diseases among Hispanic populations. His research has been continuously funded by the National Institutes of Health since 1991 and he has published over 300 professional peer-reviewed articles and reviews. He is the coeditor of the *Handbook of Pediatric Obesity*, published in 2006, coeditor of *Dietary Sugars and Health*, published in late 2014, and serves as editor-in-chief for *Pediatric Obesity*. He has been the recipient of a number of scientific awards for his research and teaching, including the Nutrition Society Medal for Research (1996), the Lilly Award for Scientific Achievement from the Obesity Society (2006), the Bar-Or Award for Excellence in Pediatric Obesity Research from the Obesity Society (2009), and the TOPS Research Achievement Award from the Obesity Society (2014). Full details on Dr. Goran's research can be found on his website at www.GoranLab.com. Outside of work, Michael is an avid tennis player, and enjoys cooking, eating, and traveling with his family.

Contributors

Jonathan A. Africa
Department of Pediatrics
University of California San Diego
San Diego, California
and
Department of Pediatric Gastroenterology
Rady Children's Hospital
San Diego, California

P. Babu Balagopal
Nemours Children's Specialty Care
and
Mayo Clinic College of Medicine
Jacksonville, Florida

Katherine N. Balantekin
Department of Psychiatry
Washington University School of Medicine
St. Louis, Missouri

Andrew James Beamish
Department of Research
Royal College of Surgeons of England
London, United Kingdom
and
Department of Gastrosurgical Research
Gothenburg University
Gothenburg, Sweden

Brooke Bell
Department of Preventive Medicine
University of Southern California
Los Angeles, California

Paige K. Berger
Department of Foods and Nutrition
University of Georgia
Athens, Georgia

Regien Biesma
Department of Epidemiology and Public Health
  Medicine
Royal College of Surgeons in Ireland
Dublin, Ireland

Leann L. Birch
Department of Foods and Nutrition
University of Georgia
Athens, Georgia

Stacy A. Blondin
Tufts University Friedman School of Nutrition
  Science and Policy
Boston, Massachusetts

Bruce Blumberg
Departments of Developmental and Cell
  Biology and Pharmaceutical Sciences
University of California
Irvine, California

Kerri N. Boutelle
Departments of Pediatrics and Psychiatry
University of California San Diego
San Diego, California

Helen Budge
School of Medicine
University of Nottingham
Nottingham, United Kingdom

Sonia Caprio
Department of Pediatrics
Yale University
New Haven, Connecticut

Katelyn A. Carr
Jacobs School of Medicine and Biomedical
  Sciences
Department of Pediatrics
University at Buffalo
Buffalo, New York

John Cawley
Departments of Policy Analysis and
  Management and Economics
Cornell University
Ithaca, New York

Deborah A. Cohen
RAND Corporation
Santa Monica, California

Noe C. Crespo
School of Nutrition and Health Promotion
College of Health Solutions
Arizona State University
Phoenix, Arizona

Tinuke Oluyomi Daniel
Department of Pediatrics
Jacobs School of Medicine and Biomedical Sciences
University at Buffalo
Buffalo, New York

Adam C. Danley
College of Medicine
Florida State University
Tallahassee, Florida

Ashlesha Datar
Center for Economic and Social Research
University of Southern California
Los Angeles, California

Terry L. Davidson
Center for Behavioral Neuroscience
and
Department of Psychology
American University
Washington, DC

Kayla de la Haye
Department of Preventive Medicine
Keck School of Medicine
University of Southern California
Los Angeles, California

William H. Dietz
Sumner M. Redstone Global Center for
    Prevention and Wellness
George Washington University
Washington, DC

Genevieve Fridlund Dunton
Department of Preventive Medicine and
    Psychology
Keck School of Medicine
University of Southern California
Los Angeles, California

Cara B. Ebbeling
New Balance Foundation Obesity Prevention
    Center
Division of Endocrinology
Boston Children's Hospital
Boston, Massachusetts

Christina D. Economos
Tufts University Friedman School of Nutrition
    Science and Policy
Boston, Massachusetts

John P. Elder
San Diego State University
and
Reducing Cancer Disparities Program
University of California, San Diego
San Diego, California

Leonard H. Epstein
Department of Pediatrics
Jacobs School of Medicine and Biomedical
    Sciences
University at Buffalo
Buffalo, New York

Myles S. Faith
Department of Counseling, School, and
    Educational Psychology
University at Buffalo
Buffalo, New York

Emily B. Ferris
Graduate School of Public Health and Health
    Policy
City University of New York
New York

David A. Fields
Department of Pediatrics
University of Oklahoma Health Sciences
    Center
Oklahoma City, Oklahoma

Alison E. Field
Department of Epidemiology
Brown University School of Public Health
Providence, Rhode Island

Jennifer O. Fisher
Temple University
Philadelphia, Pennsylvania

Jacob E. Friedman
Department of Pediatrics (Neonatology),
    Biochemistry, and Molecular Genetics
University of Colorado School of Medicine
Anschutz Medical Center
Aurora, Colorado

Ovidiu A. Galescu
Division of Translational Medicine
Eunice Kennedy Shriver National Institute of
    Child Health and Human Development
National Institutes of Health
Bethesda, Maryland

Dympna Gallagher
Department of Medicine
and
New York Obesity Research Center
Columbia University Medical Center
New York

Keith M. Godfrey
MRC Lifecourse Epidemiology Unit
University of Southampton
Southampton, United Kingdom

Michael I. Goran
Department of Preventive Medicine
Diabetes and Obesity Research Institute
Keck School of Medicine
University of Southern California
Los Angeles, California

Struan F.A. Grant
Department of Pediatrics
University of Pennsylvania School of
    Medicine
Philadelphia, Pennsylvania

Bernard Gutin
Department of Pediatrics and Physiology
Medical College of Georgia
Augusta, Georgia

Patrick C. Hanley
Division of Endocrinology and Diabetes
Children's Hospital of Philadelphia
Philadelphia, Pennsylvania

Mark Hanson
Institute of Developmental Sciences
and
NIHR Nutrition Biomedical Research Centre
University of Southampton
Southampton, United Kingdom

Sara L. Hargrave
Center for Behavioral Neuroscience and
    Department of Psychology
American University
Washington, DC

Andrew J. Hill
Academic Unit of Psychiatry and Behavioural
    Sciences
Leeds University School of Medicine
Leeds, United Kingdom

Terry T.-K. Huang
Graduate School of Public Health and Health
    Policy
City University of New York
New York, New York

Kathleen L. Keller
Pennsylvania State University, University Park,
    Pennsylvania

Jennifer Kelley
Department of Pediatrics
Vanderbilt University
Nashville, Tennessee

Tanja V. Kral
University of Pennsylvania, Philadelphia,
    Pennsylvania

Melissa Gallagher Landry
New Balance Foundation Obesity Prevention
    Center
Division of Endocrinology
Boston Children's Hospital
Boston, Massachusetts

Karen A. Lillycrop
Centre for Biological Sciences
University of Southampton
Southampton, United Kingdom

Yun Liu
Department of Nutritional Sciences
University of Michigan School of Public
    Health
Ann Arbor, Michigan

Tim Lobstein
World Obesity Federation
London, United Kingdom

Ashley A. Martin
Department of Preventive Medicine
Childhood Obesity Research Center
University of Southern California
Los Angeles, California

Shana E. McCormack
Department of Pediatrics
University of Pennsylvania School of
    Medicine
Philadelphia, Pennsylvania

Sara D. McMullin
Department of Psychiatry
Washington University School of Medicine
St. Louis, Missouri

Christopher Mulligan
Department of Pediatrics, Section of
    Nutrition
University of Colorado School of Medicine
Anschutz Medical Center
Aurora, Colorado

Robert Murray
Institute of Developmental Sciences
Academic Unit of Human Development and
    Health
University of Southampton
Southampton General Hospital
Southampton, United Kingdom

Kimberly P. Newton
Department of Pediatrics
University of California San Diego
San Diego, California
and
Department of Pediatric Gastroenterology
Rady Children's Hospital
San Diego, California

Sydney G. O'Connor
Department of Preventive Medicine
Keck School of Medicine
University of Southern California
Los Angeles, California

Shalini Ojha
Academic Division of Child Health, Obstetrics
    and Gynaecology
School of Medicine
Queen's Medical Centre
University of Nottingham
Nottingham, United Kingdom

Torsten Olbers
Department of Gastrosurgical Research
Gothenburg University
Gothenburg, Sweden

Micah L. Olson
Division of Endocrinology and Diabetes
Phoenix Children's Hospital
Phoenix, Arizona

Scott Owens
Department of Exercise Science
University of Mississippi
Oxford, Mississippi

Kathleen A. Page
Department of Internal Medicine, Division of
    Endocrinology
Diabetes and Obesity Research Institute
Keck School of Medicine
University of Southern California
Los Angeles, California

Karen E. Peterson
Department of Nutritional Sciences
University of Michigan School of Public
    Health
Ann Arbor, Michigan

Suzanne Phelan
Department of Kinesiology
California Polytechnic State University
San Luis Obispo, California

Susan Redline
Department of Medicine
Brigham and Women's Hospital
Beth Israel Deaconess Medical Center
Harvard Medical School
Boston, Massachusetts

Kyung E. Rhee
Department of Pediatrics
University of California San Diego
Rady Children's Hospital
San Diego, California

Kristie R. Ross
Department of Pediatrics
Rainbow Babies and Children's Hospital
Case Western Reserve University
Cleveland, Ohio

Sani M. Roy
Division of Endocrinology and Diabetes
Children's Hospital of Philadelphia
Philadelphia, Pennsylvania

Sarah-Jeanne Salvy
Mrs. T.H. Chan Division of Occupational
    Science and Occupational Therapy
Herman Ostrow School of Dentistry
University of Southern California
Los Angeles, California

Nicola Santoro
Department of Pediatrics
Yale University
New Haven, Connecticut

Jeffrey B. Schwimmer
Department of Pediatrics
University of California San Diego
Rady Children's Hospital
San Diego, California

Gabriel Q. Shaibi
Center for Health Promotion and Disease
    Prevention
College of Nursing and Health Innovation
Arizona State University
Phoenix, Arizona

Eleanor T. Shonkoff
Gerald J. and Dorothy R. Friedman School of
    Nutrition Science and Policy
Tufts University
Boston, Massachusetts

Bassem M. Shoucri
Department of Developmental and Cell
    Biology
University of California
Irvine, California

Alanna Soupen
School of Population Health
University of Auckland
Auckland, New Zealand

Donna Spruijt-Metz
Center for Economic and Social
    Research
Departments of Psychology and
    Preventive Medicine
University of Southern California
Los Angeles, California

Boyd Swinburn
School of Population Health
University of Auckland
Auckland, New Zealand

Michael E. Symonds
School of Medicine
Queen's Medical Centre
University Hospital
University of Nottingham
Nottingham, United Kingdom

Claudia M. Toledo-Corral
Department of Public Health
Rongxiang Xu College of Health and Human
    Services
California State University, Los Angeles
Los Angeles, California

Hillary Tolley
School of Population Health
University of Auckland
Auckland, New Zealand

Dorothy J. Van Buren
Department of Psychiatry
Washington University School of
Medicine
St. Louis, Missouri

Stefanie Vandevijvere
School of Population Health
University of Auckland
Auckland, New Zealand

Alison K. Ventura
Department of Kinesiology
California Polytechnic State University
San Luis Obispo, California

Youfa Wang
Department of Epidemiology and
Environmental Health
University at Buffalo
Buffalo, New York

Marc J. Weigensberg
Department of Pediatrics
Keck School of Medicine
University of Southern California
and
USC Institute for Integrative Health
Los Angeles, California

Elizabeth M. Widen
Departments of Medicine and Epidemiology
Institute of Human Nutrition
New York Obesity Research Center
Columbia University Medical Center
New York, New York

Cheng K. Fred Wen
Department of Preventive Medicine
University of Southern California
Los Angeles, California

Denise E. Wilfley
Department of Psychiatry
Washington University School of Medicine
St. Louis, Missouri

Jack A. Yanovski
Division of Translational Medicine
Eunice Kennedy Shriver National Institute of
Child Health and Human Development
National Institutes of Health
Bethesda, Maryland

Elizabeth L. Yu
Department of Pediatrics
University of California San Diego
Rady Children's Hospital
San Diego, California

Section I

Epidemiology of Childhood
Obesity in Different Populations

1 Epidemiology of Childhood Obesity and Associated Risk Factors

An Overview

Alison E. Field

CONTENTS

INTRODUCTION

Obesity is the most prevalent chronic health condition in children, thereby it is a major public health concern. Between the 1960s and 2012, there was an almost fourfold increase in the prevalence of overweight and obesity among both children and adolescents in the United States.[1,2] According to the 2011–2012 National Health and Nutrition Examination Survey (NHANES), approximately 34% of children and 35% of adolescents are overweight or obese.[2] Trends in preschool-age children have been slightly different. Although there has been a substantial increase in the prevalence of obesity, from less than 4% of preschool-age children in NHANES I (1971–1974) to more than 7% in 2011–2012, rates are now decreasing among preschool-age children, but continue to increase among adolescents.[3] Between 2003–2004 and 2011–2012, the prevalence of obesity among two- to five-year-old children decreased from 13.9% to 8.4%;[2] however, this decline is not seen in all subgroups. There are considerable racial and ethnic disparities in the prevalence of obesity among two- to five-year-olds. The rates are highest among Hispanics (15.2% among females, 18% among males) and African Americans (13.9% among females, 9.0% among males) and lowest among non-Hispanic whites (0.6% among females, 6.3% among males).[2]

DEFINITIONS AND AGE DIFFERENCES

Unlike adults, children should gain both weight and height due to growth. Therefore, rather than a single cutoff to demarcate overweight or obesity, age and gender-specific cutoffs are used. In the United States, most clinicians and researchers use the Centers for Disease Control and Prevention

(CDC) percentile cutoffs to define weight status. Youth with a body mass index (BMI) ≥85th percentile for age and gender are considered overweight and those with a BMI >95th percentile are considered obese. The standards used to determine percentiles come from the National Health and Examination Surveys. An alternative approach for defining obesity was developed by the International Obesity Taskforce (IOTF). Using data from six countries (Brazil, Great Britain, Hong Kong, the Netherlands, Singapore, and the United States), the taskforce determined the age and gender-specific cutoff point that best predicted having a BMI ≥25 (overweight) or ≤30 (obese) at age 18.[4] Until midadolescence, the CDC and IOTF approaches identified similar cutoffs. However, the CDC cutoffs classify some 17–20-years-olds with a BMI ≥25 as being in the healthy weight range because the 85th percentile of BMI among older adolescents is above 25 kg/m². It is therefore advisable that if using the CDC cutoffs, one should revise the algorithm to make sure that all youth with a BMI between 25 and 29.9 are classified as overweight, irrespective of their BMI percentile. Regardless of which BMI classification is used, it is important to remember that relying on BMI to classify people results in some error. Since BMI does not distinguish between muscle and fat and muscle weighs more than fat, people who are highly active and muscular may have a high BMI despite low body fat. Moreover, puberty is associated with hormonal and body composition changes. Puberty causes females to increase their weight and body fat, whereas males increase their weight and lean mass. Therefore, BMI may misclassify more postpubertal males than females.

In the 1960s, the prevalence of obesity was approximately 5% in both children (6–11 years) and adolescents of both genders. As of 2011–2012, obesity is now more common among adolescents (20.3% among males, 20.7% among females) than children (16.4% among males, 19.1% among females). The patterns among preschool-age children are more complex. In the 1980s and 1990s, the prevalence of obesity increased among preschool-age females, but not males. However, the prevalence in 2011–2012 is higher among males (9.5%) than females (7.8%). It is unclear what explains this gender difference in prevalence over time.

RACE/ETHNIC GROUP DIFFERENCES

There are large differences in the prevalence of obesity across race/ethnic groups in the United States. Currently, Asian female children and adolescents have the lowest rate of obesity and Hispanic males have the highest prevalence of obesity.[2] Although it should be noted that obesity rates are higher among some subpopulations of Asians (i.e., those from Korea and India). Research documenting differences among Hispanics of different origins (i.e., from Mexico vs. Puerto Rico) is lacking. In the 1960s, obesity rates were higher among white (14.4%) than black (9.3%) adolescent males. Among the adolescent females, whites (8.3%) and Hispanics (8.7%) had similar prevalence of obesity, which was lower than the prevalence among black females (14.4%). The issue of race/ethnic differences is described in more depth in Chapter 2.

Race and ethnic differences in obesity may reflect differences in rates of poverty and living in economically depressed neighborhoods. Although the results of studies examining the associations between socioeconomic status (SES) and obesity in youth are mixed,[5,6] studies focusing on neighborhood or community-level indicators of economic deprivation and hardship have had more consistent findings. For example, among fifth-, seventh-, and ninth-grade schoolchildren living in Los Angeles County, the prevalence of obesity was approximately 27% among those from the highest quartile of community economic hardship, but only 12.5% among those from the lowest quartile.[7] Moreover, using the 2001–2010 NHANES data, Rossen found that after controlling for levels of neighborhood deprivation, African American youth were no longer significantly more likely to be obese.[8] The reduction in association was not completely due to differences in SES since she found that higher SES was only protective for youth living in areas with low levels of neighborhood deprivation. These results suggest that African American youth are more likely than white youth from a similar SES to live in high deprivation communities with minimal resources.

RISK FACTORS

Despite a plethora of studies, relatively few factors have consistently been prospectively linked to the development of overweight or obesity. This reflects several issues. First, except for factors that do not change over time, such as race, one cannot draw any inference from cross-sectional studies. Second, many prospective studies measured dietary intake and physical activity using methods with considerable error. Third, many prospective studies using state-of-the-art diet and activity assessments are relatively small and underpowered. Fourth, obesity is a heterogeneous condition and it is unlikely that more than a few factors are risk factors for all types of obesity. Therefore, analyses predicting overall obesity may end up obscuring risk factors that are not associated with all types of obesity.

DIETARY INTAKE

It is widely accepted that dietary intake must be related to weight gain and the development of obesity. However, other than sugar-sweetened beverages and fast food,[9,10] few dietary factors have been consistently linked to obesity and the complications of obesity. A brief overview of the important findings and issues is presented here, and more details of other specific dietary contributions relevant to child obesity are covered in Chapters 6 through 11. Although there are numerous cross-sectional studies on associations between dietary intake and obesity, one cannot draw any inference on the temporal order of the association or whether the diet before the person became overweight was the same as the current diet. Thus, one must rely on prospective observational studies and clinical trials to understand how dietary intake is related to the development of obesity.

Some studies, primarily in adults, have suggested that dietary fat is predictive of weight gain and obesity, but most have not controlled for total calories. It is therefore unclear whether the association is due to fat *per se* or the fact that there are more calories per gram of fat than protein or carbohydrate. The results for low-glycemic load diets are also mixed.[11,12] There have been few clinical trials and the results have not consistently observed that a low-fat or low-glycemic load diet is superior to other dietary strategies for weight control in children or youth.[12,13]

Although it is widely believed that increasing fruit and vegetable intake should protect against weight gain and the development of obesity, there is little empirical support for a protective effect. Vegetable consumption was unrelated to weight gain among elementary schoolchildren[14] and adolescent girls in the National Growth and Health Study[15] or the Growing Up Today Study,[16] as well as among adult women in the Women's Health Study.[17] The results have been more mixed for fruit intake, with some studies finding a protective effect[15,17] and others finding no association.[16] There are several possible reasons for the lack of a consistent protective effect. First, children may need to consume high levels of fruits and vegetables for it to have a clinically meaningful effect on limiting weight gain, but few children eat a sufficient quantity to have an effect. Second, youth are adding more fruits and vegetables to their diet rather than substituting them for less healthy foods, and thus fruit and vegetable intake might be positively related to total caloric intake. Third, youth may be consuming their fruits and vegetables in high calorie preparations. For example, salads with cheese, lots of salad dressing, and bread products (i.e., croutons, tortilla strips, etc.). Fourth, fruits and vegetables may be part of a heart-healthy diet but unrelated to weight change.

It is possible that few dietary predictors of obesity have been identified because there have been relatively few large prospective studies of children or youth and there has been considerable measurement error in diet assessment methods used in those studies. A further complicating factor is that dietary intake is related to both normal growth and development and obesity during childhood and adolescence, thus making it particularly difficult to identify dietary predictors of excessive weight gain in youth.

DISORDERED EATING

As many as 24.7% of female and 8.3% of male youth report having eating episodes where they felt like they could not stop eating, even if they wanted to stop.[18] These episodes are described as loss of control (LOC) eating. If the amount of food consumed is large in a short amount of time, the episodes are considered eating binges. In both children[19] and adolescents,[20] LOC and binge eating are robust predictors of weight gain and the development of obesity. Among adults in weight loss trials, eating binges tend to reduce in frequency as weight is lost. This association has not been studied in children or adolescence.

The definition of binge eating, which requires LOC episodes where a large amount of food, larger than most people would eat in similar circumstances, is consumed in a short amount of time, makes it a difficult topic to study in adolescent males. Since adolescent males tend to eat very large quantities of food, it is hard to define what is abnormally large. Thus, there is likely considerable misclassification in observation studies of binge eating, which could bias the results toward the null.

Many cross-sectional studies have reported higher rates of emotional eating and eating in the absence of hunger among overweight and obese youth, but these associations have not been studied prospectively. However, self-reports of dieting to control weight have been found to predict BMI gain in both children[21] and adolescents.[22] Dieting is associated with binge eating and higher BMI z-scores, but the association with BMI change is independent of both these factors. It should be noted that self-reports of dieting do not necessarily mean that the individual is making a meaningful reduction in energy intake, rather it should be thought of as a proxy for concern with weight and taking some action to control weight.

PHYSICAL ACTIVITY

Although increasing physical activity is a public health goal and included in many obesity prevention interventions, there is a surprising lack of empirical support for activity protecting against weight gain. An exception would be the International Study of Childhood Obesity, Lifestyle and the Environment (ISCOLE), which found that high levels of moderate and vigorous physical activity were strongly inversely related to obesity.[23] However, data from prospective studies found a much smaller effect of activity on prevention of weight gain. Among adults it is generally found that activity is necessary for weight loss maintenance. A very high volume is needed to prevent weight gain in adults.[24] Most youth decrease their activity level as they age and interventions have had limited success at increasing activity.[25] Both the Pathways Study[26] and the Trial of Activity for Adolescent Girls[25] found that increases in activity predicted lower percentage of body fat at follow-up, but not BMI change or incidence of overweight and obesity. It is possible that the lack of protection against BMI gain and the development of obesity is due to insufficient volume of activity. An alternative explanation is that physical activity may result in decreases in fat mass/increase in lean mass but no change in weight. Since BMI cannot distinguish between lean and fat mass it is a suboptimal outcome measure to employ in studies examining the impact of physical activity. In addition, there is considerable measurement error in many of the activity assessments, other than accelerometers and other methods that directly measure activity, that would make it more difficult to observe a protective association with physical activity. For more details on the role of physical activity interventions to treat or prevent childhood obesity, see Chapter 35.

ENVIRONMENT

In the past decade, there has been a growing interest in the impact of the neighborhood and school environment on obesity and obesity risk behaviors. The built environment refers to man-made structures (including fast-food outlets, street design, etc.), green spaces, and parks. Most of the research on the impact of the environment has focused on the toxic food environment, road connectivity, the presence of sidewalks, and green space. More recently, there has been recognition that the social environment can also influence behaviors. The results have not been consistent, but the results do suggest a small impact of the built environment.[27,28] Many cross-sectional studies have examined how residential density, distance to or number of parks and green space or food outlets, and street connectivity are related to diet, physical activity, and obesity in youth. One of the largest cross-sectional studies examined associations among 122,118 youth in the United States and found that BMI percentile was positively associated with the number of fast-food outlets and grocery stores and inversely related to the number of parks and fitness centers.[29] However, one needs to be cautious when interpreting cross-sectional studies on the built environment since BMI is inversely related to SES and SES is positively related to more green space. Unfortunately, there have been relatively few prospective studies. However, Epstein et al. studied children who had been in one of four randomized trials for weight loss. They found that few supermarkets and greater parkland were predictive of bigger losses in BMI z-score at 24 months regardless of clinical trials in which they had participated.[30] Another small prospective study found that greenness, but not residential density, was predictive of changes in BMI z-score.[31]

The studies on relationships with food outlets are more mixed. Studies have observed inverse cross-sectional associations between obesity and the number of or proximity to fast-food outlets[32–34] and convenience stores.[32,34] Although it was initially thought that more large grocery stores, rather than bodegas and convenience stores, were needed in urban environments with high obesity rates, recent studies have found that the closer a child lives to a large grocery store, the higher his or her BMI will be.[35] Unfortunately, relatively few prospective studies have been conducted. However, one prospective study of 353 adolescent females found that having a convenience store within a 0.25 mile buffer of their residence predicted higher odds of being overweight or obese at the 3-year follow-up and a greater increase in BMI.[36] Most studies have examined the impact of the neighborhood environment, but among adolescents, the environment around their schools may be at least as important as the environment where they live. However, it has been much less studied.

As of 2015, three-quarters of 13- to 17-year-olds reported having or having access to a smartphone.[37] Since smartphones are equipped with global positioning system (GPS) technology, future studies of the built environment will be able to use individual-level GPS information to more accurately classify built environment exposures of adolescents and will allow for testing assumptions about the relative distance from home or school that exert an influence on youth behaviors. For further information on the role of the built environment in childhood obesity, see Chapter 17.

SEDENTARY TIME

Time spent engaged in sedentary behaviors, particularly watching television, is the most robust behavior predictor of weight gain and the development of obesity.[38] Children with televisions in their bedroom not surprisingly have been found to watch more television[39] and gain more weight. Numerous epidemiologic studies have found that the more time a child or adolescent spends watching television, the more weight he or she gains and the more likely he or she is to become obese.[40,41] Several different mechanisms have been proposed for this association, but it does not seem to be due to television time replacing time spent being active. In both epidemiologic and clinical studies, decreases in television viewing, regardless of whether they are coupled with increases in physical activity, are predictive of less weight gain or weight loss.[42]

The mechanism with the strongest empirical support is that the advertisements on television, which are mostly for foods high in sugar and fat and low in nutritional value, cue people to eat while watching television regardless of whether they are hungry.[43] They are also cued to eat these advertised foods at later times as well. Falbe et al. found that among adolescents, increases in screen time, particularly television time, predicted increases in intake of fast food, sugar-sweetened beverages, and salty snack foods.[44] The findings are even stronger among younger children. Nickelodeon, the Cartoon Network, and Disney (until 2015) channels, which are very popular with children and adolescents, show many advertisements for fast food, sugar-sweetened beverages, and sugary cereals. In fact, Nickelodeon and the Cartoon Network have partnerships with food and beverage companies, such as the Burger King Corporation and PepsiCo. Thus, it is not surprising that more than 70% of the food advertisements on Nickelodeon are for fast food.[45] The advertising pays off for these companies. Robinson et al. asked 63 preschool-age children to taste five sets of identical foods, one in McDonald's packaging and the same food in unbranded food packaging. The children were asked which one tasted better or if they tasted the same. Despite being the exact same food, such as carrots, the item in the McDonald's packing was perceived as tasting better.[46] Thus, the children had been taught that foods from McDonald's are desirable. For more information on the role of advertising and marketing in childhood obesity, see Chapter 42.

SLEEP

Children who sleep less have been found to consume more calories[47] and gain more weight than their peers who get more hours of sleep.[48–50] The associations with sleep are observed at multiple ages in childhood. For example, Gillman et al. found that infants who slept less than the recommended 12 h per day were almost two times more likely to be overweight at age 3.[49] Moreover, the gain is in fat mass, not lean mass.[51] Among adolescents, reasons for suboptimal sleep duration include screen time,[52] being woken by a cell phone,[53] and early start time for high school. The issue of sleep and childhood obesity is covered in more detail in Chapter 28.

CONCLUSION

During the past several decades, obesity rates in the United States have increased dramatically among youth, but the rates are now declining slightly among preschool-age children. It remains to be seen whether the decline among preschool-age children and the plateauing among 6- to 11-year-olds is a real change or just part of the natural fluctuation in rates. The still increasing rates among older youth are a cause for concern, as are the racial, ethnic, and neighborhood-characteristic disparities in obesity. Although it is widely accepted that genetics, dietary intake, physical activity, and screen time all contribute to the risk of excessive weight gain and the development of obesity, relatively few risk factors have been consistently identified across studies. There are several reasons for the lack of robust predictors. To study associations with factors that change over time, such as dietary intake, physical activity, sleep patterns, and screen time, one needs prospective data from clinical trials or observational studies. Unfortunately, the majority of the published papers on factors associated with childhood obesity have used a cross-sectional design. Moreover, until recently, many studies used self-report measures of dietary intake and physical activity that had considerable measurement error, thus making it harder to identify associations. Another reason for the lack of identifying robust predictors of obesity is that in children one must disentangle healthy from unhealthy weight gain, which is very difficult, particularly since dietary intake can promote both healthy and unhealthy weight gain.

The next generation of epidemiologic research on pediatric obesity should include the use of new technology that will allow for precise measures of the environment, dietary intake, and physical activity. The inclusion of electronic medical information would also greatly enhance studies. Some of these methods have been developed, but many more will need to be developed and validated for use in epidemiologic samples. Future studies should also be advised to consider obesity as a heterogeneous disease and to identify risk factors for subtypes of obesity.

REFERENCES

1. Troiano RP, Flegal KM, Kuczmarski RJ, Campbell SM, Johnson CL. Overweight prevalence and trends for children and adolescents: The National Health and Nutrition Examination Surveys, 1963 to 1991. *Arch Pediatr Adolesc Med*. 1995;149(10):1085–1091.
2. Ogden CL, Carroll MD, Kit BK, Flegal KM. Prevalence of childhood and adult obesity in the United States, 2011–2012. *JAMA*. 2014;311(8):806–814.
3. Skinner AC, Skelton JA. Prevalence and trends in obesity and severe obesity among children in the United States, 1999–2012. *JAMA Pediatr*. 2014;168(6):561–566.

4. Cole TJ, Bellizzi MC, Flegal KM, Dietz WH. Establishing a standard definition for child overweight and obesity worldwide: International survey. *BMJ*. 2000;320(7244):1240–1243.

5. Wang YF, Zhang Q. Are American children and adolescents of low socioeconomic status at increased risk of obesity? Changes in the association between overweight and family income between 1971 and 2002. *Am J Clin Nutr*. 2006;84(4):707–716.

6. Gordon-Larsen P, Adair LS, Popkin BM. The relationship of ethnicity, socioeconomic factors, and overweight in US adolescents. *Obes Res*. 2003;11(1):121–129.

7. Shih M, Dumke KA, Goran MI, Simon PA. The association between community-level economic hardship and childhood obesity prevalence in Los Angeles. *Pediatr Obes*. 2013;8(6):411–417.

8. Rossen LM. Neighbourhood economic deprivation explains racial/ethnic disparities in overweight and obesity among children and adolescents in the USA. *J Epidemiol Community Health*. 2014;68(2):123–129.

9. Pereira MA, Kartashov AI, Ebbeling CB, et al. Fast-food habits, weight gain, and insulin resistance (the CARDIA study): 15-year prospective analysis. *Lancet*. 2005;365(9453):36–42.

10. Ebbeling CB, Feldman HA, Chomitz VR, et al. A randomized trial of sugar-sweetened beverages and adolescent body weight. *N Engl J Med*. 2012;367(15):1407–1416.

11. Spieth LE, Harnish JD, Lenders CM, et al. A low-glycemic index diet in the treatment of pediatric obesity. *Arch Pediatr Adolesc Med*. 2000;154(9):947–951.

12. Mirza NM, Palmer MG, Sinclair KB, et al. Effects of a low glycemic load or a low-fat dietary intervention on body weight in obese Hispanic American children and adolescents: A randomized controlled trial. *Am J Clin Nutr*. 2013;97(2):276–285.

13. Demol S, Yackobovitch-Gavan M, Shalitin S, Nagelberg N, Gillon-Keren M, Phillip M. Low-carbohydrate (low & high-fat) versus high-carbohydrate low-fat diets in the treatment of obesity in adolescents. *Acta Paediatr*. 2009;98(2):346–351.

14. Bayer O, Nehring I, Bolte G, von Kries R. Fruit and vegetable consumption and BMI change in primary school-age children: A cohort study. *Eur J Clin Nutr*. 2014;68(2):265–270.

15. Berz JP, Singer MR, Guo X, Daniels SR, Moore LL. Use of a DASH food group score to predict excess weight gain in adolescent girls in the National Growth and Health Study. *Arch Pediatr Adolesc Med*. 2011;165(6):540–546.

16. Field AE, Gillman MW, Rosner B, Rockett HR, Colditz GA. Association between fruit and vegetable intake and change in body mass index among a large sample of children and adolescents in the United States. *Int J Obes Relat Metab Disord*. 2003;27(7):821–826.

17. Rautiainen S, Wang L, Lee IM, Manson JE, Buring JE, Sesso HD. Higher intake of fruit, but not vegetables or fiber, at baseline is associated with lower risk of becoming overweight or obese in middle-aged and older women of normal BMI at baseline. *J Nutr*. 2015;145(5):960–968.

18. Mond J, Hall A, Bentley C, Harrison C, Gratwick-Sarll K, Lewis V. Eating-disordered behavior in adolescent boys: Eating disorder examination questionnaire norms. *Int J Eat Disord*. 2014;47(4):335–341.

19. Tanofsky-Kraff M, Yanovski SZ, Schvey NA, Olsen CH, Gustafson J, Yanovski JA. A prospective study of loss of control eating for body weight gain in children at high risk for adult obesity. *Int J Eat Disord*. 2009;42(1):26–30.

20. Field AE, Sonneville KR, Micali N, et al. Prospective association of common eating disorders and adverse outcomes. *Pediatrics*. 2012;130(2):e289–295.

21. Tanofsky-Kraff M, Cohen ML, Yanovski SZ, et al. A prospective study of psychological predictors of body fat gain among children at high risk for adult obesity. *Pediatrics*. 2006;117(4):1203–1209.

22. Field AE, Austin SB, Taylor CB, et al. Relation between dieting and weight change among preadolescents and adolescents. *Pediatrics*. 2003;112(4):900–906.

23. Katzmarzyk PT, Barreira TV, Broyles ST, et al. Relationship between lifestyle behaviors and obesity in children ages 9–11: Results from a 12-country study. *Obesity (Silver Spring)*. 2015;23(8):1696–1702.

24. Mekary RA, Feskanich D, Malspeis S, Hu FB, Willett WC, Field AE. Physical activity patterns and prevention of weight gain in premenopausal women. *Int J Obes (Lond)*. 2009;33(9):1039–1047.

25. Stevens J, Murray DM, Baggett CD, et al. Objectively assessed associations between physical activity and body composition in middle-school girls: The trial of activity for adolescent girls. *Am J Epidemiol*. 2007;166(11):1298–1305.

26. Stevens J, Suchindran C, Ring K, et al. Physical activity as a predictor of body composition in American Indian children. *Obes Res*. 2004;12(12):1974–1980.

27. Duncan DT, Castro MC, Gortmaker SL, Aldstadt J, Melly SJ, Bennett GG. Racial differences in the built environment—Body mass index relationship? A geospatial analysis of adolescents in urban neighborhoods. *Int J Health Geogr*. 2012;11:11.

28. Gilliland JA, Rangel CY, Healy MA, et al. Linking childhood obesity to the built environment: A multi-level analysis of home and school neighbourhood factors associated with body mass index. *Can J Public Health*. 2012;103(9 Suppl 3):eS15–21.

29. Wasserman JA, Suminski R, Xi J, Mayfield C, Glaros A, Magie R. A multi-level analysis showing associations between school neighborhood and child body mass index. *Int J Obes (Lond)*. 2014;38(7):912–918.

30. Epstein LH, Raja S, Daniel TO, et al. The built environment moderates effects of family-based childhood obesity treatment over 2 years. *Ann Behav Med*. 2012;44(2):248–258.

31. Bell JF, Wilson JS, Liu GC. Neighborhood greenness and 2-year changes in body mass index of children and youth. *Am J Prev Med*. 2008;35(6):547–553.

32. Laska MN, Hearst MO, Forsyth A, Pasch KE, Lytle L. Neighbourhood food environments: Are they associated with adolescent dietary intake, food purchases and weight status? *Public Health Nutr*. 2010;13(11):1757–1763.

33. Leatherdale ST, Pouliou T, Church D, Hobin E. The association between overweight and opportunity structures in the built environment: A multi-level analysis among elementary school youth in the PLAY-ON study. *Int J Public Health*. 2011;56(3):237–246.

34. Prince SA, Kristjansson EA, Russell K, et al. Relationships between neighborhoods, physical activity, and obesity: A multilevel analysis of a large Canadian city. *Obesity (Silver Spring)*. 2012;20(10):2093–2100.

35. Fiechtner L, Block J, Duncan DT, et al. Proximity to supermarkets associated with higher body mass index among overweight and obese preschool-age children. *Prev Med*. 2013;56(3–4):218–221.

36. Leung CW, Laraia BA, Kelly M, et al. The influence of neighborhood food stores on change in young girls' body mass index. *Am J Prev Med*. 2011;41(1):43–51.

37. Lenhart A. Teens, social media & technology overview 2015. http://www.pewinternet.org/2015/04/09/teens-social-media-technology-2015/ Accessed August 20, 2015.

38. Falbe J, Rosner B, Willett WC, Sonneville KR, Hu FB, Field AE. Adiposity and different types of screen time. *Pediatrics*. 2013;132(6):e1497–1505.

39. Cameron AJ, van Stralen MM, Brug J, et al. Television in the bedroom and increased body weight: Potential explanations for their relationship among European schoolchildren. *Pediatr Obes*. 2013;8(2):130–141.

40. Helajarvi H, Rosenstrom T, Pahkala K, et al. Exploring causality between TV viewing and weight change in young and middle-aged adults: The cardiovascular risk in young Finns study. *PLoS One*. 2014;9(7):e101860.

41. Schuster MA, Elliott MN, Bogart LM, et al. Changes in obesity between fifth and tenth grades: A longitudinal study in three metropolitan areas. *Pediatrics*. 2014;134(6):1051–1058.

42. Epstein LH, Roemmich JN, Robinson JL, et al. A randomized trial of the effects of reducing television viewing and computer use on body mass index in young children. *Arch Pediatr Adolesc Med*. 2008;162(3):239–245.

43. Harris JL, Bargh JA, Brownell KD. Priming effects of television food advertising on eating behavior. *Health Psychol*. 2009;28(4):404–413.

44. Falbe J, Willett WC, Rosner B, Gortmaker SL, Sonneville KR, Field AE. Longitudinal relations of television, electronic games, and digital versatile discs with changes in diet in adolescents. *Am J Clin Nutr*. 2014;100(4):1173–1181.

45. Center for Science in the Public Interest. Nearly 70% of food ads on Nickelodeon are for junk. http://cspinet.org/new/201303211.html. Accessed August 16, 2015.

46. Robinson TN, Borzekowski DL, Matheson DM, Kraemer HC. Effects of fast food branding on young children's taste preferences. *Arch Pediatr Adolesc Med*. 2007;161(8):792–797.

47. Fisher A, McDonald L, van Jaarsveld CH, et al. Sleep and energy intake in early childhood. *Int J Obes (Lond)*. 2014;38(7):926–929.

48. Carter PJ, Taylor BJ, Williams SM, Taylor RW. Longitudinal analysis of sleep in relation to BMI and body fat in children: The FLAME study. *BMJ*. 2011;342:d2712.

49. Gillman MW, Rifas-Shiman SL, Kleinman K, Oken E, Rich-Edwards JW, Taveras EM. Developmental origins of childhood overweight: Potential public health impact. *Obesity (Silver Spring)*. 2008;16(7):1651–1656.

50. Nielsen LS, Danielsen KV, Sorensen TI. Short sleep duration as a possible cause of obesity: Critical analysis of the epidemiological evidence. *Obes Rev*. 2011;12(2):78–92.

51. Diethelm K, Bolzenius K, Cheng G, Remer T, Buyken AE. Longitudinal associations between reported sleep duration in early childhood and the development of body mass index, fat mass index and fat free mass index until age 7. *Int J Pediatr Obes*. 2011;6(2–2):e114–123.

52. Arora T, Hussain S, Hubert Lam KB, Lily Yao G, Neil Thomas G, Taheri S. Exploring the complex pathways among specific types of technology, self-reported sleep duration and body mass index in UK adolescents. *Int J Obes* (Lond). 2013;37(9):1254–1260.
53. Redmayne M, Smith E, Abramson MJ. The relationship between adolescents' well-being and their wireless phone use: A cross-sectional study. *Environ Health*. 2013;12:90.

2 Racial and Ethnic Disparities in Prevalence of and Risk Factors for Childhood Obesity

Claudia M. Toledo-Corral

CONTENTS

INTRODUCTION

Diversification of race and ethnicity in the United States continues to evolve and it is now projected that by 2050 non-Latino Caucasians will no longer be the majority [1]. These estimates show that the fastest migration rates will arise from Latino and Asian countries but Latinos will compose the largest racial and ethnic group [1]. Due to this racial and ethnic population shift, any existing health disparities are of increasing concern in public health and medicine. As a prime example, the rates of obesity in US children, adolescents, and adults are more pronounced in racial and ethnic groups such as Blacks and Latinos [2,3]. The risk of obesity and metabolic disease is also increasing in the Asian population, which has gone unnoticed due to the misclassification of obesity using the current body mass index (BMI) cutoffs [4]. The projected population increase in each of these racial and ethnic groups, coupled with current pediatric obesity rates in the United States, has severe implications for adult health disparity burdens including obesity and overt cardiometabolic disease.

The racial and ethnic inequalities in risk factors associated with childhood obesity can be explained as unique products of multifactorial determinants. Using the multicausational model of chronic disease (Figure 2.1), these layers are (1) inherent risk factors, such as genetics and predispositions affecting biological mechanisms; (2) culturally associated behaviors specific to body image, diet, and exercise routines; and (3) the environmental context, including socioeconomic status (SES) and the environment, which can either foster or inhibit health behaviors. Each of these risk layers can interact and have synergistic effects on childhood obesity risks. For instance, inherent risk factors intersect the behavioral and environmental components of the model, illustrating the interdependency of all three layers (Figure 2.1). Children of certain racial and ethnic groups are not only affected by multiple risk factors, but may also have more inherent risk due to poor maternal health via fetal programing (Figure 2.2). This combination of environment and genetic risk factors reflects the importance of multifaceted public health preventive measures at a family level to combat childhood obesity. As described in this chapter, racial and ethnic groups are increasingly exposed

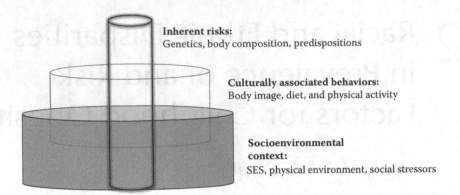

FIGURE 2.1 A multicausational model of childhood obesity risk. Race and ethnicity play a role on every level and obesity risk is maximized when all layers interact.

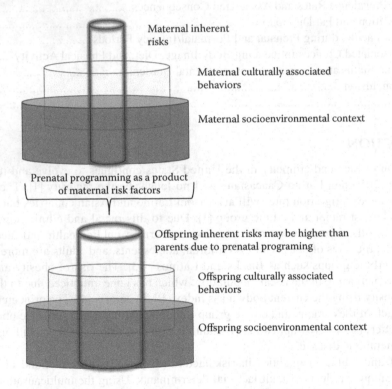

FIGURE 2.2 Transgenerational effects of multicausational model of childhood obesity risk.

to a composite of these three layers of risk factors, leading to a greater disruption in energy and hormonal balance, as well as metabolism.

As public health researchers and officials, we must consider the differences in inherent genetic or biological mechanisms, in conjunction with culturally rooted behavioral choices in environments that support and sustain gene–behavior interactions. However, categorizing race and ethnicity has numerous challenges as terms are constantly evolving and are often used interchangeably or imprecisely [5]. For US census and other government purposes, race is predominantly used for grouping individuals into populations based on observable features including skin color, facial qualities, body composition, and other inheritable traits. Ethnicity is used to group by cultural characteristics including, but not limited to, historical background, language, geographical ancestry, religious beliefs, and dietary traditions and preferences. For the purposes of this chapter, the race and ethnic categories of Asian (including Pacific Islanders), Black, non-Latino Caucasian, Latino (Caucasian), and Native American will be used, unless otherwise listed as a specific group.

BACKGROUND: PREVALENCE RATES AND ASSOCIATED CONSEQUENCES

The trends over the past decade show a stabilization of obesity rates in children ($\geq$95th BMI percentile per Centers for Disease Control [CDC] year 2000 growth curves); however, racial/ethnic disparities in childhood obesity rates are evident [2,3]. Specifically, the 2011–2012 National Health and Nutrition Examination Survey (NHANES) data revealed significant ethnic differences in childhood obesity prevalence: rates were lowest among Asian (8.6%) and non-Latino Caucasian children (14.1%) compared with Black (20.2%) and Latino children (22.4%) [2]. With the exception of Asians, at least 70% of the obesity prevalence was composed of children in the $\geq$97th BMI percentile, indicating that extreme obesity is overwhelming in these populations. In addition, 12-year US trends (1999–2010) revealed that Black and Latino children had 27% and 99% higher odds of developing obesity compared with Caucasian children [3]. Moreover, Black and Latino obese adolescents were most likely to suffer from persistent obesity (extreme or otherwise) [6]. These extreme disparities in childhood obesity rates were carried into adulthood: 90% of US obese adolescents in 1996 remained obese into the second and third decade of life [6].

Increased childhood obesity rates coincide with similar increases in cardiometabolic sequelae, such as type 2 diabetes, atherosclerosis, and fatty liver disease, in children (see Chapters 25 through 28). Overt disease in children is rare, but subclinical diseases, such as metabolic syndrome (MetS) and nonalcoholic fatty liver disease (NAFLD), show disparate rates by race and ethnicity [7,8]. For instance, MetS is a constellation of three or more risk factors including abdominal obesity, hyperglycemia, hypertension, and dyslipidemias [9]. Between 2001 and 2010, MetS affected approximately 10% of the overall US pediatric population, but Latino children and adolescents had the highest rate of 14% [7]. The most defining feature among Latino children with MetS was a high prevalence (21%) of impaired fasting glucose (defined as $\geq$100 mg/dL), suggesting early development of type 2 diabetes. The prevalence of type 2 diabetes in US youth remains low (<1%) in all racial and ethnic groups but it is still highest among Native American, Black, and Latino youth between the ages of 15 and 19 years [10]. Rates of subclinical liver disease in children also vary by race and ethnicity. A unique autopsy-based study in youth reported that the prevalence of NAFLD ($\geq$5% of hepatocytes contained macrovesicular fat) was highest among Latinos (11.8%), followed by Asians (10.2%), non-Latino Caucasians (8.6%), and Blacks (1.5%) [8]. Interestingly, MetS, NAFLD, and obesity can coincide more often in some racial and ethnic groups or can be found independently. As an example, rates of obesity, MetS, and NAFLD are highest in Latinos while Asians have lower levels of overall adiposity yet suffer from higher rates of NAFLD. To fully elucidate this racial and ethnic differences in cardiometabolic disease, further study on body composition, genetics, and metabolic adaptation to a Westernized diet is needed.

BODY COMPOSITION AND FAT DISTRIBUTION

In children, the applied use of BMI percentiles using age and sex-specific growth curves from the Centers for Disease Control and Prevention (CDC) is the simplest form of obesity assessment; however, this method has significant limitations as discussed in Chapter 1. Currently, the 2000 CDC growth curves cannot fully characterize extreme obesity as the cutoffs used for evaluation did not include a percentile beyond the 97th due to sparse data available prior to the obesity epidemic (pre-1990s). Additionally, these data were based largely on Caucasian children, which led research and public health officials to question their applicability to specific racial and ethnic groups since BMI trajectories do not account for ethnic differences in body composition. In both children and adults, the predictive value of BMI as a true measure of body fat varies between racial groups.

For example, data suggest that higher BMI thresholds for overweight and obesity should be set for Black populations, largely due to higher percentages of fat-free mass compared with other racial/ethnic groups [11]. For the Asian population, there has been ongoing discussions regarding the lowering of the thresholds for obesity diagnosis, yet no consensus has been reached [4]. Despite this, the American Diabetes Association (ADA) recently made a significant revision to its Standards of Medical Care in Diabetes, specifically with regard to screening for type 2 diabetes in Asian adults by lowering the BMI threshold for diabetic screening from 25 to 23 kg/m^2 [12]. The recommendation was supported by studies in Asians showing higher levels of visceral fat and onset of metabolic disease at lower BMI [4,13]. Collectively, recent data show that existing use of the non-race-specific BMI cutoffs may lead to either misclassification of obesity and/or lack of screening for obesity-related disease in specific racial and ethnic groups. Although no recommendations were made in the pediatric diagnosis of early diabetic disease risk, we can extrapolate that similar indications should be considered for youth.

In addition to the use of BMI, more robust measures of adiposity have been employed in numerous research studies that assess actual body fat percentage as well as body fat distribution using dual x-ray absorptiometry (DEXA) and magnetic resonance imagine (MRI) scans. These studies reveal that racial disparities in cardiometabolic disease are not necessarily a consequence of overall obesity but instead the distribution of fat depots [14–16]. In children and adults, studies have shown that increased abdominal adiposity and high prevalence of NAFLD are more common in Latino and Asian populations [8]. Interestingly, despite the low overall US obesity rate in Asian youth, fatty liver is highly prevalent; a finding that contributed to the lower BMI threshold for diabetes screening in Asian populations [12]. Other race and ethnic differences in fat distribution include intramyocellular lipid (IMCL), or fat found within skeletal muscle. Specifically, IMCL has been shown to be greater in Black and Latino youth than in Caucasians, even after controlling for total body fat [17]. These major differences in body fat distribution by ethnicity have also been associated with disease risk. Abdominal and ectopic fat distribution, such as liver, pancreatic, and muscle fat depots may explain racial differences in obesity-related disease via different underlying pathophysiology associated with each fat depot. These include unique biological mechanisms such as adipose tissue inflammation and nonesterified free fatty acid metabolism [15]. Briefly, abdominal adipose tissue in youth, specifically visceral adiposity, has been associated with markers of insulin resistance. Higher liver fat has been related to lower insulin sensitivity in both Black and Latino youth; however, Black youths' metabolism appears to be more sensitive to liver fat compared with Latino youth [14,16]. In addition to this finding, another ectopic fat depot, pancreatic fat, has been associated with prediabetes in Black adolescents [16]. To date, there is no definitive study to show that IMCL independently contributes to metabolic risk, but it may be a contributing factor as this form of ectopic fat deposition may have large effects on insulin sensitivity [18]. An examination of each of these fat depots is warranted in future studies to further clarify the ethnic-specific differences in adiposity and fat depots, and their contribution to metabolic disease.

MATERNAL RISK FACTORS DURING PRENATAL AND POSTNATAL/INFANCY PERIODS

Maternal health during the prenatal period can have profound consequences on infant growth and development as overweight and obese mothers are more likely to have obese children [19,20]. This is discussed in more detail in Chapter 12, but is introduced here as it pertains to ethnic differences. The emerging literature supports the notion of early-life programing, which is dependent on the intrauterine environment, maternal genetics, behaviors, and environment [19]. Maternal obesity, excessive gestational weight gain, and gestational diabetes mellitus (GDM) are maternal risk factors that vary by race or ethnicity and associate differently with infant birth weight [20]. When considering all three of these maternal risk factors, Caucasian and Latino mothers have nearly twice the odds of delivering an infant with high birth weight [20]. Asian mothers with only two of these risk factors (obesity and GDM) have the highest odds among all ethnicities of delivering an infant with high birth weight. Interestingly, either a high or a low birth weight has been associated with future obesity [21,22]. Of all the aforementioned risk factors, most of the literature supports GDM as an independent prenatal risk factor for future obesity working via intrauterine mechanisms [21,23,24]. Differences by race and ethnicity are evident in recent trends of increasing GDM morbidity, where Latina women showed a 66% increase from 1999 to 2008 in GDM incidence, while Asian/Pacific Islanders had the highest GDM prevalence (6.48%–10.27%) [25]. Offspring born to GDM mothers have exhibited increased levels of abdominal adiposity [26], higher risk for childhood or adolescent obesity [21,23], and even longer-term consequences of higher BMI in adulthood [24]. To further exemplify these findings in a race-specific context, a longitudinal study of overweight and obese Latino children found that offspring exposed to GDM experienced a sharper increase in total body fat during the pubertal transition compared with those without GDM exposure [27]. Collectively, these findings suggest that the ethnic GDM disparity could have profound consequences on Asian and Latino childhood obesity rates and that the intrauterine environment plays an important role in childhood obesity risk.

In addition to the prenatal period, postnatal development is vulnerable to acquired inherent risks, in combination with the mother's culturally associated rearing behavior and environment. These include rapid infant weight gain, nonexclusive breast-feeding, earlier introduction to solid and/or sugary foods, and fewer than 12 h of sleep [28,29]. An emerging body of data also shows that alterations in infant microbiota from lack of breast-feeding and antibiotic use are associated with childhood obesity [30,31]. Some of these infant-rearing behaviors have been shown to differ by race and ethnicity and by association with childhood obesity [28,29]. Compared with Caucasian children, Black and Latino children were not only more highly exposed to adverse dietary, breast-feeding patterns, and sleep patterns during infancy [28] but these risk factors were also associated with higher BMI z-score at seven years of age [29]. Postnatal exposures (i.e., during infancy), either acting individually or synergistically, may contribute to early programing of dietary preference to sugar, altered circadian rhythms, and altered microbiota that could lead to childhood obesity.

Exposure to pre- and postnatal risk factors are closely linked to cultural practices, acculturation, socioeconomic factors, and urban environment, all of which will be discussed in further detail. In the context of racial and ethnicity disparities, early-life exposures and transgenerational effects are highlighted due to the increased number and severity of obesity risk factors present in Black and Latino mothers. Presumably, these maternal risk factors will increase the inherent risk of the offspring so that their baseline risk is elevated even before birth (Figure 2.2).

CULTURALLY ASSOCIATED CHOICES INFLUENCING BODY IMAGE, DIET, AND PHYSICAL ACTIVITY

Parental and child obesity–related behavior choices can be characterized as either those rooted in ethnic/cultural beliefs of the culture of origin or those of the US (Westernized) lifestyle, or a mixture [32,33]. The level of cultural integration and associated behavioral patterns are difficult to tease apart. Therefore, the current review focuses on any adverse behaviors that stem from either traditionally held ethnic practices or Westernized practices.

Parental views of body image affect child-rearing choices that shape offspring's diet and physical activity patterns that can persist throughout their lifetime. For example, despite strong US public health messages indicating childhood obesity as an adverse health determinant, there remains a high rate of child weight misperception among mothers with lower education levels, independent of race [34,35] and mothers of various race and ethnic groups including Black, Latina, and Asian mothers [34,36,37]. Latina mothers are less likely to associate obesity with poor health [32] and often feel pressure to follow cultural traditions and endorse weight gain in their children [33]. Parental views on child weight or underestimation of the health consequences associated with obesity may translate to acceptance of obesity in children. These personal and cultural beliefs further shape parental choices and influence acculturation and adoption of a Westernized lifestyle, which includes a poor diet, lack of physical activity, and increased sedentary behavior. For example, families who are acculturated to the Westernized culture have increased rates of dietary sugar intake: 82% of Black and 74% of Latino children were already exposed to high sugar-sweetened beverages at age two compared to only 45% of Caucasians [28]. Similarly, by four years of age, 66%, 83%, and 88% of Caucasian, Black, and Latino children had some exposure to fast food [28]. This early-life familiarity with sweets and fast foods leads to increased palatability for sweets and fats, and subsequently, increased consumption. Specifically, high dietary intake of sugars can interact with coexisting risk factors-such as genetic susceptibility to obesity and/or disease risk. For example, it has been shown that high dietary sugar intake interacts with the GG genotype of the PNPLA3 gene in Latino children to increase liver fat [38]. At the same time, interactions between high dietary sugar and cortisol levels have also been associated with higher visceral fat in Latino youth [39]. These studies highlight significant health disparities that are partially attributed to the detrimental effects of diet as seen in Latino children whose genetics and high sugar intake amplify risk for obesity and NAFLD. An examination of these gene–behavior interactions has not been done in other ethnicities; however, it has been shown that on average, compared with Caucasian middle-school children, mostly all other ethnic groups, including Native American, Pacific Islanders, Black, Latino, and multiracial children, consumed more sugar-sweetened beverages [40]. Given the existing obesity risk factors already discussed, investigations of potential additive or synergistic effects of multiple risk factors are warranted.

Physical activity and sedentary behavior patterns also vary by ethnicity. Especially in immigrant groups, adolescents are not as likely to engage in sports or intense physical activity [41]. For example, moderate to vigorous physical activity was reported to be highest in non-Latino Caucasian adolescent girls compared with any other racial and ethnic group, with the lowest being in Latina girls [42]. Sedentary behavior such as television viewing has been shown to be more common in Black and Latino children, many of whom are exposed to televisions in their bedrooms [28], with an average of more than 3 h a day of television screen time [42]. Given these findings, comprehensive studies are necessary to delineate the independent and interactive effects of diet and physical lifestyle, specific cultural practices by ethnicity, and other community-level factors.

SOCIOECONOMIC STATUS AND ASSOCIATED ENVIRONMENTAL BURDENS

When addressing the racial/ethnic disparities in childhood obesity prevalence rates, low SES and associated environmental burdens cannot be overlooked. In general, low SES groups typically have little or no access to higher-quality resources and this results in poor lifestyle choices and increased disease risk [43]. Specifically, low-SES neighborhoods are burdened by neighborhood deprivation, which is characterized by scarce resources and an obesogenic environment (e.g., liquor stores, industry, lack of green space) [44,45]. These neighborhood environments have limited food choice and availability, as well as limited accessible areas for physical activity (see Chapter 17). Moreover, limitations on food access and recreation contextualize and breed obesogenic behaviors. In the United States, many racial and ethnic groups at high risk for obesity are gathered in low-SES areas, possibly accounting for the racial disparity in obesity rates. Specifically in youth, several studies have examined the contributions of race and ethnicity and socioeconomic factors. Longitudinal studies found that the disparity in adolescent obesity between Black and/or Latino versus Caucasian youth was not entirely explained by race, but instead by economic contextual factors, household demographics, and individual SES [41,46]. Interestingly, others have reported that while economic hardship was a defining factor for high childhood obesity rates in Caucasian Latino, and Asian children, in Black children this relationship was attenuated [47]. Differential effects of individual-level SES on childhood obesity, independent of contextual factors, have also been observed. For example, in a study of Caucasian and Black children followed from kindergarten to eighth grade, a higher baseline BMI z-score was associated with a higher SES in Black male students and a lower SES in Caucasian male students [48]. This study exemplifies how individual versus neighborhood SES may play a smaller role in Black children, possibly due to other stronger risk factors, such as cultural beliefs and behaviors about body image [37]. Based on these studies, low SES on the individual level and/or the neighborhood level has adverse effects on childhood obesity by race and ethnic group and should be considered when holistically examining childhood obesity risk. A more detailed review of economic factors associated with disparities in childhood obesity is provided in Chapter 4.

Low-SES communities also suffer from increased environmental injustices exposing residents to disproportionate burdens of chemical exposures and social–environmental stressors that contribute to ill health, including obesity [49]. Although this is discussed in further detail in Chapters 18 through 20, this topic is briefly covered in this chapter as it pertains to the childhood obesity risk in low-SES minority children residing in urban cnvironments. Toxic chemical exposures in the air, soil, and water have only recently been implicated as possible determinants in childhood obesity. Although the mechanisms behind how pollutants contribute to childhood obesity are not well understood, there is a consensus that exposures during early development may have the biggest impact on obesity during childhood. For example, one study found that compared with maternal exposure in the lowest tertile of ambient air polycyclic aromatic hydrocarbons (PAH), maternal exposure in the highest tertile carried a greater relative risk of 2.26 for offspring obesity at seven years of age [50]. In a separate study of children 6–18 years of age, increased PAH metabolites from urine were independently associated with higher BMI and waist circumference, and simultaneous exposure to environmental tobacco smoke further increased obesity risk [51]. Finally, a longitudinal analysis from the Children's Health Study (CHS) found that maternal smoking during pregnancy predicted increased BMI in children and interacted with in utero air pollution exposure [52]. At the same time, additional findings from the CHS found that vehicular traffic contributed to higher BMI in children [52,53]. This modest body of evidence suggests that chemical exposures during prenatal and early life may affect neurological, metabolic, and behavioral alterations that may increase metabolic vulnerability and obesity.

In addition to environmental pollution exposure, low-SES minority children residing in the urban landscape are chronically exposed to psychosocial burdens that impact stress levels and contribute to obesity risk. Such community-level stressors include violence, noise, and lack of green space and are thought to contribute to mental stress levels by the decreased sense of safety, decreased social interaction, and decreased physical activity [54]. Conversely, quiet and greener neighborhoods lend themselves to increased social interaction and a sense of community among its members. Physiologically, chronic exposure to the community-level psychosocial stress can alter the hypothalamic–pituitary–adrenal axis [54–56]. Consequently, alterations in cortisol concentrations and diurnal patterns have been associated with community stressors including cumulative exposure to violence [54,55] and loss of green space [56], both of which are common in low-SES communities that are composed of largely Black or Latino populations. Collectively, these studies support the current postulations that the physical and social environment contribute and foster obesogenic behaviors, particularly in low-SES neighborhoods.

SUMMARY/CONCLUSION

In the United States, racial and ethnic minority children bear a disproportionate burden of multiple childhood obesity risk factors that encompass heritable traits, pre- and postnatal exposures, culturally associated habits and behaviors, and lower socioeconomic environments with increased chemical and social stressors. Asian children appear to have more of the inherent risk factors while Black and Latino groups suffer from a constellation of risk factors that are likely interdependent and/or work synergistically to increase obesity risk. Consequently, childhood obesity prevention methods should engage ethnic-specific and/or culturally sensitive interventions that involve family-level and community-level transformation toward a healthy lifestyle.

REFERENCES

1. Colby SL, Ortman JM. Projections of the size and composition of the US population: 2014 to 2060. https://www.census.gov/content/dam/Census/library/publications/2015/demo/p25-1143.pdf.
2. Ogden CL, Carroll MD, Kit BK, Flegal KM. Prevalence of childhood and adult obesity in the United States, 2011–2012. *JAMA*. 2014;311(8):806–14.
3. Ogden CL, Carroll MD, Kit BK, Flegal KM. Prevalence of obesity and trends in body mass index among US children and adolescents, 1999–2010. *JAMA*. 2012;307(5):483–90.
4. WHO Expert Consultation. Appropriate body-mass index for Asian populations and its implications for policy and intervention strategies. *Lancet*. 2004;363(9403):157–63.
5. Ma IWY, Khan NA, Kang A, Zalunardo N, Palepu A. Systematic review identified suboptimal reporting and use of race/ethnicity in general medical journals. *J Clin Epidemiol*. 2007;60(6):572–8.
6. Gordon-Larsen P, The NS, Adair LS. Longitudinal trends in obesity in the United States from adolescence to the third decade of life. *Obesity (Silver Spring)*. 2010;18(9):1801–4.
7. Miller JM, Kaylor MB, Johannsson M, Bay C, Churilla JR. Prevalence of metabolic syndrome and individual criterion in US adolescents: 2001–2010 National Health and Nutrition Examination Survey. *Metab Syndr Relat Disord*. 2014;12(10):527–32.
8. Schwimmer JB, Deutsch R, Kahen T, Lavine JE, Stanley C, Behling C. Prevalence of fatty liver in children and adolescents. *Pediatrics*. 2006;118(4):1388–93.
9. Cruz ML, Goran MI. The metabolic syndrome in children and adolescents. *Curr Diab Rep*. 2004;4(1):53–62.
10. Pettitt DJ, Talton J, Dabelea D, Divers J, Imperatore G, Lawrence JM, et al. Prevalence of diabetes in U.S. youth in 2009: The SEARCH for diabetes in youth study. *Diabetes Care*. 2014;37(2):402–8.
11. Heo M, Faith MS, Pietrobelli A, Heymsfield SB. Percentage of body fat cutoffs by sex, age, and race-ethnicity in the US adult population from NHANES 1999–2004. *Am J Clin Nutr*. 2012;95(3):594–602.
12. American Diabetes Association. Standards of medical care in diabetes—2015: Summary of revisions. *Diabetes Care*. 2015;38(Suppl 1):S4–S4.
13. Hsu WC, Araneta MRG, Kanaya AM, Chiang JL, Fujimoto W. BMI cut points to identify at-risk Asian Americans for type 2 diabetes screening. *Diabetes Care*. 2015;38(1):150–8.
14. Alderete TL, Toledo-Corral CM, Desai P, Weigensberg MJ, Goran MI. Liver fat has a stronger association with risk factors for type 2 diabetes in African-American compared with Hispanic adolescents. *J Clin Endocrinol Metab*. 2013;98(9):3748–54.
15. Alderete TL, Toledo-Corral CM, Goran MI. Metabolic basis of ethnic differences in diabetes risk in overweight and obese youth. *Curr Diab Rep*. 2014;14(2):455.
16. Toledo-Corral CM, Alderete TL, Hu HH, Nayak K, Esplana S, Liu T, et al. Ectopic fat deposition in prediabetic overweight and obese minority adolescents. *J Clin Endocrinol Metab*. 2013;98(3):1115–21.
17. Maligie M, Crume T, Scherzinger A, Stamm E, Dabelea D. Adiposity, fat patterning, and the metabolic syndrome among diverse youth: The EPOCH study. *J Pediatr*. 2012;161(5):875–80.
18. Brumbaugh DE, Crume TL, Nadeau K, Scherzinger A, Dabelea D. Intramyocellular lipid is associated with visceral adiposity, markers of insulin resistance, and cardiovascular risk in prepubertal children: The EPOCH study. *J Clin Endocrinol Metab*. 2012;97(7):E1099–105.
19. Wahlqvist ML, Krawetz SA, Rizzo NS, Dominguez-Bello MG, Szymanski LM, Barkin S, et al. Early-life influences on obesity: From preconception to adolescence. *Ann NY Acad Sci*. 2015;1347(1):1–28.
20. Bowers K, Laughon SK, Kiely M, Brite J, Chen Z, Zhang C. Gestational diabetes, pre-pregnancy obesity and pregnancy weight gain in relation to excess fetal growth: Variations by race/ethnicity. *Diabetologia*. 2013;56(6):1263–71.
21. Gillman MW, Rifas-Shiman S, Berkey CS, Field AE, Colditz GA. Maternal gestational diabetes, birth weight, and adolescent obesity. *Pediatrics*. 2003;111(3):e221–6.
22. Reynolds RM. Glucocorticoid excess and the developmental origins of disease: Two decades of testing the hypothesis—2012 Curt Richter Award Winner. *Psychoneuroendocrinology*. 2013;38(1):1–11.
23. Kubo A, Ferrara A, Windham GC, Greenspan LC, Deardorff J, Hiatt RA, et al. Maternal hyperglycemia during pregnancy predicts adiposity of the offspring. *Diabetes Care*. 2014;37(11):2996–3002.
24. Lawlor DA, Lichtenstein P, Långström N. Association of maternal diabetes mellitus in pregnancy with offspring adiposity into early adulthood: Sibling study in a prospective cohort of 280,866 men from 248,293 families. *Circulation*. 2011;123(3):258–65.
25. Bardenheier BH, Imperatore G, Gilboa SM, Geiss LS, Saydah SH, Devlin HM, et al. Trends in gestational diabetes among hospital deliveries in 19 U.S. states, 2000–2010. *Am J Prev Med*. 2015;49(1):12–9.

26. Crume TL, Ogden L, West NA, Vehik KS, Scherzinger A, Daniels S, et al. Association of exposure to diabetes in utero with adiposity and fat distribution in a multiethnic population of youth: The Exploring Perinatal Outcomes among Children (EPOCH) Study. *Diabetologia*. 2011;54(1):87–92.

27. Davis JN, Gunderson EP, Gyllenhammer LE, Goran MI. Impact of gestational diabetes mellitus on pubertal changes in adiposity and metabolic profiles in Latino offspring. *J Pediatr*. 2013;162(4):741–5.

28. Taveras EM, Gillman MW, Kleinman K, Rich-Edwards JW, Rifas-Shiman SL. Racial/ethnic differences in early-life risk factors for childhood obesity. *Pediatrics*. 2010;125(4):686–95.

29. Taveras EM, Gillman MW, Kleinman KP, Rich-Edwards JW, Rifas-Shiman SL. Reducing racial/ethnic disparities in childhood obesity: The role of early life risk factors. *JAMA Pediatr*. 2013;167(8):731–8.

30. Koleva PT, Bridgman SL, Kozyrskyj AL. The infant gut microbiome: Evidence for obesity risk and dietary intervention. *Nutrients*. 2015;7(4):2237–60.

31. Azad MB, Bridgman SL, Becker AB, Kozyrskyj AL. Infant antibiotic exposure and the development of childhood overweight and central adiposity. *Int J Obes* (Lond). 2014;38(10):1290–8.

32. Baker EH, Altman CE. Maternal ratings of child health and child obesity, variations by mother's race/ethnicity and nativity. *Matern Child Health J*. 2015;19(5):1000–9.

33. Lindsay AC, Sussner KM, Greaney ML, Peterson KE. Latina mothers' beliefs and practices related to weight status, feeding, and the development of child overweight. *Public Health Nurs*. 2011;28(2):107–18.

34. Paeratakul S, White MA, Williamson DA, Ryan DH, Bray GA. Sex, race/ethnicity, socioeconomic status, and BMI in relation to self-perception of overweight. *Obes Res*. 2002;10(5):345–50.

35. Dorsey RR, Eberhardt MS, Ogden CL. Racial/ethnic differences in weight perception. *Obesity (Silver Spring)*. 2009;17(4):790–5.

36. Yao N-L, Hillemeier MM. Weight status in Chinese children: Maternal perceptions and child self-assessments. *World J Pediatr*. 2012;8(2):129–35.

37. Moore SE, Harris CL, Watson P, Wimberly Y. Do African American mothers accurately estimate their daughters' weight category? *Ethn Dis*. 2008;18(2 Suppl 2):S2–211–4.

38. Davis JN, Lê K-A, Walker RW, Vikman S, Spruijt-Metz D, Weigensberg MJ, et al. Increased hepatic fat in overweight Hispanic youth influenced by interaction between genetic variation in PNPLA3 and high dietary carbohydrate and sugar consumption. *Am J Clin Nutr*. 2010;92(6):1522–7.

39. Gyllenhammer LE, Weigensberg MJ, Spruijt-Metz D, Allayee H, Goran MI, Davis JN. Modifying influence of dietary sugar in the relationship between cortisol and visceral adipose tissue in minority youth. *Obesity (Silver Spring)*. 2014;22(2):474–81.

40. Richmond TK, Spadano-Gasbarro JL, Walls CE, Austin SB, Greaney ML, Wang ML, et al. Middle school food environments and racial/ethnic differences in sugar-sweetened beverage consumption: Findings from the Healthy Choices study. *Prev Med*. 2013;57(5):735–8.

41. Gordon-Larsen P, Harris KM, Ward DS, Popkin BM. Acculturation and overweight-related behaviors among Hispanic immigrants to the US: The National Longitudinal Study of Adolescent Health. *Soc Sci Med*. 2003;57(11):2023–34.

42. Carson V, Staiano AE, Katzmarzyk PT. Physical activity, screen time, and sitting among U.S. adolescents. *Pediatr Exerc Sci*. 2015;27(1):151–9.

43. Pampel FC, Krueger PM, Denney JT. Socioeconomic disparities in health behaviors. *Annu Rev Sociol*. 2010;36(1):349–70.

44. Rossen LM. Neighbourhood economic deprivation explains racial/ethnic disparities in overweight and obesity among children and adolescents in the U.S.A. *J Epidemiol Community Health*. 2014;68(2):123–9.

45. Hsieh S, Klassen AC, Curriero FC, Caulfield LE, Cheskin LJ, Davis JN, et al. Fast-food restaurants, park access, and insulin resistance among Hispanic youth. *Am J Prev Med*. 2014;46(4):378–87.

46. Powell LM, Wada R, Krauss RC, Wang Y. Ethnic disparities in adolescent body mass index in the United States: The role of parental socioeconomic status and economic contextual factors. *Soc Sci Med*. 2012;75(3):469–76.

47. Shih M, Dumke KA, Goran MI, Simon PA. The association between community-level economic hardship and childhood obesity prevalence in Los Angeles. *Pediatr Obes*. 2013;8(6):411–7.

48. Banks GG, Berlin KS, Rybak TM, Kamody RC, Cohen R. Disentangling the longitudinal relations of race, sex, and socioeconomic status, for childhood body mass index trajectories. *J Pediatr Psychol*. 2015;pii:jsv062.

49. Evans GW, Kim P. Multiple risk exposure as a potential explanatory mechanism for the socioeconomic status-health gradient. *Ann NY Acad Sci*. 2010;1186(1):174–89.

50. Rundle A, Hoepner L, Hassoun A, Oberfield S, Freyer G, Holmes D, et al. Association of childhood obesity with maternal exposure to ambient air polycyclic aromatic hydrocarbons during pregnancy. *Am J Epidemiol*. 2012;175(11):1163–72.

51. Kim H-W, Kam S, Lee D-H. Synergistic interaction between polycyclic aromatic hydrocarbons and environmental tobacco smoke on the risk of obesity in children and adolescents: The U.S. National Health and Nutrition Examination Survey 2003–2008. *Environ Res.* 2014;135:354–60.

52. McConnell R, Shen E, Gilliland FD, Jerrett M, Wolch J, Chang C-C, et al. A longitudinal cohort study of body mass index and childhood exposure to secondhand tobacco smoke and air pollution: The Southern California Children's Health Study. *Environ Health Perspect.* 2015;123(4):360–6.

53. Jerrett M, McConnell R, Wolch J, Chang R, Lam C, Dunton G, et al. Traffic-related air pollution and obesity formation in children: A longitudinal, multilevel analysis. *Environ Health.* 2014;13(1):49.

54. Do DP, Diez-Roux AV, Hajat A, Auchincloss AH, Merkin SS, Ranjit N, et al. Circadian rhythm of cortisol and neighborhood characteristics in a population-based sample: The Multi-Ethnic Study of Atherosclerosis. *Health Place.* 2011;17(2):625–32.

55. Aiyer SM, Heinze JE, Miller AL, Stoddard SA, Zimmerman MA. Exposure to violence predicting cortisol response during adolescence and early adulthood: Understanding moderating factors. *J Youth Adolesc.* 2014;43(7):1066–79.

56. Roe JJ, Thompson CW, Aspinall PA, Brewer MJ, Duff EI, Miller D, et al. Green space and stress: Evidence from cortisol measures in deprived urban communities. *Int J Environ Res Public Health.* 2013;10(9):4086–103.

3 Global Perspectives of Childhood Obesity

Prevalence, Contributing Factors, and Prevention

Youfa Wang

CONTENTS

INTRODUCTION

The childhood obesity epidemic has become a serious public health problem in many countries worldwide [1–4]. During recent years, the prevalence of overweight and obesity has been increasing dramatically in many developing countries, particularly in urban settings and among high socio-economic status (SES) groups [1–4]. Although current understanding of the health consequences of overweight/obesity is predominately based on adult studies, increasing evidence suggests that childhood obesity has a number of immediate, intermediate, and long-term health consequences, as reviewed in other chapters in this book.

This chapter describes the current prevalence and time trends of childhood obesity worldwide. It also discusses the methods for defining childhood overweight/obesity, the factors that have contributed to the current epidemic, and the large differences in the prevalence across countries and population groups worldwide. Understanding the differences in the methods (e.g., body mass index [BMI] cutoff points) used to define childhood overweight/obesity is important to appropriately interpret the reported results regarding overweight/obesity rates and related risk factors. The related recommendations and practices for defining childhood overweight/obesity are complex and inconsistent, and much more complex than those for adults. Recently, the World Health Organization (WHO) has called on country leaders worldwide to exert joint efforts to fight against the childhood obesity epidemic [3]. A broad comprehension of the global childhood obesity epidemic will aid understanding of its causes and guide the development of effective intervention programs and policies to address this threat to public health.

CLASSIFICATIONS OF CHILDHOOD OBESITY

Various measures and references have been used to define overweight/obesity in children and adolescents. This has affected prevalence estimates reported over time as well as across populations and studies, which could result in problems in making comparisons of results across studies and countries. The consensus developed since the 1990s is to use BMI (=weight [kg]/height [m]^2) cutoff points to define overweight/obesity both in adults and in children, as research shows that BMI is a good indirect measure of adiposity [4–9]. However, BMI varies substantially by age and gender during childhood and in adolescence. Thus, unlike in adults, age-gender-specific BMI cutoff points should be used in children and adolescents. For adults, BMI of 23, 25, 27, 28, and 30 kg/m^2 are widely used to define overweight/obesity, respectively [8], and the lower cutoff points are used more in Asian populations than in other populations as research shows that with the same level BMI, some Asian population groups have lower percentage body fat and higher obesity-associated health risks.

Since the 1990s, when more attention became focused on childhood obesity, different references based on weight-for-height indexes, such as BMI and weight-for-height, skinfold thickness measures, and waist circumference, have been used to classify body weight status for children [6,9]. Applications of these measures varied considerably across studies and countries [4–9]. For example, in the United States, two sets of sex-age-specific 85th and 95th BMI percentiles have been used. Other countries, such as China, France, the United Kingdom, Singapore, and the Netherlands, have developed their own BMI references using local data. The WHO has published different recommended references since the 1990s. The corresponding BMI cutoff points differ considerably. A global reference would help facilitate international comparisons and monitor the global obesity epidemic. A few references (some are called *standards*) have been developed and recommended for international use, including those endorsed by the WHO and the International Obesity Task Force (IOTF) [5–8], and these are discussed in the next section.

IOTF BMI REFERENCE

The IOTF endorses a series of sex-age-specific BMI cutoff points for children aged 2–18 years for international use [5]. It was developed based on large data sets from six countries: Brazil, Britain, Hong Kong, the Netherlands, Singapore, and the United States. The cutoff points are linked to adult BMI cutoff points, which are established risk indicators for adverse health outcomes. It is also simple to use and consistent for children and adolescents. However, there are also some concerns about the IOTF reference [10]. The concerns include that only six populations were included in the study and there were differences in maturation status within the populations.

THE 2006 WHO GROWTH STANDARDS FOR PRESCHOOL CHILDREN

In 2006, the WHO released new growth standards for children from birth to 60 months (five years old) [11]. In order to establish growth standards for different races/ethnicities, the Multicentre Growth Reference Study (MGRS) recruited affluent, breast-fed, and healthy infants/children whose mothers did not smoke during or after delivery from six cities in Brazil, Ghana, India, Norway, Oman, and the United States. These standards included anthropometric indicators such as height-for-age (length-for-age), weight-for-age, weight-for-height (weight-for-length), and BMI-for-age. A BMI z-score ≥2 was recommended to classify "obesity" and a BMI z-score ≥1 to classify "overweight."

THE 2007 WHO GROWTH REFERENCE FOR SCHOOL-AGE CHILDREN AND ADOLESCENTS

In 2007, the WHO released another set of growth references for children and adolescents aged 5–19 years [12]. To our knowledge, these have not been widely used. The references were derived based on the same US data set as the 1978 WHO/National Center for Health Statistics (NCHS) growth references, but used different growth curve smoothing techniques. The references included three indicators: BMI-for-age, weight-for-age, and height-for-age. Overweight/obesity cutoff points were based on BMI-for-age z-scores. A z-score of 1 was found to be equivalent to a BMI-for-age 25.4 for boys and 25.0 for girls in 19-year-olds. As these values are equal or close to the WHO BMI cutoff points of 25 used in adults, it was recommended to use a z-score of 1 to classify "overweight" and a z-score ≥ 2 to classify "obesity." BMI-for-age z-scores <-2 and <-3 were set as the cutoff points for thinness and severe thinness, respectively.

BMI REFERENCES USED IN THE UNITED STATES

Two sets of different BMI 85th and 95th percentiles have been used in the United States to classify children's weight status. In 2000, the US NCHS and the Centers for Disease Control and Prevention (CDC) updated growth charts using data from five national health examination surveys from 1963 to 1994. The resultant 2000 CDC Growth Charts provided new BMI percentiles [13] and recommended the use of sex- and age-specific 85th and 95th BMI percentiles to classify childhood overweight/obesity, respectively, in children over two years old. Before the release of the 2000 CDC Growth Charts, the sex-age specific 85th and 95th percentiles developed by Dr. Aviva Must and her colleagues, based on the First National Health and Nutrition Examination Survey (NHANES, 1971–1974) data, were used in the United States and many other countries to classify childhood overweight/obesity [6,14]. The BMI cutoff points of the two sets of percentiles differ.

It is worth noting that to examine the time trends in prevalence estimates of overweight/obesity based on BMI cutoff points is useful, but is limited as it cannot reveal details about shifts in adiposity measures or in distribution over time. For example, we examined changes over time in various adiposity measures among US adolescents [15]. Specifically, the measures that we focused on included BMI, waist circumference, and triceps skinfold thickness. We used the NHANES III (1988–1994) and NHANES 1999–2004 data. We found the overall means of BMI, waist circumference, and triceps skinfold thickness increased significantly over time in adolescents (aged 12–19 years) and noted sex differences. During the study period, the overweight/obese US adolescents had gained more adiposity, especially central adiposity as reflected by waist circumference. Our analysis indicates that an examination that solely focuses on changes over time in overweight/obesity rates is unable to capture such complex patterns. However, to our knowledge, little similar research has been carried out to examine the situation for other populations.

GLOBAL PREVALENCE AND TREND OF CHILDHOOD OVERWEIGHT AND OBESITY

Numerous data have demonstrated that childhood obesity has become a global public health crisis with, based on the current prevalence, increasing trends and related health consequences. There are still large variations in the rates of overweight/obesity across countries and across population groups within most countries (e.g., by SES, region, ethnicity, and gender) [1,2,16–19]. This is potentially explained by the many related biological, behavioral, social, economic, and environmental factors.

The prevalence is highest in Western and industrialized countries, but is still low in some developing countries, predominately in Africa and Southeast Asia. The prevalence also varies by age, SES, and gender within countries. The WHO Americas and Eastern Mediterranean regions have higher prevalence of overweight/obesity (30%–40%) than the European (20%–30%), Southeast Asian, Western Pacific, and African regions (10%–20% in the latter three). It is estimated that about 43 million children (35 million in developing countries) were overweight or obese, and 92 million were at risk of overweight in 2010. The global overweight/obesity prevalence has increased dramatically since 1990, for example, in preschool-age children, from approximately 4% in 1990 to 7% in 2010. If this trend continues, the prevalence may reach 9% or 60 million people in 2020. However, some research also indicates that in some European countries and for some young children populations in the United States, the prevalence of childhood overweight/obesity has leveled off or shown signs of declining [20]. This may be due to the efforts made in those countries to address the epidemic.

RECENT PREVALENCE AND LARGE BETWEEN-COUNTRY DIFFERENCES

Available data show that the combined prevalence of overweight/obesity (briefly called *combined prevalence*) is substantial in many regions and countries around the world, but large variations exist. Our previous study that projected the combined prevalence for 2006 yielded a range from 17% in Southeast Asia to 40% in the Americas [1]. In general, combined prevalence is much higher in developed countries than in developing countries. There are also considerable age and gender differences in many populations. Based on our estimations and the findings of others, approximately 26% of school-age children in European countries were overweight or obese in 2006 and 5% were obese. In the Americas, these figures were 28% and 10%, respectively.

There are large between-country variations in the prevalence across and within world regions. Combined prevalence is high in Western and industrialized countries, such as the United States, Canada, some European countries, some countries in South America, some nations in the Middle East, some nations in North Africa, and in the Asia-Pacific region (e.g., in Indonesia and in New Zealand) [21]. According to a recent study examining combined prevalence by WHO region [21], the region of the Americas (approximately 25%–30%) and the Eastern Mediterranean region (approximately 20%–40%) had higher prevalence than the Southeast Asian and Western Pacific regions including nations such as India, Malaysia, Vietnam, China, Australia, South Korea, and Japan. In contrast, the WHO African region had the lowest prevalence rate (about 10%). There were also differences between countries within the same WHO region. In the Eastern Mediterranean region, the combined prevalence in Egypt and Kuwait was about 30% and 45% among girls, respectively, while the prevalence was only 14% among Iranian girls. Self-reported information in a 2001–2002 international school survey of 11-, 13-, and 15-year-olds from 35 countries in Europe and North America ($n = 162,305$) showed large variations in the adolescent overweight prevalence in these countries, which ranged from 3.5% in Lithuanian girls to 31.7% in boys from Malta [21].

TIME TRENDS IN THE PREVALENCE OF CHILDHOOD OBESITY

Substantial data have been collected in many developed countries over the past two decades allowing for the examination of time trends of obesity in both adults and young people, but data are limited for developing countries. Nonetheless, some studies have examined the trends over time worldwide [1,17–19]. We studied the global trends in childhood obesity based on data from approximately 70 countries [1]. We found the combined prevalence of overweight/obesity had increased in almost all countries for which data were available. Russia and Poland during the 1990s were exceptions to this trend. From the 1970s to the end of the 1990s, the combined prevalence doubled or tripled in several large countries in North America (i.e., Canada and the United States), the Western Pacific Region (i.e., Australia), and Europe (i.e., Finland, France, Germany, Italy, and Spain).

A recent comprehensive study estimated the global, regional, and national prevalence of overweight/obesity in children and adults during 1980–2013 using data collected from a large number of countries [17]. It reported that the prevalence had increased substantially in children in developed countries: in 2013, 23.8% (22.9%–24.7%) of boys and 22.6% (21.7%–23.6%) of girls were overweight or obese. The figure had also increased in children and adolescents in developing countries between 1980 and 2013: for boys from 8.1% (7.7%–8.6%) to 12.9% (12.3%–13.5%); and for girls, from 8.4% (8.1%–8.8%) to 13.4% (13.0%–13.9%). A large variation in the prevalence across countries was observed. The study concluded that obesity had become a major global health challenge, and no national success stories had been reported in the past three decades. Urgent global actions are needed to help countries to effectively intervene. The study's conclusions are consistent with those from our previous study based on findings from approximately 70 countries, which reported the trend and variation in obesity and overweight rates across countries and also projected that the prevalence of childhood obesity would continue to increase if no effective programs were implemented [1].

Another recent study examined time trends in the combined prevalence in preschool-age children aged 0–5 years from 1990 to 2010 and projected worldwide rates for 2015 and 2020 (Table 3.1) [18]: 43 million children (35 million in developing countries) were estimated to be overweight or obese in 2010, and 92 million were at risk of overweight. This represents an estimated increase in global combined prevalence from 4.2% in 1990 to 6.7% in 2010. If such trends continue, these numbers

TABLE 3.1
Time Trends in the Combined Prevalence (%) of Overweight and Obesity in Preschool-Age Children Age 0–5 Years Old

UN Region and Subregion	1990	1995	2000	2005	2010	2015	2020
Global	4.2	4.6	5.1	5.8	6.7	7.8	9.1
Developing countries	3.7	4.0	4.5	5.2	6.1	7.2	8.6
Developed countries[c]	7.9	8.8	9.7	10.6	11.7	12.9	14.1
Africa	4.0	4.7	5.7	6.9	8.5	10.4	12.7
Eastern	3.9	4.4	5.1	5.8	6.7	7.6	8.7
Middle	2.5	3.4	4.7	6.4	8.7	11.7	15.5
Northern	6.1	8.0	10.3	13.3	17.0	21.4	26.6
Southern	10.2	9.5	8.8	8.2	7.6	7.0	6.5
Western	2.2	2.9	3.8	4.9	6.4	8.3	10.6
Asia[f]	3.2	3.4	3.7	4.2	4.9	5.7	6.8
Eastern	4.8	4.9	5.0	5.1	5.2	5.3	5.4
South Central	2.3	2.6	2.9	3.2	3.5	3.9	4.3
Southeastern	2.1	2.6	3.1	3.8	4.6	5.6	6.7
Western	3.0	4.5	6.8	10.1	14.7	21.0	29.1
Latin America and Caribbean	6.8	6.8	6.8	6.9	6.9	7.0	7.2
Caribbean	4.6	5.1	5.6	6.2	6.9	7.6	8.3
Central America	4.8	5.3	5.9	6.5	7.2	8.0	8.8
South America	8.0	7.7	7.4	7.1	6.8	6.5	6.3
Oceania[g]	2.9	3.1	3.2	3.3	3.5	3.6	3.8

Source: de Onis, M., et al., *American Journal of Clinical Nutrition*, 92, 1257–1264, 2010.

Note: All surveys included both boys and girls. Cross-sectional data on the prevalence of overweight and obesity were obtained from national nutrition surveys. A total of 450 nationally representative surveys were available from 144 countries. Of the 450 surveys, 413 were conducted in developing countries and 37 in developed countries. About 38% of the surveys (171 surveys) were conducted between 1991 and 1999, 16% (70 surveys) were conducted before 1991, and 46% (209 surveys) after 1999. Linear mixed-effects models were fit to estimate prevalence rates and numbers of affected children by region from 1990 to 2020. Overweight and obese statuses were defined based on >2 SDs (standard deviations) from the weight-for-height median.

[a] Including Europe, North America, Australia, New Zealand, and Japan.

[b] Excluding Japan.

[c] Excluding Australia and New Zealand.

may reach 9.1% (or approximately 60 million children) in 2020. For developing countries alone, the combined prevalence was estimated at 6.1% in 2010 and is expected to rise, perhaps as high as 8.6% by 2020. Rates in 2010 were lower in Asia than in Africa (4.9% vs. 8.5%), but a much larger number of children are affected (17.7 million vs. 13.3 million) in Asia compared with Africa. The study concluded that effective interventions starting as early as infancy were necessary to reverse anticipated trends.

In some developing countries, the prevalence of child overweight/obesity has increased tremendously over the past two decades, with the combined prevalence within some subregions and population groups reaching levels of prevalence on par with some industrialized countries. This is especially the case in countries that are in the midst of rapid social economic transitions such as China, Brazil, and Mexico. China, in particular, is illustrative of dramatic increases in obesity and overweight prevalence that outpace rates observed in industrialized countries. The next section provides two examples of the largest developed and developing countries in the world, the United States and China.

Trend in the United States

Since the late 1970s, the prevalence of overweight/obesity (BMI ≥85th percentile) in children has increased for all ages between 2 and 19 years, but the increase in obesity (BMI ≥95th percentile) leveled off in some age groups in recent years [22–24]. Between NHANES II (1976–1980) and 2003–2004, the average annual rate of increase in obesity prevalence was approximately 0.5% in children aged 2–19 years [22]. During this period, the prevalence of overweight only increased from 7.2% to 13.9% in children aged 2–5 years, but almost tripled in children aged 6–11 years (from 6.5% to 18.8%). In adolescents (12–19 years), the prevalence more than tripled, increasing from 5.0% to 17.4%. In contrast, data from NHANES 2007–2008 show a decrease in the prevalence of obesity among children aged 2–5 years, from 13.9% in NHANES 2003–2004 to 10.4%. During the same time period, the prevalence in both children aged 6–11 years and adolescents was only slightly increased. In 2009–2010, the national prevalence of obesity (16.9%) was similar to that in 2007–2008; and it was 12.0%, 18.0%, and 18.4% in children aged 2–5, 6–11, and 12–19 years, respectively [23]. In 2011–2012, 8.1% of infants and toddlers had high weight for recumbent length, and 16.9% of 2- to 19-year-olds were obese. A more recent study reported that there was no significant change from 2003–2004 through 2011–2012 in high weight for recumbent length among infants and toddlers and obesity in 2- to 19-year-olds [24].

Trend in China

Good nationally representative data collected in China have allowed for the examination of national time trends in childhood obesity [25,26]. Data from large nationwide school–based surveys showed that by 2005, the combined prevalence in urban areas reached 32.5% in boys and 17.6% in girls aged 7 years or older [26], which was similar to that in some industrialized countries. The Chinese National Survey on Students Constitution and Health Association has conducted these surveys every five years since 1985. Remarkably, the combined prevalence of overweight/obesity in boys and girls has increased approximately 10-fold since 1985, and is currently about 15%.

FACTORS THAT HAVE CONTRIBUTED TO THE GLOBAL CHILDHOOD OBESITY EPIDEMIC AND THE LARGE VARIATIONS IN THE PREVALENCE AND TRENDS ACROSS COUNTRIES

Obesity is a result of positive energy balance (=energy intake > energy expenditure), while many factors affect people's eating and physical activity (PA). The factors are more complex for children than for adults due to the many differences between them [3,4,27]. These global patterns of the obesity epidemic (e.g., consistent increasing trends in a large number of countries, large variations in the prevalence and in the increasing trends across countries, and decline or leveling off in some developed countries) also provide useful insights into the causes of the problem.

The increase in childhood obesity worldwide is a result of many changes in society due, in particular, to social and economic development and policies in the areas of agriculture, transport, urban planning, the environment, food processing, distribution and marketing, and education. These factors have contributed to unhealthy eating, lack of PA, and increasing sedentary behaviors in children, which result in excessive weight gain. There has been a global shift in diet toward increased intake of energy-dense foods that are high in fat and sugars but low in other healthy micronutrients and a trend toward decreased PA levels due to the increasingly sedentary nature of recreation activities, changing modes of transportation, and urbanization [3].

Rapid economic development and urbanization have contributed to nutrition transition and thus affected people's lifestyle (e.g., the shift from under nutrition to over nutrition, energy-dense diets have replaced traditional diets, and sedentary lifestyles) [18]. Many developing countries have experienced rapid economic development and urbanization during the past two to three decades, partially related to the expansion of global trade and the development of technologies.

Over the past decade, there has been a growing interest in studying the impact of environment factors including neighborhood and school environment, on obesity risk and related health behaviors in children. The built environment refers to man-made structures (such as food outlets, grocery stores, street design, green spaces, and parks). Most of the research was conducted in high-income countries; and it has reported some mixed results. It has also been recognized that the social environment can also influence behaviors.

Research shows that time spent engaged in sedentary behaviors, particularly watching television, is positively related to weight gain and the development of obesity [4]. Children with televisions in their bedroom watch more television and gain more weight. Growing evidence from multiple countries, in particular, medium- and high-income countries, suggests that sedentary behaviors are prevalent among children.

Family and parental SES is another important factor affecting children's risk of developing obesity. The obesity–SES relation is complex and seems to have changed over time, and it varies by gender, age, and country [2]. The reported mixed results are due, in part, to the complex relationship between SES and obesity. The other reason for mixed results is that various different measures have been used to measure SES, such as the use of family income and education levels. In general, research shows that low-SES individuals in industrialized countries and high-SES individuals in developing countries were at greater risk of obesity when compared with referent groups [2]. In developing countries, higher-SES groups (families) have greater access to energy-dense diets and sedentary lifestyles than their lower-SES counterparts. On the contrary, in developed countries, the low-SES groups (families) have greater access to energy-dense diets, including food items such as processed food and fast food, but less access to healthier diets consisting of adequate fresh vegetables and fruits than their high-SES counterparts. A recent large study using data from 78 countries reported that the prevalence of obesity and overweight among young children in the wealthiest quintile was on average 1.31 times higher than the poorest quintile [28]. Maternal education was associated with improved childcare practices related to health and nutrition and, therefore, seems to affect children's obesity risk [28].

As an example, one recent study [29] used data collected from 5844 children from local study sites (i.e., cities, not nationally representative) in 12 countries (Australia, Brazil, Canada, China, Colombia, Finland, India, Kenya, Portugal, South Africa, the United Kingdom, and the United States). It showed that sedentary behaviors were common among the children studied, although there are large differences across countries (Table 3.2). These children had an average of 8.6 h of daily total sedentary time, and 54.2% of the children failed to meet screen-time guidelines (i.e., had >2 h of screen time/day). In all study sites, boys reported higher screen time, were less likely to meet screen-time guidelines, and had higher BMI z-scores than girls. In 9 of the 12 sites, girls had significantly more total sedentary time than boys. Participants from the China site (Tianjin City, one of the four largest cities in China) engaged in the highest amount of sedentary time (9.4 h/day), but had the second lowest screen-time score (about 1.9 h/day). This indicates that children in cities or/and high-SES groups in developing countries such as China already are similarly, or even more,

TABLE 3.2
Prevalence (%) of Overweight and Obesity and Sedentary Time of Participants (n = 5844) in The International Study of Childhood Obesity, Lifestyle, and the Environment

Site Country (City)	World Bank Ranking (Income)	Parental Higher Education[a] (n, [%])	Sample Size (% Boys)	Overweight/ Obese[b] (n, [%])	Sedentary Time (h/day, Mean [SD])	Screen-Time Score[d] (Mean [SD])	Not Meeting Screen-Time Guidelines[e] (n, [%])
All sites		3406 (58.3)	5844 (45.6)	1888 (32.3)[c]	8.6 (1.2)	2.6 (1.8)	3158 (54.2)
1. Australia (Adelaide)	High	364 (80.2)	454 (46.0)	169 (37.2)	7.9 (1.0)	2.8 (1.8)	266 (58.6)
2. Brazil (São Caetano do Sul)	Upper middle	172 (40.3)	427 (48.0)	195 (45.7)	8.3 (1.4)	3.7 (2.3)	309 (72.4)
3. Canada (Ottawa)	High	458 (91.2)	502 (41.6)	154 (30.7)[c]	8.5 (1.0)	2.4 (1.9)	227 (45.2)
4. China (Tianjin)	Upper middle	240 (49.3)	487 (52.0)	204 (41.9)[c]	9.4 (1.1)	1.9 (1.7)	164 (33.7)
5. Colombia (Bogotá)	Upper middle	281 (33.6)	836 (49.3)	192 (23.0)[c]	8.3 (1.1)	2.9 (1.5)	552 (66.0)
6. Finland (Helsinki, Espoo, Vantaa)	High	331 (73.2)	452 (46.9)	110 (24.3)	8.8 (1.2)	2.7 (1.7)	257 (56.9)
7. India (Bangalore)	Lower middle	448 (83.0)	540 (45.6)	173 (32.0)	8.6 (1.1)	1.8 (1.3)	169 (31.3)
8. Kenya (Nairobi)	Low	298 (64.2)	464 (45.9)	90 (19.4)	8.2 (1.1)	2.4 (1.7)	246 (53.0)
9. Portugal (Porto)	High	116 (21.1)	547 (43.0)	250 (45.7)[c]	9.2 (1.0)	2.3 (1.5)	265 (48.5)
10. South Africa (Cape Town)	Upper middle	91 (29.7)	306 (40.0)	80 (26.1)	8.2 (1.1)	3.1 (2.1)	191 (62.4)
11. The United Kingdom (Bath, Northeast Somerset)	High	294 (72.2)	407 (42.8)	111 (27.3)	8.3 (1.0)	2.9 (1.7)	275 (67.6)
12. The United States (Baton Rouge)	High	313 (74.2)	422 (41.0)	160 (37.9)	8.7 (1.0)	3.1 (2.3)	247 (58.5)

Source: LeBlanc, A. G., et al., *PLoS One*, 10(6), e0129622, 2015.

Note: BMI, body mass index; SD, standard deviation.

a Number (%) of sample who had had at least one parent complete more than high school education (i.e., > some college/university).

b Number (%) with WHO BMI z-score classification overweight or obese.

c Sites where boys had significantly higher values than girls (*p* < .05).

d Screen-time score = ([hours of TV on weekdays × 5] + [hours of TV on weekend days × 2] + [hours of video games and computers on weekdays × 5] + [hours of video games and computers on weekend days × 2])/7.

e Number (%) of children not meeting guidelines of ≤2 h of screen time/day.

sedentary than children in many other industrialized countries. This help explains why obesity rates have increased so rapidly in these developing countries; and in urban areas or/and high-SES groups, the obesity prevalence has reached a level similar to that in industrialized countries. The study reported that the prevalence of overweight/obesity ranged from 19% (in the city from Kenya) to almost 46% (in the two cities from Brazil and Portugal).

PREVENTION OF CHILDHOOD OBESITY: GLOBAL IMPLICATIONS

A large number of studies have been conducted regarding childhood obesity prevention and treatment, though the majority are conducted in high-income countries and very little is known about other countries [30–32]. Nevertheless, lessons learned in high-income countries are useful for middle- and low-income countries. The growing obesity problem is societal, and thus it demands a population-based multisectoral, multidisciplinary, and culturally relevant approach, and international collaborations are needed [3]. Unlike most adults, children do not have much power to choose the environment in which they live and the food they eat. Further, they also have a limited ability to understand the long-term consequences of their behaviors. Therefore, special attention and efforts are needed to help them to develop desirable lifelong habits for preventing obesity.

More research is needed in developing countries, as the reported studies are predominately conducted in developed countries. We, and others, have reviewed various interventions conducted in countries worldwide to determine what programs are successful and where more research is needed for childhood obesity prevention [30–34]. A large number of studies have been conducted to study childhood obesity prevention, and mixed results are reported [30,31]. Nevertheless, adequate evidence has been accumulated that supports the possibility that interventions, especially school-based programs, could be effective in preventing childhood obesity. Meanwhile, even if some of the interventions cannot reduce obesity, they may still result in other beneficial changes in other health outcomes, such as lowered blood pressure and improved blood lipid profile, as shown by our recent systematic reviews and meta-analyses [30,31,35,36].

In the most comprehensive systematic review and meta-analysis on childhood obesity prevention studies reported thus far, we evaluated the effectiveness of various childhood obesity prevention programs [30,31]. The findings would help various stakeholders to understand the effectiveness of obesity prevention programs for children and offer insights for future research and intervention development. We assessed 139 studies conducted in multiple settings in high-income countries over the past three decades, focusing on adiposity-related outcomes and strength of evidence (SOE). Our study showed that the SOE varied by intervention strategy and setting. There was at least moderate SOE for school-based intervention and about 50% of schools reported statistically significant desirable effects for adipose-related measures. The SOE for the effectiveness of interventions in settings other than schools and homes was insufficient mainly due to the small number of published research found.

Both healthy eating and PA should be the targets in obesity prevention, though some researchers have argued that it may be more feasible and effective to target the control of energy intake, by using national policies, regulations, programs, etc. Recently, top experts in the childhood obesity research field argued that nutrition policies are needed to tackle child obesity; and such policies need to promote healthy growth, availability of healthy foods in the home and to protect children from inducements to be inactive or to overconsume foods of poor nutritional quality. A public health effort is needed to protect children from the marketing of sedentary activities and energy-dense, nutrient-poor foods and beverages. The governance of food supply and food markets should be improved and commercial activities need be monitored and regulated [33].

CONCLUSIONS

Over the past decade, rich data from both industrialized and developing countries have demonstrated that obesity has become a serious global public health problem. Recently, the WHO has called on countries to take actions to combat the epidemic [3]. The combined prevalence has tripled in many countries worldwide since the 1980s and the number of people and families affected is expected to continue to rise. Obesity development during childhood has many short- and long-term health and financial consequences for individuals, families, and society. Obesity is already responsible for 2%–8% of health-care costs and 10%–13% of deaths in parts of Europe, and it is projected to be even worse in the United States, reaching 17% of deaths in 2030 [37]. Children are the key target to focus on to control the obesity epidemic.

The obesity burden is huge at present, and will become worse in the future. The many profound changes in society, living environments, and individual behavioral patterns of the past two to three decades have contributed to the epidemic. Economic growth, modernization, urbanization, the globalization of food markets and service have fueled lifestyle shifts, including overconsumption of food and reduced PA in people's daily lives [1–4]. Compared with adults, children are often more sensitive to changes in their living and social environments.

Childhood obesity is a serious public threat in many industrialized and developing countries worldwide and the problem is expected to continue to grow. The epidemic calls for timely and effective population-based approaches to face its challenges. Obesity is largely preventable. However, once developed, it is difficult to cure. Obesity has many health and financial consequences for individuals, their families, and society. Therefore, the prevention of childhood obesity should take high national priority in many countries. The development of effective population-based intervention programs for the prevention and management of obesity in children is crucial to combat the epidemic of obesity and noncommunicable chronic diseases.

ACKNOWLEDGMENTS

This work is supported in part by research grants from the US National Institute of Health, the Eunice Kennedy Shriver National Institute of Child Health and Human Development (NICHD), and the Office of Behavioral and Social Sciences Research (OBSSR) (grant numbers are 1R01HD064685–01A1 and 1U54 HD070725). I want to thank Professors Hyun-Jung Lim and Liang Wang and Miss Huiru Chang for their assistance in helping prepare this chapter.

REFERENCES

1. Wang Y. and Lobstein T. Worldwide trends in childhood overweight and obesity. *International Journal of Pediatric Obesity*, 2006, 1, 11–25.
2. Wang Y. and Lim H. The global childhood obesity epidemic and the association between socioeconomic status and childhood obesity. *International Review of Psychiatry*, 2012, 24(3), 176–188.
3. World Health Organization (WHO). Childhood overweight and obesity. http://www.who.int/dietphysicalactivity/childhood/en, accessed November 11, 2015.
4. Lobstein T., Baur L., Uauy R., and IASO International Obesity Task Force. Obesity in children and young people: A crisis in public health. *Obesity Reviews*, 2004, 5 Suppl 1, 4–104.
5. Cole T. J., Bellizzi M. C., Flegal K. M., and Dietz W. H. Establishing a standard definition for child overweight and obesity worldwide: International survey. *British Medical Journal*, 2000, 320, 1240–1243.
6. Wang Y. Epidemiology of childhood obesity–methodological aspects and guidelines: What is new? *International Journal of Obesity*, 2004, 28 Suppl 3, S21–28.
7. World Health Organization (WHO). *Physical Status: The Use and Interpretation of Anthropometry. Report of a WHO Expert Committee.* World Health Organization Technical Report Series, 854, pp. 1–452, Geneva: WHO, 1995.
8. World Health Organization (WHO). Obesity: Preventing and managing the global epidemic. Report of a WHO consultation. World Health Organization Technical Report Series, 894, pp. i–xii, 1–253, Geneva: WHO, 2000.
9. Wang Y., Moreno L. A., Caballero B., and Cole T. J. Limitations of the current World Health Organization growth references for children and adolescents. *Food and Nutrition Bulletin*, 2006, 27(4 Suppl Growth Standard), S175–188.
10. Wang Y. and Wang J. Q. A comparison of international references for the assessment of child and adolescent overweight and obesity in different populations. *European Journal of Clinical Nutrition*, 2002, 56, 973–982.

11. World Health Organization (WHO). The WHO child growth standards. 2006. http://www.who.int/childgrowth/en/, accessed November 11, 2015.

12. de Onis M., Onyango A. W., Borghi E., Siyam A., Nishida C., and Siekmann J. Development of a WHO growth reference for school-aged children and adolescents. *Bulletin of the World Health Organization*, 2007, 85, 660–667.

13. Kuczmarski R. J., Ogden C. L., Grummer-Strawn L. M., et al. CDC growth charts: United States. *Advance Data*, 2000, 314, 1–27.

14. Must A., Dallal G. E., and Dietz W. H. Reference data for obesity: 85th and 95th percentiles of body mass index (wt/ht2) and triceps skinfold thickness. *American Journal of Clinical Nutrition*, 1991, 53(4), 839–846.

15. Beydoun M. A. and Wang Y. Socio-demographic disparities in distribution shifts over time in various adiposity measures among American children and adolescents: What changes in prevalence rates could not reveal. *International Journal of Pediatric Obesity*, 2011, 6(1), 21–35.

16. Due P., Damsgaard M. T., Rasmussen, M., et al. Socioeconomic position, macroeconomic environment and overweight among adolescents in 35 countries. *International Journal of Obesity*, 2009, 33, 1084–1093.

17. Ng M., Fleming T., Robinson M., et al. Global, regional, and national prevalence of overweight and obesity in children and adults during 1980–2013: A systematic analysis for the Global Burden of Disease Study 2013. *Lancet*, 2014, 384(9945), 766–781.

18. de Onis M., Blossner M., and Borghi, E. Global prevalence and trends of overweight and obesity among preschool children. *American Journal of Clinical Nutrition*, 2010, 92, 1257–1264.

19. Tzioumis E. and Adair L. S. Childhood dual burden of under- and overnutrition in low- and middle-income countries: A critical review. *Food and Nutrition Bulletin*, 2014, 35(2), 230–243.

20. Wang Y., Baker J. L., Hill J. O., and Dietz W. H. Controversies regarding reported trends: Has the obesity epidemic leveled off in the United States? *Advances in Nutrition*, 2012, 3(5), 751–752.

21. Ahrens W., Moreno L. A., and Pigeot, I. *Childhood Obesity: Prevalence Worldwide Epidemiology of Obesity in Children and Adolescents*, 1st edn, pp. 219–235, New York: Springer, 2011.

22. Wang Y. and Beydoun M. A. The obesity epidemic in the United States–gender, age, socioeconomic, racial/ethnic, and geographic characteristics: A systematic review and meta-regression analysis. *Epidemiologic Reviews*, 2007, 29, 6–28.

23. Ogden C. L., Carroll M. D., Kit B. K., and Flegal K. M. Prevalence of obesity and trends in body mass index among US children and adolescents, 1999–2010. *JAMA*, 2012, 307, 483–490.

24. Ogden C. L., Carroll M. D., Kit B. K., and Flegal K. M. Prevalence of childhood and adult obesity in the United States, 2011–2012. *JAMA*, 2014, 311(8), 806–814.

25. Wang Y., Mi J., Shan X. Y., Wang Q. J., and Ge K. Y. Is China facing an obesity epidemic and the consequences? The trends in obesity and chronic disease in China. *International Journal of Obesity* (London), 2007, 31(1), 177–188.

26. Ji C. Y. and Cheng T. O. Epidemic increase in overweight and obesity in Chinese children from 1985 to 2005. *International Journal of Cardiology*, 2009, 132, 1–10.

27. Institute of Medicine (IOM). Early childhood obesity prevention: Policies goals, recommendations, and potential actions. 2011. https://iom.nationalacademies.org/Reports/2011/Early-Childhood-Obesity-Prevention-Policies/Recommendations.aspx, accessed October 23, 2015.

28. Black R. E., Victora C. G., Walker S.P., et al; Maternal and Child Nutrition Study Group. Maternal and child undernutrition and overweight in low-income and middle-income countries. *Lancet*, 2013, 382(9890), 427–451.

29. LeBlanc A. G., Katzmarzyk P. T., Barreira T.V., et al; ISCOLE Research Group. Correlates of total sedentary time and screen time in 9–11 year-old children around the world: The international study of childhood obesity, lifestyle and the environment. *PLoS One*, 2015, 10(6), e0129622.

30. Wang Y., Wu Y., Wilson R. F., Bleich S., Cheskin L., Weston C., Showell N., Fawole O., Lau B., and Segal J. *Childhood Obesity Prevention Programs: Comparative Effectiveness Review and Meta-Analysis*. Rockville, MD: Agency for Healthcare Research and Quality (US), 2013.

31. Wang Y., Cai L., Wu Y., et al. What childhood obesity prevention programmes work? A systematic review and meta-analysis. *Obesity Reviews*, 2015, 16(7), 547–565.

32. Showell N. N., Fawole O., Segal J., Wilson R. F., Cheskin L. J., Bleich S. N., Wu Y., Lau B., and Wang Y. A systematic review of home-based childhood obesity prevention studies. *Pediatrics*, 2013, 132(1), e193–200.

33. Lobstein T., Jackson-Leach R., Moodie M. L., Hall K. D., Gortmaker S. L., Swinburn B. A., James P., Wang Y., and McPherson K. Child and adolescent obesity: Part of a bigger picture. *Lancet*, 2015, 385(9986), 2510–2520.

34. van Hoek E., Feskens E. J., Bouwman L. I., and Janse A. J. Effective interventions in overweight or obese young children: Systematic review and meta-analysis. *Childhood Obesity*, 2014, 10(6), 448–460.

35. Cai L., Wu Y., Wilson R., Segal J. B., Kim M., and Wang Y. Effect of childhood obesity prevention programs on blood pressure: A systematic review and meta-analysis. *Circulation*, 2014a, 129(18), 1832–1839.

36. Cai L., Wu Y., Cheskin L., Wilson R. F., and Wang Y. The effect of childhood obesity prevention programs on blood lipids: A systematic review and meta-analysis. *Obesity Reviews*, 2014b, 15(12), 933–944.

37. Wang Y., Beydoun M. A., Liang L., Caballero B., and Kumanyika S. K. Will all Americans become overweight or obese? Estimating the progression and cost of the US obesity epidemic. *Obesity (Silver Spring)*, 2008, 16(10), 2323–2330.

4 Economic Considerations in Childhood Obesity

John Cawley and Ashlesha Datar

CONTENTS

INTRODUCTION

This chapter discusses the economic aspects of childhood obesity. The first three sections discuss the economic causes and correlates of obesity in children and youth. The first section starts with a discussion of the recent literature on the impact of federal food assistance programs that provide subsidized food for low-income families. The next section discusses the evidence on how food prices, in particular the prices of energy-dense, nonnutritious foods and beverages relative to the prices of more nutritious foods and beverages, are related to children's dietary intake and body weight outcomes. The third section describes the current evidence on how macroeconomic conditions, in particular economic downturns that are characterized by high unemployment rates, are related to children's dietary intake and body weight outcomes. The fourth section discusses the evidence on one important economic consequence of obesity: higher medical care costs. Finally, the last section discusses what is known from economic evaluations of antiobesity interventions. The method of cost effectiveness has been used to estimate which programs give society the greatest "bang for the buck." This section lists which interventions have been found to be cost saving, which are cost-effective (i.e., costly but considered good value), and which are not cost-effective (the benefits are small relative to the costs).

FOOD ASSISTANCE AND NUTRITION PROGRAMS

There are four large federal food assistance and nutrition programs (FANP) in the United States that have the potential to substantially influence children's diets and obesity. A shared goal of these programs is to promote adequate nutritional intake in their specific target populations (all of them low income). We describe each of these programs briefly (for detailed eligibility and benefits, see Aussenberg and Colello [1]) and summarize the current research findings about their impacts on children's diets and obesity.

Empirical estimation of the effects of FANP is challenging because participation in these programs is nonrandom. Therefore, much of the literature has compared the outcomes of participants with nonparticipants, conditional on observable characteristics (see the discussion in Meyerhoefer and Yang [2]). A much smaller literature, which is the focus of our review, has sought to estimate causal effects by addressing selection into the programs using quasi-experimental methods that leverage, for example, variation in program rollout, policy variation, or longitudinal data.

The largest of the four food assistance programs is the Supplemental Nutrition Assistance Program (SNAP), formerly called the Food Stamp Program, which provides low-income households (i.e., those with gross income below 130% of the federal poverty line and who also have low assets) with electronic benefit transfer cards that can be used to purchase groceries. In 2014, the program served 46.5 million individuals, with average monthly benefits of $125 per person [3].

Studies of the effect of SNAP on child BMI find varying effects [2–8]. For example, Gibson [6] examined longitudinal data from the National Longitudinal Survey of Youth 1979 Child Sample and found that SNAP participation led to a reduction in overweight for 5- to 11-year-old boys but an increase in overweight for 5- to 11-year-old girls. Schmeiser [7] analyzed the same data but used the method of instrumental variables to estimate causal effects and found that SNAP participation reduced BMI for most gender-age groups. Yet another study, Kreider et al. [8], addressed selection into and measurement error of SNAP using the National Health and Nutrition Examination Survey (NHANES) data and found that positive or negative effects of SNAP on child BMI could not be ruled out. It is perhaps unsurprising that research has found mixed results regarding the effect of SNAP on child weight, given that there are no nutritional requirements for the types of foods and beverages that can be purchased with SNAP vouchers.

The second largest food assistance and nutrition program is the Special Supplemental Nutrition Program for women, infants, and children (WIC). Only children under age five years and pregnant (or recently postpartum) women in low-income households (i.e., income no higher than 185% of the federal poverty line) are eligible. The program provides nutritious food supplements, nutrition education, and access to health services. WIC benefits can be used to purchase infant formula and a limited range of food items such as milk, cereal, and juice. In 2014, WIC served 8.3 million individuals, of whom 10% were pregnant women, 13% were postpartum or breast-feeding women, 24% were infants, and 53% were children [9].

Much of the literature on WIC's impact has focused on birth outcomes, especially birth weight, which is an important predictor of later-life health. On the one hand, high birth weight (>4000 g) has been hypothesized to "program" an increased risk of later obesity [10,11]. On the other hand, the "developmental origins of disease" literature proposes that undernutrition during fetal life and infancy is associated with higher risk of coronary heart disease (CHD), type 2 diabetes, stroke, hypertension, and other chronic diseases. The general finding in the WIC literature is that women who participate in WIC are less likely than nonparticipants to have low birth weight babies [4,12–16]. Based on the "fetal programing hypothesis," this finding implies a reduction in the likelihood of CHD and related chronic diseases in adulthood. Given WIC's focus on providing nutritious food supplements in early childhood, the program has tremendous potential for reducing child BMI and obesity, but unfortunately there has been no rigorous evaluation of these impacts yet.

The National School Lunch Program (NSLP) and the School Breakfast Program (SBP) provide free and reduced-price meals to low-income children at public and private schools. The NSLP and SBP serve meals to 30.4 million and 13.6 million students, respectively [9]. Meals served as part of these programs are subject to nutritional regulations. In response to concerns about the nutritional quality of school meals, the 2010 Healthy, Hunger-Free Kids Act made major changes to nutrition standards for school meals. Updated program rules have imposed both minimum and maximum calorie rules. The new rules also include stronger requirements for daily and weekly food group servings, including weekly requirements for a variety of vegetables (such as dark green, red/orange, and starchy), restrictions on the fat content of milk, and a phased-in requirement to use only whole grains. The act also gave the US Department of Agriculture (USDA) authority to set nutritional standards for all "competitive foods" sold in schools during the school day.

Research on the NSLP has used data that were collected prior to the 2012–2013 implementation of the Healthy, Hunger-Free Kids Act, so any benefits of that legislation will not yet be evident.

Findings regarding the impact of NSLP participation on children's diet quality are mixed. Gleason and Suitor [17] used data from the School Nutrition and Dietary Assessment Study and compared observations of dietary intake for a student across multiple days that varied by whether the student did or did not receive a school lunch, and found mixed evidence on nutrition intake. NSLP participation increased the consumption of fat, protein, and six types of vitamins and minerals, but there was no overall impact on total calories eaten at lunch or over a 24 h period. Therefore, not surprisingly, evidence on the relationship between NSLP participation and childhood obesity is also mixed. Schanzenbach [18] and Millimet et al. [19] analyzed longitudinal data on a national sample of children and found that NSLP participants became comparatively heavier as their exposure to school lunches increased, conditional on their BMI at school entry. Mirtcheva and Powell [20] used longitudinal data on children participating in the Panel Study of Income Dynamics (PSID) and found that NSLP had no effect on body weight. In contrast, Gundersen et al. [21] addressed selection and measurement problems in NSLP using NHANES data and found that receipt of free or reduced-price lunch substantially reduced obesity rates. Thus, every possible relationship has been found between school lunch receipt and child weight.

The evidence on the impact of SBP participation is more consistent and encouraging. Bhattacharya et al. [22] found that SBP participation improved dietary quality as measured by the Healthy Eating Index and several measures of diet (vitamin intake, folate, anemia, and high cholesterol) based on the results of blood serum tests. Millimet et al. [19] found that school breakfast participation was associated with a lower risk of childhood obesity. Some states have statutes requiring participation in the SBP for schools that have a critical mass of students (which varies across states, typically between 10% and 40%) eligible for free or reduced-price meals. Frisvold [23] used these thresholds to estimate the impact of SBP for schools near the thresholds. He found that SBP participation improved the nutritional content of breakfast. Finally, evidence from the only randomized experiment conducted on this question found protective effects of SBP participation. Crepinsek et al. [24] analyzed data from a USDA-sponsored, large, randomized-controlled trial of Universal Free Breakfast (UFB) and found that students who attended a school randomly assigned to receive UFB were more likely to consume a nutritionally substantive breakfast, although the program had no impact on 24 h dietary intakes or the probability of skipping breakfast.

The NSLP and SBP programs have enormous potential to influence children's diets and obesity due to their tremendous reach. It will be important to evaluate whether improvements to the nutritional standards for school meals since 2012–2013 have been successful at reducing childhood obesity.

FOOD PRICES

Understanding how food prices influence food consumption and body weight is important because food taxes and subsidies represent potential policy tools for preventing and reducing obesity. Adults' food and beverage purchases appear to respond to changes in price, with price elasticities (i.e., the percentage change in purchases of a good associated with a 1% change in its price) ranging from −0.27 to −0.81 [25]. When elasticities are estimated separately by category of food, food away from home (e.g., restaurant meals), soft drinks, juice, and meat purchases are most responsive to price. However, while consumers buy less of the foods that become relatively more expensive, they may also switch to buying more of the foods that have become relatively less expensive, with little net change in weight (see the review in [26]). Several studies have investigated the relationship between prices of specific food groups—such as meat, fruits/vegetables, and fast food—and childhood obesity. This literature has found that higher prices for fast food and lower prices for fruits and vegetables are associated with lower child BMI [27–30]. More recently, Wendt and Todd [31] estimated the association of food prices with children's BMI using retail food prices from the USDA's Quarterly Food-at-Home Price Database (QFAHPD). It found that lower prices for soda, starchy vegetables, and sweet snacks were associated with higher child BMI. It speculated that consumer responses to price reductions (subsidies) are similar in magnitude to price increases (taxes), though of course in the opposite direction.

Research has also found variation in price responsiveness by household income and weight status. The estimated effects are larger among children in lower-income households, which is consistent with economic theory [32]. Studies also found that price responsiveness is higher among overweight and obese individuals. For example, Sturm et al. [33] found a negative and statistically significant effect of state soda taxes on BMI among children at or above the 85th percentile.

Overall, this literature suggests that, while children's dietary behaviors and body weight outcomes may be responsive to prices of nutritious and less-nutritious foods, the magnitude of those relationships is small [34], and therefore small taxes or subsidies are unlikely to produce meaningful changes in body weight outcomes in children. More research is needed to examine if larger taxes on unhealthy foods and/or subsidies for healthy foods would be effective.

ECONOMIC FLUCTUATIONS

Social scientists have had a long-standing interest in examining how fluctuations in macroeconomic conditions can influence health behaviors and outcomes [35–40]. It is argued that declines in working hours during recessions reduce stress levels and make more time available for positive health behaviors such as exercise and healthy eating [41]. Also, resulting reductions in income may force cutbacks of unhealthy behaviors such as smoking and consumption of alcohol, sugared soft drinks, and restaurant food. Research on adults has found mixed results; some researchers have found that economic downturns are associated with higher body weight [42] and reductions in the consumption of fruits and vegetables [43,44], whereas others have found that economic downturns are associated with a lower probability of obesity [37] and reductions in fat intake [35].

The relationship between economic fluctuations and children's health behaviors and outcomes has received less attention. Economic downturns can affect children through household-specific shocks (e.g., income shocks and stress resulting from parents' job loss, home foreclosure) that might lead to changes in households' consumption and expenditure patterns related to diet and activity behaviors. Two recent studies suggest that the Great Recession may have been associated with adverse diet and BMI outcomes among children. Ng et al. [45] analyzed the Nielsen Homescan data and found that the caloric purchases of households with children increased slightly in areas with higher unemployment rates; Oddo et al. [46] analyzed children's statewide fitness data from California and found that the recession was associated with an increase in BMI z-score and the risk of overweight and obesity. In contrast, a growing literature suggests that decreases in maternal work, induced by economic downturns, are associated with better dietary behaviors and lower obesity in children [47–50]. Research examining the effects among adolescents and teenagers [51] has found interesting gender differences: increases in the state unemployment rate are associated with higher BMI in female teenagers but lower BMI in male teenagers, possibly because teenage males are more physically active than females during downturns.

MEDICAL CARE COSTS OF CHILDHOOD OBESITY

Estimates of the medical care costs of childhood obesity are useful for several reasons. First, they give a sense of the burden on the health-care system (and, more generally, the economy) imposed by childhood obesity. Second, such estimates are necessary to calculate the cost effectiveness of programs designed to prevent or treat childhood obesity. Third, they provide information about the extent of external costs, which are the costs that are paid by people other than the decision maker. The vast majority of the medical care costs of children in the United States are paid by private health insurance companies or public health insurance programs such as Medicaid and the State Children's Health Insurance Program (SCHIP). Neither the premiums paid in private group health insurance nor the taxes that fund Medicaid and SCHIP are indexed to weight, and as a result those who are not obese subsidize the medical care costs of those who are obese. Such external costs impose deadweight loss (inefficiency) on society, and they represent an economic rationale for government intervention.

Ideally, we would like to know the causal effect of obesity on medical care costs for youth. However, causal effects are difficult to measure in this context. It would, of course, be unethical to conduct a randomized controlled trial (RCT) that made youth obese in order to measure the resulting increase in their medical care costs. We could conduct an RCT for a weight loss intervention and measure the extent to which medical care costs fall with the resulting weight loss, but the method of weight loss could have a direct effect on medical care costs, independent of weight loss. For example, bariatric surgery or prescription weight loss drugs could result in complications or side effects that raise medical care costs, or a more nutritious diet or physically active lifestyle could have health benefits (aside from weight loss) that lower costs.

Given these complexities, there is little evidence on the causal effect of childhood obesity on medical care costs. Instead, numerous studies have measured the correlation of childhood obesity and medical care costs; that is, the extent to which the medical care costs of overweight or obese youth exceed those of healthy-weight youth. These correlations could be quite different from the causal effect if obese youths have comorbidities or behaviors that also affect health-care costs.

Trasande and Chatterjee [52] estimated the extent to which childhood obesity is associated with higher expenditures on outpatient visits, prescription drugs, and emergency room visits. They examined data for youths aged 6–19 years in the Medical Expenditure Panel Study (MEPS) for 2002–2005, with all medical expenditures converted to year 2005 dollars. Youth were classified as overweight or obese based on weight and height that were proxy reported by parents (for those aged 6–17 years) or self-reported (for youths aged 18–19). The MEPS consisted of up to six interviews over two years. The authors estimated that children who were obese in both years of the MEPS had $194 higher outpatient visit expenditures, $114 higher prescription drug expenditures, and $12 higher emergency room expenditures, per year than children who were normal weight or underweight in at least one of the 2 years. Children who were overweight in both years of the MEPS, or overweight in one year and obese in the other, had $79 higher outpatient visit expenditures, $64 higher prescription drug expenditures, and $25 higher emergency room expenditures, per year compared with children who were normal weight or underweight in at least one of the two years. The authors estimated that overweight and obesity combined cost the United States $14.1 billion annually in additional outpatient visits, prescription drugs, and emergency room visits.

Trasande et al. [53] estimated the hospital costs associated with childhood obesity. They examined data for children aged 2–19 years in the 1999–2005 National Inpatient Sample, which samples 20% of community hospitals each year. Hospital charges were converted to costs using hospital-specific cost-to-charge ratios from the Centers for Medicare and Medicaid Services, and were expressed in year 2005 dollars. BMI and weight were not observed; the authors identified obese youths using ICD-9 codes that indicated obesity was a primary or secondary diagnosis (which presumably results in a high degree of false negatives). Among hospitalizations with obesity as a secondary diagnosis, the most common primary diagnoses were affective disorders (e.g., depression, bipolar disorder, and anxiety disorder), pregnancy-associated conditions, asthma, and diabetes mellitus. Obesity as a secondary diagnosis was associated with, on average, a 0.85 day longer length of hospital stay and $727 higher hospitalization costs. For pregnancy-related conditions, the increase in hospitalization costs was $2319; for affective disorders, $1031; and for asthma, $1479. The authors estimated that the total costs of hospitalizations of youths with any diagnosis of obesity totaled $237.6 million in 2005. Note that this does not represent the *additional* costs associated with obesity—these are the *total* costs of hospitalizations for any youth assigned an ICD-9 code for obesity. Some of these youths might still have been hospitalized (albeit at lower cost) if they were healthy weight. This is also almost certainly an underestimate given that many hospital stays for obese youths will not receive an ICD-9 code for obesity.

Finkelstein et al. [54] reviewed the literature on the medical care costs of obesity and estimated that the incremental lifetime medical cost of an obese child relative to a normal-weight child who maintains normal weight throughout adulthood is $19,000 in year 2006 dollars. If one takes into account the likelihood of eventual weight gain among normal weight youth, the incremental lifetime costs are lowered to $12,660.

One interesting question is whether the duration of childhood obesity matters. That is, do children who have been obese for a longer period have higher medical care costs than those who have been obese for a shorter period? This question is difficult to answer using US data; the MEPS has only up to 2 years of data on each individual. However, Au [55], using data from the Longitudinal Study of Australian Children for 2004, 2006, and 2008, found that the duration of childhood overweight (classified using BMI based on measurements of weight and height) does raise medical care costs, but only starting at age 8–9 years.

There is general consensus that the medical care costs of obesity are smaller for children than adults [56]. For example, Ma and Frick [57] estimated models of medical care expenditures using the MEPS data for 2006 and found that obese adults spent $1548 more and obese children $264 more per capita than healthy-weight adults or children. In terms of annual medical expenditures for the United States, Trasande et al. [53] estimated that childhood obesity is associated with $14.1 billion higher costs (in 2005 dollars) per year, while Cawley et al. [58] estimated that adult obesity raises medical care costs by $315.8 billion (in 2010 dollars) per year. Thus, one of the greatest costs of childhood obesity is that it increases the risk of adult obesity, which is quite expensive.

The increase in the medical care costs of obesity with age also implies that the cost effectiveness of interventions to prevent or reduce childhood obesity will be much greater the more durable the weight loss or prevention of weight gain [56]. Programs with benefits that dissipate rapidly will generate far lower savings than programs that cause weight loss that persists into adulthood.

COST EFFECTIVENESS OF INTERVENTIONS TO PREVENT AND REDUCE CHILDHOOD OBESITY

The method of cost effectiveness analysis allows decision makers to compare the benefits per unit cost (or "bang for the buck") of various interventions. One challenge is that the benefits from each program must be expressed in the same units; the most common such unit is the quality-adjusted life year saved or QALY. An intervention is generally considered cost-effective if it costs less than $50,000 per QALY saved (although this threshold is debatable and somewhat controversial). Other studies measure all benefits in terms of disability-adjusted life years (DALY) averted.

There exist estimates of the cost effectiveness of several US interventions to prevent and reduce childhood obesity. One of the most cost-effective such programs is the Coordinated Approach to Child Health (CATCH), a comprehensive intervention in elementary schools that promotes healthy eating and physical activity; it costs $900 per QALY saved [59].

Planet Health, a comprehensive intervention in middle schools that also promotes healthy eating and physical activity, is cost effective for girls (for whom it costs $4305 per QALY saved) but is not effective for boys [60].

Not all interventions measure program benefits in terms of QALYs and DALYs. One recent study evaluated the cost effectiveness of FitKid, an after-school program for third graders that promoted physical activity and healthy snacks, as well as academic enrichment and tutoring [61]. The outcome of focus was percentage body fat, rather than QALYs or DALYs. Based on a randomized controlled experiment, Wang et al. estimated that students who attended 40% or more of the intervention reduced percentage body fat by 0.76%, at a cost of $317 per student. Although the use of body fat as an outcome has its advantages—relative to measuring BMI, it does not penalize students who gain muscle through physical activity—it has the disadvantage of complicating comparisons with other cost effectiveness studies.

Facilitating comparisons of different programs is the goal of Assessing the Cost Effectiveness of Obesity (ACE Obesity), an ambitious project in Australia that seeks to estimate the cost effectiveness of all major antiobesity interventions in that country using a consistent methodology.

The extent to which each intervention reduced future morbidity and mortality was expressed as DALYs. A review of the project [62] classified such projects as either cost saving, cost-effective (i.e., costs less than $50,000 AUD per DALY), or not cost-effective (i.e., costs more than $50,000 AUD per QALY).

The list of cost-saving interventions to prevent or treat childhood obesity include (see Ananthapavan et al. [62], table 1)

- A family-based general practitioner program targeted to obese children
- A multifaceted targeted school-based program for overweight and obese children
- A school-based education program to reduce television watching
- A multifaceted school-based program to promote good nutrition and physical activity
- A school-based education program to reduce consumption of sugar-sweetened beverages
- Reducing advertising of unhealthy food and beverages to children
- Front-of-pack traffic light nutrition labeling
- A tax on unhealthy foods and beverages

The list of cost-effective interventions includes (see Ananthapavan et al. [62], table 1)

- Orlistat medication for obese adolescents
- A family-based general practitioner program targeted at overweight and moderately obese children

The list of interventions that were deemed not cost effective includes (see Ananthapavan et al. [62], table 1)

- Walking school bus
- TravelSMART (a program that works with primary schools to promote safe and active ways to travel to school)
- Active after-schools communities program

A recent study [63] estimated the net savings associated with a variety of policies to address childhood obesity in the United States. Using published estimates of program effects and costs, and a microsimulation model, it estimated that three policies would save more in medical expenditures than they cost: (1) an excise tax on sugar-sweetened beverages; (2) elimination of the tax deduction for advertising unhealthy food to children; and (3) nutrition standards for food and beverages sold in schools outside of meals. In contrast, bariatric surgery for adults was found to be a much more expensive way to reduce BMI, leading the authors to conclude that investment in prevention, rather than treatment, should be prioritized.

This relates to the old adage "prevention is cheaper than cure." This is not a universal rule, but is something that can be determined on a case-by-case basis using cost effectiveness analysis. The Ananthapavan et al. [62] review finds considerable heterogeneity; for both primary prevention programs and treatment programs, some specific interventions are cost saving, others are costly but cost-effective, and some are not cost-effective. In other words, prevention is sometimes, but not always, cheaper than cure; one must check the evidence from cost effectiveness analysis.

CONCLUSION

Economic research on child and youth obesity has yielded important insights. Research on the economic causes of obesity has found that school lunches may promote childhood obesity, while school breakfasts may prevent it, that people are responsive to the prices of food but that existing food taxes may be too small to have any detectable impact on weight, and that the impact of the macroeconomy on obesity is ambiguous. Research on the economic consequences of obesity indicates that childhood obesity raises health-care costs in the United States by at least $14.1 billion annually, but perhaps its greatest cost is that it increases the probability of adult obesity, which is extraordinarily expensive ($315.8 billion per year in the United States). Finally, the method of cost effectiveness provides vitally important information about which interventions work, and which provide the greatest "bang for the buck," which is important because there will always be a limited budget devoted to the prevention and reduction of childhood obesity. While not every method of prevention has been shown to be cheaper than treatments, in general the most cost-effective interventions are prevention programs for children. Using the results of cost effectiveness analysis to guide policymaking will ensure that those limited budgets achieve the greatest possible prevention and reduction of childhood obesity.

REFERENCES

1. Aussenberg RA, Colello KJ. Domestic food assistance: Summary of programs. Congressional Research Service Report. 2015. 7-5700 R42353. https://www.fas.org/sgp/crs/misc/R42353.pdf. Accessed January 7, 2016.
2. Meyerhoefer C, Yang M. The relationship between food assistance and health: A review of the literature and empirical strategies for identifying program effects. *Appl Econ Perspect Pol.* 2011; 33(3): 304–344.
3. U.S. Department of Agriculture (USDA). Supplemental nutrition assistance program (SNAP). 2015. http://www.fns.usda.gov/pd/supplemental-nutrition-assistance-program-snap. Accessed July 29, 2015.
4. Currie J. U.S. food and nutrition programs. In Moffitt, RA. (Ed.), *Means-Tested Transfer Programs in the United States*, pp. 291–363, Chicago, IL: University of Chicago Press, 2003.
5. Hoynes H, Schanzenbach DW. U.S. food and nutrition programs. In Moffitt, RA. (Ed.), *Economics of Means-Tested Transfer Programs*, Chicago, IL: University of Chicago Press, 2015.
6. Gibson D. Long-term food stamp program participation is differentially related to overweight in young girls and boys. *J Nutr.* 2004; 134(2): 372–379.
7. Schmeiser MD. The impact of long-term participation in the supplemental nutrition assistance program on child obesity. *Health Econ.* 2012; 21(4): 386–404.
8. Kreider B, Pepper JV, Gundersen C, Jolliffe D. Identifying the effects of SNAP (food stamps) on child health outcomes when participation is endogenous and misreported. *J Amer Statist Assoc.* 2012; 107(499): 958–975.
9. U.S. Department of Agriculture (USDA). Child nutrition tables. 2015. http://www.fns.usda.gov/pd/child-nutrition-tables. Accessed July 29, 2015.
10. Barker DJ. Maternal nutrition, fetal nutrition, and disease in later life. *Nutrition.* 1997; 13(9): 807–813.
11. Yu ZB, Han SP, Zhu GZ, et al. Birth weight and subsequent risk of obesity: A systematic review and meta-analysis. *Obes Rev.* 2011; 12(7): 525–542.
12. Bitler M, Currie J. Does WIC work? The effects of WIC on pregnancy and birth outcomes. *J Policy Anal Manage.* 2005; 24 (1): 73–91.
13. Joyce T, Racine A, Yunzal-Butler C. Reassessing the WIC effect: Evidence from the pregnancy nutrition surveillance system. *J Policy Anal Manage.* 2008; 27(2): 277–303.
14. Joyce T, Gibson D, Colman S. The changing association between prenatal participation in WIC and birth outcomes in New York City. *J Policy Anal Manage.* 2005; 24(4): 661–685.
15. Figlio D, Hamersma S, Roth J. Does prenatal WIC participation improve birth outcomes? New evidence from Florida. *J Public Econ.* 2009; 93(1): 235–245.
16. Currie J, Rajani I. Within-mother estimates of the effects of WIC on birth outcomes in New York City. Working paper no. w20400. Cambridge, MA: National Bureau of Economic Research, 2014.
17. Gleason PM, Suitor CW. Eating at school: How the national school lunch program affects children's diets. *Am J Agric Econ.* 2003; 85(4): 1047–1061.
18. Schanzenbach DW. Do school lunches contribute to childhood obesity? *J Hum Resour.* 2009; 44(3): 684–709.
19. Millimet DL, Tchernis R, Husain M. School nutrition programs and the incidence of childhood obesity. *J Hum Resour.* 2010; 45(3): 640–654.
20. Mirtcheva DM, Powell LM. National school lunch program participation and child body weight. *East Econ J.* 2013; 39(3): 328–345.

21. Gundersen C, Kreider B, Pepper J. The impact of the national school lunch program on child health: A nonparametric bounds analysis. *J Econom.* 2012; 166(1), 79–91.

22. Bhattacharya J, Currie J, Haider SJ. Breakfast of champions? The school breakfast program and the nutrition of children and families. *J Hum Resour.* 2006; 41(3): 445–466.

23. Frisvold DE. Nutrition and cognitive achievement: An evaluation of the school breakfast program. Discussion paper no. 1402-12. Madison, WI: Institute for Research on Poverty, 2012.

24. Crepinsek MK, Singh A, Bernstein LS, McLaughlin JE. Dietary effects of universal-free school breakfast: Findings from the evaluation of the school breakfast program pilot project. *J Am Diet Assoc.* 2006; 106(11): 1796–1803.

25. Andreyeva T, Long MW, Brownell KD. The impact of food prices on consumption: A systematic review of research on the price elasticity of demand for food. *Am J Public Health.* 2010; 100(2): 216–222.

26. Cawley J. An economy of scales: A selective review of obesity's economic causes, consequences, and solutions. *J Health Econ.* 2015; 43: 244–268.

27. Auld MC, Powell LM. Economics of food energy density and adolescent body weight. *Economica.* 2009; 76: 719–740.

28. Powell LM, Bao YJ. Food prices, access to food outlets and child weight. *Econ Hum Biol.* 2009; 7: 64–72.

29. Sturm R, Datar A. Body mass index in elementary school children, metropolitan area food prices and food outlet density. *Public Health.* 2005; 119(12): 1059–1068.

30. Sturm R, Datar A. Food prices and weight gain during elementary school: 5-year update. *Public Health.* 2008; 122(11): 1140–1143.

31. Wendt M, Todd JE. *The Effect of Food and Beverage Prices on Children's Weights.* ERR-118. Washington, DC: U.S. Department of Agriculture, Economic Research Service, 2011.

32. Lakdawalla D, Philipson T, Bhattacharya J. Welfare-enhancing technological change and the growth of obesity. *Amer Econ Rev Papers Proceedings.* 2005; 95(2): 253–257.

33. Sturm R, Powell LM, Chriqui JF, Chaloupka FJ. Soda taxes, soft drink consumption, and children's body mass index. *Health Aff (Milwood).* 2010; 29(5), 1052–1058.

34. Powell LM, Chaloupka FJ. Food prices and obesity: Evidence and policy implications for taxes and subsidies. *Milbank Q.* 2009; 87: 229–257.

35. Ruhm CJ. Are recessions good for your health? *Q J Econ.* 2000; 115(2): 617–650.

36. Ruhm CJ. Good times make you sick. *J Health Econ.* 2003; 22(4): 637–658.

37. Ruhm CJ. Healthy living in hard times. *J Health Econ.* 2005; 24(2): 341–363.

38. Ruhm CJ. A healthy economy can break your heart. *Demography.* 2007; 44(4): 829–848.

39. Gerdtham UG, Ruhm CJ. Deaths rise in good economic times: Evidence from the OECD. *Econ Hum Biol.* 2006; 4(3): 298–316.

40. Granados JAT. Recessions and mortality in Spain, 1980–1997. *Eur J Popul.* 2005; 21(4): 393–422.

41. Catalano R, Goldman-Mellor S, Saxton K, et al. The health effects of economic decline. *Annu Rev Public Health.* 2011; 32: 431–450.

42. Bockerman P, Johansson E, Helakorpi S, Prattala R, Vartiainen E, Uutela A. Does a slump really make you thinner? Finnish micro-level evidence 1978–2002. *Health Econ.* 2007; 16(1): 103–107.

43. Asgeirsdottir TL, Corman H, Noonan K, Reichman NE. Lifecycle effects of a recession on health behaviors: Boom, bust, and recovery in Iceland. *Econ Hum Biol.* 2016; 20: 90–107.

44. Dave DM, Kelly IR. How does the business cycle affect eating habits? *Soc Sci Med.* 2012; 74(2): 254–262.

45. Ng SW, Slining MM, Popkin BM. Turning point for US diets? Recessionary effects or behavioral shifts in foods purchased and consumed. *Am J Clin Nutr.* 2014; 99(3): 609–616.

46. Oddo VM, Nicholas LH, Bleich SN, Jones-Smith JC. The impact of changing economic conditions on overweight risk among children in California from 2008 to 2012, *J Epidemiol Community Health.* 2016. doi: 10.1136/jech-2015-207117. [Epub ahead of print].

47. Datar A, Nicosia N, Shier V. Maternal work and children's diet, activity, and obesity. *Soc Sci Med.* 2014; 107: 196–204.

48. Anderson PM, Butcher KF, Levine PB. Maternal employment and overweight children. *J Health Econ.* 2003; 22(3): 477–504.

49. Fertig AR, Glomm G, Tchernis R. The connection between maternal employment and childhood obesity: Inspecting the mechanisms. *Rev Econ Househ.* 2009; 7(3): 227–255.

50. Courtmanche C. Longer hours and larger waistlines? The relationship between work hours and obesity. *Forum Health Econ Policy.* 2009; 12(2): 1–31.

51. Arkes J. How the economy affects teenage weight. *Soc Sci Med.* 2009; 68(11): 1943–1947.

52. Trasande L, Chatterjee S. The impact of obesity on health service utilization and costs in childhood. *Obesity (Silver Spring)*. 2009; 17(9): 1749–1754.

53. Trasande L, Liu Y, Fryer G, Weitzman M. Effects of childhood obesity on hospital care and costs, 1999–2005. *Health Aff (Millwood)*. 2009; 28(4):w751–760.

54. Finkelstein EA, Graham WC, Malhotra R. Lifetime direct medical costs of childhood obesity. *Pediatrics*. 2014; 133(5): 854–862.

55. Au N. The health care cost implications of overweight and obesity during childhood. *Health Serv Res*. 2012; 47(2): 655–676.

56. Finkelstein EA, Trogdon JG. Public health interventions for addressing childhood overweight: Analysis of the business case. *Am J Public Health*. 2008; 98(3): 411–415.

57. Ma S, Frick KD. A simulation of affordability and effectiveness of childhood obesity interventions. *Acad Pediatr*. 2011; 11(4): 342–350.

58. Cawley J, Meyerhoefer C, Biener A, Hammer M, Wintfeld N. Savings in medical expenditures associated with reductions in body mass index among adults with obesity, by diabetes status. *Pharmacoeconomics*. 2015; 33: 707–722.

59. Brown HS, III, Pérez A, Li YP, Hoelscher DM, Kelder SH, Rivera R. The cost effectiveness of a school-based overweight program. *Int J Behav Nutr Phys Act*. 2007; 4: 47.

60. Wang LY, Yang Q, Lowry R, Wechsler H. Economic analysis of a school-based obesity prevention program. *Obes Res*. 2003; 11: 1313–1324.

61. Wang, LY, Gutin B, Barbeau P, et al. Cost effectiveness of a school-based obesity prevention program. *J Sch Health*. 2008; 78(12): 619–624.

62. Ananthapavan J, Sacks G, Moodie M, Carter R. Economics of obesity: Learning from the past to contribute to a better future. *Int J Environ Res Public Health*. 2014; 11(4): 4007–4025.

63. Gortmaker SL, Wang YC, Long MW, et al. Three interventions that reduce childhood obesity are projected to save more than they cost to implement. *Health Aff (Milwood)*. 2015; 34(11): 1932–1939.

5 Assessment of Body Composition and Fat Distribution in Infants, Children, and Adolescents

Elizabeth M. Widen and Dympna Gallagher

CONTENTS

INTRODUCTION

With the increasing global prevalence of overweight and obesity, pediatric body composition continues to be of high interest to clinicians, researchers, and the general public. Measurement of body composition and fat distribution, and changes in these factors among infants, children, and adolescents, can provide more information about nutritional status than simple anthropometric measurements alone and may provide important insights about later size and health that can be used to guide nutritional interventions and clinical practice. Assessing body composition and body composition changes in this population is, however, challenged by several factors, including the limited number of methods that can be used continuously from infancy through adolescence, physical challenges (excessive movement, crying, equipment designed only for a specific range of body sizes), and lack of validation studies.

From birth through adolescence, body composition changes considerably with more marked changes during infancy and puberty. These changes include gains in overall mass (weight) and stature (recumbent length and height) with concomitant changes in fat mass (FM) and fat-free mass (FFM), which include muscle, body water, organs, and other components. After birth, dynamic changes in body composition occur. Weight loss occurs during the first 24 h period, but weight is relatively stable in the periods 25–48 and 48–72 h [1]. Some have reported weight loss of 4%–10% in the first 2 weeks [2]. These changes are attributable to loss of body water rather than FM [3]. Total body water (TBW), or the hydration of FFM, declines rapidly from a peak of about ~0.80 [4] at birth, to values around ~0.78–0.79 from 1 to 12 months [5], eventually stabilizing at adult values

(~0.73) in adolescence [6]. FFM (as a proportion of body weight) increases during infancy [5,7], while the proportion of FM decreases. Percentage body fat varies by ethnicity, sex, and age, with some studies reporting higher body fat than others at specific ages (e.g., at 3 months, %fat in Butte's study was greater than the %fat in Fomon's study) and at pubertal stage [5,7–9].

Although total body composition, namely FM and FFM, is often measured, body fat distribution is more closely linked to later health; specifically, evidence suggests that visceral fat is more positively associated with cardiometabolic health and disease risk compared with subcutaneous fat [10]. While there is substantial variability in visceral and subcutaneous fat deposition by age, sex, and ethnicity, some general trends are apparent [9]. In infancy, subcutaneous adipose tissue is the predominant depot, as there is minimal intra-abdominal adipose tissue [11]. Visceral adipose tissue increases with age, but accumulation slows down over time and is affected by many factors including gender and pubertal staging; however, to date, no reports have examined visceral fat changes from infancy through adolescence in a single cohort, thus understanding of these factors that drive changes is somewhat limited [9,12]. Taken together, more work is needed to establish population-specific reference data with the most advanced body composition assessment methods.

There are several available methods for estimating total and regional body composition. Here, we provide a brief review of the most commonly used methods to assess body composition in infants, children, and adolescents and describe other methods that are forthcoming (Table 5.1).

ANTHROPOMETRY

Anthropometric measurements include body weight, circumferences of specific regions (typically head, arm, waist, or hip), skeletal breadths, physical length (recumbent length in infants <2 years and stature or height ≥2 years), and skinfold thickness. Weight and length are most often used to determine body mass index (kg/m^2) or relative size based on a reference population (e.g., body mass index z-scores by the Centers for Disease Control and Prevention or the World Health Organization growth charts, which provide information on weight relative to height and are often used as a proxy for adiposity). Circumferences and skeletal breadths are used to determine body proportions. Typically, measured circumferences include mid-upper arm, waist, hip, and thigh circumference, and head circumference (frontooccipital, measured in infants and young children). Waist circumference is often used as an indicator of visceral adipose tissue. In children (7–16 years), waist circumference was positively correlated with visceral adipose tissue assessed by magnetic resonance imaging (MRI) ($R^2 = .64$, $p < .0001$) [13]. However, in infants aged 3 and 12 months, waist circumference was not correlated with visceral adipose tissue assessed by MRI ($R^2 = .16$) [14], suggesting that waist circumference is not an appropriate indicator of visceral adiposity in younger children. The measurement site selected for waist circumference has important implications for use in research and clinical practice [15–17]. Commonly used sites for waist circumference include (1) the measured midpoint between the palpated iliac crest and the lowest rib along the midaxillary line; (2) the umbilicus; (3) the narrowest waist; (4) the lowest rib; (5) the iliac crest; or (6) immediately above the iliac crest. In prepubertal children, the lowest rib measurements (boys: $r = .76$, $p < .001$; girls: $r = .73$, $p < .001$) were more strongly correlated with visceral adipose tissue than midpoint and iliac crest waist circumference measures in both boys and girls [15]. However, in pubertal children, measures at the rib, crest, and midpoint were similarly correlated with visceral adipose tissue [15]. For reproducibility in longitudinal studies, measurement using bony landmarks is strongly recommended, such as the midpoint between the iliac crest and lowest rib.

Skinfold thickness is typically measured with Harpenden, Lange, or Holtain calipers. Common skinfold measurement sites include triceps, biceps, subscapular, suprailiac, and midthigh; at each of these sites, bony landmarks are used to standardize measurements. The caliper is applied to a double layer of fat and skin and measurement is obtained after the reading has stabilized; in young infants the reading should be obtained at approximately 30 s, while in older infants and in children/adolescents, the reading should stabilize in a much shorter period (i.e., 3 s). After each

TABLE 5.1

Summary of Methods to Measure Body Composition from Infancy through Adolescence

	Method(s)	Age and Size	Body Components	Pros/Cons
Air Displacement Plethysmography (ADP)	PEA POD	0–6 months (<8 kg)	Body volume from which estimates of FM and FFM are derived	Pro: • Noninvasive and quick measurement. Con: • Infants >8 kg cannot be measured. • Density constants may not be appropriate for study population.
	BOD POD with attachment	2–6 years (<25 kg)		Pro: • Noninvasive and quick measurement. Con: • Movement and crying limits usability of measures.
	BOD POD	> 6 years (<250 kg)		Pro: • Noninvasive and quick measurement. Con: • Density constants may not be appropriate for population.
	Dual-energy x-ray absorptiometry (DXA)	>0	Fat mass Lean mass Bone mineral content	Pro: • Provides total and regional (arms, legs, trunk, android, gynoid) estimates of body composition (fat mass, fat-free mass, and bone). Con: • Challenging to limit movement in some younger children. • Radiation exposure. • Measurement error (especially smaller sizes) .
Anthropometry	Weight/height; skinfolds; circumferences and skeletal breadth	>0	Relative size (BMI, ponderal index, waist-to-hip ratio); Subcutaneous adipose tissue (skinfold) Estimate body composition with prediction equations	Pro: • Can be used from birth through adulthood. • Provides information on body size, proportions, and regional adiposity. • Equations can be applied to estimate body fat in select populations and age groups. Con: • Equations may not be available for population of interest. • Specialized training needed.

(Continued)

TABLE 5.1 (CONTINUED)
Summary of Methods to Measure Body Composition from Infancy through Adolescence

	Method(s)	Age and Size	Body Components	Pros/Cons
Imaging	Magnetic resonance imaging (MRI)	>0	Adipose tissue, muscle volume	Pro: • Can be used from birth through adulthood. • Quantify tissue in vivo. Con: • Challenging to limit movement in some younger children.
	Quantitative magnetic resonance (QMR)	0–12 kg (infant) <80 kg (adolescent) <250 kg (adult)	FM FFM Free water mass Total water mass	Pro: • No radiation exposure. • Movement does not appear to affect estimates in infants. Con: • System not widely available. • Further information on validity needed for adolescent and infant systems.
Hydrometry	TBW by dilution	>0	TBW from which estimates of FM and FFM are derived	Pro: • High accuracy and precision. Con: • Challenges associated with (1) insuring that full dose has been ingested in infants and (2) collection of some physiologic samples such as urine.

Note: FM, fat mass; FFM, fat-free mass; TBW, total body water.

measurement, the tissue should be allowed to normalize before obtaining replicates. Typically, one replicate is obtained and a third measurement is conducted if differences exceed 1–3 mm, which depends on skinfold site and child age.

While skinfold thickness measures can be used to assess regional adiposity (e.g., trunk) or general distribution (e.g., trunk-to-limbs ratio), values are often used in prediction equations along with other anthropometric measures (i.e., height, weight, circumferences) and age to estimate body fat or lean mass [6]. These equations, however, are prone to error at the individual level and are most useful for specific age groups (consistent with the populations where validation was performed). Furthermore, the racial/ethnic composition of the source population for the prediction equation may not be generalizable to the study population of interest. For example, the Slaughter equation was developed in prepubescent (Tanner stages 1 and 2; male %fat: 19.0% ± 8.1% [mean ± standard deviation (SD), all such values]; female %fat: 23.2% ± 6.6%), pubescent (Tanner stage 3; male %fat: 17.3% ± 7.3%; female %fat: 23.7% ± 6.8%), and postpubescent (Tanner stage 4 and 5; male %fat: 14.0% ± 6.2%; female %fat: 23.6% ± 6.0%) black and white males and females. The equation utilizes the sum of the triceps and the calf or subscapular skinfold thickness to estimate body fatness [18]. Body fat estimates with the Slaughter equation were compared with dual-energy x-ray absorptiometry (DXA) based on estimates in two populations: (1) white, black, Hispanic, or Asian children aged 5–18 years from New York City ($n = 1169$), and (2) black and white children aged 5–17 years from Bogalusa, Louisiana ($n = 6725$) [19]. Although body fat estimates with the Slaughter equation were highly correlated with DXA estimates overall ($r = .90$), there were differences depending on the level of body fatness with greater accuracy among nonobese children [19]. Among children with lower skinfold values (<15 mm for boys and <20 mm for girls), the difference between Slaughter and DXA %fat was minimal (<1%); but among heavier children, body fat was overestimated by 12% among boys and by 6% among girls with thicker skinfold thickness values (sum of subscapular and triceps skinfold ≥50 mm for boys and ≥60 mm for girls) [19].

Due to low cost and portability, anthropometric measures can be obtained in most research settings assuming standardization of measurement devices, including scale calibration up to the highest participant weight with certified calibration weights, and standardization within and between observers, but there are limitations. First, training in a similar population in terms of age and body size is necessary to achieve optimal within and between observer variability, particularly for skinfold measurements. Second, infants and young children need to be calm and cooperative during measures to minimize error, which may be challenging in hungry, thirsty, or otherwise distressed subjects.

DENSITOMETRY

Densitometry methods for estimating body composition include hydrostatic weighing (underwater weighing), which estimates body density, and air displacement plethysmography (ADP), which estimates body volume from which body density is derived (e.g., density = mass/volume) and body composition is estimated. For FFM estimation, the assumed density of FFM changes from infancy through adolescence until chemical maturation (i.e., adult values) and is also subject to between-individual variability [5,7,20]. In addition, there is variation in the density of FFM by age and race/ethnicity; in general, the density of FFM is greater in blacks than whites [21]. As participant cooperation is necessary to follow directions and hold breath for hydrostatic weighing, this method is not recommended for infants, toddlers, and younger children. Thus, this section will focus on ADP, which estimates body volume by applying the principles of Boyle's and Poison's gas laws. The PEA POD and the BOD POD (Cosmed USA) are currently available ADP systems for measuring infants and children. For both systems, the subject is placed inside the enclosed test chamber and the amount of air displaced by the subject is measured. For infants 1–8 kg (approximately 6 months of age), the PEA POD estimates body fat by applying sex- and age-specific density constants and residual thoracic lung volume estimates [4,7]. The PEA POD was validated against deuterium dilution estimates of body fat in infants, where the mean difference in percentage body fat between methods was very small ($-0.07 \pm 3.39\%$, $p = .9$) and the values were highly correlated ($R^2 = .76$) [22]. The limits of agreement in Bland–Altman analysis were narrower than other methods previously used in infants, but were still wide (-6.84% to 6.71% body fat) [22]. This suggests that there may be biological contributions (FFM hydration) or other individual differences (i.e., feeding, crying, sweating, water turnover) contributing to the error [22].

The BOD POD is used for estimating body composition in children (≥ 2 years) and adults up to 250 kg. Measurements include body weight, body volume, body density, FM, FFM, and thoracic gas volume (if not estimated). A pediatric adaptor seat for young children aged 2–6 years (and 12–27 kg) is available for use for the BOD POD GS system (November 2007 and thereafter); the seat is similar to a high chair with a small tray and is accompanied with a pediatric calibration cylinder (20.02 L). The BOD POD pediatric adaptor system was validated against the four-compartment (4C) model (Lohman) in 31 children aged 2–6 years, where bone mineral content was estimated by DXA (described in DXA section), total body water (TBW) was assessed with deuterium dilution (described in the TBW section), and body volume was estimated by ADP and body mass [23]. Compared with the 4C model, the coefficient of variation was 3.5% for percentage body fat. Based on the Bland–Altman plot, there appeared to be no bias between the %fat estimates between the BOD POD with pediatric option and the 4C %fat estimates [23]. However, one %fat estimate was substantially lower than 2SD from the mean and two others were adjacent to 2SD from the mean [23], and unfortunately, information on subjects with aberrant %fat values was not provided. This indicates that the BOD POD with the pediatric option may considerably underestimate %fat in some circumstance and, therefore, limit the validity of %fat estimates in this population. Obtaining satisfactory participant cooperation represented by limited movement and minimal crying was problematic in this report (i.e., several subjects' data were unacceptable due to crying [23]), thus, this challenge may be important to consider for planning body composition assessment in younger children. This report corroborates other reports in infants aged 6–48 months [24] and children aged 3–5 years [25] comparing the BOD POD with pediatric option with DXA or D_2O-derived body fat estimates that indicated that the ADP with pediatric option was invalid in younger children. In children aged 5–18 years, BOD POD estimates of body fat have been compared with the 4C model as the criterion method [26,27]. In 30 children aged 11–17 (mean 14 years), ADP estimates of body fat were highly correlated with 4C ($r \geq .95$), and the ADP estimates that applied Lohman equations [28] were more similar to 4C than Siri-derived estimates [26]. In another report of 25 children aged 9–14, the regression between ADP FM and 4C FM did not differ from the line of identity (R^2: .97; intercept, kg: 0.88 ± 0.64; slope: 1.036 ± 0.38) and no bias was observed in residual plots ($p = .1$) [27]; however, two outliers were beyond the limits of agreement and the limits of agreement were wide, which suggests that ADP may not be accurate in some instances in this population [27].

ADP is a safe and noninvasive method for body composition assessment in infants, children, and adolescents, which does not require sedation; however, there are some challenges in using this method in this population. First, ADP is not appropriate for use in children >8 kg (~6 months) and ADP has not been validated in children from 6 months to 2 years. Furthermore, obtaining participant cooperation of children aged 2–6 years may be challenging and, as such, data may not be usable. The age and sex-specific density constants for FFM and thoracic gas volume estimates may not be appropriate for the study population of interest. In particular, the FFM constants may not reflect the dynamic changes in body water occurring during infancy.

DUAL-ENERGY X-RAY ABSORPTIOMETRY

DXA uses two x-rays, one that detects bone and the other that estimates fat and lean soft tissue based on an algorithm. Several systems are available for use in pediatric populations that have instrument-specific software and pediatric-specific algorithms. The system and software used for measurements impact body composition estimates [29], thus, for longitudinal studies, use of the same system and software over time is advised.

In infants, one study has compared DXA with ADP in infancy; 84 infants, who were full term at birth, were measured at 6 months of age [30]. In this report, DXA and ADP were highly correlated, but compared with ADP, DXA estimates of percentage body fat were higher by an average of 4.4% and FFM estimates were lower by an average of 166 g [30]. Several studies have compared body fat estimates from DXA with the 4C model, as the criterion method, in children [6,31]. Among a sample of children ($n = 411$) aged 6–18 years of black ($n = 89$, 21.7%), Hispanic ($n = 74$, 18.0%), white ($n = 153$, 37.2%), Asian American ($n = 47$, 11.4%), and "other" ($n = 48$, 11.7%) ancestry, DXA (Lunar DPX/DPX-L) was found to overestimate percentage body fat, compared with 4C [31]. While the estimates were correlated with each other ($R^2 = .85$), DXA overestimated percentage body fat with a mean difference of 1.012% ($p < .001$) between methods [31]. Agreement, however, varied by subjects' body fat; among subjects with higher percentage body fat, DXA overestimated body fat, while among subjects with less fat, DXA underestimated body fat compared with 4C [31]. In obese children and adolescents aged 5–21 years (mean 10.7 years), DXA was found to overestimate FM by 0.9 kg and underestimate lean mass by 1 kg, compared with 4C estimates, and the limits of agreement were wide (i.e., ~4 kg) [32]. Based on a study of 176 multiethnic children and adolescents aged 5–17, prediction models can be applied to DXA total body fat to estimate total adipose tissue and subdepots, including subcutaneous, intermuscular, and visceral adipose tissue [33]. Simple methods to derive estimates of visceral fat with DXA software have not been validated in pediatric populations against criterion methods. One study compared DXA estimates of skeletal muscle, derived from an adult prediction model, with reference estimates by MRI in children aged 5–17 (BMI < 35 kg/m^2) [34]. The adult model was found to be valid for Tanner 5 children, but for ≤Tanner 4 children, the adult model overestimated skeletal muscle and, thus, a pediatric prediction formula for estimating skeletal muscle in children at or below Tanner 4 was developed [34].

The advantages of this system include short measurement time (varies by height of participant), good precision, ability to estimate regions (arms, legs, and trunk) and for the whole body or any specific region, the separation of body into fat, bone, and bone-free lean. There are limitations; the DXA system exposes subjects to radiation (whole body scan, 1–5 μSv), where 5 μSv is equivalent to 25% of the radiation dose of a chest x-ray (20 μSv) [3]. Radiation exposure requires females of child-bearing potential to have a pregnancy test before the DXA test. The DXA system is expensive (>$70,000), younger children need to be sleeping or tightly wrapped in a sheet to limit movement, and finally, the dynamic changes in FFM hydration and bone changes during growth may introduce error.

IMAGING

MAGNETIC RESONANCE IMAGING

MRI can be used to estimate total-body and regional adipose tissue volume (i.e., visceral, subcutaneous, bone mineral adipose tissue), skeletal muscle, and the volume of other lean tissues [6,35]. Other depots and tissues that can be quantified include organ mass, such as high metabolic rate organs, including spleen, liver, and kidney, and brain mass [6,36,37]. Multiple cross-sectional images are assessed from which tissue volumes are reconstructed, which are converted to tissue mass by applying known assumed densities [38]. Tissue volume is measured, rather than mass as in other methods, which needs to be considered when making comparisons between MRI and other assessment methods. Assumptions regarding the composition and density of tissues are made to derive estimates of mass, and these vary with age from infancy until adult levels are attained [6]. The advantages of MRI include the ability to test all ages provided they can remain motionless for 15–20 min in a confined magnet, no radiation exposure, detailed and high-quality images, and the ability to discern specific tissue subdepots and regional body composition. There are limitations. First, MRI access is limited to radiology facilities as these highly specialized instruments that are costly to purchase and maintain must be operated by certified radiology technicians and study-specific protocols must be developed and implemented. The costs associated with MRI scanning time (e.g., $550 for a 30 min block; variable by institution) and postprocessing for image analysis are high; postprocessing analyses are dependent on scan protocol and specific measurement. MRI requires the subject to be completely motionless, thus, infants and younger children need to be asleep for measurements. Sedation for nonclinical research studies is not recommended. Yet, the scanning time in younger subjects is relatively fast due to their smaller size (i.e., <10 min for infants) [6]. Although MRI has acceptable reproducibility ~2%–~4% for adipose tissue volume estimates in infants [11,35,39] and 17.4% for internal adipose tissue [11], further validation of body composition estimates in children from infancy through adolescence is needed [3].

QUANTITATIVE MAGNETIC RESONANCE

Quantitative magnetic resonance (QMR) is a nonimaging method that estimates whole body FM but not the distribution of lean tissue mass, TBW, and free water (water not bound to tissues) based on the magnetic properties of tissues and water. There are several QMR analyzers that are size and age specific. EchoMRI-Infants can be used to assess body composition in infants up to 12 kg and validation of this analyzer is currently in progress. Thus far, the system shows high precision and reproducibility for estimating FM, lean mass, and body water [3]. Another QMR analyzer (EchoMRI-AH) was compared with deuterium dilution and the 4C model for infants and children up to 50 kg. This analyzer overestimated body fat by ~10% when compared with 4C and underestimated body fat by ~4%, when compared with deuterium dilution in children ≥6 years. Subsequently, the equations were redeveloped to account for this bias [40]. The EchoMRI-Adolescent was developed for children/adolescents up to 80 kg, but information on its validity is lacking. The system has many strengths including that it does not use ionizing radiation, several systems sizes are available for different ages and body sizes, and finally, the measurement time is short ~4 min and the subject does not need to remain still during the measurement. The primary disadvantage is that these systems are very expensive to purchase (EchoMRI, LLC, Houston, TX: http://www.echomri.com) and currently are only available in select research facilities.

HYDROMETRY (TOTAL BODY WATER)

As mentioned in the introduction of this chapter, TBW, or the hydration of FFM, changes markedly from infancy through adolescence. FFM hydration peaks at birth (~0.8) and declines thereafter, eventually plateauing at adult values of ~0.73 in adolescence [5–7,41]. TBW is estimated with hydrometry, where naturally occurring isotopes, ^{2}H or ^{18}O, are measured in physiologic samples (blood, saliva, or urine) at baseline and then measurements are obtained after dosage with a stable isotope and an equilibrium period [41]. Labeled water, as ^{2}H$_2$O (deuterium) or H$_2$^{18}O (Oxygen 18), is administered, typically via a syringe or a small cup. After equilibrium, follow-up physiologic samples are obtained, from which TBW is estimated [7]. Body fat estimates can be derived from TBW measurement; however, due to high between-individual variability and dynamic changes in the hydration of FFM, especially in infancy, this method may not be appropriate for estimating body fat in some circumstances (i.e., newborn period) [42].

Hydrometry is accurate and precise for measuring TBW (coefficient of variation (CV) 1%–2% [41]); however, estimates of body fat may be prone to error due to the rapid and variable changes in hydration of FFM in this population. Other limitations include (1) spillage due to regurgitation during oral dose administration in younger children and infants; (2) challenges in obtaining saliva or urine samples when phlebotomy is not practical or appropriate; (3) time involved for equilibrium (range 3–4+ h) depending on dose administration route and estimation method; and finally

(4) difficulties because hydrometry is based on the assumption of no feeding during the equilibration period, which may not be feasible in infants or younger children.

BIOELECTRICAL IMPEDANCE

Bioelectrical impedance (BIA) is based on the principles of the electrical conductivity of various tissues, where the impedance or resistance to the delivered electrical current is measured. From the resistance and other factors (age, sex, etc.), prediction equations are applied to estimate TBW from which estimates of FM and FFM are derived. The applicability of BIA is limited for use in infants and younger children due to the wide variability in the hydration of FFM, which underlie BIA estimates, thus impacting the accuracy of body composition estimates. Recently, an equation that leverages BIA estimates (resistance) and anthropometry for use in 2-year-olds was found to strongly predict DXA FFM estimates in 2-year-old New Zealanders [43]; however, more work is needed to extend the age and applicability to other populations. In older children, body composition estimates derived from BIA should use prediction equations that account for age, sex, and pubertal stage; unfortunately, appropriate prediction equations are often not available. Furthermore, it is important to determine if the BIA device has been validated against gold-standard methods in a population similar to the study population in age, race, and pubertal stage, or alternatively, if other specific prediction equations are available that may be more appropriate and can be used with the raw BIA values [6,44,45].

FOUR-COMPARTMENT METHODS

The 4C model is considered the gold-standard method for assessing body composition (FM) in general and is often appropriate for assessment in children. The 4C model typically uses estimates of total body water by dilution, total body bone mineral content by DXA, body volume by ADP or hydrostatic weighing, and body weight to estimate FM. The Lohman equation is often used for ages 1–16 years, where Bd is body density in grams per cubic centimeter, W is TBW in liters, BMC is total bone mineral content (BMC by DXA × 1.22) [28], and FM (kg) = (2.749/Bd − 0.714 W + 1.146 bmc—2.0503).

SUMMARY

There are many widely available methods that can be applied to assess body composition and its distribution in infants, children, and adolescents, but few of these methods can be applied across the full life course. As pediatric body composition becomes more widely used and methods are further refined and developed, understanding of the assumptions and limitations of available methods is of utmost importance. As we gain a greater understanding of the dynamic changes in body composition in this period, standards for body composition by age, sex, and race/ethnicity need to be established in order to ensure that body composition measurements can be clearly interpreted by clinicians and patient populations.

REFERENCES

1. Hull HR, Thornton JC, Ji Y, Paley C, Rosenn B, Mathews P, et al. Higher infant body fat with excessive gestational weight gain in overweight women. *American Journal of Obstetrics and Gynecology*. 2011;205(3):211.e1–7.
2. Noel-Weiss J, Courant G, Woodend AK. Physiological weight loss in the breastfed neonate: A systematic review. *Open Medicine: A Peer-Reviewed, Independent, Open-Access Journal*. 2008;2(4):e99–e110.
3. Toro-Ramos T, Paley C, Pi-Sunyer FX, Gallagher D. Body composition during fetal development and infancy through the age of 5 years. *European Journal of Clinical Nutrition*. 2015;69(12):1279–89.
4. Fomon SJ, Nelson SE. Body composition of the male and female reference infants. *Annual Review of Nutrition*. 2002;22:1–17.

5. Fomon SJ, Haschke F, Ziegler EE, Nelson SE. Body composition of reference children from birth to age 10 years. *The American Journal of Clinical Nutrition*. 1982;35(5 Suppl):1169–75.

6. Sopher A, Shen W, Pietrobelli A. Pediatric body composition methods. In Heymsfield SB, Lohman TG, Wang ZM, Going SB (eds), *Human Body Composition*, pp. 129–39, 2nd Edn. Champaign, IL: Human Kinetics, 2005.

7. Butte NF, Hopkinson JM, Wong WW, Smith EO, Ellis KJ. Body composition during the first 2 years of life: An updated reference. *Pediatric Research*. 2000;47(5):578–85.

8. Freedman DS, Wang J, Thornton JC, Mei Z, Pierson RN, Jr., Dietz WH, et al. Racial/ethnic differences in body fatness among children and adolescents. *Obesity*. 2008;16(5):1105–11.

9. Staiano AE, Katzmarzyk PT. Ethnic and sex differences in body fat and visceral and subcutaneous adiposity in children and adolescents. *International Journal of Obesity*. 2012;36(10):1261–9.

10. Wajchenberg BL. Subcutaneous and visceral adipose tissue: Their relation to the metabolic syndrome. *Endocrine Reviews*. 2000;21(6):697–738.

11. Harrington TA, Thomas EL, Modi N, Frost G, Coutts GA, Bell JD. Fast and reproducible method for the direct quantitation of adipose tissue in newborn infants. *Lipids*. 2002;37(1):95–100.

12. Slyper AH. Childhood obesity, adipose tissue distribution, and the pediatric practitioner. *Pediatrics*. 1998;102(1):e4.

13. Brambilla P, Bedogni G, Moreno LA, Goran MI, Gutin B, Fox KR, et al. Crossvalidation of anthropometry against magnetic resonance imaging for the assessment of visceral and subcutaneous adipose tissue in children. *International Journal of Obesity*. 2006;30(1):23–30.

14. De Lucia Rolfe E, Modi N, Uthaya S, Hughes IA, Dunger DB, Acerini C, et al. Ultrasound estimates of visceral and subcutaneous-abdominal adipose tissues in infancy. *Journal of Obesity*. 2013;2013:951954.

15. Bosy-Westphal A, Booke CA, Blocker T, Kossel E, Goele K, Later W, et al. Measurement site for waist circumference affects its accuracy as an index of visceral and abdominal subcutaneous fat in a Caucasian population. *The Journal of Nutrition*. 2010;140(5):954–61.

16. Hitze B, Bosy-Westphal A, Bielfeldt F, Settler U, Monig H, Muller MJ. Measurement of waist circumference at four different sites in children, adolescents, and young adults: Concordance and correlation with nutritional status as well as cardiometabolic risk factors. *Obesity Facts*. 2008;1(5):243–9.

17. Wang J, Thornton JC, Bari S, Williamson B, Gallagher D, Heymsfield SB, et al. Comparisons of waist circumferences measured at 4 sites. *The American Journal of Clinical Nutrition*. 2003;77(2):379–84.

18. Slaughter MH, Lohman TG, Boileau RA, Horswill CA, Stillman RJ, Van Loan MD, et al. Skinfold equations for estimation of body fatness in children and youth. *Human Biology*. 1988;60(5):709–23.

19. Freedman DS, Horlick M, Berenson GS. A comparison of the Slaughter skinfold-thickness equations and BMI in predicting body fatness and cardiovascular disease risk factor levels in children. *The American Journal of Clinical Nutrition*. 2013;98(6):1417–24.

20. Eriksson B, Lof M, Eriksson O, Hannestad U, Forsum E. Fat-free mass hydration in newborns: Assessment and implications for body composition studies. *Acta Paediatrica*. 2011;100(5):680–6.

21. Wagner DR, Heyward VH. Measures of body composition in blacks and whites: A comparative review. *The American Journal of Clinical Nutrition*. 2000;71(6):1392–402.

22. Ma G, Yao M, Liu Y, Lin A, Zou H, Urlando A, et al. Validation of a new pediatric air-displacement plethysmograph for assessing body composition in infants. *The American Journal of Clinical Nutrition*. 2004;79(4):653–60.

23. Fields DA, Allison DB. Air-displacement plethysmography pediatric option in 2–6 years old using the four-compartment model as a criterion method. *Obesity*. 2012;20(8):1732–7.

24. Rosendale RP, Bartok CJ. Air-displacement plethysmography for the measurement of body composition in children aged 6–48 months. *Pediatric Research*. 2012;71(3):299–304.

25. Crook TA, Armbya N, Cleves MA, Badger TM, Andres A. Air displacement plethysmography, dual-energy x-ray absorptiometry, and total body water to evaluate body composition in preschool-age children. *Journal of the Academy of Nutrition and Dietetics*. 2012;112(12):1993–8.

26. Gately PJ, Radley D, Cooke CB, Carroll S, Oldroyd B, Truscott JG, et al. Comparison of body composition methods in overweight and obese children. *Journal of Applied Physiology*. 2003;95(5):2039–46.

27. Fields DA, Goran MI. Body composition techniques and the four-compartment model in children. *Journal of Applied Physiology*. 2000;89(2):613–20.

28. Lohman TG. Assessment of body composition in children. *Pediatric Exercise Science*. 1989;1(1):19–30.

29. Barbour LA, Hernandez TL, Reynolds RM, Reece MS, Chartier-Logan C, Anderson MK, et al. Striking differences in estimates of infant adiposity by new and old DXA software, PEAPOD and skin-folds at 2 weeks and 1 year of life. *Pediatric Obesity*. 2015, doi: 10.1111/ijpo.12055.

30. Fields DA, Demerath EW, Pietrobelli A, Chandler-Laney PC. Body composition at 6 months of life: Comparison of air displacement plethysmography and dual-energy x-ray absorptiometry. *Obesity*. 2012;20(11):2302–6.

31. Sopher AB, Thornton JC, Wang J, Pierson RN, Jr., Heymsfield SB, Horlick M. Measurement of percentage of body fat in 411 children and adolescents: A comparison of dual-energy x-ray absorptiometry with a four-compartment model. *Pediatrics*. 2004;113(5):1285–90.

32. Wells JC, Haroun D, Williams JE, Wilson C, Darch T, Viner RM, et al. Evaluation of DXA against the four-component model of body composition in obese children and adolescents aged 5–21 years. *International Journal of Obesity*. 2010;34(4):649–55.

33. Bauer J, Thornton J, Heymsfield S, Kelly K, Ramirez A, Gidwani S, et al. Dual-energy x-ray absorptiometry prediction of adipose tissue depots in children and adolescents. *Pediatric Research*. 2012;72(4):420–5.

34. Kim J, Shen W, Gallagher D, Jones A, Jr., Wang Z, Wang J, et al. Total-body skeletal muscle mass: Estimation by dual-energy x-ray absorptiometry in children and adolescents. *The American Journal of Clinical Nutrition*. 2006;84(5):1014–20.

35. Olhager E, Thuomas KA, Wigstrom L, Forsum E. Description and evaluation of a method based on magnetic resonance imaging to estimate adipose tissue volume and total body fat in infants. *Pediatric Research*. 1998;44(4):572–7.

36. Hsu A, Heshka S, Janumala I, Song MY, Horlick M, Krasnow N, et al. Larger mass of high-metabolic-rate organs does not explain higher resting energy expenditure in children. *The American Journal of Clinical Nutrition*. 2003;77(6):1506–11.

37. Fox KR, Peters DM, Sharpe P, Bell M. Assessment of abdominal fat development in young adolescents using magnetic resonance imaging. *International Journal of Obesity and Related Metabolic Disorders: Journal of the International Association for the Study of Obesity*. 2000;24(12):1653–9.

38. Snyder WSC, Cook MJ, Nasset,ES, Karhaussen LR, Howells GP, Tipton IH, *Report of the Task Group on Reference Men*. Oxford, UK: International Commission on Radiological Protection, 1975.

39. Bauer JS, Noel PB, Vollhardt C, Much D, Degirmenci S, Brunner S, et al. Accuracy and reproducibility of adipose tissue measurements in young infants by whole body magnetic resonance imaging. *PloS One*. 2015;10(2):e0117127.

40. Andres A, Gomez-Acevedo H, Badger TM. Quantitative nuclear magnetic resonance to measure fat mass in infants and children. *Obesity*. 2011;19(10):2089–95.

41. Schoeller DA. Hydrometry. In Heymsfield SB, Lohman TG, Wang ZM, Going SB (eds), *Human Body Composition*, pp. 35–49, 2nd Edn. Champaign, IL: Human Kinetics, 2005.

42. Hashimoto K, Wong WW, Thomas AJ, Uvena-Celebrezze J, Huston-Pressley L, Amini SB, et al. Estimation of neonatal body composition: Isotope dilution versus total-body electrical conductivity. *Biological Neonate*. 2002;81:170–175.

43. Rush EC, Bristow S, Plank LD, Rowan J. Bioimpedance prediction of fat-free mass from dual-energy x-ray absorptiometry in a multi-ethnic group of 2-year-old children. *European Journal of Clinical Nutrition*. 2013;67(2):214–7.

44. Demerath EW, Fields DA. Body composition assessment in the infant. *American Journal of Human Biology: The Official Journal of the Human Biology Council*. 2014;26(3):291–304.

45. Kyle UG, Earthman CP, Pichard C, Coss-Bu JA. Body composition during growth in children: Limitations and perspectives of bioelectrical impedance analysis. *European Journal of Clinical Nutrition*. 2015;69(12):1298–305.

Section II

Nutritional Factors Contributing to Childhood Obesity

6 The Influence of Daily Eating Patterns on Weight Status

A Review of the Evidence on Breakfast Consumption, Snacking, and Eating Frequency

Stacy A. Blondin and Christina D. Economos

CONTENTS

INTRODUCTION

Among the myriad factors contributing to overweight and obesity among children, the timing and distribution of energy intake across daily eating occasions (henceforth referred to as "daily eating patterns") have been recognized as variables influencing weight status during childhood and adolescence (Table 6.1) [1]. Although daily eating patterns at the individual level are influenced by biological factors, including hunger and satiety cues and circadian rhythm, they are also influenced by environmental factors, such as social norms, culture, media exposure, family routines, and institutional settings and schedules [1–4]. Children in today's society typically distribute their time across a wide variety of settings and activities [5], which vary in structure and opportunity for energy intake and expenditure. Taking a closer look at temporal shifts in eating patterns and the coincidence of these trends with rising obesity rates could shed light on modifiable behavioral changes that may alter energy balance.

Because of the salience of daily eating patterns to children's everyday lives and variability observed across cultures in timing and composition of eating occasions, related hypotheses have been generated and tested over the past half century. In this chapter, we will review evidence on the respective relationships between breakfast, snacking, and eating frequency on weight status among children. We will present prevalence and trends estimates of children's daily eating and results of studies investigating potential links between daily eating patterns and weight status. Prevalence

TABLE 6.1

Percentage Skipping Breakfast and Percentage of Total Energy Consumed at Breakfast by Age Group and Gender

Age-Gender Group (years)	% Skipping (NHANES 2009–2010)	% Total Energy (NHANES 2011–2012)
Males		
2–5	6	21
6–11	13	19
12–19	26	15
Females		
2–5	5	19
6–11	14	18
12–19	25	15

Source: WWEIA Data Table D1.14. Food Surveys Research Group, Beltsville Human Nutrition Research Center, Agricultural Research Service, USDA. WWEIA Data Tables, NHANES 2009–2010.

and trends estimates presented are from US data, which have been most comprehensively and consistently collected, while associational evidence includes international studies to maximize the number of quality studies included. In the discussion section, we will consider some of the intricacies, nuances, and limitations of the extant research and priorities for future directions in related research.

Before providing an overview of the extant peer-reviewed literature addressing these topics, it is important to recognize that humans consume food episodically over the course of a day. While it is theoretically possible to feed an individual at a continuous rate in a laboratory or health-care setting intravenously, consuming food constantly throughout the day is practically impossible. Free-living individuals usually consume food in discrete bouts, often described as eating episodes or eating occasions [6]. In modern societies, eating episodes/occasions are generally dichotomized into two categories: meals and snacks. Meals, which are generally larger and consist of a greater diversity of foods and food groups, typically include breakfast, lunch, and dinner [7–9]. Though the timing, relative importance, and composition of meals varies among and within countries, families, and individuals [10], meals are generally consumed at a roughly fixed time of day and are often eaten in the company of others. Snacks, on the other hand, are commonly defined as *any food(s) consumed outside the boundaries of typical mealtimes*. While the Dietary Guidelines for Americans includes meal and snack patterns, frequency, and quality under the umbrella of a wide variety of "eating behaviors," [1] precise and standardized definitions of each are lacking for research purposes, and the lines between the two are considerably subjective and ambiguous. Though idiosyncratic patterns have generated increased attention in recent years [11], the majority of the US population consumes three meals and at least one snack per day [1]. Though little change in daily eating patterns has been observed in recent years (2005–2010) [1], trends over the past 40 years indicate shifts in meal frequency, type, and timing among adults [6].

Research on daily eating patterns in children has predominantly focused on breakfast and snacking, as two distinct behaviors that may independently influence weight status. Total daily eating episodes/occasions, which incorporate both snacking and breakfast but encompass eating frequency more generally, have also been considered in association with adiposity outcomes. Each of these topics will be discussed independently and conjointly in the sections that follow.

BREAKFAST

PREVALENCE AND TRENDS

Though the content, timing, and size of the breakfast meal vary considerably within and between cultures [12], according to the English definition, the only requisite is its ordinal position as the first meal of the day [13]. Despite the universality of the breakfast meal and its colloquial—and increasingly scientific—recognition as the "most important meal of the day," consumption trends in the United States suggest incongruity between adage, evidence, and behavior. In fact, the most recent prevalence estimates based on nationally representative What We Eat in America (WWEIA) and National Health and Nutrition Evaluation Survey (NHANES) 2009–2010 data suggest that breakfast skipping increases as children age, from 6% of males and 5% of females ages 2–5 years to 26% and 25%, respectively, ages 12–19 years, and that these prevalence estimates have remained stable since 2005 [1]. Though estimates have not been compared for 2011–2012 data, previous evidence consistently suggests that breakfast skipping may be more prevalent in children from lower socioeconomic backgrounds [14]. Another recent analysis, using data from a nationally representative sample of US students in 6th–10th grades, recruited using a multistage stratified design by census region, found that adolescents consumed breakfast approximately 5 days per week and were more likely to eat breakfast on weekends than weekdays [15]. In this study, significant interactions were found by gender, age, and race/ethnicity, with girls reporting eating breakfast less frequently than boys, older children less frequently than younger, and African American and Hispanic children less frequently than white and other race/ethnicities. Based on the same data, breakfast consumption on weekdays increased from 2001–2002 to 2005–2006, whereas breakfast eating on weekends did not change significantly over time. Among boys, breakfast eating on weekdays increased from 2001 to 2009, and, among girls, breakfast eating on weekdays increased across all three time points [15].

The majority of evidence suggests that breakfast consumption among children and adolescents is positively associated with daily nutrient intake and diet quality [1,14,16]. According to the most recent NHANES data, the breakfast meal contributes a higher nutrient-to-energy ratio for shortfall nutrients (fiber, calcium, vitamin D, potassium, and iron) and lower nutrient-to-energy ratio for nutrients to limit (sodium, saturated fat, added sugar) than any other eating occasion among Americans 2 years and older (Figure 6.1). This is especially true for calcium, vitamin D, and iron. For males and females ages 2–19 years, breakfast contributed approximately 17% of total energy intake (337 kcals) on average [1]. Though research also suggests that

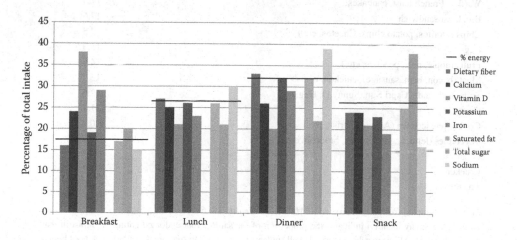

FIGURE 6.1 Percentage of daily nutrient intake relative to energy intake by eating occasion for children 2–19 years. (Adapted from DGAC 2015 Figure D1.40 using original data sourced from What We Eat in America, NHANES 2009–2010.)

breakfast consumption is positively associated with energy intake [14], more evidence is needed to confirm these findings.

Trend data from 1965 to 1991 suggest that children increased consumption of low-fat milk, ready-to-eat cereals, and juices, and decreased consumption of high-fat milk, whole-grain breads, and eggs across the latter half of the twentieth century [17]. Cross-sectional 2001–2002 NHANES data showed that ready-to-eat cereal (RTEC), milk, 100% fruit juice, and breads, bagels, roll, and muffins were among the most commonly reported foods consumed at breakfast (at least 20% of participants reported), with no differences reported by age group [18]. Breakfast composition did appear to differ between meals consumed at home and away from the home, with RTEC and milk more commonly consumed at home. Although not from a nationally representative sample, data on breakfast type and location collected from a large, ethnically diverse sample of 4th–6th grade children provides some insight into more recent patterns [19] (Table 6.2); across all locations, cereal, milk, water, 100% fruit juice, bread, and muffins/donuts were most commonly consumed. An earlier analysis of NHANES data collected from 1999 to 2006 showed that 35.9% of children and 25.4% of adolescents consumed RTEC for breakfast, and that diet quality was positively associated with RTEC consumption [20]. In this study, RTEC consumers had lower intakes of total fat and cholesterol and higher intakes of total carbohydrate, dietary fiber, and several micronutrients compared with breakfast skippers and other breakfast consumers. RTEC consumers also had the highest mean adequacy ratio (MAR) for micronutrients, which was the lowest for breakfast skippers.

TABLE 6.2
Students' Consumption of Breakfast Item Categories by Location ($n = 651$)

Category	(%)
Ate at any location	87.6
Cereal	32.5
Milk, yogurt, or cheese	31.7
Water	29.0
100% fruit juice (Juicy Juice)	27.5
Bread (bagel, toast, or roll)	21.0
Muffin, donut, pastry, cake, or pie	18.9
Waffles, French toast, pancakes	17.9
Breakfast sandwich	17.6
Chips (Doritos, potato chips, Cheetos, etc.)	17.5
Eggs	15.3
Fruits (apple, pear, peaches, etc.)	14.6
Meat (bacon, ham, sausage), chicken, or fish	13.7
Soda, lemonade, Capri Sun, Sunny D, Hug, etc.	12.6
Candy	11.7
Coffee, tea, iced tea (Arizona, Brisk, etc.)	10.7
Vegetables (lettuce, green beans, broccoli, etc.)	5.7
Other	4.3
Cracker	1.2
Pretzel	0.2

Source: Adapted from Lawman et al., *BMC Public Health*, 14, 604, 2014.

Note: Ate at any location indicates the proportion of the sample that endorsed eating breakfast in that location. All three schools provided all students with access to free breakfast before school hours. Category descriptions are presented as they were shown to participants.

RELATIONSHIP BETWEEN BREAKFAST CONSUMPTION AND CHILDHOOD OVERWEIGHT AND OBESITY

Regular breakfast consumption among children has been recognized as a daily eating pattern that is possibly protective against overweight and obesity [21]. Large-scale observational studies using nationally representative samples have consistently supported inverse associations between breakfast consumption and adiposity outcomes [20,22–26], as have a systematic review and meta-analysis of European [27] and Asian/Pacific [28] studies, which included studies with cross-sectional designs. A National Evidence Library (NEL) systematic review conducted by the US Department of Agriculture (USDA) in 2010 including 15 non-cross-sectional international studies (one randomized controlled trial [RCT], one non-RCT, and 13 prospective cohort studies) published between 2000 and 2010 [21] found moderate strength of evidence for increased risk of overweight and obesity among children who do not eat breakfast, with a stronger association observed among adolescents. This review supported a 2005 review of 16 studies published between 1970 and 2004, which also reported a generally positive association between breakfast skipping and childhood adiposity despite higher daily energy intake relative to skippers [14]. Between the years 2010 and 2015, 12 additional non-cross-sectional studies were published, including 10 longitudinal, 1 case control, and 1 experimental study ([29], Table 6.3). Eight of the ten longitudinal studies along with the case control and experimental study reported inverse associations between breakfast consumption and adiposity. The sole experimental study investigated breakfast in combination with a nutrition education program; it found that, after one school year, children in the intervention group experienced reductions in body mass index (BMI) while those in the control group (education alone) experienced increases in BMI. Overall, effect sizes and likelihood/risk estimates for these studies ranged considerably, and the variety of adiposity indices used renders cross-study comparison challenging. Regardless, the magnitudes of several estimates were notable, particularly in the two studies with the longest follow-up time [30,31], which may better reflect the long-term impact of breakfast consumption throughout development. One reported a 3.74 kg/m^2 mean difference in waist circumference and 1.31 cm mean difference in BMI [31], while the other reported a 2.18 times greater risk of central adiposity among breakfast skippers compared with consumers [30]. The results achieved in the experimental study are especially promising. In the experimental group, the prevalence of overweight dropped 10.2% among boys (31.5–21.3) and 7.7% among girls (21.7–14), while the prevalence of obesity dropped 2.4% (7.9–5.5) among boys and 0.8% among girls (4.7–3.9) [32]. Although the remaining studies reported relatively smaller effect sizes, even these could have meaningful implications at the population level. Together, the results of these studies, in combination with previous reviews and cross-sectional studies reporting similar findings, support some role for breakfast consumption in the prevention of overweight and obesity among children. However, methodological limitations, discussed in the conclusion, render casual conclusions elusive.

SNACKING

PREVALENCE AND TRENDS

In the United States, the majority of studies considering nationally representative samples report notable increases in snack consumption among children over the past four decades [33–37]. According to the most recent National Health and Nutrition Examination Survey (NHANES) data (2009–2010), the vast majority (96% ages 2–19 years) of children consume at least one snack per day, approximately half of whom consumed two or three per day [1]. On average, children who consume snacks do so 2.2 times per day [38]. Repeat cross-sectional analysis of NHANES (1977–1978 to 2003–2006) investigating trends in snacking behavior over time indicates that the prevalence of snacking among all children increased from 74% to 98% overall, with the average number of snacks consumed per day nearly doubling within each age group. The most substantial increases were observed from 1989 to 1994 and 1994 to 2006 [37]. Children ages 2–6 years consumed the

TABLE 6.3
Original Research Studies Reporting Associations between Breakfast Consumption/Skipping and Adiposity Outcomes among Children and Adolescents 2010–2015

First Author, Year Location Study Name	Design, Follow-up	Sample	Exposure (Definition and Measurement)	Outcome(s) (Definition and Measurement)	Key Findings (Based on Fully-Adjusted Regression Models)
Smith, 2010 Australia CDAH	Longitudinal, 21 years	n = 2184 (53% female) Age at baseline: 7–15.0 years	Breakfast consumption defined as usual breakfast consumption before school (at baseline) and as eating a snack, small meal, or large meal 6–9 a.m. (at follow-up), categorized into four childhood to adulthood breakfast behavior trajectory groups. Child reported. Assessed by a single-item response on a FFQ at baseline and meal pattern chart at follow-up.	Mean difference in continuous BMI and waist circumference (measured height and weight and waist circumference).	Participants who reported skipping breakfast in childhood and adulthood had larger waist circumference (β = 3.74, CI: 0.83, 6.65) and higher BMIs (β = 1.31, CI: 0.03, 2.59) than those who reported eating breakfast at both time points.
Haerens, 2010 Belgium Longitudinal Eating and Activity study	Longitudinal, 3 years	n = 3716 (48% female; 98% Belgian) Age at baseline: 10.0 years	Breakfast defined as the number of week and weekend days on which children reported consuming breakfast (never, 1–2 weekend days, 1–5 weekdays). Child reported. Assessed by a supplementary FFQ question asking participants to mark the number of week and weekend days they had breakfast.	BMI z-score (self-reported height and weight). Flemish reference standards.	Breakfast consumption frequency was inversely associated with BMI z-score across four measurement time points (β = −0.03, SE = 0.012, $p < .01$).
Laska, 2012 MN, United States IDEA/ECHO	Longitudinal, 2 years	n = 693 (51% female; 86% white) Age at baseline: 14.6 years	Breakfast consumption frequency defined as the percentage of recall days on which participants reported eating a meal called breakfast containing ≥50 cal. Child reported. Assessed by three telephone-administered 24 h dietary recalls (telephone administered) and operationalized as proportion of recalls reporting eating breakfast.	Continuous BMI (measured height and weight) and percentage body fat (digital BIA scale).	Breakfast consumption was inversely associated with BMI and percentage cross-sectionally among males (BMI: β = −5.08, SE = 1.53, p = .001; PBF: β = −8.82, SE = 2.81, p = .002) and females (BMI: β = −4.33, SE = 1.62, p = .008; PBF: β = −7.30, SE = 2.22, p = .001) but not longitudinally.
Tin, 2012 Hong Kong, China	Longitudinal, 2 years	n = 68,606 (51% female; 100% Chinese) Age at baseline: 9.9 years	Breakfast consumption defined as usually eating breakfast at "home," "fast food/cafe/restaurant," or "some other place" (breakfast skipping defined as eating "no breakfast at all"). Child reported. Assessed by questionnaire.	Mean difference in continuous BMI (measured height and weight).	Compared with eaters, baseline breakfast skippers experienced a greater increase in BMI in the subsequent 2 years (β = 0.11, CI: 0.07, 0.16, $p < .001$). The effect was stronger among children who also skipped lunch and children who watched ≤2 h of television per day.

Chang, 2013 United States ECLS-K	Longitudinal, 3 years	n = 6220 (51% female; 66% white, 15% Hispanic, 8% African American) Age at baseline: 11.2 years	Breakfast consumption defined as positive response to the prompt: "At least some of the family eats breakfast together." Parent reported. Assessed by computer-assisted telephone or personal interview.	Likelihood of change in weight trajectory group for nine mutually exclusive weight trajectory groups based on BMI (measured height and weight), category (healthy, overweight, obese), CDC growth charts	Children who consumed breakfast were more likely to revert from being overweight in the fifth grade to being normal weight in the eighth grade, compared with those who did not (OR: 1.02, CI: 1.0, 1.03). There were no significant changes across other weight trajectory groups.
Drenowatz, 2013 Germany	Longitudinal, 1 year	n = 1495 (49% female; 22% migration background) Age at baseline: 7.0 years	Breakfast consumption defined as frequency of child having breakfast before school. Parent reported. Assessed by questionnaire.	Likelihood of weight gain compared with loss, defined by a ≥ 5 percentage point increase or decrease in age- and sex-specific BMI percentile (measured height and weight). German reference standards.	Increased odds for weight gain were observed with a lack of regular breakfast consumption (OR = 1.04, CI: 1.03, 1.04).
Quick, 2013 MN, United States Project EAT I-III	Longitudinal, 10 years	n = 1643 (54% female) Age at baseline: 15.0 years	Breakfast consumption defined as frequency of breakfast consumption in the past week. Child reported. Assessed by FFQ with a supplementary question on breakfast consumption frequency.	Ten-year incidence of overweight (self-reported height and weight, validated by measured height and weight among a subsample). CDC growth charts	Females with higher breakfast consumption frequency during adolescents experienced lower incidence of overweight at 10-year follow-up (OR = 0.91, CI:0.86, 0.97).
Carlson et al., 2012 San Diego County, United States MOVE Project	Longitudinal, 2 years	n = 254 (56% female; 39% white, 48% Latino) Age at baseline: 6.7 years	Breakfast consumption defined as the number of times per week the child ate breakfast with his or her family. Parent reported. Assessed by questionnaire.	BMI z-score (measured height and weight) and percentage of body fat (BIA, PBF calculated using Schaefer equation). CDC growth charts.	Increased number of days/week breakfast eaten with family was associated with decreased BMI z-score ($\beta = -0.04$, CI: -0.07–0.02, $p = .027$) and PBF ($\beta = -0.35$, CI: -0.69, -0.02, $p = .039$).
Kupers, 2014 Netherlands GECKO Drenthe Cohort	Longitudinal, 3 years	n = 1,366 (50% female; 93% Dutch) Age at baseline: 2.1 years	Breakfast consumption defined as the weekly frequency ("How often does your child eat breakfast weekly?"), categorized as "eating breakfast daily" (7/week) or "not eating breakfast daily" (<7/week). Parent reported. Assessed by questionnaire.	Risk of being overweight at age 5 based on BMI z-score (measured height and weight). Dutch reference growth charts (1997) and Cole's BMI category cutoff for overweight status.	Skipping breakfast was not associated with adiposity status cross-sectionally at 2 years or 5 years, or over time (OR: 0.72, CI: 0.15, 3.49).

(Continued)

TABLE 6.3 (CONTINUED)
Original Research Studies Reporting Associations between Breakfast Consumption/Skipping and Adiposity Outcomes among Children and Adolescents 2010–2015

First Author, Year Location Study Name	Design, Follow-up	Sample	Exposure (Definition and Measurement)	Outcome(s) (Definition and Measurement)	Key Findings (Based on Fully-Adjusted Regression Models)
Wennberg, 2014 Sweden Northern Swedish Cohort	Longitudinal, 27 years	$n = 889$ Age at baseline: 16 years	Breakfast consumption determined by participants' response to the question: "What did you have for breakfast this morning?" and underlining of commonly consumed breakfast items. Responses dichotomized into "Eating breakfast" and "Poor breakfast habits" (breakfast skippers and participants who only reported a beverage or something sweet, $n = 88$) at age 16. Child-reported. Assessed by questionnaire (classroom at age 16, reunion/mail at age 43).	Risk of central obesity at follow-up (measured waist circumference, defined as ≥80 cm for women or ≥94 cm for men). IDFG guidelines.	Participants with poor breakfast habits were at increased risk of central obesity (OR: 2.18, CI: 1.31, 3.60).
Zurriaga, 2011 Spain OBICE	Case-control	$n = 1188$ (44% female), 437 cases, 751 controls Mean age: 8.8 years	Breakfast consumption measured as frequency of breakfast consumption per week, dichotomized as regular breakfast consumption vs. not. Assessed by two questionnaires asking about frequency of breakfast consumption: one completed by the participants' pediatrician and the other by the children's families as part of a FFQ.	Risk of childhood obesity defined as BMI >95th age-sex BMI percentile (measured height and weight). Fundacion Orbegozo-Sobradillo tables.	Regular breakfast consumption was associated with reduced risk of obesity (OR: 0.5, CI: 0.26, $p = .042$).
Campos Pastor, 2012 Spain NEP	Cluster randomized trial, one school year	$n = 256$ (50% female) Mean age: 13.9 years	Daily breakfast (consisting of a dairy product, fruit, cereal, nuts, and a sandwich with protein filling, either tuna or ham and totaling 275–350 cal) provided by the school in combination with the NEP program compared with NEP only.	Continuous BMI (measured height and weight) and prevalence of overweight/obesity, waist circumference (measured), and fat mass/lean mass measured via BIA. Cole's BMI cutoffs.	Males and females in the intervention group experienced reductions in BMI ($p < .001$) and in waist circumference among females only ($p < .001$). Prevalence of overweight dropped 10.2 percentage points among boys (31.5–21.3) and 7.7% among girls (21.7–14) and the prevalence of obesity dropped 2.4% (7.9–5.5) among boys and 0.8% among girls (4.7–3.9). BMI and waist circumference significantly decreased among children who were normal weight or overweight at baseline ($p = .001$), whereas only BMI decreased among children who were obese at baseline ($p = .02$).

Note: BIA, bioelectrical impedance analysis; BMI, body mass index; CDC, Centers for Disease Control and Prevention; CI, confidence interval; FFQ, food frequency questionnaire; NEP, Nutrition Education Program; OBIDF, International Diabetes Federation; OR, odds ratio; PBF, percent body fat.

greatest number of snacks per day (2.75) and were also the group with the largest increase occurring from 1977 to 2006 (~1.41 additional snacks per day). While energy-dense, nutrient-poor snack foods and beverages are widely available across diverse settings where young people spend time, including schools, corner stores, and recreational facilities [39–41], most snacking occurs in the home [35,37,41]. Since more than two-thirds of calories are consumed in the home, the vast majority of which come from food purchased from stores [1], enabling and encouraging healthy choices at the point-of-purchase could go a long way toward improving the home food environment and diet quality. Such policy efforts, some already underway, include ingredient regulation (e.g., sodium and *trans* fat), nutrition facts panel updates (added sugars, percentage daily value footnote), and front-of-package labeling.

With regard to snack composition, desserts and sweetened beverages contributed the greatest number of calories to total energy consumed from snacks, despite an observed decrease in dessert consumption from 2003 to 2006 [37]. The second main source of energy from snacking was salty snacks, such as crackers, chips, popcorn, and pretzels, which experienced the largest increase in the past three decades and accounted for the largest increases in snacking occasions through 2006 [37]. While a more recent subgroup analysis of NHANES data from the years 2003–2010 reported no changes in the percentage of daily energy derived from sweet and salty snacks in the full sample, significant declines were observed among children of select race/ethnicity and/or weight-status categories [43]. Specifically, among overweight and obese adolescents, the percentage consuming sweet snacks declined significantly over the study period (59% vs. 50%) and was significantly lower than the healthy-weight adolescents in both time periods (2003–2006: 59% vs. 65%; 2007–2010: 50% vs. 64%). In the most recent survey year, overweight/obese adolescents consumed significantly fewer calories from salty snacks than healthy-weight adolescents (253 vs. 295 kcal). Among white children aged 2–5 years and 6–11 years who were overweight/obese, calories from salty snacks declined significantly (age 2–5 years: 192 vs. 134 kcal; age 6–11: 273 vs. 200 kcal). Among black children aged 12–19 years and at a healthy weight, calories from salty snacks also declined significantly (343 vs. 283 kcal). With respect to sweet snacks, significant declines in calories consumed were observed among white children aged 2–5 years who were at a healthy weight (217 vs. 184 kcal) [43]. Assuming overweight and obese children did not underreport consumption, these results suggest that improvements in snack quality, especially among those at highest risk, may be improving and possibly contributing to the leveling trends in obesity and the 201 kcal/day reduction in total calorie intake observed from 2003–2004 to 2009–2010 among 2- to 18-year-olds [44].

Coinciding with the increase in snacking occasions has been an increase in the percentage of energy derived from snacks. In fact, children consumed approximately 168 more calories a day from snacking from 1977–1978 to 2003–2006, reaching 27% of total daily intake in 2006 [37], an estimate which has remained relatively stable since, with 26% of energy (516 kcals) coming from snacks among 2- to 19-year-olds, according to 2011–2012 NHANES data [45]. Consistent with the increase in snacking calories, the largest increase in total energy was found among children ages 2–6 years, who consumed 182 cal more per day over the three decades observed [37]. NHANES 2011–2012 estimates show that 2- to 5-year-old males and females continue to consume 30% and 31% of energy from snacks (relative to roughly 24.5% among 6–11 and 12–19-year-old children) [45]. The increase in calories from snacks paralleled a 113 total calorie increase per day from 1977 to 2006 [37]. Although a small decline in calories per snacking event was observed from 1994 to 2006 among all age groups, the increased energy per snack from 1977 to 2006 was significant, and grams of food consumed per snack event also increased significantly from 1977 to 2003 in all age groups (~50 g more per snack). NHANES 2009–2010 data support these estimates, with nearly 500 cal to daily energy intake, equating to roughly one-quarter of total energy intake (498 kcals; 25.7%) coming from snacks. Independent of beverages consumed as snacks, snack foods contributed 20% (379 kcals) of total daily energy in children. Moreover, total energy intake increased with snacking frequency, with children reporting four or more snacking occasions per day consuming an average 19% more total energy compared with nonsnackers [40]. Given the overall leveling in obesity rates in recent years, the stable contribution of snacks to total calories suggests that children are consuming less at meals and/or increasing physical activity levels in order to keep calories at a steady or lower rate. A possible decrease in caloric beverage consumption, a behavior possibly not falling into either the meal or snack category, could also be responsible.

RELATIONSHIP WITH WEIGHT STATUS

Despite the observed trends in snacking behavior over the past several decades, whether the observed changes in frequency, type, and contribution of snacks to total daily energy intake has contributed to rising obesity rates is a research question lacking a definitive answer. The most recent review of evidence on the relationship between snacking and weight status among children and adolescents was published in 2013 (Larson and Story) and included 2 case control, 23 cross-sectional, and 7 longitudinal studies published internationally between January 2000 and December 2011 [41]. The exclusion of studies with exposure variables that could independently impact adiposity, such as dietary pattern scores/categories, consumption venue, advertisement source, and/or particular foods, left 15 cross-sectional and 2 longitudinal studies looking exclusively at snacking frequency, snack timing, and/or percentage energy from snacks. Of the 15 cross-sectional studies, 3 reported positive associations (one only for snacks consumed after dinner), 8 found no association, and 4 reported negative associations (one only among males in urban areas) between snacking behavior and adiposity outcomes. One of the longitudinal studies found no association, while the other reported an inverse association between snacking frequency and risk of excess adiposity. The five remaining longitudinal studies reported on either dietary pattern adherence ($n = 3$) or consumption of specific snack foods ($n = 2$), which may independently impact weight status. Two measured adherence to an empirically derived snacking pattern and found null associations; one reported a positive association between adherence to a pattern that combined energy intake and expenditure indices (snacking + sedentary pattern, characterized by energy-dense snacks and television watching). Finally, two found no association between energy-dense snack consumption and adiposity outcomes. Taken together, the results from the longitudinal studies included in the review suggest little evidence for a favorable or adverse impact on adiposity even among those consuming poor-quality snacks.

In light of these inconsistent findings, researchers have continued to investigate the relationship between snacking and adiposity among children. Table 6.4 provides details on studies published since 2012. As with the recent studies on breakfast, the majority took place outside the United States, representing seven unique countries (Norway, China, Korea, Italy, Japan, Greece, and the United States). Overall, findings were evenly split by direction of impact, with three reporting null associations [40,46,47], three reporting inverse associations [48–50], and three reporting positive associations between snacking and adiposity outcomes [51–53]. The majority of the studies were cross-sectional. The two longitudinal studies both reported positive associations between snack consumption and BMI, detailed as follows [51,52].

The first sampled 1504 children (474 first graders and 1030 fourth graders) in Korea participating in the Obesity and Metabolic Disorders Cohort in Childhood registry, which collected data on physical activity, dietary intake, and socioeconomic status through self-administered questionnaires, and measured height and weight annually for 2 years [51]. Dietary intake was recorded for 2 weekdays and 1 weekend day by a 24 h dietary recall, with the frequency of skipping meals and snack intake reported. Physical activity was measured via self-report and quantified as days with moderate physical activity of more than 30 min duration or vigorous physical activity of more than 20 min duration. In a cross-sectional analysis, BMI of first and fourth graders was positively associated with frequent snack consumption ($p = .049$). BMI increased in both groups over time; however, in longitudinal analyses, controlling for energy intake and physical activity, frequent snack consumption ($p = .010$) predicted change in BMI only among fourth graders. The second longitudinal study published since 2012 analyzed data collected from 45,392 participants in the twenty-first-century Longitudinal Survey in Newborns in Japan to identify time-dependent and independent

TABLE 6.4

Original Research Studies Reporting Associations between Snacking Behavior and Adiposity Outcomes among Children and Adolescents, Published 2012–2015

First Author, Year Location Study Name	Design, Follow-up	Sample	Exposure (Definition and Measurement)	Outcome(s) (Definition and Measurement)	Key Findings
Grydeland, 2012 Norway The HEIA	Cross-sectional	n = 1103 (50% female) Mean age: 11.2 years	Intake of snacks assessed by four questions; "how often do you eat chocolate/candy, salty snacks, cookies and buns/cakes/pastry," with seven response categories ranging from "never/seldom" to "twice a day or more." All variables were recorded into frequency of intake per week and summed. Child reported. Internet-based questionnaire.	Risk of overweight (measured height and weight). IOTF BMI cutoffs.	Snack frequency was not associated with weight status (β: 0.97; CI: 0.92, 1.03; p = .30).
Guo, 2012 China	Cross-sectional	n = 4,262 (49% female) Mean age: 11.04 years	Frequency of snacking defined as: "never or occasionally," "less than once a week," "1–3 days per week," "4–6 days per week," and "everyday." Child-reported. Questionnaire.	Risk of overweight and obesity (measured height and weight). IOTF BMI cutoffs	Participants who never or occasionally consumed snacks were at increased risk of excess adiposity (OR overweight: 1.074; CI: 0.904, 1.276; p = 0.418; OR obese: 1.348; CI: 1.039, 1.748, p = 0.025).
Jelastopula, 2012 Greece	Cross-sectional	n = 200 (54% female) Mean age: 11.2 years +/−0.8	Snacking frequency defined as having an afternoon snack daily, sometimes, or never. Child-reported. In-person interviews using a 24-item questionnaire.	Overweight and obesity, mean BMI, and waist circumference (measured height and weight). IOTF BMI cutoffs.	Rates of overweight and obesity were significantly higher among children who never consumed an afternoon snack (44.7% overweight and 25.5% obese) compared with children who consumed an afternoon snack daily (25% overweight and 2.5% obese) (p < .001). Daily afternoon snack consumption was associated with significantly lower BMI (β: −3.020 kg/cm²; CI: −4.410, −1.629; p < .001). Consuming a snack daily and sometimes were inversely associated with waist circumference (β: −5.65; CI: −9.28, −2.02; p = .002; β:−4.12; CI: −7.1, −1.13; p = .007). *(Continued)*

TABLE 6.4 (CONTINUED)
Original Research Studies Reporting Associations between Snacking Behavior and Adiposity Outcomes among Children and Adolescents, Published 2012–2015

First Author, Year Location Study Name	Design, Follow-up	Sample	Exposure (Definition and Measurement)	Outcome(s) (Definition and Measurement)	Key Findings
Lee, 2014 Korea Obesity and Metabolic Disorders in Children registry	Longitudinal, 2 years	$n = 1504$ Age at baseline: 7.3 years and follow-up:10.0 years	Meal skipping and snack intake. Child-reported. 24 h recalls administered on 2 weekdays and 1 weekend day.	Mean BMI change (measured height and weight).	At 2-year follow-up, snack consumption was positively associated with increase in BMI among fourth graders (β: 0.278; CI: 0.066, 0.490; $p = .010$) but not among first graders. No association was found between meal skipping and BMI change over 2 years among first or fourth graders.
Bo, 2014 Italy	Cross-sectional	$n = 400$ (48% female) Mean age: 12.1 years	Percentage of total daily calorie intake from snacks (<15%, 15%–20%, >20%), daily snacking frequency (1, 2, ≥3), and timing of consuming the most caloric snack (morning, afternoon, evening). Parent reported. 24 h dietary recall and a 19-item FFQ.	Mean BMI, BMI percentile, overweight/ obesity (measured height and weight). Italian growth charts (overweight/obesity defined as BMI ≥85th percentile based on age- and gender-specific BMI).	Proportion of daily calories derived from snacks, snacking frequency, and evening snacking were positively associated with mean BMI, BMI percentile, and overweight/obesity status. Children consuming 15%–20% and >20% of kcals from snacks had significantly higher risk of overweight/obesity compared with those consuming <15% of daily kcals from snacks (RR: 1.35; CI: 0.58, 3.15; $p = .49$ and RR: 2.32; CI: 1.10, 4.89; $p = .03$, respectively). Relative to children consuming one snack/day, those consuming two snacks were at higher risk of overweight or obesity (RR: 2.20; CI 0.92, 5.27; $p = .08$), with those consuming ≥3 snacks at greatest risk (RR: 4.17; CI: 1.60, 10.9; $p = .004$). Children consuming the most energy-dense snack in the evening were at higher risk for overweight/ obesity compared with those consuming it in the morning (RR: 3.12; CI: 1.17, 8.34; $p = .02$).
Hauser, 2014 MA, United States	Cross-sectional	$n = 820$ (51.7% female) Mean age: 7.6 years	Number of snacks consumed per day. Parent reported. Survey questionnaire.	Overweight (defined as BMI >85th percentile) and obesity (BMI >95th percentile), based on measured height and weight. CDC growth charts.	Snack servings/day did not vary significantly between normal and overweight children (mean [SD] of 1.84[1.0] vs. 1.71[0.9], respectively; $p = .082$).

Franchetti, 2014 Japan Twenty-first century Longitudinal Survey in Newborns	Longitudinal, 5.5 years	$n = 45{,}392$ (48% female) Age at baseline: 0 years (birth) and follow-up: 4.5 years for breakfast and snack consumption variables and 5.5 years for BMI	Consumption of breakfast, lunch, dinner, and snacks classified as regular, irregular, or no consumption. Parent reported. Questionnaires.	Mean BMI, overweight (≥85th percentile) and obesity (≥95th percentile) (parental reported height and weight at birth).	Irregular snack consumption at age 4.5 was associated with lower BMI at age 5.5 (β: −0.047; CI: −0.083, −0.010; $p = .01$) when compared with regular snack consumption.
Grigorakis, 2015 Greece	Cross-sectional	$n = 124{,}113$ (49.2% female) Mean age: 9.9 years	Snack consumption at school during the school day or in the afternoon between lunch and dinner (yes/no) and type of snacks usually consumed (fruits or fruit juice, toast or sandwich, dairy products, salty snacks, and sweets). Child reported with assistance of teachers. Seven-day diet recall questionnaire (closed-question multiple choice format), validated.	Central obesity defined as waist-to-hip ratio ≥0.5 (measured waist and hip circumferences).	Children with central obesity reported less frequent snack consumption and lower total meal frequency ($p < .001$) compared with children without central obesity. Snack consumption was inversely associated with risk of central obesity, such that children who habitually consumed snacks throughout the day (compared with those not consuming snacks) had a 30% lower probability of being centrally obese (OR: 0.70; CI: 0.67, 0.74).
Gugger, 2015 United States	Cross-sectional	$n = 2985$ (2–18 years)	Frequency of snacking and nutrient contribution from snacks. One-day 24 h recall from NHANES 2011–2012.	BMI (body weight and height measured), categorized into overweight/obese status.	Total energy intake increased with snacking frequency; children consuming four or more snacks/day consumed on average 19% more total energy compared with nonsnackers. However, snacking frequency was not associated with overweight/obesity.

Note: BIA, bioelectrical impedance analysis; BMI, body mass index; CDC, Centers for Disease Control and Prevention; CI, confidence interval; FFQ, food frequency questionnaire; HEIA, HEalth In Adolescence; IOTF, International Obesity Task Force; NHANES, National Health and Nutrition Examination Survey; OR, odds ratio; PBF, percent body fat; RR, relative risk.

demographic, social, and lifestyle factors that affect change in BMI across 5.5 years [52]. Snack consumption was classified into regular, irregular, or no consumption. In final, longitudinal models, irregular snack consumption was inversely associated with BMI ($\beta = -0.047$, $p = .01$, CI: -0.083, -0.010). Though this study did not control for physical activity or energy intake, it did include television hours, sleep duration, and regular meal consumption in regression models. Notably, both studies took place in Asian countries and neither study measured snack composition nor quality. Nonetheless, their findings add to the existing body of evidence.

The recent cross-sectional studies included in Table 6.4 reported null findings in Norway [47] and the United States [40,46], inverse findings in China [48] and Greece [49,50], and positive in Italy [53]. In addition to studies measuring snacking behavior directly, three studies published since 2013 have investigated associations between empirically derived snacking patterns and adiposity outcomes. Two used longitudinal data, one reporting null [54] associations between snacking and adiposity outcomes across eight European countries and the other, conducted in Bogota, Columbia, reporting a positive association [55]. A third cross-sectional analysis of NHANES data reported inverse associations with several of the empirically derived snacking patterns in the United States, despite snacking pattern adherence also being associated with increased energy intake [56]. As a whole, the disparate nature and findings of these studies make it difficult to draw general conclusions about the relationship between snacking and weight status among children.

EATING FREQUENCY

PREVALENCE AND TRENDS

Although breakfast consumption and snacking behavior may contribute to and, therefore, correlate with increased *eating frequency*, the latter term has been used to encompass all daily eating occasions, regardless of size or composition. Consequently, eating frequency has been considered independently of breakfast and snacking behavior as an exposure variable. Nationally representative US trend data from children aged 2–18 years suggest that the number of daily eating and drinking occasions has increased from 3.9 to 5.1 between 1977–1978 and 2005–2010. Total daily energy intake increased by a net 108 kcal/day over the same time frame (with the greatest increase of 173 kcal/day occurring between 1989–1991 and 1994–1998 and a modest decline of 85 kcal/day occurring between 1994–1998 and 2005–2010), and evidence suggests that changes in daily eating patterns may have contributed [57–59].

Changes in the number of eating occasions accounted for a 2 kcal/day decrease per year from the late 1970s to the early 1990s but were followed by an increase of 69 kcal/day per year through 1998. Between 1977–1978 and 1989–1991, changes in the average portion size per eating occasion accounted for 5 additional kcal/day/year of the annualized increase in total energy intake and a decrease of 31 kcal/day/year of the decline in energy between 1994–1998 and 2005–2010. Changes in the number of eating occasions, on the other hand, accounted for 2 fewer kcal/day/year between 1977–1978 and 1989–1991 but an additional 69 kcal/day/year between 1989–1991 and 1994–1998. The energy density of foods increased over this time period, from 2.0 kcal/g/eating occasion in 1977–1978 to 2.19 kcal/g/eating occasion in 2005–2010. These changes reflect larger increases in the total daily energy from foods (111 kcal/day increase) relative to beverages (4 kcal/day decrease) over the past 30 years, with the number of daily eating occasions responsible for the largest portion of increase of 19 kcal/day/year in total energy intake and a decrease in portion size per eating occasion accounting for a 13 kcal/day/year decrease in the annualized change [60].

RELATIONSHIP BETWEEN EATING FREQUENCY AND WEIGHT STATUS

The first study to investigate the relationship between eating frequency and weight outcomes among children was conducted in the late 1960s, in which participants from a school-based sample were assigned to a three or seven meal-per-day condition. Although the two groups had similar total energy intake, children assigned to the three daily meals group gained more weight compared with those assigned to seven meals per day [61]. Since this seminal study, the majority of research has used cross-sectional study designs. A meta-analysis of these studies published in 2013 (Kaisari et al.) systematically assessed the association between eating frequency and excess adiposity in children and adolescents [62]. The analysis included 21 cross-sectional studies representing a total sample size of 18,849 subjects and reported an inverse association between eating frequency and overweight/obesity status. Specifically, children and adolescents who had a higher number of eating episodes per day had a 22% lower probability of being overweight or obese compared with those who had fewer episodes. However, after stratifying the results by sex, the inverse association only held among boys, suggesting possible differences in dietary patterns and behaviors and their effect on overweight/obesity, though the authors caution that publication bias and the significant heterogeneity observed in the results of the selected studies warrant caution in interpreting these findings.

Three longitudinal studies have also investigated the relationship between eating frequency and weight status among children. The first found a positive association between eating frequency and change in BMI z-score among girls (8–12 years at baseline, 11–19 at follow-up) [63], the second reported an inverse association between eating frequency and increase in BMI over 10 years (9–10 years at baseline, 19–20 at follow-up) [64], and the third found a positive association cross-sectionally at baseline and longitudinally at 6- but not 12-month follow-up [65]. A fourth longitudinal study [66], looking specifically at *meal* frequency in a sample of Norwegian children, reported increased odds of overweight among children who no longer consumed regular meals in seventh grade compared with fourth grade (OR: 3·1; CI: 1.1, 9.0), controlling for sex, socioeconomic status, and physical activity, but not after controlling for fourth-grade weight status (OR: 2.8; CI: 0.7, 11.6). A recent cross-sectional study examined the associations of eating frequency with metabolic risk factors in British children and adolescents and found that eating frequency was positively associated with BMI z-score in adolescents only ($p = .004$), controlling for total energy intake and physical activity levels. Although eating frequency was inversely associated with total cholesterol and LDL-cholesterol concentrations ($p = .01$ and .04, respectively) among children, no associations were detected for BMI [67]. On the other hand, an analysis of data collected from a population-based sample of 16-year-old boys and girls ($n = 6247$) participating in the Northern Finland Birth Cohort 1986 found that adolescents who ate five meals/day (compared with those consuming fewer) were at lower risk for overweight/obesity (OR for boys: 0.47, CI: 0.34, 0.65; OR for girls: 0.57, CI: 0.41, 0.79) and abdominal obesity (OR for boys: 0.32, CI: 0.22, 0.48; OR for girls: 0.54, CI: 0.39, 0.75), after adjusting for later childhood factors [68]. A subsequent analysis suggested that the five meal/day pattern attenuated children's genetic predisposition toward overweight/obesity, though more research is needed to confirm these findings and to explore interindividual response differences more generally [69].

DISCUSSION AND CONCLUSION

Based on the evidence presented in this chapter for each of the three main daily eating pattern-related exposure variables (i.e., breakfast, snacking, and eating frequency) and adiposity-related outcomes among children and adolescents, the evidence supporting a protective effect of breakfast consumption on childhood obesity is most comprehensive and consistent. On the other hand, associations between snacking and eating frequency are less consistently significant and unidirectional. In relating and discussing the relative strength of evidence, it is important to underscore the methodological challenges and limitations of extant literature, inherent and common among all three bodies of literature [66].

First and foremost, the majority of studies on daily eating patterns have employed observational designs and, therefore, regardless of the consistency of results, preclude causal inference. While longitudinal designs address issues of temporality and reverse causality, stronger study designs are needed to overcome the potential for residual confounding by unobservable or unmeasured variables. However, because prescribed daily eating patterns are difficult to assign and adhere to, in addition to presenting ethical challenges among children, natural experiments and/or innovative methods of data collection and analysis could compensate, in part, for these methodological challenges.

Regardless of study design, a first priority in eating pattern research is developing standardized operational definitions and assessment methods for the daily eating behaviors of interest (i.e., breakfast, snack, eating occasion) [70] and adiposity outcomes of interest (i.e., continuous BMI, BMI percentile, or BMI z-score and reference population/cutoffs). Acknowledging this weakness in current methodology, the Scientific Report of the 2015 Dietary Guidelines Advisory Committee recognized the standardized exposure and outcome assessment methods and the development of operational definitions for meals and snacks as priorities for future research in this area due to the disparate and sometimes conflicting definitions currently in use, which impede comparison across studies [1].

In addition to stronger study designs and the application of standardized primary exposure and outcome definitions, findings from observational studies could be strengthened by employing more precise, valid, and standardized measurements of confounding, effect modifying, and mediating variables. In this regard, two are of top priority: total energy intake and energy expenditure (i.e., physical activity). Because these are the two most proximal determinants of energy balance and possibly associated with or determinants of daily eating patterns, failing to test each as potential confounding and mediating variables renders results less useful. Previous studies have linked breakfast consumption with increased energy intake and/or physical activity, but few have thoroughly investigated the relationship between these outcomes and weight status [71]. Second to energy intake and expenditure, the measurement of meal and snack composition and quality is of utmost priority. Without this information, it is impossible to know whether it is the eating occasion/ frequency or content that is impacting adiposity outcomes. Breakfast, in particular, may be a proxy for better overall diet quality and/or linked with other positive health behaviors that are protective against obesity. To this end, controlling for overall diet quality would also be useful. Longitudinal studies should also control for a baseline measure of adiposity. Beyond these essential variables, considering differences by sex, race/ethnicity, and socioeconomic status could shed light on potential factors that could modify the relationship between daily eating patterns and adiposity outcomes. Findings from these analyses could optimally direct the targeting of public health messaging and interventions toward specific subgroups. Finally, in drawing conclusions about existing and future research as a whole, potential publication and funding biases need to be considered and taken into account. Conclusive evidence on associations between the timing and distribution of energy intake across daily eating occasions and adiposity outcomes among children could lend itself to targeted public health messaging, interventions, and campaigns. In the meantime, efforts aimed at improving the quality of foods consumed at every eating occasion, regardless of time of day, place, or quantity consumed, should be continued and prioritized in the fight against childhood obesity.

REFERENCES

1. US Department of Agriculture and US Department of Health and Human Services. Scientific report of the 2015 Dietary Guidelines for Americans Advisory Committee. 2015. Available at http://health.gov/dietaryguidelines/2015-scientific-report/
2. Williams JW, Canterford L, Toumbourou JW, Patton GC, Catalano RF. Social development measures associated with problem behaviours and weight status in Australian adolescents. *Prev Sci* 2015;16(6):822–831.
3. Gurnani M, Birken C, Hamilton J. Childhood obesity: Causes, consequences, and management. *Pediatr Clin North Am* 2015;62(4):821–840.
4. Gluckman P, Nishtar S, Armstrong T. Ending childhood obesity: A multidimensional challenge. *Lancet* 2015;385(9973):1048–1050.

5. Institute of Medicine (IOM). *Accelerating Progress in Obesity Prevention: Solving the Weight of the Nation.* Washington, DC: National Academies Press, 2012.

6. Kant AK, Graubard BI. Within-person comparison of eating behaviors, time of eating, and dietary intake on days with and without breakfast: NHANES 2005–2010. *Am J Clin Nutr* 2015;102(3):661–670.

7. de Graaf C. Effects of snacks on energy intake: An evolutionary perspective. *Appetite* 2006;47(1):18–23.

8. Gatenby SJ. Eating frequency: Methodological and dietary aspects. *Br J Nutr* 1997;77(S1):S7–S20.

9. Miller R, Benelam B, Stanner S, Buttriss J. Is snacking good or bad for health: An overview. *Nutr Bull* 2013;38(3):302–322.

10. Leonard WR. The global diversity of eating patterns: Human nutritional health in comparative perspective. *Physiol Behav* 2014;134:5–14.

11. Horne JA. Human REM sleep: Influence on feeding behaviour, with clinical implications. *Sleep Med* 2015;16(8):910–916.

12. Wollan M. Rise and shine: What kids around the world eat for breakfast. *New York Times*, October 8, 2014.

13. Merriam-Webster Dictionary. Breakfast. 2015. Available at http://www.merriam-webster.com/dictionary/breakfast#. Accessed June 15, 2016.

14. Rampersaud GC, Pereira MA, Girard BL, Adams J, Metzl JD. Breakfast habits, nutritional status, body weight, and academic performance in children and adolescents. *J Am Diet Assoc* 2005;105(5):743–760.

15. Blondin SA, Anzman–Frasca S, Djang HC, Economos CD. Breakfast consumption and adiposity among children and adolescents: An updated review of the literature. *Pediatric Obesity* 2016; doi: 10.1111/ijpo.12082. [Epub ahead of print].

16. Iannotti RJ, Wang J. Trends in physical activity, sedentary behavior, diet, and BMI among US adolescents, 2001–2009. *Pediatrics* 2013;132(4):606–614.

17. Deshmukh-Taskar PR, Radcliffe JD, Liu Y, Nicklas TA. Do breakfast skipping and breakfast type affect energy intake, nutrient intake, nutrient adequacy, and diet quality in young adults? NHANES 1999–2002. *J Am Coll Nutr* 2010;29(4):407–418.

18. Siega-Riz AM, Popkin BM, Carson T. Trends in breakfast consumption for children in the United States from 1965–1991. *Am J Clin Nutr* 1998;67(4):748S–756S.

19. Beltsville Human Nutrition Research Center, Food Surveys Research Group. Breakfast in America, 2001–2002: Most frequently reported foods and beverages at breakfast. 2002. Available at https://www.ars.usda.gov/SP2UserFiles/Place/80400530/pdf/DBrief/1_Breakfast_2001_2002.pdf. Accessed November 22, 2008.

20. Lawman HG, Wilson DK. Associations of social and environmental supports with sedentary behavior, light and moderate-to-vigorous physical activity in obese underserved adolescents. *Int J Behav Nutr Phys Act* 2014;11:92.

21. Deshmukh-Taskar PR, Nicklas TA, O'Neil CE, Keast DR, Radcliffe JD, Cho S. The relationship of breakfast skipping and type of breakfast consumption with nutrient intake and weight status in children and adolescents: The National Health and Nutrition Examination Survey 1999–2006. *J Am Diet Assoc* 2010;110(6):869–878

22. Dietary Guidelines Advisory Committee. Report of the Dietary Guidelines Advisory Committee on the Dietary Guidelines for Americans, 2010, to the Secretary of Agriculture and the Secretary of Health and Human Services. Washington, DC, Dietary Guidelines Advisory Committee, 2010.

23. O'Neil CE, Nicklas TA, Fulgoni III VL. *Nutrient Intake, Diet Quality, and Weight Measures in Breakfast Patterns Consumed by Children Compared with Breakfast Skippers: NHANES 2001–2008.* New Delhi, India: AIMS Public Health, 2015.

24. Gregori D, Vecchio M. Is breakfast associated with an increase of body weight in children? An international comparison based on the OBEY-AD Study (621.4). *FASEB J* 2014;28(1 Suppl):621.4.
25. Huang CJ, Hu HT, Fan YC, Liao YM, Tsai PS. Associations of breakfast skipping with obesity and health-related quality of life: Evidence from a national survey in Taiwan. *Int J Obes* (Lond) 2010;34(4):720–725.
26. Hallstrom L, Vereecken CA, Labayen I, Ruiz JR, Le Donne C, Cuenca Garcia M, et al. Breakfast habits among European adolescents and their association with sociodemographic factors: The HELENA (Healthy Lifestyle in Europe by Nutrition in Adolescence) study. *Public Health Nutr* 2012;15(10):1879–1889.
27. Papoutsou S, Briassoulis G, Wolters M, Peplies J, Iacoviello L, Eiben G, et al. No breakfast at home: Association with cardiovascular disease risk factors in childhood. *Eur J Clin Nutr* 2014;68(7):829–834.
28. Szajewska H, Ruszczyński M. Systematic review demonstrating that breakfast consumption influences body weight outcomes in children and adolescents in Europe. *Crit Rev Food Sci Nutr* 2010;50(2):113–119.
29. Horikawa C, Kodama S, Yachi Y, Heianza Y, Hirasawa R, Ibe Y, et al. Skipping breakfast and prevalence of overweight and obesity in Asian and Pacific regions: A meta-analysis. *Prev Med* 2011;53(4):260–267.
30. Wennberg M, Gustafsson PE, Wennberg P, Hammarström A. Poor breakfast habits in adolescence predict the metabolic syndrome in adulthood. *Public Health Nutr* 2015;18(1):122–129.
31. Smith KJ, Gall SL, McNaughton SA, Blizzard L, Dwyer T, Venn AJ. Skipping breakfast: Longitudinal associations with cardiometabolic risk factors in the Childhood Determinants of Adult Health Study. *Am J Clin Nutr* 2010;92(6):1316–1325.
32. Campos Pastor MM, Serrano Pardo MD, Fernandez Soto ML, Luna Del Castillo JD, Escobar-Jimenez F. Impact of a "school-based" nutrition intervention on anthropometric parameters and the metabolic syndrome in Spanish adolescents. *Ann Nutr Metab* 2012;61(4):281–288.
33. Jahns L, Arab L, Carriquiry A, Popkin BM. The use of external within-person variance estimates to adjust nutrient intake distributions over time and across populations. *Public Health Nutr* 2005;8(1):69–76.
34. Frazao E. *The American Diet. Health and Economic Consequences: An Economic Research Service Report.* Washington, DC: European Respiratory Society, 1995.
35. Adair PM, Pine CM, Burnside G, Nicoll AD, Gillett A, Anwar S, et al. Familial and cultural perceptions and beliefs of oral hygiene and dietary practices among ethnically and socio-economicall diverse groups. *Community Dent Health* 2004;21(1 Suppl):102–111.
36. Nielsen SJ, Siega-Riz AM, Popkin BM. Trends in food locations and sources among adolescents and young adults. *Prev Med* 2002;35(2):107–113.
37. Piernas C, Popkin BM. Trends in snacking among U.S. children. *Health Aff (Millwood)* 2010;29(3):398–404.
38. Gugger C, Bidwai S, Joshi N, Holschuh N, Albertson A. Nutrient contribution of snacking in Americans: Results from the National Health and Nutrition Examination Survey 2011–2012. *FASEB J* 2015;29(1 Suppl):587.14.
39. Poti JM, Slining MM, Popkin BM. Solid fat and added sugar intake among US children: The role of stores, schools, and fast food, 1994–2010. *Am J Prev Med* 2013;45(5):551–559.
40. Folliard J, Duncan-Goldsmith D. Opportunities to improve snacks and beverages in schools. *J Acad Nutr Diet* 2013;113(9):1145–1151.
41. Larson N, Story M. A review of snacking patterns among children and adolescents: What are the implications of snacking for weight status? *Child Obes* 2013;9(2):104–115.

42. Deming D, Briefel R, Reidy K. Infant feeding practices and food consumption patterns of children participating in WIC. *J Nutr Educ Behav* 2014;46(3):29–37.
43. Bleich SN, Wolfson JA. US adults and child snacking patterns among sugar-sweetened beverage drinkers and non-drinkers. *Prev Med* 2015;72:8–14.
44. Slining MM, Popkin BM. Trends in intakes and sources of solid fats and added sugars among US children and adolescents: 1994–2010. *Pediatr Obes* 2013;8(4):307–324.
45. United States Department of Agriculture Agricultural Research Service. What we eat in America data Tables 2011–2012, Table 25: Snacks. 2015. Available at http://www.ars.usda.gov/Services/docs.htm?docid=18349. Accessed June 15, 2016.
46. Hauser SI, Economos CD, Nelson ME, Goldberg JP, Hyatt RR, Naumova EN, et al. Household and family factors related to weight status in first through third graders: A cross-sectional study in Eastern Massachusetts. *BMC Pediatr* 2014;14(1):167.
47. Grydeland M, Bergh IH, Bjelland M, Lien N, Andersen LF, Ommundsen Y, et al. Correlates of weight status among Norwegian 11-year-olds: The HEIA study. *BMC Public Health* 2012;12:1053.
48. Guo X, Zheng L, Li Y, Yu S, Sun G, Yang H, et al. Differences in lifestyle behaviors, dietary habits, and familial factors among normal-weight, overweight, and obese Chinese children and adolescents. *Int J Behav Nutr Phys Act* 2012;9(1):120.
49. Grigorakis DA, Georgoulis M, Psarra G, Tambalis KD, Panagiotakos DB, Sidossis LS. Prevalence and lifestyle determinants of central obesity in children. *Eur J Nutr* 2015:1–9.
50. Jelastopulu E, Kallianezos P, Merekoulias G, Alexopoulos EC, Sapountzi-Krepia D. Prevalence and risk factors of excess weight in school children in West Greece. *Nurs Health Sci* 2012;14(3):372–380.
51. Lee HH, Park HA, Kang JH, Cho YG, Park JK, Lee R, et al. Factors related to body mass index and body mass index change in Korean children: Preliminary results from the obesity and metabolic disorders cohort in childhood. *Korean J Fam Med* 2012;33(3):134–143.
52. Franchetti Y, Ide H. Socio-demographic and lifestyle factors for child's physical growth and adiposity rebound of Japanese children: A longitudinal study of the 21st century longitudinal survey in newborns. *BMC Public Health* 2014;14:334.
53. Bo S, De Carli L, Venco E, Fanzola I, Maiandi M, De Michieli F, et al. Impact of snacking pattern on overweight and obesity risk in a cohort of 11- to 13-year-old adolescents. *J Pediatr Gastroenterol Nutr* 2014;59(4):465–471.
54. Pala V, Lissner L, Hebestreit A, Lanfer A, Sieri S, Siani A, et al. Dietary patterns and longitudinal change in body mass in European children: A follow-up study on the IDEFICS multicenter cohort. *Eur J Clin Nutr* 2013;67(10):1042–1049.
55. Shroff MR, Perng W, Baylin A, Mora-Plazas M, Marin C, Villamor E. Adherence to a snacking dietary pattern and soda intake are related to the development of adiposity: A prospective study in school-age children. *Public Health Nutr* 2014;17(07):1507–1513.
56. Nicklas TA, O'Neil CE, Fulgoni VL. Relationship between snacking patterns, diet quality and risk of overweight and abdominal obesity in children. *Int J Child Health Nutr* 2013;2(3):189–200.
57. Dwyer T, Sallis JF, Blizzard L, Lazarus R, Dean K. Relation of academic performance to physical activity and fitness in children. *Pediatr Exer Sci* 2001;13(3):225–237.
58. Toschke AM, Küchenhoff H, Koletzko B, Kries R. Meal frequency and childhood obesity. *Obes Res* 2005;13(11):1932–1938.
59. Macdiarmid J, Loe J, Craig L, Masson L, Holmes B, McNeill G. Meal and snacking patterns of school-aged children in Scotland. *Eur J Clin Nutr* 2009;63(11):1297–1304.
60. Duffey KJ, Popkin BM. Causes of increased energy intake among children in the US, 1977–2010. *Am J Prev Med* 2013;44(2):e1–e8.

61. Fabry P, Hejda S, Cerny K, Osancova K, Pechar J. Effect of meal frequency in school-children: Changes in weight-height proportion and skinfold thickness. *Am J Clin Nutr* 1966;18(5):358–361.

62. Kaisari P, Yannakoulia M, Panagiotakos DB. Eating frequency and overweight and obesity in children and adolescents: A meta-analysis. *Pediatrics* 2013;131(5):958–967.

63. Thompson O, Ballew C, Resnicow K, Gillespie C, Must A, Bandini L, et al. Dietary pattern as a predictor of change in BMI z-score among girls. *Int J Obes* 2006;30(1):176–182.

64. Ritchie LD. Less frequent eating predicts greater BMI and waist circumference in female adolescents. *Am J Clin Nutr* 2012;95(2):290–296.

65. Evans E, Jacques P, Dallal G, Sacheck J, Must A. The role of eating frequency on relative weight in urban school-age children. *Pediatr Obes* 2015;10(6):442–447.

66. Stea TH, Vik FN, Bere E, Svendsen MV, Oellingrath IM. Meal pattern among Norwegian primary-school children and longitudinal associations between meal skipping and weight status. *Pub Health Nutr* 2015;18(2):286–291.

67. Murakami K, Livingstone MBE. Associations of eating frequency with adiposity measures, blood lipid profiles and blood pressure in British children and adolescents. *Br J Nutr* 2014;111(12):2176–2183.

68. Jaaskelainen P, Magnussen CG, Pahkala K, Mikkila V, Kahonen M, Sabin MA, et al. Childhood nutrition in predicting metabolic syndrome in adults: The cardiovascular risk in Young Finns Study. *Diabetes Care* 2012;35(9):1937–1943.

69. Jääskeläinen A, Schwab U, Kolehmainen M, Pirkola J, Järvelin M, Laitinen J. Associations of meal frequency and breakfast with obesity and metabolic syndrome traits in adolescents of Northern Finland Birth Cohort 1986. *Nutr Metab Cardiovasc Dis* 2013;23(10):1002–1009.

70. O'Neil CE, Byrd-Bredbenner C, Hayes D, Jana L, Klinger SE, Stephenson-Martin S. The role of breakfast in health: Definition and criteria for a quality breakfast. *J Acad Nutr Diet* 2014;12(114):S8–S26.

71. Amigo-Vázquez I, Busto-Zapico R, Errasti-Pérez JM, Peña-Suárez E. Skipping breakfast, sedentarism and overweight in children. *Psychol Health Med* 2016:1–8.

7 Portion Sizes in Childhood Obesity

Kathleen L. Keller, Tanja V. Kral, and Jennifer O. Fisher

CONTENTS

INTRODUCTION

Large portion sizes of palatable, energy-dense foods were first suggested to be a part of the obesogenic food environment almost two decades ago [1]. Today's children and adults have ubiquitous exposure to large food and beverage portion sizes in the marketplace, from large single-serving containers and family-value multiple-serving containers found in grocery and convenience stores to food and beverage offerings at fast-food and full-service restaurants [2,3]. The appeal of large food portions to consumers, including families with young children, is enhanced by aggressive marketing efforts for foods high in sugar and fat, as well as by pricing incentives for the purchase of larger portion sizes (i.e., value pricing) [4].

Population-based intake data show increases in portion sizes consumed by US children and adults over the past 40 years [5,6]. Increases in the average portion size consumed have been seen across many different types of categories of foods, with the largest increases seen for pizza, burgers, Mexican food, soft drinks, and salty snacks. Secular trends toward larger portion sizes have not only been seen for foods consumed at restaurants where portions tend to be largest, but also at home. Increases in portion size have also been seen for snacks high in solid fats and added sugars, which are frequently consumed by children [7]. Trends toward large portion sizes in combination with more frequent eating have produced increases in energy intake in the US population over the period when obesity began to emerge as a threat to public health in the United States and worldwide [8]. These and other epidemiological data fueled concerns that large portion sizes have played a causal role in the childhood obesity epidemic [9]. While providing population-representative "signals," it is important to note that epidemiological studies do not provide causal evidence of portion-size effects on excessive energy intake.

EFFECTS OF PORTION SIZE ON CHILDREN'S FOOD AND ENERGY INTAKE

Much of the research on food portion size in children has focused on preschoolers (age 3–5 years), but has also included children ranging in age from 2 to 9 years. Controlled experiments conducted in laboratory settings have demonstrated that increasing the portion size of palatable energy dense entrées increased children's intake of those foods by 25%–60% [10]. Increases were observed, despite the fact that children, on average, consumed only two-thirds of the larger portions and reported awareness of the changes in entrée portion size. Further, increased entrée intakes were not accompanied by appreciable decreases in children's intake of other foods served at the meal. Consequently, offering larger entrée portions produced increases in total meal-energy intake ranging from 13% to 39% [10]. Studies of portion size conducted outside the laboratory have observed similar effects on intake, although not of the same magnitude [11]. Not all studies, however, have observed portion-size effects and the reasons for these inconsistencies remain unclear [12,13]. In general, however, experimental evidence of portion-size effects in children is consistent with that observed in adults [14].

When faced with larger portion sizes, children tend to increase the average size of each bite taken without appreciable changes to the number of bites taken [15,16]. An increase in the size of bites taken as an effect of larger portions has also been reported in adults [17–19]. In addition, a similar pattern was observed when children aged 4–6 years were allowed to serve themselves a main dish that varied in portion size [20]. Children served themselves larger spoonfuls when there was a greater amount of the main dish available in the serving dish. Collectively, these studies suggest that visual cues conveying information about size and food availability influence subsequent serving and eating behaviors. However, whether there are particular visual parameters (e.g., width of portion) to which children attend that explain these changes in behavior remains unclear [21].

In addition to amorphous foods (e.g., those that can be piled), effects have been demonstrated for unit foods (e.g., those with a distinct shape such as sandwiches and chicken nuggets), possibly due to "unit bias," as described by Geirer and Rozin [22], where consumption occurs in units and therefore is driven by unit size. Intake-promoting effects of large portions have also been seen with packaged snack foods and beverages. Finally, while most of the research demonstrating intake-promoting effects has involved energy-dense foods, several studies of young children suggest that the effects of portion size are separate to those of food-energy density [13,23], where the combination of the two has an additive effect on energy consumed at snacks [23] and meals [24]. For example, decreasing the energy density of a lunch entrée by 25% significantly reduced energy intake of the entrée by 25% in 3- to 5-year-old children. However, decreasing the portion size of the entrée by 25% did not significantly affect children's energy intake at lunch [13]. Another experiment [24] showed that when serving 5- to 6-year-old children different portions of an entrée that also differed in energy density (1.3 vs. 1.8 kcal/g), the effect of portion size and energy density were independent but additive.

Given the evidence of intake-promoting effects of portion size, some have investigated whether portion size can be used strategically to increase the intake of healthful foods, such as fruits and vegetables [25]. A number of studies have examined portion size influences on fruit and vegetable intake before and at meals [26–29]. In general, these studies have found that increasing entrée size increases entrée intake and decreases side dish intake (i.e., fruit and vegetable intake) [29]. Alternatively, doubling the portion size of fruit or vegetable side dishes offered to children at meals has produced modest increases in the consumption of those foods, especially fruit, without appreciable changes to energy intake, increasing the relative proportion of meal energy consumed from those healthful foods [26,27]. It is important to point out, however, that the increases observed in those studies were small in absolute terms and food waste was considerable. For instance, a within-subject experimental study of 30 children aged 4–6 years demonstrated increases of 70% and 34% in fruit and vegetable intakes, respectively, at a meal when 75 g portion sizes of each food were doubled to 150 g. In absolute terms, however, offering twice as much only increased intake by ~1/4 c for fruit (41 g increase) and even less for vegetables (12 g increase). These observations underscore the point that increasing portion size may not be an effective stand-alone strategy for promoting vegetable intake in particular, but may compliment other strategies to promote food acceptance in early development, such as repeated exposure and modeling [30,31].

Most experimental studies of food portion size have focused on short-term energy intake at a meal. While the effects on long-term intake among children are not well characterized, the findings of several studies suggest that children do not fully compensate for the intake-promoting effects of larger portions at subsequent eating occasions. One study of 59 low-income Hispanic and African

American 5-year-olds doubled the portion size of three main entreés and an afternoon snack served across a 24 h period [32]. Daily energy intake was 140 kcal greater or 12% higher in the large portion condition than the reference condition. These findings are consistent with several adult studies that demonstrated increases in energy intake over periods ranging from 2 [33] to 11 days [34] when portion sizes of all foods offered were increased.

Taken as a whole, research to date suggests that large portion sizes have intake-promoting effects on children's eating that may promote excessive energy intake. The extent to which large portion sizes are truly obesogenic for children, however, remains unclear. Experimental studies on portion size have failed to observe an association between children's susceptibility to portion size and weight status [15,16,32,35,36]. Long-term experimental studies of food portion size effects on weight outcomes in children are not possible for ethnical reasons. A few cross-sectional observational studies have documented associations between portion size and child weight status [37–39]. For instance, a study of 784 French children aged 3–11 years found that portion size of pastries consumed was positively related to overweight in 3- to 6-year-old children, while portion size of liquid dairy products was negatively associated with overweight in 7 to 11-year-old children [38]. Observational findings, however, are difficult to interpret because of the inherent confound that heavier children may require larger portions due to greater energy needs. Longitudinal research is needed to understand the relationship between portion size and growth over time taking into account children's initial weight and energy requirements.

DEVELOPMENTAL AND INDIVIDUAL DIFFERENCES IN HOW MUCH IS ENOUGH

The first study of food portion size in young children suggested developmental shifts in children's responsiveness to portion size such that intakes among older children were affected by portion size but those of younger children were not [40]. Those findings are consistent with the notion that children become more susceptible to food cues in the environment and less responsive to internal hunger and fullness cues with age. Indeed, caloric compensation (i.e., adjustments in intake in response to changes in the caloric content of a preload) at meals has been shown to decrease [41] and eating in the absence of hunger (i.e., children's susceptibility to eating when satiated in response to the presence of palatable snack foods) has been shown to increase with age during middle childhood [42]. However, subsequent research demonstrated portion-size effects on meal energy among children as young as 2 years of age [15]. These contradictory findings raise questions about the extent to which children's responses to food portion size are governed by biological versus situational and learned components acquired through experience. It is interesting to note that children's perceptions of the amount of fullness produced by a given food are shaped by familiarity with the foods [43]. The extent to which children's familiarity with foods influences their expectations of fullness and behavior at meals remains unknown. Research is needed to understand how experience influences what children "learn" about the satiating value of foods and food portion sizes.

Dimensions of appetite regulation show significant heritability, including eating rate, eating in the absence of hunger, and satiety responsiveness [44]. There is some suggestion that these heritable traits influence children's susceptibility to overconsume large portion sizes. In one study, 34 obese and 66 normal-weight African American children were seen in four experimental conditions where all foods at the meal were increased by 150%, 200%, and 250% over a reference condition [35]. Children with lower levels of satiety responsiveness showed greater increases in intake with exposure to large portion sizes. This is similar to one of the first portion-size studies that showed that children who exhibited greater levels of eating in the absence of hunger also showed the largest increases in intake when the portion size of an entrée served at a lunch meal was doubled [16]. It is possible that the relationship between portion size and subsequent eating behaviors may partially be mediated by the brain's response to visual portion size cues. Recent work suggests that brain responses to large portions of food, particularly in regions involved in inhibitory control (e.g., the inferior frontal gyrus) and reward processing (e.g., the ventral tegmental area), may influence the relationship between portion size and subsequent eating behaviors. English and colleagues found that 7- to 10-year-old children who were rated as faster eaters showed greater activation in brain reward centers to large portions of food, while children who had lower activation in inhibitory control regions in response to large portions tended to be rated as more emotional and fussy eaters [45]. Additional neuroimaging studies might help to elucidate the mechanisms of portion size on children's eating behaviors.

ROLE OF PORTION SIZE IN OBESITY PREVENTION AND TREATMENT

Experimental studies of food portion size in children have produced fairly consistent evidence of causal effects on short-term intake. The controlled nature of these studies, however, precludes generalizability to more naturalistic settings in which young children typically eat, such as at home, childcare, school, and restaurants. These settings likely differ in numerous ways that may influence children's response to food portion size, including children's familiarity with foods and portions offered as well as social influences on eating. For example, it is well known that social models (e.g., peers, teachers) can influence children's acceptance of novel and disliked foods [31]. Similarly, social models can facilitate intake in a manner that increases portion sizes and energy consumed [46]. In addition to modeling influences, there is increasing evidence that parents shape portion sizes selected and consumed by young children through their feeding styles and practices. For instance, children of indulgent feeders (i.e., those who show warmth and acceptance in conjunction with a lack of monitoring of child's behaviors) have been observed to serve and consume larger portions of energy-dense entrées [47]. In addition, an observational study of 154 low-income Hispanic and African American caregivers observed that parents who served themselves larger portions, served their preschool-age children larger portions which, in turn, was closely aligned with the amount that children consumed [48]. Qualitative data reveal that maternal decisions about portion sizes of meals and snacks offered to children are influenced by a variety of factors including the child's general appetite (e.g., picky eating), preferences, hunger at the time of eating, as well as the perceived healthfulness of the foods and the nutrient needs of the child [49,50].

The most effective method of conveying information to caregivers regarding appropriate portion sizes is unclear, because children and caregivers often inaccurately estimate food portions [51,52]. This is true for the numeric information about portion size on food labels as well as for estimating the portion sizes of foods served and consumed [53–55]. For example, in a study of 120, 8- to 13-year-olds, 39.7% of respondents incorrectly classified the portion size of food images presented on a computer [56]. Complicating poor estimation is the belief held by many adults that the amount they consume represents an average or "medium" portion size [57]. While numeric presentations of portion size (e.g., household measures) are not easily understood, the effectiveness of alternative strategies is unclear. For instance, household items are often used to convey information about portion size in clinical settings (e.g., a deck of cards to approximate 3 oz. of meat). While such aids may improve portion size estimation [58], the effectiveness of these types of aids for communicating information about appropriate portion sizes to caregivers is not known. It is clear that caregivers use a variety of strategies to determine portion sizes offered to young children. In a qualitative study of child snacking, for instance, low-income mothers of preschool-age children portioned snacks by using small containers, subdividing large portions, buying prepackaged snacks, and using hand measurement estimations, measuring cups, and scales [49]. However, the effectiveness of such strategies to convey information about portion size and support healthful portion sizes for young children is unclear.

A number of studies suggest that manipulating subtle size-related cues of the immediate eating environment may shape portion sizes offered to and selected by young children. It has been known for some time that package size influences the amount of food that adults serve themselves from containers holding multiple servings [59]. Similarly, the portion sizes of individually packaged servings also appear to influence the amount consumed by adults [60,61]. Reducing the unit size of foods (e.g., smaller cookies) has also been shown to reduce portion sizes consumed by children [62]. More recent studies, including studies of children, indicate that other size-related cues in the eating environment may influence portion sizes selected and consumed. For instance, the use of smaller plates, particularly those with wide and color-contrasted borders, may support smaller portion sizes by encouraging smaller servings [63]. A study of 42 predominantly African American elementary school–age children evaluated children's self-served portion sizes and intake of an entrée and side dishes in a school setting using either child- or adult-size dishware, which represented a 100% increase in the surface area of plates and volume of bowls across conditions [64]. Children were served more energy when using adult-size dishware. Adult-size dishware promoted energy intake indirectly, where every additional calorie served resulted in a 0.43 kcal increase in total energy intakes at lunch. Similarly, using smaller serving utensils may result in smaller portions served without undue burden on caregivers. A small pilot intervention found that the use of smaller plates, along with education about appropriate portion sizes, reduced portions served by caregivers of young children [65]. Another suggested approach to promote appropriate portion sizes during the preschool years is the rule of thumb to offer one tablespoon of food for every year of life. A nutrient content analysis of recommendations for tablespoon per year of age found this strategy met intakes of most vitamins and minerals though it appeared to underestimate the estimated energy needs for children aged 2–5 years [66].

CONCLUSIONS AND PRIORITIES FOR RESEARCH

Young children's appetites are thought to be strongly driven by internal cues of hunger and fullness (as reviewed in other chapters in this book). At the same time, numerous lines of evidence highlight environmental influences on children's eating. Evidence to date suggests that young children's intake at meals and snacks, particularly of highly palatable, energy-dense foods, closely approximates the portion sizes routinely offered to them. Indeed, a recent Cochrane review of 72 studies, published between 1978 and July 2013, concluded that people consume more food when larger portion sizes, package sizes, and tableware are used [14]. While highly controlled studies have characterized an intake-promoting role of large portions on children's eating, links to weight status remain weak. Longitudinal data are needed to understand the role of portion size in appetite regulation beyond a single day as well as its role in trajectories for growth. An important research need is to understand how to encourage healthy, age-appropriate portion sizes in children. It is unclear whether helping children focus on internal satiety cues is sufficient or effective given the ubiquitous food cues in the modern environment. Recent research on the formation of child feeding habits suggests research opportunities to help caregivers offer smaller portion sizes and engage in healthy portion-size behaviors, such as the use of small plates [67,68]. Another important line of inquiry for research is to identify optimal snack portion sizes. Secular data point to increases in the frequency of eating among both children and adults. There are currently few data to understand the optimal portion size and energy content of snacks relative to meals for young children. Conveying recommendations to the public and to parents of young children regarding appropriate portion sizes is yet another area for research. In particular, research is needed to identify easy to understand and actionable guidance for caregivers of young children.

REFERENCES

1. Hill JO, Peters JC. Environmental contributions to the obesity epidemic. *Science*. 1998;280(5368):1371–4.
2. Young LR, Nestle M. The contribution of expanding portion sizes to the US obesity epidemic. *Am J Public Health*. 2002;92(2):246–9.
3. Young LR, Nestle M. Portion sizes and obesity: Responses of fast-food companies. *J Public Health Policy*. 2007;28(2):238–48.

4. Vinci DM, Philipp SF. Perceived value in food selection when dining out: Comparison of African Americans and Euro-Americans. *Percept Mot Skills*. 2007;104(3 Pt 2):1088–96.
5. Piernas C, Popkin BM. Food portion patterns and trends among U.S. children and the relationship to total eating occasion size, 1977–2006. *J Nutr*. 2011;141(6):1159–64.
6. Nielsen SJ, Popkin BM. Patterns and trends in food portion sizes, 1977–1998. *JAMA*. 2003;289(4):450–3.
7. Piernas C, Popkin BM. Trends in snacking among U.S. children. *Health Aff (Millwood)*. 2010;29(3):398–404.
8. Piernas C, Popkin BM. Snacking increased among U.S. adults between 1977 and 2006. *J Nutr*. 2010;140(2):325–32.
9. Sahoo K, Sahoo B, Choudhury AK, Sofi NY, Kumar R, Bhadoria AS. Childhood obesity: Causes and consequences. *J Family Med Prim Care*. 2015;4(2):187–92.
10. Fisher JO, Kral TV. Super-size me: Portion size effects on young children's eating. *Physiol Behav*. 2008;94(1):39–47.
11. Ramsay S, Safaii S, Croschere T, Branen LJ, Wiest M. Kindergarteners' entrée intake increases when served a larger entrée portion in school lunch: A quasi-experiment. *J Sch Health*. 2013;83(4):239–42.
12. Johnson SL, Ross ES, Grunwald G, Burger K, Fisher JO. Increasing entrée portion size does not always increase children's energy intake at a meal. *FASEB J*. 2008:A459.1.
13. Leahy KE, Birch LL, Fisher JO, Rolls BJ. Reductions in entrée energy density increase children's vegetable intake and reduce energy intake. *Obesity (Silver Spring)*. 2008;16(7):1559–65.
14. Hollands GJ, Shemilt I, Marteau TM, Jebb SA, Lewis HB, Wei Y, et al. Portion, package or tableware size for changing selection and consumption of food, alcohol and tobacco. *Cochrane Database Syst Rev*. 2015;9:CD011045.
15. Fisher JO. Effects of age on children's intake of large and self-selected food portions. *Obesity (Silver Spring)*. 2007;15(2):403–12.
16. Orlet Fisher J, Rolls BJ, Birch LL. Children's bite size and intake of an entrée are greater with large portions than with age-appropriate or self-selected portions. *Am J Clin Nutr*. 2003;77(5):1164–70.
17. Burger KS, Fisher JO, Johnson SL. Mechanisms behind the portion size effect: Visibility and bite size. *Obesity (Silver Spring)*. 2011;19(3):546–51.
18. Spiegel TA, Kaplan JM, Tomassini A, Stellar E. Bite size, ingestion rate, and meal size in lean and obese women. *Appetite*. 1993;21(2):131–45.
19. Almiron-Roig E, Tsiountsioura M, Lewis HB, Wu J, Solis-Trapala I, Jebb SA. Large portion sizes increase bite size and eating rate in overweight women. *Physiol Behav*. 2015;139:297–302.
20. Fisher JO, Birch LL, Zhang J, Grusak MA, Hughes SO. External influences on children's self-served portions at meals. *Int J Obes* (Lond). 2013;37(7):954–60.
21. English L, Lasschuijt M, Keller KL. Mechanisms of the portion size effect: What is known and where do we go from here? *Appetite*. 2015;88:39–49.
22. Geier AB, Rozin P, Doros G. Unit bias: A new heuristic that helps explain the effect of portion size on food intake. *Psychol Sci*. 2006;17(6):521–5.
23. Looney SM, Raynor HA. Impact of portion size and energy density on snack intake in preschool-aged children. *J Am Diet Assoc*. 2011;111(3):414–8.
24. Fisher JO, Liu Y, Birch LL, Rolls BJ. Effects of portion size and energy density on young children's intake at a meal. *Am J Clin Nutr*. 2007;86(1):174–9.
25. Kim SA, Moore LV, Galuska D, Wright AP, Harris D, Grummer-Strawn LM, et al. Vital signs: Fruit and vegetable intake among children—United States, 2003–2010. *MMWR Morb Mortal Wkly Rep*. 2014;63(31):671–6.
26. Kral TV, Kabay AC, Roe LS, Rolls BJ. Effects of doubling the portion size of fruit and vegetable side dishes on children's intake at a meal. *Obesity (Silver Spring)*. 2010;18(3):521–7.
27. Mathias KC, Rolls BJ, Birch LL, Kral TV, Hanna EL, Davey A, et al. Serving larger portions of fruits and vegetables together at dinner promotes intake of both foods among young children. *J Acad Nutr Diet*. 2012;112(2):266–70.
28. Spill MK, Birch LL, Roe LS, Rolls BJ. Eating vegetables first: The use of portion size to increase vegetable intake in preschool children. *Am J Clin Nutr*. 2010;91(5):1237–43.
29. Savage JS, Fisher JO, Marini M, Birch LL. Serving smaller age-appropriate entrée portions to children aged 3–5 y increases fruit and vegetable intake and reduces energy density and energy intake at lunch. *Am J Clin Nutr*. 2012;95(2):335–41.
30. Birch LL, Doub AE. Learning to eat: Birth to age 2 y. *Am J Clin Nutr*. 2014;99(3):723S–8S.
31. Blissett J, Fogel A. Intrinsic and extrinsic influences on children's acceptance of new foods. *Physiol Behav*. 2013;121:89–95.

32. Fisher JO, Arreola A, Birch LL, Rolls BJ. Portion size effects on daily energy intake in low-income Hispanic and African American children and their mothers. *Am J Clin Nutr.* 2007;86(6):1709–16.

33. Rolls BJ, Roe L, Meengs JS. Larger portion sizes lead to a sustained increase in energy intake over 2 days. *J Am Diet Assoc.* 2006;106(4):543–9.

34. Rolls BJ, Roe LS, Meengs JS. The effect of large portion sizes on energy intake is sustained for 11 days. *Obesity (Silver Spring).* 2007;15(6):1535–43.

35. Mooreville M, Davey A, Orloski A, Hannah EL, Mathias KC, Birch LL, et al. Individual differences in susceptibility to large portion sizes among obese and normal-weight children. *Obesity (Silver Spring).* 2015;23(4):808–14.

36. Kral TV, Remiker AM, Strutz EM, Moore RH. Role of child weight status and the relative reinforcing value of food in children's response to portion size increases. *Obesity (Silver Spring).* 2014;22(7):1716–22.

37. Huang TTK, Howarth NYC, Lin BH, Roberts SB, McCrory MA. Energy intake and meal portions: Associations with BMI percentile in US children. *Obes Res.* 2004;12(11):1875–85.

38. Lioret S, Volatier JL, Lafay L, Touvier M, Maire B. Is food portion size a risk factor of childhood over-weight? *Eur J Clin Nutr.* 2009;63(3):382–91.

39. McConahy KL, Smiciklas-Wright H, Birch LL, Mitchell DC, Picciano MF. Food portions are positively related to energy intake and body weight in early childhood. *J Pediatr.* 2002;140(3):340–7.

40. Rolls BJ, Engell D, Birch LL. Serving portion size influences 5-year-old but not 3-year-old children's food intakes. *J Am Diet Assoc.* 2000;100(2):232–4.

41. Johnson SL, Taylor-Holloway LA. Non-Hispanic white and Hispanic elementary school children's self-regulation of energy intake. *Am J Clin Nutr.* 2006;83(6):1276–82.

42. Fisher JO, Cai G, Jaramillo SJ, Cole SA, Comuzzie AG, Butte NF. Heritability of hyperphagic eating behavior and appetite-related hormones among Hispanic children. *Obesity (Silver Spring).* 2007;15(6):1484–95.

43. Hardman CA, McCrickerd K, Brunstrom JM. Children's familiarity with snack foods changes expectations about fullness. *Am J Clin Nutr.* 2011;94(5):1196–201.

44. Faith MS, Carnell S, Kral TV. Genetics of food intake self-regulation in childhood: Literature review and research opportunities. *Hum Hered.* 2013;75(2–4):80–9.

45. English LK, Lasschuijt, M., Wilson, S., Fisher, J.O., Savage, J., Rolls, B.J., Keller, K.L. Appetitive traits are associated with the neural response to food portion size in children. Paper presented at Obesity Week, Los Angeles, CA, 2015.

46. Salvy SJ, Howard M, Read M, Mele E. The presence of friends increases food intake in youth. *Am J Clin Nutr.* 2009;90(2):282–7.

47. Fisher JO, Birch LL, Grusak MA, Hughes SO. How much is enough: Effects of portion and serving spoon size on the amount of children's self-served entrée portion and intake. *Obesity.* 2008;15:A203.

48. Johnson SL, Hughes SO, Cui X, Li X, Allison DB, Liu Y, et al. Portion sizes for children are predicted by parental characteristics and the amounts parents serve themselves. *Am J Clin Nutr.* 2014;99(4):763–70.

49. Blake CE, Fisher JO, Ganter C, Younginer N, Orloski A, Blaine RE, et al. A qualitative study of parents' perceptions and use of portion size strategies for preschool children's snacks. *Appetite.* 2015;88:17–23.

50. Johnson SL, Goodell LS, Williams K, Power TG, Hughes SO. Getting my child to eat the right amount: Mothers' considerations when deciding how much food to offer their child at a meal. *Appetite.* 2015;88:24–32.

51. Foster E, Matthews JN, Lloyd J, Marshall L, Mathers JC, Nelson M, et al. Children's estimates of food portion size: The development and evaluation of three portion size assessment tools for use with children. *Br J Nutr.* 2008;99(1):175–84.

52. Wrieden WL, Longbottom PJ, Adamson AJ, Ogston SA, Payne A, Haleem MA, et al. Estimation of typical food portion sizes for children of different ages in Great Britain. *Br J Nutr.* 2008;99(6):1344–53.

53. Huizinga MM, Carlisle AJ, Cavanaugh KL, Davis DL, Gregory RP, Schlundt DG, et al. Literacy, numeracy, and portion-size estimation skills. *Am J Prev Med.* 2009,36(4):324–8.

54. Rothman RL, Housam R, Weiss H, Davis D, Gregory R, Gebretsadik T, et al. Patient understanding of food labels: The role of literacy and numeracy. *Am J Prev Med.* 2006;31(5):391–8.

55. Vanderlee L, Goodman S, Sae Yang W, Hammond D. Consumer understanding of calorie amounts and serving size: Implications for nutritional labelling. *Can J Public Health.* 2012;103(5):e327–31.

56. Baranowski T, Baranowski JC, Watson KB, Martin S, Beltran A, Islam N, et al. Children's accuracy of portion size estimation using digital food images: Effects of interface design and size of image on computer screen. *Public Health Nutr.* 2011;14(3):418–25.

57. Young LR, Nestle M. Variation in perceptions of a medium food portion: Implications for dietary guidance. *J Am Diet Assoc.* 1998;98(4):458–9.

58. Byrd-Bredbenner C, Schwartz J. The effect of practical portion size measurement aids on the accuracy of portion size estimates made by young adults. *J Hum Nutr Diet*. 2004;17(4):351–7.
59. Wansink B. Can package size accelerate usage volume? *J Market*. 1996;60:1–14.
60. Raynor HA, Van Walleghen EL, Niemeier H, Butryn ML, Wing RR. Do food provisions packaged in single-servings reduce energy intake at breakfast during a brief behavioral weight-loss intervention? *J Am Diet Assoc*. 2009;109(11):1922–5.
61. Stroebele N, Ogden LG, Hill JO. Do calorie-controlled portion sizes of snacks reduce energy intake? *Appetite*. 2009;52(3):793–6.
62. Marchiori D, Waroquier L, Klein O. "Split them!" smaller item sizes of cookies lead to a decrease in energy intake in children. *J Nutr Educ Behav*. 2012;44(3):251–5.
63. McClain AD, van den Bos W, Matheson D, Desai M, McClure SM, Robinson TN. Visual illusions and plate design: The effects of plate rim widths and rim coloring on perceived food portion size. *Int J Obes* (Lond). 2014;38(5):657–62.
64. DiSantis KI, Birch LL, Davey A, Serrano EL, Zhang J, Bruton Y, et al. Plate size and children's appetite: Effects of larger dishware on self-served portions and intake. *Pediatrics*. 2013;131(5):e1451–8.
65. Small L, Bonds-McClain D, Vaughan L, Melnyk B, Gannon A, Thompson S. A parent-directed portion education intervention for young children: Be Beary Healthy. *J Spec Pediatr Nurs*. 2012;17(4):312–20.
66. Ramsay SA, Branen LJ, Johnson SL. How much is enough? Tablespoon per year of age approach meets nutrient needs for children. *Appetite*. 2012;58(1):163–7.
67. Gardner B. A review and analysis of the use of "habit" in understanding, predicting and influencing health-related behaviour. *Health Psychol Rev*. 2015;9(3):277–95.
68. Gardner B, Sheals K, Wardle J, McGowan L. Putting habit into practice, and practice into habit: A process evaluation and exploration of the acceptability of a habit-based dietary behaviour change intervention. *Int J Behav Nutr Phys Act*. 2014;11:135.

8 Role of Satiety Responsiveness in Childhood Obesity

Myles S. Faith and Adam C. Danley

CONTENTS

INTRODUCTION

This chapter summarizes the literature on *satiety responsiveness* (SR) and its relation to childhood obesity. SR is a form of self-regulation specific to the domain of food intake [1]. Emerging evidence indicates that this is a behavioral mechanism through which young children overconsume calories and gain excess body weight. As described in the fourth section, studies from around the world find that poorer SR is correlated with a risk factor for childhood obesity. Despite this evidence, there has been limited clinical research focused on SR as an intervention target.

This chapter is organized into six sections. In the first two sections, we define SR as a construct and discuss how it is operationalized in studies with children. The third section addresses the extent to which SR is a familial trait and the extent to which genes and home environmental factors contribute to individual differences in this trait. The fourth section reviews evidence for an association between SR and excess child body weight. Cross-sectional and prospective studies from different countries are described. In the fifth section, SR as a potential intervention focus is discussed. It is argued that, to date, a "first generation" of studies has been conducted that includes (1) satiety training laboratory experiments and (2) preliminary intervention studies. These have set the stage for what is needed now: a second generation of treatment and prevention studies guided by basic behavioral science and targeting more diverse populations. The chapter concludes with ideas for future research.

DEFINING SR AS A CONSTRUCT

SR refers to a child's ability to recognize and adjust eating in response to internal feelings of fullness [2,3]. In colloquial parlance, some children are better "in touch" with feelings of fullness and are more capable of self-regulating their eating in response to what was recently consumed. Children who are better at SR eat proportionally less following a filling meal while those poorer in the trait will continue to eat without compensating for prior food intake. For example, if a child "overconsumed" at a midmorning snack (perhaps eating an extra 150 kcal from graham crackers), then the perfectly compensating child would make up for it by eating 150 kcal less at lunch. Such a child has strong SR. Peers with poorer SR would not compensate as well and would overeat (relative to their energy needs) at lunch. And because obesity in early childhood can result from small but sustained energy imbalances (perhaps as little as ~50 kcal/day [4]), poorer SR should promote excess weight gain over time. In fact, as discussed later, data from many studies support this prediction. Thus, SR as a construct can be considered a form of self-regulation specific to the domain of food intake. It is highly relevant to children's everyday living and food choices.

OPERATIONALLY DEFINING SR IN SCIENTIFIC RESEARCH

Most research has assessed SR using the parent-report Child Eating Behaviour Questionnaire (CEBQ) [5]. The instrument has a five-item SR subscale, with higher scores reflecting greater SR (Table 8.1). The CEBQ was developed in the United Kingdom by Wardle and colleagues, using a population-based sample of young twins [5]. The instrument has been used in population-based, community, clinical, and convenience samples across the world [6–10]. Hence, this tool has had a major impact. It also has strong psychometric properties, including reliability and validity [5,11]. As discussed in the next section, a comparable tool for infants has been developed and validated—the Baby Eating Behaviour Questionnaire [12].

SR can also be assessed by a laboratory-preloading paradigm that tests *energy (caloric) compensation*. Specifically, this protocol assesses children's ability to adjust *ad libitum* meal intake following low- versus high-calorie preload snacks (i.e., fixed amounts of a food/drink). The protocol is grounded in the premise that children should eat proportionally less food at an *ad libitum* meal ~20 min following the higher- compared with the lower-energy preload. This adjustment reflects "compensation." A particular formula has been used to define compensation ability, that is, the percentage compensation index (COMPX%) [13–15]:

$$COMPX(\%) = \frac{Meal_{low} - Meal_{high}}{Preload_{high} - Preload_{low}}(100) \tag{8.1}$$

where:
$Meal_{low}$ = energy intake from the lunch meal following the low-energy preload
$Meal_{high}$ = energy intake from the lunch meal following the high-energy preload
$Preload_{high}$ = energy consumed from the high-energy preload intake
$Preload_{low}$ = energy consumed from the low-energy preload intake

The COMPX% index is a continuous measure. It is scaled such that 100% reflects "perfect" compensation, with progressively lower scores reflecting the tendency to *overeat* following the high-energy preload relative to the low-energy preload (*undercompensation*). Progressively higher scores

---

TABLE 8.1
The SR Subscale of the Child Eating Behavior Questionnaire

1. My child has a big appetite*
2. My child leaves food on his/her plate at the end of a meal
3. My child gets full before his/her meal is finished
4. My child gets full up easily
5. My child cannot eat a meal if s/he has had a snack just before

Response options: never = 0, rarely = 1, sometimes = 2, often = 3, always = 4.
* Reverse scored.

---

reflect the tendency to *undereat* following the high-energy relative to the low-energy preload (*over-compensation*). Hence, lower scores should put children at greater risk for obesity or excess weight gain. An illustration of the formula can be found in the Appendix to this chapter.

In sum, there are two established research methods to assess SR: a brief parent-report questionnaire or a laboratory-preloading paradigm. The latter is considered by some to be a gold-standard assessment, because it is a direct behavioral measurement obtained under controlled laboratory conditions. On the other hand, this very strength is perhaps its greatest limitation. Specifically, it is an intensive protocol that requires much preparation, research staff, and food preparations, and also might not be feasible in younger subjects (e.g., less than 4 years of age). Compared with the parent-report CEBQ, it cannot be implemented on a much broader scale such as population-based research. Even for a smaller-scale clinical intervention that might need to prescreen for youth poorer in SR, the questionnaire may be more feasible. That said, these are two strong measures of the SR construct.

ASSOCIATION BETWEEN SR AND CHILD ADIPOSITY

Studies from many nations have shown that poorer SR, as measured by the parent-report CEBQ, is associated with increased child body mass index (BMI) or obesity status. In one of the first studies conducted, Carnell and Wardle [16] examined a population-based twin study of >10,000 children aged 8–11 years residing in the United Kingdom, as well as a separate community-based sample of 3–5-year-old children ($n = 572$). Poorer SR was associated with greater BMI z-score in both the younger ($r = -0.22$, $p < .001$) and the older samples ($r = -0.19$, $p < .001$). In a population-based study of >4000 children aged 4 years old participating in the "Generation R" study (Rotterdam, the Netherlands), poorer parent-report SR was associated with a higher child BMI z-score ($r = -.236$, $p < .001$) [17]. In logistic regression models, children who scored high on SR were significantly less likely to be overweight (OR = 0.63) or obese (OR = 0.43). Sleddens et al. [18] examined 135 Dutch children, who were 6 and 7 years of age, from seven primary schools in the Netherlands. Using a translated version of the CEBQ, they found that poorer parent-reported SR was correlated cross-sectionally with higher child BMI z-score (standardized $\beta = 0.24$, $p = .006$). Similar findings have been reported using pediatric samples from Canada, Portugal, and Brazil, among other nations [10,15–17,19–21].

SR also has been linked to greater food intake at meals. Specifically, poorer SR at age 2 years predicted greater total energy intake from a standardized lunch meal provided at children's homes at age 4 years ($r = .43$, $p = .011$) [22]. Lower SR also predicted prospectively greater child BMI z-score ($r = -.42$, $p = .012$).

Interestingly, the link between poorer SR and child overweight appears to emerge in infancy. Recent studies from the United Kingdom have examined infants' SR using the Baby Eating Behaviour Questionnaire [12] (Table 8.2), a three-item parent-report questionnaire that evaluates infants' propensity to eat in response to fullness. In fact, poorer infant SR at 3 months of age has been associated with significantly greater increases in body weight in the period from 3 to 15 months in a sample of ~1500 infant twins [23]. Interestingly, greater infant standardized weight at 3 months of age was associated with poorer SR at age 15 months as well. These findings support a

---

TABLE 8.2

The SR Subscale of the Baby Eating Behavior Questionnaire

1. My baby found it difficult to manage a complete feed.
2. My baby got full before taking all the milk I thought she or he should have.
3. My baby got full up easily.

Response options: never = 0, rarely = 1, sometimes = 2, often = 3, always = 4

bidirectional association between SR and overweight. These are compelling data in need of replication; they suggest that the association between SR and obesity risk emerges in early life. If true, this opens the door to a novel obesity prevention target in the first year of life.

With respect to laboratory experiments, several experiments report poorer energy compensation among heavier children. Johnson and Birch reported a significant negative association ($r = -.37$) between COMPX% and adiposity in 3–5-year-olds, but among girls only [15]. Thus, heavier girls tended to undercompensate relative to normal-weight girls. Birch and Fisher found that poorer compensation predicted greater 24 h energy intake, which in turn predicted relative weight, in a sample of 4–6-year-old girls [24]. A study of 9–14-year-old boys also reported poorer compensation ability among obese children, compared with normal-weight children [25]. Finally, we found in two independent samples that undercompensation (i.e., a lower COMPX% score) was associated with greater child body fat as measured by dual-energy x-ray absorptiometry [14,26].

FAMILIAL ORIGINS OF SR

Behavioral genetics studies indicate that SR, whether assessed by the CEBQ or COMPX%, has a familial component. That is, the trait is correlated among family members. The familial association likely reflects both genetic and environmental influences, although studies have differed with respect to specific heritability estimates depending on how SR was measured. Carnell et al. [6] studied 5435 twin pairs, ages 8–11 years old, whose SR was assessed by the CEBQ [5]. Results indicated that 63% of the variance in SR was due to genetic factors, with the remaining variance accounted for by environmental factors. In a UK population-based twin cohort, the heritability of SR was estimated to be 72% [27]. However a different conclusion was reached by Faith and colleagues [14] who assessed SR using a laboratory-based preloading paradigm [15,28]. They studied a sample of sixty-nine 4–7-year-old same-sex twins recruited from the New York metropolitan area. In this investigation, heritability was estimated to be 0% (i.e., no genetic influence), with all the familial resemblance apparently due to environmental factors. The inconsistent findings between this study and others may be due to measurement issues (i.e., parent-report vs. laboratory observation), age differences (i.e., 8 years and older and infants vs. 4–7 years old), and/or sample size differences (i.e., hundreds of child participants vs. less than 70).

In sum, there is a familial influence on SR although the magnitude of genetic influence is unclear. That said, family membership does matter and there is a resemblance among siblings. Interestingly, no study to date has examined parent–child correlations for the trait. This information could inform novel family-based treatments that attempt to improve SR in both parents and children.

SR AS A NOVEL INTERVENTION TARGET

There has been limited intervention research targeting SR in children. However, there have been pertinent laboratory-based experiments and preliminary intervention studies over the past 15 years. We call these studies *Generation-1 SR Training Studies*. These consist of (1) satiety scaling experiments and (2) preliminary SR intervention protocols. Arguably, these studies provide proof of principle that SR can be ameliorated with the right training procedures. We summarize these next.

SATIETY SCALING EXPERIMENTS

There is evidence that young children can scale feelings of fullness quantitatively on a continuum, beyond a mere "hungry versus full" dichotomy. This has been studied through experiments using novel pictorial stimuli—or silhouettes—that challenge children to scale how full they feel.

In 2002, we developed the first sex-specific satiety silhouettes for young children for scaling fullness on an ordinal scale [29]. We tested if children—with minimal training—could learn to scale feelings of fullness using this tool. Specifically, children could point to one of five silhouettes, each of which had bellies filled with differing amounts of bubbles to represent fullness (Figure 8.1).

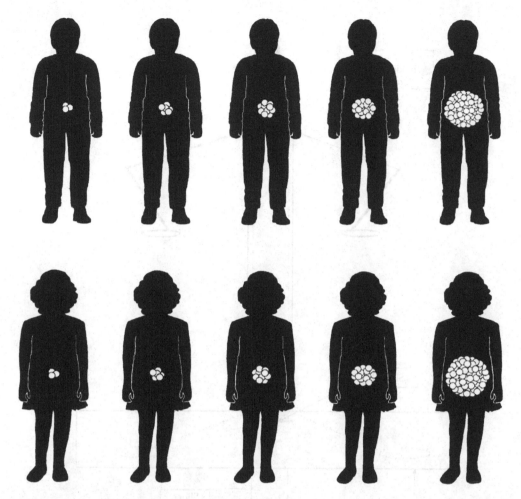

FIGURE 8.1   Satiety silhouettes. (From Faith et al., *Physiology & Behavior*, 76(2):173–8, 2002.)

To validate this instrument, we used an imagined eating paradigm in which children were asked to rate how full they would feel in a situation associated with minimal fullness (i.e., before dinner), moderate fullness (i.e., when interrupted in the middle of dinner, or following a small snack), and high fullness (i.e., after a meal). Children did this following a brief training requiring them to discriminate familiar food-related stimuli (e.g., utensils, foods) with varying amounts of objects, as well as to discriminate everyday objects that differed in how empty versus how full they were. Children provided responses and were given feedback during this training.

Following training and during the satiety-scaling challenge, children reported significantly higher fullness levels with the silhouettes across the three imagined eating scenarios. Specifically, average imagined fullness scores were least before dinner, higher for the interrupted meal or following a snack, and highest after dinner. Qualitative data collected in this study further attested to children's understanding of the experience of fullness. For example, when children were asked to define "fullness," responses fell into the following categories: the time to stop eating (55%); the time their stomach would be hurting (20%); the time following dinner when ready for bed (10%); after eating a lot (10%); and when they could no longer speak (5%). Integrating all results from this project, we concluded that "young children may be more capable of quantitatively reporting feelings of satiety than is commonly believed, if appropriate experimental materials are used" [29, p. 173].

Keller et al. [30] next developed a satiety silhouette that consisted of a cardboard doll ("Freddie") with a sliding, retractable ruler that slides along the length of the doll's belly (Figure 8.2). Children

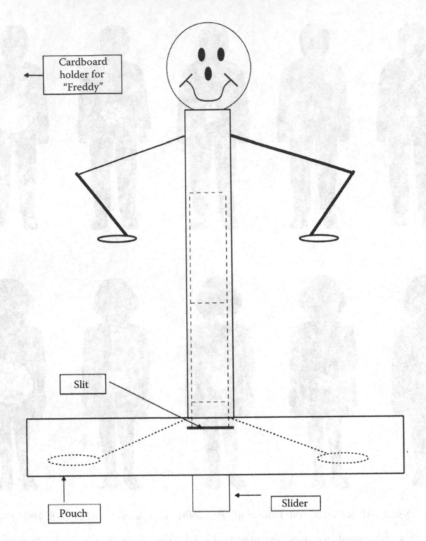

FIGURE 8.2　Satiety silhouettes. (From Keller et al., *Appetite*, 47(2):233–43, 2006.)

were instructed to slide the ruler higher up to communicate a greater sensation of fullness following an imagined or actual eating situation. By measuring the distance (i.e., how far the ruler has been moved, in millimeters), one can quantify satiety on a more refined level than the scale originally developed by Faith et al. [29].

"Freddie" was used in an initial study with 4–5-year-old children, who first received training procedures using everyday objects to orient them to the concept of differential fullness. For example, for one training activity ("A Day at the Beach"), investigators poured incremental amounts of sand into clear 16 oz. plastic cups, which simulated pails. The researchers filled up differing amounts representing a small amount of fullness (one-third full), medium fullness (two-thirds full), or large fullness (completely full). Following this and other training activities, children were challenged to rate their fullness with "Freddie" as they imagined eating incremental portions of french fries and fruit salad. Results supported the hypothesis that children can scale feelings of fullness quantitatively. Seventy-two percent of children (8/11) could successfully scale fullness in response to incremental portions of fries, and 90% (10/11) could successfully scale fullness for fruit salad. The authors concluded that "children can be trained to use an analogue scale to quantify differences [in fullness sensations] in proportion sizes of food" [30, p. 233]. In one follow-up study with 5–6-year-old children studied in a preschool setting, participants successfully used "Freddie" to scale fullness in response to actual food (i.e., 15 mL portions of strawberry yogurt) [31].

Recently, Bennett and Blissett [32] developed satiety silhouettes that were used with children aged 5 to 9 years of age. They developed the "Teddy the Bear" rating system, a five-level ordinal scale depicting five bears with incrementally greater dark bubbles over their bellies to represent incremental fullness (Figure 8.3). Thus, their ordinal scale was more similar to that of Faith et al. [29] than Keller et al. [30] Across three studies, children successfully scaled fullness levels during both imagined and actual eating situations. For example, in one of the studies, children rated how full a fictitious teddy bear would feel both before and after a large meal. In fact, children assigned a higher fullness rating following the imagined meal compared with before. In another one of the studies, children rated their own hunger/fullness levels before an actual snack provided in a school setting. Results indicated that higher fullness levels before the snack predicted significantly less meal intake ($r = -.418$, $p = .006$). The authors concluded on page 47 that "the scale may be useful for interventions focusing on improving children's awareness of hunger and satiety in order to foster healthier eating behavior as well as teaching children at risk for overweight/obesity about the appropriate timing of the initiation and termination of eating episodes."

In sum, evidence from three studies indicates that—with minimal training—children can use different pictorial silhouettes to communicate quantitatively how full they feel. These tools are yet to be used in intervention studies *per se*, which might be an opportunity for future research.

PRELIMINARY SR INTERVENTIONS

Using a prepost design, Johnson [33] tested a 6-week intervention designed to foster awareness of internal hunger and satiety cues. Participants were thirty-one 3- and 4-year-old children enrolled in two Denver day-care facilities, of whom 25 completed the program. Intervention components included discussion of hunger and fullness sensations through play skits and videos (e.g., *Winnie the Pooh and the Honey Jar*); training children to assess their own fullness levels throughout the day by putting their hand on their belly and communicating their satiety (i.e., hungry vs. a little full vs. very full); and pointing to special constructed dolls to communicate how full they feel. The three dolls had clear glass jars as their bellies with varying amounts of salt inside. Specifically, they contained no salt (i.e., empty stomach), a little salt (i.e., a little full), or a lot of salt (i.e., very full). During midmorning snacks, children were prompted at least twice to see if they were still hungry and wanted more food. Additionally, they were prompted to report their fullness levels with the dolls after their snack. The primary outcome was the laboratory-based COMPX% index, as described previously in this chapter. Results indicated that the intervention successfully improved children's SR. When looking to the breakdown of responders, 68% of children showed improvements in COMPX% scores, 16% stayed the same from baseline, and 16% showed deteriorations. The findings were encouraging.

Boutelle et al. [34] developed an 8-week "children's appetite awareness training" intervention to reduce overeating in 8–12-year-old overweight children. Youth were trained to recognize and eat in response to internal hunger and satiety cues, using the metaphor of a gas tank in a car. Additionally, children received experiential exercises to identify hunger/fullness levels and had behavioral assignments to hone these skills. The latter included laboratory meals during which members were challenged to recognize and rate hunger levels. Results indicated that this intervention significantly reduced children's objective and subjective binge-eating episodes, as assessed by a standardized clinical interview. The treatments did not significantly reduce BMI or BMI z-score, although this was not the primary study aim and the intervention duration of 8 weeks may not have been long enough.

In sum, there is proof of concept from two intervention studies that children's eating regulation can be improved following age-appropriate interventions targeting SR. These investigations, along with the prior satiety scaling experiments, provide a strong foundation for future intervention studies. This is discussed next.

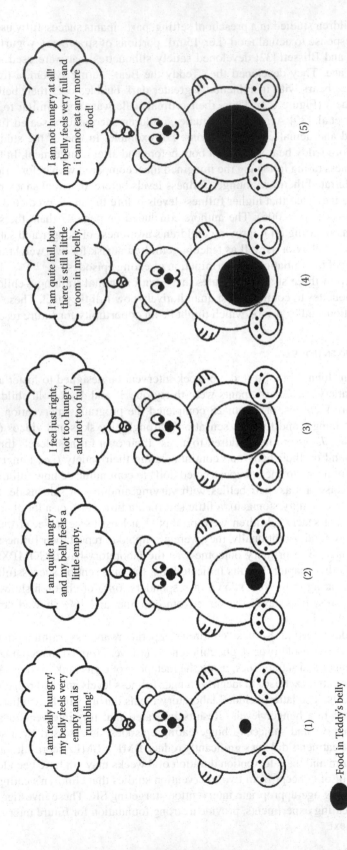

FIGURE 8.3   Satiety silhouettes. (From Bennett and Blissett *Appetite*. 78:40–8, 2014.)

RESEARCH GAPS AND OPPORTUNITIES FOR "GENERATION 2 SR INTERVENTION STUDIES"

Given the current state of the science, the timing arguably is right for a second generation of SR interventions for obese or obese-prone youth. Table 8.3 summarizes opportunities for future research, although this list is by no means exhaustive. These opportunities fall into the categories of measurement, sampling, setting, technology, and dose and timing.

SUMMARY

SR is an important type of food intake self-regulation in early childhood. Poorer SR is associated with increased child BMI, body fat, and obesity status. It is associated with increased weight gain in infants. The epidemiological and laboratory studies are compelling. Looking forward, a critical question is whether SR training represents a novel strategic target for childhood obesity prevention and/or treatment. Might interventions training children to "flex their SR muscles" prove effective to improving eating self-regulation and obesity status? Would there be important effect modifiers of such treatments (e.g., child sex, age, or family attributes)? What might be the optimal intervention dose for such approaches, and could innovative technologies support such training? The answers are currently unknown.

That said, "first-generation" experimental and preliminary intervention studies have been encouraging. There is proof of concept. Young children can be trained to scale satiety using

---

TABLE 8.3
Research Opportunities for Generation 2 SR Training Studies

1. **Measurement Opportunities:** Include a broader range of measures that potentially could be secondary outcomes and/or mediators through which the treatment works. Examples include measures of
   a. Global self-regulation from the child development literature
   b. Global self-control
   c. Impulsivity
   d. Executive function parameters (e.g., working memory, task flexibility)
   e. Biological markers of self-regulation or appetite, including genetic markers
2. **Sampling Opportunities:** Study more diverse population attributes. Examples include diversity with respect to
   a. Race/ethnicity
   b. Age (e.g., preschool vs. middle childhood vs. adolescents)
   c. Family membership (e.g., parent involvement in SR training)
   d. Risk status (e.g., children who are high vs. low in obesity risk, or high vs. low in SR based on initial prescreening of children)
3. **Setting Opportunities:** Examining a broader range of settings in which treatments could be provided including
   a. Preschool/school settings
   b. Home-based training
   c. Community settings
   d. Combination of settings
4. **Technology Opportunities:** Leverage new technologies to foster SR. Examples include
   a. The "manometer." This device incorporates a universal eating monitor-type to provide real-time feedback on children's eating rate during the course of a meal, and assesses child satiety during the course of the meal. (For details and intervention results, see [35].)
5. **Dose and Timing Opportunities:** Determine the optimal treatment dosage and timing to detect potential intervention effects. Opportunities include experimental variations in
   a. Number of treatment sessions
   b. Number of booster sessions
   c. Follow-up duration

age-appropriate silhouettes, as demonstrated in different laboratories. Two initial SR interventions successfully improved child eating outcomes [33,34]. These provide a foundation for what might evolve into a second generation of SR intervention studies that use larger samples and more comprehensive measurement batteries, assess markers of self-regulation, and examine more diverse samples of children. Advances in basic behavioral and biological research should strengthen such intervention studies.

APPENDIX

To illustrate the COMPX% formula and its calculation, consider an experiment in which children consume a low-energy preload of 3 kcal and a high-energy preload of 159 kcal, across two laboratory visits. Imagine a child within this study who consumes exactly 456 kcal at lunch following the low-energy preload and 300 kcal at lunch following the high-energy preload. Plugging these values into the formula yields [(456 − 300) / (159 − 3)] * 100, or COMPX = 100%. Had this child consumed 800 kcal rather than 300 kcal following the high-energy preload (with all else the same), this would have yielded [(456 − 800) / (159 − 3)] * 100, or COMPX% = −220.51%. But had this child consumed only 150 kcal following the high-energy preload (with all else the same), this would have yielded [(456 − 150) / (159 − 3)]*100, or COMPX% = 196.15%.

REFERENCES

1. Faith MS, Carnell S, Kral TV. Genetics of food intake self-regulation in childhood: Literature review and research opportunities. *Human Heredity*. 2013;75(2–4):80–9.
2. Carnell S, Wardle J. Appetitive traits in children: New evidence for associations with weight and a common, obesity-associated genetic variant. *Appetite*. 2009;53(2):260–3.
3. Carnell S, Wardle J. Appetitive traits and child obesity: Measurement, origins and implications for intervention. *The Proceedings of the Nutrition Society*. 2008;67(4):343–55.
4. Goran MI. Metabolic precursors and effects of obesity in children: A decade of progress, 1990–1999. *The American Journal of Clinical Nutrition*. 2001;73(2):158–71.
5. Wardle J, Guthrie CA, Sanderson S, Rapoport L. Development of the children's eating behaviour questionnaire. *Journal of Child Psychology and Psychiatry, and Allied Disciplines*. 2001;42(7):963–70.
6. Carnell S, Haworth CM, Plomin R, Wardle J. Genetic influence on appetite in children. *International Journal of Obesity* (London). 2008;32(10):1468–73.
7. Daniels LA, Mallan KM, Battistutta D, Nicholson JM, Meedeniya JE, Bayer JK, et al. Child eating behavior outcomes of an early feeding intervention to reduce risk indicators for child obesity: The NOURISH RCT. *Obesity (Silver Spring)*. 2014;22(5):E104–11.
8. Mallan KM, Liu WH, Mehta RJ, Daniels LA, Magarey A, Battistutta D. Maternal report of young children's eating styles: Validation of the Children's Eating Behaviour Questionnaire in three ethnically diverse Australian samples. *Appetite*. 2013;64:48–55.
9. Svensson V, Lundborg L, Cao Y, Nowicka P, Marcus C, Sobko T. Obesity related eating behaviour patterns in Swedish preschool children and association with age, gender, relative weight and parental weight–factorial validation of the Children's Eating Behaviour Questionnaire. *The International Journal of Behavioral Nutrition and Physical Activity*. 2011;8:134.
10. dos Passos DR, Gigante DP, Maciel FV, Matijasevich A. Children's eating behaviour: Comparison between normal and overweight children from a school in Pelotas, Rio Grande do Sul, Brazil. *Revista Paulista de Pediatria: Orgao oficial da Sociedade de Pediatria de Sao Paulo*. 2015;33(1):42–9.
11. Carnell S, Wardle J. Measuring behavioural susceptibility to obesity: Validation of the child eating behaviour questionnaire. *Appetite*. 2007;48(1):104–13.
12. Llewellyn CH, van Jaarsveld CH, Johnson L, Carnell S, Wardle J. Development and factor structure of the Baby Eating Behaviour Questionnaire in the Gemini birth cohort. *Appetite*. 2011;57(2):388–96.
13. Faith MS, Keller KL, Johnson SL, Pietrobelli A, Matz PE, Must S, et al. Familial aggregation of energy intake in children. *The American Journal of Clinical Nutrition*. 2004;79(5):844–50.
14. Faith MS, Pietrobelli A, Heo M, Johnson SL, Keller KL, Heymsfield SB, et al. A twin study of self-regulatory eating in early childhood: Estimates of genetic and environmental influence, and measurement considerations. *International Journal of Obesity* (London). 2012;36(7):931–7.

15. Johnson SL, Birch LL. Parents' and children's adiposity and eating style. *Pediatrics*. 1994;94(5):653–61.

16. Carnell S, Wardle J. Appetite and adiposity in children: Evidence for a behavioral susceptibility theory of obesity. *The American Journal of Clinical Nutrition*. 2008;88(1):22–9.

17. Jansen PW, Roza SJ, Jaddoe VW, Mackenbach JD, Raat H, Hofman A, et al. Children's eating behavior, feeding practices of parents and weight problems in early childhood: Results from the population-based Generation R Study. *The International Journal of Behavioral Nutrition and Physical Activity*. 2012;9:130.

18. Sleddens EF, Kremers SP, Thijs C. The children's eating behaviour questionnaire: Factorial validity and association with Body Mass Index in Dutch children aged 6–7. *The International Journal of Behavioral Nutrition and Physical Activity*. 2008;5:49.

19. Viana V, Sinde S, Saxton JC. Children's Eating Behaviour Questionnaire: Associations with BMI in Portuguese children. *The British Journal of Nutrition*. 2008;100(2):445–50.

20. Webber L, Hill C, Saxton J, Van Jaarsveld CH, Wardle J. Eating behaviour and weight in children. *International Journal of Obesity* (London). 2009;33(1):21–8.

21. Spence JC, Carson V, Casey L, Boule N. Examining behavioural susceptibility to obesity among Canadian pre-school children: The role of eating behaviours. *International Journal of Pediatric Obesity: IJPO: An official journal of the International Association for the Study of Obesity*. 2011;6(2–2):e501–7.

22. Mallan KM, Nambiar S, Magarey AM, Daniels LA. Satiety responsiveness in toddlerhood predicts energy intake and weight status at four years of age. *Appetite*. 2014;74:79–85.

23. van Jaarsveld CH, Llewellyn CH, Johnson L, Wardle J. Prospective associations between appetitive traits and weight gain in infancy. *The American Journal of Clinical Nutrition*. 2011;94(6):1562–7.

24. Birch LL, Fisher JO. Mothers' child-feeding practices influence daughters' eating and weight. *The American Journal of Clinical Nutrition*. 2000;71(5):1054–61.

25. Bellissimo N, Desantadina MV, Pencharz PB, Berall GB, Thomas SG, Anderson GH. A comparison of short-term appetite and energy intakes in normal weight and obese boys following glucose and whey-protein drinks. *International Journal of Obesity* (London). 2008;32(2):362–71.

26. Kral TV, Allison DB, Birch LL, Stallings VA, Moore RH, Faith MS. Caloric compensation and eating in the absence of hunger in 5- to 12-year-old weight-discordant siblings. *The American Journal of Clinical Nutrition*. 2012;96(3):574–583.

27. Llewellyn CH, van Jaarsveld CH, Johnson L, Carnell S, Wardle J. Nature and nurture in infant appetite: Analysis of the Gemini twin birth cohort. *The American Journal of Clinical Nutrition*. 2010;91(5):1172–9.

28. Birch LL, Birch D, Marlin DW, Kramer L. Effects of instrumental consumption on children's food preference. *Appetite*. 1982;3(2):125–34.

29. Faith MS, Kermanshah M, Kissileff HR. Development and preliminary validation of a silhouette satiety scale for children. *Physiology & Behavior*. 2002;76(2):173–8.

30. Keller KL, Assur SA, Torres M, Lofink HE, Thornton JC, Faith MS, et al. Potential of an analog scaling device for measuring fullness in children: Development and preliminary testing. *Appetite*. 2006;47(2):233–43.

31. Kissileff HR, Keller KL, Lofink HL, Torres M, Thornton JC. Ratings of fullness after ad libitum meals are not predicted from ratings of fullness during interrupted meals in pre-school children. *Appetite*. 2010;51:376.

32. Bennett C, Blissett J. Measuring hunger and satiety in primary school children: Validation of a new picture rating scale. *Appetite*. 2014;78:40–8.

33. Johnson SL. Improving Preschoolers' self-regulation of energy intake. *Pediatrics*. 2000;106(6):1429–35.

34. Boutelle KN, Zucker NL, Peterson CB, Rydell SA, Cafri G, Harnack L. Two novel treatments to reduce overeating in overweight children: A randomized controlled trial. *Journal of Consulting and Clinical Psychology*. 2011;79(6):759–71.

35. Ford AL, Bergh C, Sodersten P, Sabin MA, Hollinghurst S, Hunt LP, et al. Treatment of childhood obesity by retraining eating behaviour: Randomised controlled trial. *BMJ*. 2010;340:b5388.

9 Food Reward and Appetite Regulation in Children

Kathleen A. Page

CONTENTS

OVERVIEW OF BRAIN REGULATION OF APPETITE AND EATING BEHAVIOR

Eating is necessary for survival, and humans have powerful biological systems that help to maintain an adequate nutrient supply [1]. These systems involve cross talk between the brain and the rest of the body. The body sends messages to the brain about its energy needs, and the brain responds to these needs through a number of pathways that regulate food intake, energy expenditure, and energy storage in a biological process called *energy homeostasis* [2–4]. The hypothalamus is the central orchestrator of energy homeostasis. Its interactions with other brain regions and with the periphery help to ensure an adequate energy supply. The arcuate nucleus (ARC) and ventral medial nucleus (VMN) in the hypothalamus have a high density of neurons that respond to peripheral hormones, including leptin, insulin, and ghrelin [5]. The ARC contains two subsets of neurons that play opposing roles in appetite regulation. Pro-opiomelanocorticotropin (POMC) neurons are anorexigenic (i.e., suppress appetite), whereas neurons that coexpress neuropeptide Y (NPY) and agouti-related peptide (AgRP) are orexigenic (i.e., stimulate appetite) [3]. Arcuate POMC and NPY/AgRP neurons send projections to other areas in the hypothalamus, including the dorsomedial (DMN) and paraventricular (PVN) nuclei of the hypothalamus and the lateral hypothalamic area (LHA), as well as other brain regions involved in regulating energy homeostasis [5]. POMC is cleaved into anorexigenic peptides, including α-melanocyte stimulating hormone (MSH) and cocaine- and amphetamine-regulated transcript (CART). When POMC neurons are activated, α-MSH is released into the PVN, where it acts on melanocortin-3 and 4 receptors to promote satiety. In contrast, NPY/AgRP neurons activate orexigenic signaling via NPY receptors and inhibit anorexigenic signaling via melanocortin receptors [5–7].

While the hypothalamus primarily regulates the homeostatic drive to eat, other brain regions, such as the ventral tegmental area (VTA), striatum, orbitofrontal cortex, amygdala, hippocampus, and insula, control motivation-reward systems associated with the hedonic drive to eat. Dopamine and opioid are neurotransmitters that play an important role in the regulation of hedonic feeding behavior. Dopamine receptors, D_1 and D_2, are located in various brain regions, including the nucleus

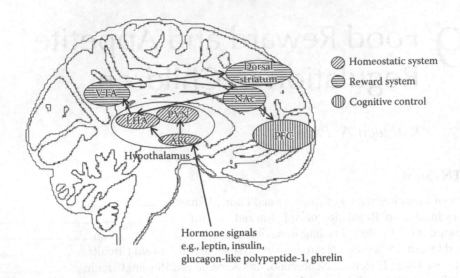

Hormone signals
e.g., leptin, insulin,
glucagon-like polypeptide-1, ghrelin

FIGURE 9.1 Central nervous system regulation of eating behavior. Figure shows communication between the homeostatic, reward, and cognitive brain regions that control food intake. The hypothalamus is the central regulator of energy homeostasis. Hypothalamic nuclei, including the ARC, PVN, and LHA, integrate satiety-related hormone signals from the periphery and communicate these signals to brain reward circuits. The mesolimbic dopaminergic neurons in the VTA project to the dorsal striatum and NAc to regulate the reward value of food. Cortical regions, including the PFC, help regulate impulse control and inhibit the motivation for rewarding signals arising from the dopaminergic reward circuitry.

accumbens (NAc), dorsal striatum, and prefrontal cortex (PFC). The reward-associated mesolimbic dopamine pathway includes dopamine neurons that originate in the VTA and project to the NAc, which sends signals to other limbic brain regions, including the hypothalamus, amygdala, and hippocampus and higher cortical circuits [7,8]. The opioid system is also important in regulating the perception of pleasure associated with eating. Opioid receptors are located throughout the brain, including the VTA and NAc. Activation of opiate receptors in the NAc results in a disinhibition of the neurons in the LHA, which in turn stimulates feeding behavior [8].

Cortical regions, including the PFC, regulate impulse control and inhibit the motivation for rewarding stimuli like palatable food [9]. These homeostatic, hedonic, and cortical brain regions are tightly interconnected and form an integrated network that regulates feeding behavior (Figure 9.1).

HORMONES INVOLVED IN REGULATION OF APPETITE AND REWARD

The body produces a number of hormones that help regulate appetite. Long-term energy stores are reflected by circulating levels of leptin, a hormone that is secreted by adipose tissue in proportion to body fat mass [3,8]. Insulin is produced by the β-cells in the pancreas, and plasma insulin, like leptin levels, parallel overall levels of adiposity [5]. Insulin and leptin act on neurons located in the hypothalamus, particularly in the ARC, to suppress appetite. In addition, both insulin and leptin decrease reward signals that are triggered by the striatum and other components of the brain reward circuitry [3,5,10].

During periods of hunger, the stomach produces the hormone, ghrelin, which stimulates food intake. Ghrelin levels rise before consuming a meal and decline after eating, which suggests that ghrelin plays an important role in hunger and meal initiation [5,11,12]. Ghrelin activates NPY/AgRP neurons and inhibits POMC neurons located in the ARC nucleus of the hypothalamus [12]. In addition, ghrelin stimulates the reactivity of the striatum and other reward-related brain regions, which drives food-seeking behavior [13–15]. After a meal is consumed, the gut releases appetite-suppressing hormones, including glucagon-like polypeptide-1 (GLP-1) and polypeptide YY (PYY), which provide satiety signals to the hypothalamus and hindbrain to reduce food intake [16–19].

FOOD REWARD AND ITS ROLE IN FEEDING BEHAVIOR

The drive to eat palatable foods, typically those rich in fat and sugar, has a strong biological basis and exposure to palatable foods can stimulate eating even in the absence of an energy deficit. This is likely because food (particularly energy-dense food) is a natural reward that influences neurochemical systems to reinforce food intake [20,21]. The neurobiological basis for food reward has been demonstrated in a number of studies, which show that foods dense in sugar and fat can stimulate the release of neurotransmitters, including dopamine, opioids, serotonin, and cannabinoids, that enhance feelings of pleasure and reward [9,22,23]. The involvement of dopamine in food reward has been associated with the motivational salience or "wanting" of food as opposed to the "liking" of food, which is thought to primarily involve opioid signaling within the NAc [24]. Neuroimaging studies in children and adults have shown that exposure to palatable food cues, including the sight and smell of food, leads to the activation of reward-related circuitry and an increased subjective "wanting" of the food [25–31]. The current environment with ubiquitous exposure to palatable food and food-related cues is likely promoting food-seeking behavior. This may be particularly relevant to children and adolescents, who are the target audience of many food-related advertisements [32].

CHILDHOOD OBESITY: EFFECTS ON NEUROENDOCRINE APPETITE AND REWARD CIRCUITS

Emerging evidence suggests that high levels of adiposity may promote overeating behavior due to obesity-associated alterations in the neural pathways that regulate appetite, reward, and cognitive inhibitory control. Neuroimaging studies provide a way to noninvasively study the neural circuitry involved in the regulation of feeding behavior in humans. A commonly used paradigm for probing body-weight-related differences in neural circuitry is to expose people to pictures of highly palatable food items (and nonfood objects as a control). The majority of work in this area has shown that obese individuals compared with lean individuals exhibit greater activation in reward-related brain areas in response to food cues [28,29,31,33,34]. To date, findings in the small number of neuroimaging studies performed in children are in keeping with the results observed in adults [25,30,35]. Greater brain activation within reward-relevant regions has also been shown to predict weight gain in adolescent girls [36] supporting the theory that hyperresponsivity to food cues may be a risk factor for overeating [9,36–38].

Additional work has shown that obesity is related to hyporesponsiveness in the hypothalamus after the consumption of food [39,40] or glucose drinks [40–42], suggesting that appetite signaling in response to nutrient ingestion may be disrupted by obesity. Obese adults compared with lean adults also exhibited less postprandial activation in the dorsolateral PFC, a region involved in cognitive inhibitory control [43,44]. Additional evidence from preclinical and clinical studies suggests that obese individuals have a reduction in dopamine signaling, including decreases in striatal dopamine receptor (D2R) density and in dopamine release [45–47]. These findings are in keeping with functional magnetic resonance imaging (fMRI) studies showing that obese adolescent girls have a reduction in the striatal response to the receipt of food [48,49]. Some posit that a weakened reward response to food consumption could stimulate overeating in an effort to compensate for the reward deficit. This mismatch between the high expectations associated with the food cue and the weakened reward response to food consumption could perpetuate a vicious cycle of overeating and obesity [48,50,51].

Taken together, current evidence suggests that obesity is associated with an enhanced sensitivity to conditioned food stimuli that predict reward (e.g., the smell of apple pie or the sight of chocolate cake), but a decreased sensitivity to satiety and reward signaling after actual food consumption, as well as impairments in cognitive inhibitory control over appetitive behavior. Future work is necessary to determine whether these obesity-associated alterations in neural circuitry are reflective of adaptations to the obese state or if they antecede and possibly play a role in the development of obesity.

ENERGY-DENSE DIETS: EFFECTS ON NEUROENDOCRINE APPETITE AND REWARD CIRCUITS

Most of what we know about the effects of consuming diets rich in sugar and fat comes from experimental studies in animal models with limited studies in children. Mounting evidence suggests that consuming a high-fat diet can cause inflammatory damage within the hypothalamus, which leads to impaired leptin and insulin signaling and an increased susceptibility to obesity [52,53]. Chronic consumption of high-fat, high-sugar diets has also been shown to affect the reward centers in the brain, including a reduction in the expression of D2R [46] and decreased dopamine content in the striatum [54]. Moreover, when rats are given repeated but intermittent access to foods high in sugar, fat, or both, they develop binge-eating behavior and alterations in the reward circuitry [20,45,55].

Currently, there are few human studies on the effects of chronic intake of energy-rich diets on brain circuits involved in the regulation of feeding behavior. However, one fMRI study showed that normal-weight adolescents who reported frequent ice cream consumption had lower activation in the striatum in response to the receipt of small tastes of milk shake [56]. These findings support animal studies suggesting that chronic exposure to energy-dense foods can lead to a reduction in dopamine signaling [55]. Another fMRI study reported that adolescents who habitually consumed the soft drink, Coke, when compared with nonsoft drink consumers, had greater brain activation to Coke logo ads in the posterior cingulate and decreased activation in the ventrolateral PFC when anticipating the receipt of Coke. The investigators interpreted these findings to suggest that habitual soft drink consumption may promote increased responsiveness within brain regions encoding salience toward brand-specific cues, as well as hyporesponsiveness within inhibitory brain regions while anticipating intake of the soft drink [57]. Thus, it appears that consumption of diets high in fat and/or sugar could lead to alterations in the brain circuitry that regulate reward and cognitive control over feeding behavior.

DIFFERENT TYPES OF SUGAR: EFFECTS OF FRUCTOSE VERSUS GLUCOSE ON NEUROENDOCRINE AND APPETITE RESPONSES

Fructose and glucose are both monosaccharides with the same number of calories, but their differential effects on the neuroendocrine circuits involved in appetite and reward processing may affect feeding behavior [58–61]. When compared with glucose, fructose may be a weak suppressor of appetite due to attenuated stimulation of the purported satiety hormones, insulin, leptin, and GLP-1 [19,62–64]. Moreover, fructose is sweeter than glucose and, in contrast to glucose, very little fructose circulates in the bloodstream due to the complete extraction of fructose into the liver [65]. These differences in fructose versus glucose may help explain their differential effects on brain appetite and reward pathways. Animal studies have shown that the central administration of fructose activates appetite-signaling pathways in the hypothalamus and increases food intake, whereas glucose inhibits hypothalamic appetite-signaling pathways and decreases food intake [61]. Similarly, neuroimaging studies in humans also show differential brain responses to glucose compared with fructose ingestion [58,60]. Relative to fructose, ingestion of drinks containing glucose resulted in a greater reduction in hypothalamic cerebral blood flow (CBF), a marker of neural activation in healthy young adults [59]. The acute ingestion of fructose relative to glucose was also shown to increase brain activation to food cues in the orbitofrontal cortex, visual cortex, and ventral striatum (brain regions involved in attention and reward processing) and led to greater hunger and motivation for immediate food rewards [58]. These studies provide potential insights into epidemiological evidence linking fructose consumption to overeating behavior in healthy adults [66,67]. However, future work is necessary to determine the neuroendocrine effects in children of consuming different types of sugar as well as the effects of obesity and other metabolic conditions on these responses and the long-term effects of fructose intake on neuroendocrine pathways. Moreover, future studies are necessary to determine neuroendocrine and appetite responses to combinations of fructose and glucose, such as high-fructose corn syrup or sucrose, as they are commonly consumed in the real world.

DEVELOPMENTAL PROGRAMING: EFFECTS OF PRENATAL ENVIRONMENT ON NEUROENDOCRINE APPETITE AND REWARD CIRCUITS

Human and animal studies provide compelling evidence that the nutritional and metabolic conditions that an individual is exposed to *in utero* can shape long-term susceptibility to obesity and other metabolic diseases [5,68,69]. Epidemiological and cross-sectional studies show an association between fetal exposure to maternal overnutrition (through maternal obesity, diabetes, or high-fat feeding during pregnancy) and increased risk for obesity during childhood and adult life [70–72]. While some of this risk is likely attributable to genetic susceptibility, studies in siblings demonstrate that the risk is in excess of genetic factors alone. For example, children who were born after their mother developed diabetes (i.e., these children were exposed to diabetes *in utero*) were at higher risk for developing obesity and diabetes than their siblings who were born before their mother developed diabetes [73–75]. Other studies demonstrated that offspring who were born after their mothers lost a significant amount of weight via bariatric surgery had a lower risk for developing obesity than their siblings who were born before maternal surgery [76,77]. These data show a disproportionate risk of obesity in siblings born to the same mother under different *in utero* conditions and provide support for independent effects of the intrauterine environment on programing risk for obesity [78].

Animal models are helping to uncover potential mechanisms that underlie these early-life programing effects [5,78–81]. For example, preclinical studies show that fetal or newborn exposure to various models of maternal overnutrition can "program" hypothalamic appetite circuitry to favor orexigenic pathways in offspring. These changes in brain appetite circuitry lead to increased food intake and obesity in offspring [79,82–85]. In addition to affecting hypothalamus appetite circuits, fetal exposure to maternal high-fat, high-sugar feeding during pregnancy has also been shown to disrupt the development of brain reward pathways and increase the offspring's preference for energy-dense food [86–88].

Lactation has also been identified as a critical period for developmental programing [86,89–92]. Studies in mice have shown that maternal high-fat feeding during lactation causes a reduction in the number of projections from POMC neurons to the PVN in the hypothalamus and a predisposition for obesity and diabetes in offspring [91]. Additional studies have shown that exposure to high-fat, high-sugar diets during lactation leads to hyperphagia and a preference for energy-dense foods in offspring [86,89,92].

CONCLUSIONS

In light of the current childhood obesity epidemic and the high rates of relapse associated with current obesity treatments, it is important to understand the neural systems that regulate feeding behavior and how these systems are affected by environmental factors. Future work is needed to determine the effects of specific interventions, such as diet and physical activity, on neural pathways implicated in feeding behavior. These studies are particularly relevant during childhood and adolescence because these are critical time periods when the brain is highly plastic and susceptible to metabolic and external influences. Moreover, preventive measures that begin early in pregnancy and continue throughout lactation may be important for improving the metabolic health of offspring and reducing the rising rates of childhood obesity.

REFERENCES

1. Zheng H, Lenard NR, Shin AC, Berthoud H-R. Appetite control and energy balance regulation in the modern world: Reward-driven brain overrides repletion signals. *Int J Obes (Lond)*. 2009;33 Suppl 2:S8–13.

2. Levin BE. Metabolic sensing neurons and the control of energy homeostasis. *Physiol Behav.* 2006;89(4):486–9.

3. Morton GJ, Meek TH, Schwartz MW. Neurobiology of food intake in health and disease. *Nat Rev Neurosci.* 2014;15(6):367–78.

4. Schwartz MW, Woods SC, Porte D, Seeley RJ, Baskin DG. Central nervous system control of food intake. *Nature.* 2000;404(6778):661–71.

5. Bouret S, Levin BE, Ozanne SE. Gene-environment interactions controlling energy and glucose homeostasis and the developmental origins of obesity. *Physiol Rev.* 2015;95(1):47–82.

6. Morton GJ, Schwartz MW. The NPY/AgRP neuron and energy homeostasis. *Int J Obes Relat Metab Disord.* 2001;25 Suppl 5:S56–62.

7. Tulloch AJ, Murray S, Vaicekonyte R, Avena NM. Neural responses to macronutrients: Hedonic and homeostatic mechanisms. *Gastroenterology.* 2015;148(6):1205–18.

8. Morton GJ, Cummings DE, Baskin DG, Barsh GS, Schwartz MW. Central nervous system control of food intake and body weight. *Nature.* 2006;443(7109):289–95.

9. Volkow ND, Wang G-J, Baler RD. Reward, dopamine and the control of food intake: Implications for obesity. *Trends Cogn Sci.* 2011;15(1):37–46.

10. Figlewicz DP, Benoit SC. Insulin, leptin, and food reward: Update 2008. *Am J Physiol Regul Integr Comp Physiol.* 2009;296(1):R9–19.

11. Cowley MA, Smith RG, Diano S, Tschöp M, Pronchuk N, Grove KL, et al. The distribution and mechanism of action of ghrelin in the CNS demonstrates a novel hypothalamic circuit regulating energy homeostasis. *Neuron.* 2003;37(4):649–61.

12. Horvath TL, Diano S, Sotonyi P, Heiman M, Tschöp M. Mini review: Ghrelin and the regulation of energy balance: A hypothalamic perspective. *Endocrinology.* 2001;142(10):4163–9.

13. Goldstone A, Prechtl C, Scholtz S, Miras A, Chhina N, Durighel G, et al. Ghrelin mimics fasting to enhance human hedonic, orbitofrontal cortex, and hippocampal responses to food. *Am J Clin Nutr.* 2014;99:1319–30.

14. Malik S, McGlone F, Bedrossian D, Dagher A. Ghrelin modulates brain activity in areas that control appetitive behavior. *Cell Metab.* 2008;7(5):400–9.

15. Wren AM, Seal LJ, Cohen MA, Brynes AE, Frost GS, Murphy KG, et al. Ghrelin enhances appetite and increases food intake in humans. *J Clin Endocrinol Metab.* 2001;86(12):5992.

16. Batterham RL, Ffytche DH, Rosenthal JM, Zelaya FO, Barker GJ, Withers DJ, et al. PYY modulation of cortical and hypothalamic brain areas predicts feeding behaviour in humans. *Nature.* 2007;450(7166):106–9.

17. van Bloemendaal L, IJzerman RG, Ten Kulve JS, Barkhof F, Konrad RJ, Drent ML, et al. GLP-1 receptor activation modulates appetite- and reward-related brain areas in humans. *Diabetes.* 2014;63(12):4186–96.

18. De Silva A, Salem V, Long CJ, Makwana A, Newbould RD, Rabiner EA, et al. The gut hormones PYY 3-36 and GLP-1 7-36 amide reduce food intake and modulate brain activity in appetite centers in humans. *Cell Metab.* 2011;14(5):700–6.

19. Kong M-F, Chapman I, Goble E, Wishart J, Wittert G, Morris H, et al. Effects of oral fructose and glucose on plasma GLP-1 and appetite in normal subjects. *Peptides.* 1999;20(5):545–51.

20. Avena NM, Bocarsly ME, Hoebel BG. Animal models of sugar and fat bingeing: Relationship to food addiction and increased body weight. *Methods Mol Biol.* 2012;829:351–65.

21. Gugusheff JR, Ong ZY, Muhlhausler BS. The early origins of food preferences: Targeting the critical windows of development. *FASEB J.* 2015;29(2):365–73.

22. Liang N-C, Hajnal A, Norgren R. Sham feeding corn oil increases accumbens dopamine in the rat. *Am J Physiol Regul Integr Comp Physiol.* 2006;291(5):R1236–9.

23. Rada P, Avena NM, Hoebel BG. Daily bingeing on sugar repeatedly releases dopamine in the accumbens shell. *Neuroscience.* 2005;134(3):737–44.

24. Castro DC, Cole SL, Berridge KC. Lateral hypothalamus, nucleus accumbens, and ventral pallidum roles in eating and hunger: Interactions between homeostatic and reward circuitry. *Front Syst Neurosci.* 2015;9:90.

25. Bruce AS, Martin LE, Savage CR. Neural correlates of pediatric obesity. *Prev Med.* 2011;52 Suppl 1:S29–35.

26. Holsen LM, Zarcone JR, Thompson TI, Brooks WM, Anderson MF, Ahluwalia JS, et al. Neural mechanisms underlying food motivation in children and adolescents. *NeuroImage.* 2005;27(3):669–76.

27. Killgore WDS, Yurgelun-Todd DA. Developmental changes in the functional brain responses of adolescents to images of high and low-calorie foods. *Dev Psychobiol.* 2005;47(4):377–97.

28. Luo S, Romero A, Adam TC, Hu HH, Monterosso J, Page KA. Abdominal fat is associated with a greater brain reward response to high-calorie food cues in hispanic women. *Obesity*. 2013;21(10):2029–36.

29. van der Laan LN, de Ridder DTD, Viergever MA, Smeets PAM. The first taste is always with the eyes: A meta-analysis on the neural correlates of processing visual food cues. *NeuroImage*. 2011;55(1):296–303.

30. van Meer F, van der Laan LN, Adan RAH, Viergever MA, Smeets PAM. What you see is what you eat: An ALE meta-analysis of the neural correlates of food viewing in children and adolescents. *NeuroImage*. 2015;104:35–43.

31. Wang G-J, Volkow ND, Telang F, Jayne M, Ma J, Rao M, et al. Exposure to appetitive food stimuli markedly activates the human brain. *NeuroImage*. 2004;21(4):1790–7.

32. Boyland EJ, Halford JCG. Television advertising and branding: Effects on eating behaviour and food preferences in children. *Appetite*. 2013;62:236–41.

33. Martens MJ, Born JM, Lemmens SG, Karhunen L, Heinecke A, Goebel R, et al. Increased sensitivity to food cues in the fasted state and decreased inhibitory control in the satiated state in the overweight. *Am J Clin Nutr*. 2013;97(3):471–9.

34. Rothemund Y, Preuschhof C, Bohner G, Bauknecht H-C, Klingebiel R, Flor H, et al. Differential activation of the dorsal striatum by high-calorie visual food stimuli in obese individuals. *NeuroImage*. 2007;37(2):410–21.

35. Bruce AS, Holsen LM, Chambers RJ, Martin LE, Brooks WM, Zarcone JR, et al. Obese children show hyperactivation to food pictures in brain networks linked to motivation, reward and cognitive control. *Int J Obes (Lond)*. 2010;34(10):1494–500.

36. Yokum S, Ng J, Stice E. Attentional bias to food images associated with elevated weight and future weight gain: An fMRI study. *Obesity (Silver Spring)*. 2011;19(9):1775–83.

37. Carnell S, Gibson C, Benson L, Ochner CN, Geliebter A. Neuroimaging and obesity: Current knowledge and future directions. *Obes Rev*. 2012;13(1):43–56.

38. Stice E, Burger KS, Yokum S. Reward region responsivity predicts future weight gain and moderating effects of the TaqIA Allele. *J Neurosci*. 2015;35(28):10316–24.

39. Del Parigi A, Gautier J-F, Chen K, Salbe AD, Ravussin E, Reiman E, et al. Neuroimaging and obesity: Mapping the brain responses to hunger and satiation in humans using positron emission tomography. *Ann N Y Acad Sci*. 2002;967:389–97.

40. Gautier J-F, Del Parigi A, Chen K, Salbe AD, Bandy D, Pratley RE, et al. Effect of satiation on brain activity in obese and lean women. *Obes Res*. 2001;9(11):676–84.

41. Liu Y, Gao JH, Liu HL, Fox PT. The temporal response of the brain after eating revealed by functional MRI. *Nature*. 2000;405(6790):1058–62.

42. Matsuda M, Liu Y, Mahankali S, Pu Y, Mahankali A, Wang J, et al. Altered hypothalamic function in response to glucose ingestion in obese humans. *Diabetes*. 1999;48(9):1801–6.

43. Le DSN, Pannacciulli N, Chen K, Salbe AD, Del Parigi A, Hill JO, et al. Less activation in the left dorsolateral prefrontal cortex in the reanalysis of the response to a meal in obese than in lean women and its association with successful weight loss. *Am J Clin Nutr*. 2007;86(3):573–9.

44. Le DSNT, Pannacciulli N, Chen K, Del Parigi A, Salbe AD, Reiman EM, et al. Less activation of the left dorsolateral prefrontal cortex in response to a meal: A feature of obesity. *Am J Clin Nutr*. 2006;84(4):725–31.

45. Geiger BM, Haburcak M, Avena NM, Moyer MC, Hoebel BG, Pothos EN. Deficits of mesolimbic dopamine neurotransmission in rat dietary obesity. *Neuroscience*. 2009;159(4):1193–9.

46. Johnson PM, Kenny PJ. Dopamine D2 receptors in addiction-like reward dysfunction and compulsive eating in obese rats. *Nat Neurosci*. 2010;13(5):635–41.

47. Wang GJ, Volkow ND, Logan J, Pappas NR, Wong CT, Zhu W, et al. Brain dopamine and obesity. *Lancet*. 2001;357(9253):354–7.

48. Stice E, Spoor S, Ng J, Zald DH. Relation of obesity to consummatory and anticipatory food reward. *Physiol Behav*. 2009;97(5):551–60.

49. Stice E, Spoor S, Bohon C, Small DM. Relation between obesity and blunted striatal response to food is moderated by TaqIA A1 allele. *Science*. 2008;322(5900):449–52.

50. Volkow ND, Wang G-J, Baler RD. Reward, dopamine and the control of food intake: Implications for obesity. *Trends Cogn Sci*. 2011;15(1):37–46.

51. Wang GJ, Volkow ND, Thanos PK, Fowler JS. Imaging of brain dopamine pathways: Implications for understanding obesity. *J Addict Med*. 2009;3(1):8–18.

52. Dorfman MD, Thaler JP. Hypothalamic inflammation and gliosis in obesity. *Curr Opin Endocrinol Diabetes Obes*. 2015;22(5):325–30.

53. Thaler JP, Yi C-X, Schur EA, Guyenet SJ, Hwang BH, Dietrich MO, et al. Obesity is associated with hypothalamic injury in rodents and humans. *J Clin Invest*. 2012;122(1):153–62.

54. Davis JF, Tracy AL, Schurdak JD, Tschöp MH, Lipton JW, Clegg DJ, et al. Exposure to elevated levels of dietary fat attenuates psychostimulant reward and mesolimbic dopamine turnover in the rat. *Behav Neurosci*. 2008;122(6):1257–63.

55. Bello NT, Lucas LR, Hajnal A. Repeated sucrose access influences dopamine D2 receptor density in the striatum. *Neuroreport*. 2002;13(12):1575–8.

56. Burger KS, Stice E. Frequent ice cream consumption is associated with reduced striatal response to receipt of an ice cream-based milkshake. *Am J Clin Nutr*. 2012;95(4):810–7.

57. Burger KS, Stice E. Neural responsivity during soft drink intake, anticipation, and advertisement exposure in habitually consuming youth: Neural response to soft drinks. *Obesity (Silver Spring)*. 2014;22(2):441–50.

58. Luo S, Monterosso JR, Sarpelleh K, Page KA. Differential effects of fructose versus glucose on brain and appetitive responses to food cues and decisions for food rewards. *Proc Natl Acad Sci U S A*. 2015;112(20):6509–14.

59. Page KA, Chan O, Arora J, Belfort-Deaguiar R, Dzuira J, Roehmholdt B, et al. Effects of fructose vs glucose on regional cerebral blood flow in brain regions involved with appetite and reward pathways. *JAMA*. 2013;309(1):63–70.

60. Wölnerhanssen BK, Meyer-Gerspach AC, Schmidt A, Zimak N, Peterli R, Beglinger C, et al. Dissociable behavioral, physiological and neural effects of acute glucose and fructose ingestion: A pilot study. *PloS One*. 2015;10(6):e0130280.

61. Cha SH, Wolfgang M, Tokutake Y, Chohnan S, Lane MD. Differential effects of central fructose and glucose on hypothalamic malonyl–CoA and food intake. *Proc Natl Acad Sci U S A*. 2008;105(44):16871–5.

62. Teff KL, Elliott SS, Tschöp M, Kieffer TJ, Rader D, Heiman M, et al. Dietary fructose reduces circulating insulin and leptin, attenuates postprandial suppression of ghrelin, and increases triglycerides in women. *J Clin Endocrinol Metab*. 2004;89(6):2963–72.

63. Havel PJ. Dietary fructose: Implications for dysregulation of energy homeostasis and lipid/carbohydrate metabolism. *Nutr Rev*. 2005;63(5):133–57.

64. Curry DL. Effects of mannose and fructose on the synthesis and secretion of insulin. *Pancreas*. 1989;4(1):2–9.

65. Tappy L, Lê K-A. Metabolic effects of fructose and the worldwide increase in obesity. *Physiol Rev*. 2010;90(1):23–46.

66. Bray GA. Potential health risks from beverages containing fructose found in sugar or high-fructose corn syrup. *Diabetes Care*. 2013;36(1):11–2.

67. Malik VS, Hu FB. Fructose and cardiometabolic health: What the evidence from sugar-sweetened beverages tells us. *J Am Coll Cardiol*. 2015;66(14):1615–24.

68. Nicholas LM, Morrison JL, Rattanatray L, Zhang S, Ozanne SE, McMillen IC. The early origins of obesity and insulin resistance: Timing, programming and mechanisms. *Int J Obes* (Lond). 2016;40(2):229–38.

69. Paes ST, Gonçalves CF, Terra MM, Fontoura TS, Guerra M de O, Peters VM, et al. Childhood obesity: A (re) programming disease? *J Dev Orig Health Dis*. 2015;1–6.

70. Gillman MW, Rifas-Shiman S, Berkey CS, Field AE, Colditz GA. Maternal gestational diabetes, birth weight, and adolescent obesity. *Pediatrics*. 2003;111(3):e221–6.

71. Hillier TA, Pedula KL, Schmidt MM, Mullen JA, Charles M-A, Pettitt DJ. Childhood obesity and metabolic imprinting the ongoing effects of maternal hyperglycemia. *Diabetes Care*. 2007 Sep 1;30(9):2287–92.

72. Page KA, Romero A, Buchanan TA, Xiang AH. Gestational diabetes mellitus, maternal obesity, and adiposity in offspring. *J Pediatr*. 2014;164(4):807–10.

73. Dabelea D, Hanson RL, Lindsay RS, Pettitt DJ, Imperatore G, Gabir MM, et al. Intrauterine exposure to diabetes conveys risks for type 2 diabetes and obesity: A study of discordant sibships. *Diabetes*. 2000;49(12):2208–11.

74. Lawlor DA, Lichtenstein P, Långström N. Association of maternal diabetes mellitus in pregnancy with offspring adiposity into early adulthood: Sibling study in a prospective cohort of 280,866 men from 248,293 families. *Circulation*. 2011;123(3):258–65.

75. Sobngwi E, Boudou P, Mauvais-Jarvis F, Leblanc H, Velho G, Vexiau P, et al. Effect of a diabetic environment in utero on predisposition to type 2 diabetes. *Lancet*. 2003;361(9372):1861–5.

76. Kral JG, Biron S, Simard S, Hould F-S, Lebel S, Marceau S, et al. Large maternal weight loss from obesity surgery prevents transmission of obesity to children who were followed for 2 to 18 years. *Pediatrics*. 2006;118(6):e1644–9.

77. Smith J, Cianflone K, Biron S, Hould FS, Lebel S, Marceau S, et al. Effects of maternal surgical weight loss in mothers on intergenerational transmission of obesity. *J Clin Endocrinol Metab.* 2009;94(11):4275–83.
78. Alfaradhi MZ, Ozanne SE. Developmental programming in response to maternal overnutrition. *Front Genet.* 2011;2:27.
79. Franke K, Harder T, Aerts L, Melchior K, Fahrenkrog S, Rodekamp E, et al. "Programming" of orexigenic and anorexigenic hypothalamic neurons in offspring of treated and untreated diabetic mother rats. *Brain Res.* 2005;1031(2):276–83.
80. Plagemann A. Maternal diabetes and perinatal programming. *Early Hum Dev.* 2011;87(11):743–7.
81. Ross MG, Desai M. Developmental programming of offspring obesity, adipogenesis, and appetite. *Clin Obstet Gynecol.* 2013;56(3):529–36.
82. Davidowa H, Plagemann A. Insulin resistance of hypothalamic arcuate neurons in neonatally overfed rats. *Neuroreport.* 2007;18(5):521–4.
83. Rajia S, Chen H, Morris MJ. Maternal overnutrition impacts offspring adiposity and brain appetite markers-modulation by postweaning diet. *J Neuroendocrinol.* 2010;22(8):905–14.
84. Ralevski A, Horvath TL. Developmental programming of hypothalamic neuroendocrine systems. *Front Neuroendocrinol.* 2015;39:52–58.
85. Steculorum SM, Bouret SG. Maternal diabetes compromises the organization of hypothalamic feeding circuits and impairs leptin sensitivity in offspring. *Endocrinology.* 2011;152(11):4171–9.
86. Bayol SA, Farrington SJ, Stickland NC. A maternal "junk food" diet in pregnancy and lactation promotes an exacerbated taste for "junk food" and a greater propensity for obesity in rat offspring. *Br J Nutr.* 2007;98(4):843–51.
87. Muhlhausler BS, Ong ZY. The fetal origins of obesity: Early origins of altered food intake. *Endocr Metab Immune Disord Drug Targets.* 2011;11(3):189–97.
88. Vucetic Z, Kimmel J, Totoki K, Hollenbeck E, Reyes TM. Maternal high-fat diet alters methylation and gene expression of dopamine and opioid-related genes. *Endocrinology.* 2010;151(10):4756–64.
89. Gugusheff JR, Vithayathil M, Ong ZY, Muhlhausler BS. The effects of prenatal exposure to a "junk food" diet on offspring food preferences and fat deposition can be mitigated by improved nutrition during lactation. *J Dev Orig Health Dis.* 2013;4(5):348–57.
90. Patel MS, Srinivasan M, Laychock SG. Metabolic programming: Role of nutrition in the immediate postnatal life. *J Inherit Metab Dis.* 2009;32(2):218–28.
91. Vogt MC, Paeger L, Hess S, Steculorum SM, Awazawa M, Hampel B, et al. Neonatal insulin action impairs hypothalamic neurocircuit formation in response to maternal high-fat feeding. *Cell.* 2014;156(3):495–509.
92. Wright TM, Fone KCF, Langley-Evans SC, Voigt JPW. Exposure to maternal consumption of cafeteria diet during the lactation period programmes feeding behaviour in the rat. *Int J Dev Neurosci.* 2011;29(8):785–93.

10 Food Reinforcement and Childhood Obesity

*Katelyn A. Carr, Tinuke Oluyomi Daniel,
and Leonard H. Epstein*

CONTENTS

INTRODUCTION

Children are often drawn to sweet and fatty treats such as cake and ice cream. We can imagine a typical child, Johnny, who is willing to walk several blocks for an ice-cream cone. Food reinforcement describes how motivated one is to obtain food and is measured by observing how strongly a behavioral response is supported by the reinforcer, that is, how much work a child will perform to obtain an ice-cream cone. What choice might Johnny make if he could walk to the store to buy ice cream or eat a piece of fruit at home? Would he engage in the extra work for the ice cream, or settle for the easily available fruit? This choice could help us determine how reinforcing ice cream is for Johnny. Increased food reinforcement is associated with obesity in infants [1], in addition to obesity and weight gain in children [2] and adolescents [3]. The strong association between obesity and food reinforcement impacts research in childhood obesity and should be considered in weight-loss programs for children.

DEVELOPMENT OF FOOD REINFORCEMENT

Food reinforcement is innate and present at birth [4] and is biologically preestablished to increase the behaviors it rewards. While some foods require multiple feeding attempts for an infant or child to find them acceptable, sugary and fatty foods do not require prior learning, and only a taste of these foods by infants may develop into preferences that continue into adulthood [5]. Infants show stereotypical and automatic responses to specific tastes, with sweet foods eliciting a smile prior to bottle or breast-feeding [6]. As an infant or toddler, Johnny may have first tasted ice cream, activating primary brain reward centers signaling a pleasant taste and laying the groundwork for his high motivation to eat ice cream. Infants who have an increased bottle sucking rate gain more weight at 12 and 24 months [4]. This research suggests that even in infants, motivation to eat is present at early ages and may represent initial problems with high food reinforcement. While food is intrinsically rewarding, there are individual differences in the motivation to eat, which are characterized by the concept of food reinforcement [7].

MEASURING FOOD REINFORCEMENT IN CHILDREN

Food reinforcement is assessed in the laboratory by allowing children to play a computer game for food [7]. Reinforcing value is the quantitative measure of a person's food reinforcement or their motivation to obtain food [7]. In the game, each mouse click corresponds to a unit of work, and the number of clicks corresponding to a portion of food, or the behavioral cost of the food, can be manipulated. To measure reinforcing value, the work required to earn a portion of food needs to increase in difficulty, so that there are a range of maximum work values to distinguish between individuals with high and low food reinforcement. Each time a portion of food is earned, the work required for the next portion increases in a progressive schedule of reinforcement. In addition to a behavioral task in which children click a button for access to food, a questionnaire has also been developed and used in children [2]. A series of questions asks a child to indicate whether he or she prefers to click a handheld counter for food or for an alternative activity. The alternative activity remains at a constant, low behavioral cost (i.e., 20 clicks), while the preferred food increases in behavioral cost until the child is no longer willing to click for the food and chooses the alternative reinforcer.

The reinforcing value of food can be measured in an absolute sense, with no available alternatives, or in a relative sense, with an available alternative. While candy may be highly reinforcing to children, when ice cream is available, the motivation to eat candy may be low compared with ice cream. While most studies examine the relative reinforcing value of food, there may be important developmental considerations for measuring absolute food reinforcement, that is, if a young child is unable to consider two options simultaneously. Alternative reinforcers can include other types of food or nonfood activities. To measure relative reinforcing value, the alternative has an increasing behavioral cost (i.e., the work for each food portion increases) that matches the target reinforcer. The alternative can also be held at a constant behavioral cost to measure substitution between the food and alternative. Substitution describes a situation in which the behavioral cost of the food becomes too high and the child switches to the lower-costing alternative. Both the reinforcing value of food and the nonfood alternatives are important, as having high food reinforcement may be offset by having high reinforcing value for nonfood alternatives [8], such as children foregoing food and enjoying an alternative, such as reading or puzzles. Substitution may be especially important when trying to help a child decrease their energy intake by switching to lower-calorie, or low energy-dense healthy foods, from their usual intake of high-fat, high-sugar, energy-dense foods.

In our laboratory, research on food reinforcement in 8- to 12-year-old children uses the same procedure as adults [8,9]. A slot machine–type game is played in which various shapes change with a click of the mouse and matching shapes indicate a point is earned. Generally, the relative reinforcing value of food is measured with the available alternative being a nonfood reinforcer, such as reading materials or puzzles [8]. The game is structured to have very low reinforcing value itself, that is, children and adults do not want to play the game without the promise of a reward. This paradigm has recently been extended to preschoolers [10] and 9- to 12-month-old infants [1] by establishing developmentally appropriate measures. When measuring food reinforcement in preschoolers, task novelty may increase responding, so computer monitors are masked and only a small sound indicates that the child earned a portion of food [10]. The only study that has examined food reinforcement in preschool-age children looked at the relative reinforcing value of a target food versus an alternative food [10]; no research has examined the relative reinforcing value of food versus nonfood activities in children this age.

To measure food reinforcement in infants, our laboratory has set up a different series of reinforcement schedules. With older children, we traditionally double the work requirements after each reinforcer is earned; while with infants the work requirements only increase by one response across schedules (e.g., FR1,1,2,2,3,3 … 15,15) to control for the limited attention span and physical abilities of infants [1]. Infants need to first learn the button-reward contingency prior to measuring the reinforcing value of food, which is accomplished by using an audio clip of a cartoon-type sound when they properly click the mouse button. When the infant has learned the contingency, the experimenter then places a plate of food on the table and encourages the child to press the button to receive a food portion. Both the experimenter and the mother will observe the child to determine when the child no longer wants to play for food. The research in infants assesses the absolute reinforcing value of food and an alternative activity (e.g., 10 s blowing bubbles) in separate sessions. Pilot work has been done to assess relative reinforcing value with two concurrently available activities, but has not been successful in developing a task appropriate for infants. A reinforcing ratio can be calculated by determining the proportion of responses for food versus the total responses for both food and the alternative activity.

FOOD REINFORCEMENT IS ASSOCIATED WITH ENERGY INTAKE, OBESITY, AND WEIGHT GAIN IN CHILDREN

Studies in 8- to 12-year-old children have shown greater responding for food in overweight (body mass index [BMI] percentile ≥85) versus nonoverweight children [8], and a significant positive correlation between responding for food and greater BMI z-scores in preschoolers [10]. Higher food reinforcement is also related to greater energy intake in the laboratory for children [8] and preschoolers [10] and usual energy intake in children [11]. Recent research has examined differences in the reinforcing value of snack foods in children with different flavor profiles [11], with sweet-tasting or high-sugar foods having higher food reinforcement than savory or salty-tasting foods [11]. However, the reinforcing value of these different foods was highly correlated and loaded onto one factor in a factor analysis, rather than representing three different values [11].

Research has also shown that food reinforcement is associated with weight gain in children [2] and adolescents [3]. In adults, increased food reinforcement leads to increased energy intake [12], which can produce excess weight gain. In a sample of 7- to 10-year-old children, responses on the food reinforcement questionnaire showed that the higher reinforcing value of food predicted greater weight gain, BMI gain, and fat gain in children after 1 year [2]. This has been replicated in adolescents, as those with higher food reinforcement had greater weight gain over 2 years [3]. Johnny's high food reinforcement has led to overconsumption of food and enough weight gain for him to be considered obese.

FACTORS THAT ACUTELY INFLUENCE FOOD REINFORCEMENT

Sensitization and Satiation

The reinforcing value of a food can change over time, either growing, reducing, or staying the same with the effect depending in part on the dose and individual sensitivities. The increase in the reinforcing value with repeated exposure is called *sensitization*, and may describe why the motivation to eat some foods increases with repeated eating bouts. The opposite of sensitization is *satiation*, or a decrease in reinforcing value with repeated consumption. Temple and colleagues have shown that the reinforcing value of food can increase with repeated exposure to preferred snack foods based on dose and obesity status, as the reinforcing value of larger doses of preferred food sensitizes for obese persons, while the reinforcing value of large doses of preferred foods is reduced with repeated exposures for leaner persons [13,14]. Adults who gained the most weight over a year were also more likely to show a pattern of sensitization to food than those who gained less weight [15]. Research on how trajectories of reinforcing value shift over time is just beginning, but it may help illuminate both how the reinforcing value of food develops and, perhaps, methods of reducing the reinforcing value of food. To date, only snack foods, rather than entrées, have been studied and there is no research on the optimal intervals between eating bouts to enhance either sensitization or satiation.

Restriction and Deprivation

Research shows that food reinforcement and the motivation to eat increases as a function of food deprivation, as individuals are often willing to work harder to obtain food and consume larger quantities of food when hungry [16]. Restriction is a common practice that parents use to control the types of foods their children consume, in addition to the portion sizes of those foods [17]. Usual restriction practices attempt to control intake of high-fat, high-sugar foods, including snacks such as ice cream and potato chips. Fisher and colleagues [17] studied preschool-age children in a day-care setting, and showed that the restriction of a snack food acutely increased energy intake for that food. For 2 weeks, the children were offered two foods during their normal snack time, one of which was offered for 5 min and then removed. The restricted food had greater consumption and more requests for it from the children during the snack period. This research was recently extended, showing that food reinforcement moderated this effect, as children with higher food reinforcement consumed more of the restricted food than other children [18]. Due to Johnny's weight gain, his parents may attempt to control his energy intake by restricting ice cream to the weekend. However, this may only increase his attempts to eat ice cream and how much he wants to eat when it is available.

FACTORS THAT MODERATE THE EFFECT OF FOOD REINFORCEMENT IN CHILDREN

Alternative Reinforcers

Overweight or obese children are more motivated to work for food and have higher response rates in a food-reinforcement task than their lean peers [8]. Not only do obese children respond more for food than lean children, but they also responded less for the nonfood alternative than their lean peers [8]. Typically, when given the option to work to obtain either a preferred or less preferred food, a child will choose to work for the preferred food [19]. However, when the behavioral cost of the preferred food is increased (i.e., when the child has to work harder to obtain the preferred option), he or she opts for the less preferred alternative, which has a lower behavior cost [19]. Problems of high reinforcing value are compounded when alternatives are less reinforcing, which may prevent children from being able to both decrease energy intake *and* find alternative activities to engage in that are unrelated to food. In adults, having alternative reinforcers that are similar to the reinforcing value of food is protective against weight gain over 1 year [20], and a recent study in adolescents has shown that 42.4% of children at risk for weight gain with high food reinforcement did not gain weight over 2 years [3], suggesting some protective factors are present in children that may moderate the impact of food reinforcement on weight changes.

Reinforcement Pathology

While high food reinforcement predicts increased energy intake and BMI [8], individuals with the highest energy intake and BMI often are also low in self-control, specifically in delay of gratification [21]. *Delay of gratification* describes the preference for a choice between smaller immediate rewards and larger delayed rewards, made famous through Walter Mischel's marshmallow task [22]. This task offered children one marshmallow now or two marshmallows later and measured how long the children were able to wait for the larger reward. A more recent and precise approach to measure delay of gratification is the delay discounting task, in which choices are made between small immediate rewards and large delayed rewards across increasing time points [23]. The term *reinforcement pathology* describes an individual with both high food reinforcement and high delay discounting [21,23]. Adults with reinforcement pathology consume more calories during a buffet-style eating task [24] and are more obese [25].

Reinforcement pathology may be especially important to consider in children, as the ability to delay gratification is not fully developed until late in adolescence/early adulthood [26], leading to an increased difficulty with delaying gratification in children [27,28]. In children, difficulty in delaying gratification is associated with weight gain [29,30] and diminished weight-loss treatment success [31]. A recent study examined discordant for weight (i.e., one lean and one obese) adolescent sibling pairs [32], and found that siblings with larger differences in both delay discounting and food reinforcement also had the greatest differences in BMI z-score [32]. This study suggests reinforcement pathology may be a primary behavioral processes contributing to obesity in children, and highlights the importance of considering a child's ability to delay gratification for food as well as their food reinforcement when helping children regulate energy intake.

INTERVENTION APPROACHES TARGETING FOOD REINFORCEMENT

The research reviewed so far paints a clear picture of the association between high food reinforcement, increased energy intake, and weight gain in children and adults. When designing interventions to help children lose weight, food reinforcement, and the processes that influence it, should be an important consideration. Reducing the reinforcing value of unhealthy foods for children with high food reinforcement could facilitate the regulation of energy intake. However, food is a primary reinforcer and present at birth, so reducing food reinforcement is a difficult task. To date, methods for reducing food reinforcement involve targeting behaviors that moderate the influence of food reinforcement on energy intake and BMI. Intervention approaches that manipulate these factors can be incorporated into obesity treatment to reduce the impact of high food reinforcement in obese children.

Manipulating the Behavioral Cost of Food

Children's attempts to gain access to food are related to both their food preferences and the effort required to obtain the various food choices, as constraints on the preferred food encourages a switch to the less preferred alternative [19]. This suggests that increasing the behavioral cost of preferred but unhealthy foods and keeping the behavioral cost of healthy foods low may help to improve food choices. Even if the child still finds the unhealthy food highly reinforcing, manipulating behavioral cost may be one way to attenuate the effect of higher food reinforcement. Previous research shows that fruits and vegetables, in addition to nonfood activities, are acceptable alternatives, or substitutes, when the unhealthy snack increased in behavioral cost [33]. Thus, interventions that require children to work harder to obtain unhealthy foods may help encourage substitution of unhealthy foods with healthier low-calorie foods.

One common practice in weight-loss programs is advising families to use stimulus control [34]. This strategy involves removing or hiding unhealthy foods in the home and making healthy foods and activities more accessible. Families may hide their cookies in a high cabinet and place a bowl of fruit on the kitchen table. Some may even hide their televisions or place their sneakers by the door to make exercise more accessible. These types of strategies involve increasing the behavioral cost of participating in unhealthy behaviors and lessening the behavioral cost of the healthy habits, to encourage participation in these new, healthier behaviors.

Strategies to Lessen Impact of Food Deprivation and Restriction

A necessary component of weight-loss programs is the requirement to maintain a negative energy balance by reducing normal energy intake. This makes it unlikely for a child to be able to regulate their body weight without some periods of food deprivation or restriction of unhealthy but reinforcing foods, which may cause an increase in the motivation to eat [35]. This becomes especially problematic if a child eats unhealthy foods when they are deprived, potentially increasing the reinforcing value of those foods. While short-term food restriction does not increase the reinforcing value of a food [16], restriction increases consumption of the restricted food especially in children who are high in food reinforcement [18].

Interventions may make use of strategic food deprivation and restriction procedures to lessen their acute effects on food reinforcement. For example, allowing children limited but frequent choice of unhealthy foods in a portion-controlled manner may be useful in reducing the effect of food restriction. Reducing periods of food deprivation with healthy low-calorie snacks, or scheduling them to occur prior to a healthy meal, may attenuate the effect of food deprivation of the reinforcing value of food or increase the reinforcing value of healthy foods.

Using Food Variety to Increase Reinforcing Value of Healthy Foods

Food variety increases energy intake [36] and responding for food [37], and may be used to increase the reinforcing value and consumption of healthier foods and reduce the consumption of unhealthy foods. Increasing the variety of healthy low-calorie foods, such as fruits, vegetables and low-fat dairy, while reducing the variety of unhealthy foods that children have access to during snacks and meals could significantly improve their eating habits. Research shows that reducing the variety of unhealthy food increases the efficacy of family-based weight-loss interventions for both children and their parents [38].

Providing Reinforcing Alternatives to Food

The decision to eat is often a choice between food and some other behavioral alternative or reinforcer, and the value of food may depend on the alternatives concurrently available [39]. Providing children with reinforcing nonfood alternatives may reduce choices for food-related activities and energy intake. The availability of cognitively enriching activities (e.g., books, musical instruments) predicted greater success in a weight-loss treatment among children with low food reinforcement [31]. This suggests that finding reinforcing nonfood alternatives may be difficult for obese children as research also shows that obese individuals find food more reinforcing than other pleasurable sedentary activities [40].

Improving Ability to Delay Gratification

Targeting improvements in children's ability to delay gratification may be another way to curb the effect of high food reinforcement. Obese children often have difficulty delaying gratification for food [41], and interventions that incorporate training on how to resist the immediate gratification of food may benefit children attempting weight loss. Mischel and colleagues [22,42,43] have an extensive program of research on techniques to improve children's delay of gratification, including teaching children to divert attention away from tempting foods and imagining the tempting foods as abstract nonconsumable objects (e.g., a scoop of chocolate ice cream resembles mud) [22].

A new technique to help individuals delay gratification, episodic future thinking, has been shown to decrease energy intake and impulsivity in children [44]. Episodic future thinking involves vividly imagining or preexperiencing autobiographical details while mentally simulating a future event [45]. This technique is thought to increase the value of delayed outcomes during decision making [46] and steer individuals toward choices with long-term benefits [47]. The ability to think about episodic future events emerges between 3 and 5 years old [48], so children can be taught to imagine themselves in the future as a technique to delay gratification when they are tempted to make a less healthy food choice.

CONCLUSION

Food reinforcement is an important factor to consider in childhood obesity and interventions to both prevent obesity and help children lose weight. There are multiple factors that impact food reinforcement and these can be used to improve weight-loss interventions. We might help Johnny lose weight by teaching him delay of gratification techniques, offering a large variety of healthy foods, ensuring the availability of nonfood alternative reinforcers in his home that are more accessible than food, and allowing a small number of portion-controlled unhealthy foods. Combining a variety of techniques that target food reinforcement may be especially important to help children regulate their energy intake.

REFERENCES

1. Kong KL, Feda DM, Eiden RD, Epstein LH. Origins of food reinforcement in infants. *The American Journal of Clinical Nutrition.* 2015;101(3):515–22.
2. Hill C, Saxton J, Webber L, Blundell J, Wardle J. The relative reinforcing value of food predicts weight gain in a longitudinal study of 7–10-y-old children. *The American Journal of Clinical Nutrition.* 2009;90(2):276–81.
3. Epstein LH, Yokum S, Feda DM, Stice E. Food reinforcement and parental obesity predict future weight gain in non-obese adolescents. *Appetite.* 2014;82:138–42.
4. Stunkard AJ, Berkowitz RI, Schoeller D, Maislin G, Stallings VA. Predictors of body size in the first 2 years of life: A high-risk study of human obesity. *International Journal of Obesity and Related Metabolic Disorders.* 2004;28(4):503–13.
5. Nicklaus S, Boggio V, Chabanet C, Issanchou S. A prospective study of food preferences in childhood. *Food Quality and Preference.* 2004;15:805–18.
6. Steiner JE, Glaser D, Hawilo ME, Berridge KC. Comparative expression of hedonic impact: Affective reactions to taste by human infants and other primates. *Neuroscience and Biobehavioral Reviews.* 2001;25(1):53–74.
7. Epstein LH, Leddy JJ, Temple JL, Faith MS. Food reinforcement and eating: A multilevel analysis. *Psychological Bulletin.* 2007;133(5):884–906.
8. Temple JL, Legierski CM, Giacomelli AM, Salvy S-J, Epstein LH. Overweight children find food more reinforcing and consume more energy than do nonoverweight children. *The American Journal of Clinical Nutrition.* 2008;87(5):1121–7.
9. Epstein LH, Wright SM, Paluch RA, Leddy J, Hawk LW, Jaroni JL, et al. Food hedonics and reinforcement as determinants of laboratory food intake in smokers. *Physiology & Behavior.* 2004;81(3):511–7.
10. Rollins BY, Loken E, Savage JS, Birch LL. Measurement of food reinforcement in preschool children: Associations with food intake, BMI, and reward sensitivity. *Appetite.* 2014;72:21–7.
11. Epstein LH, Carr KA, Scheid JL, Gebre E, O'Brien A, Paluch RA, et al. Taste and food reinforcement in non-overweight youth. *Appetite.* 2015;91:226–32.
12. Epstein LH, Carr KA, Lin H, Fletcher KD, Roemmich JN. Usual energy intake mediates the relationship between food reinforcement and BMI. *Obesity (Silver Spring).* 2012;20(9):1815–9.
13. Temple JL, Bulkley A, Badawy R, Krause N, McCann S, Epstein LH. Differential effects of daily snack food intake on food reinforcement in obese and non-obese women. *The American Journal of Clinical Nutrition.* 2009;90(2):304–13.
14. Clark EN, Dewey AM, Temple JL. Effects of daily snack food intake on food reinforcement depend on body mass index and energy density. *The American Journal of Clinical Nutrition.* 2010;91(2):300–8.
15. Temple JL. Factors that influence the reinforcing value of foods and beverages. *Physiology & Behavior.* 2014;136:97–103.
16. Raynor HA, Epstein LH. The relative-reinforcing value of food under differing levels of food deprivation and restriction. *Appetite.* 2003;40(1):15–24.
17. Fisher JO, Birch LL. Restricting access to palatable foods affects children's behavioral response, food selection, and intake. *The American Journal of Clinical Nutrition.* 1999;69(6):1264–72.
18. Rollins BY, Loken E, Savage JS, Birch LL. Effects of restriction on children's intake differ by child temperament, food reinforcement, and parent's chronic use of restriction. *Appetite.* 2014;73:31–9.
19. Smith JA, Epstein LH. Behavioral economic analysis of food choice in obese children. *Appetite.* 1991;17(2):91–5.
20. Carr KA, Lin H, Fletcher KD, Epstein LH. Food reinforcement, dietary disinhibition and weight gain in nonobese adults. *Obesity (Silver Spring).* 2014;22(1):254–9.
21. Carr KA, Daniel TO, Lin H, Epstein LH. Reinforcement pathology and obesity. *Current Drug Abuse Reviews.* 2011;4(3):190–6.
22. Mischel W, Shoda Y, Rodriguez ML. Delay of gratification in children. *Science.* 1989;244(4907):933–8.
23. Epstein LH, Salvy S-J, Carr KA, Dearing KK, Bickel WK. Food reinforcement, delay discounting and obesity. *Physiology & Behavior.* 2010;100(5):438–45.

24. Rollins BY, Dearing KK, Epstein LH. Delay discounting moderates the effect of food reinforcement on energy intake among non-obese women. *Appetite*. 2010;55(3):420–5.

25. Epstein LH, Jankowiak N, Fletcher KD, Carr KA, Nederkoorn C, Raynor HA, et al. Women who are motivated to eat and discount the future are more obese. *Obesity (Silver Spring)*. 2014;22(6):1394–9.

26. Blakemore SJ, Choudhury S. Development of the adolescent brain: Implications for executive function and social cognition. *Journal of Child Psychology and Psychiatry*. 2006;47(3–4):296–312.

27. Green L, Fry AF, Myerson J. Discounting of delayed rewards: A life-span comparison. *Psychological Science*. 1994;5(1):33–6.

28. Steinberg L, Graham S, O'Brien L, Woolard J, Cauffman E, Banich M. Age differences in future orientation and delay discounting. *Child Development*. 2009;80:28–44.

29. Francis LA, Susman EJ. Self-regulation and rapid weight gain in children from age 3 to 12 years. *Archives of Pediatric and Adolescent Medicine*. 2009;163(4):297–302.

30. Seeyave DM, Coleman S, Appugliese D, Corwyn RF, Bradley RH, Davidson NS, et al. Ability to delay gratification at age 4 years and risk of overweight at age 11 years. *Archives of Pediatric and Adolescent Medicine*. 2009;163(4):303–8.

31. Best JR, Theim KR, Gredysa DM, Stein RI, Welch RR, Saelens BE, et al. Behavioral economic predictors of overweight children's weight loss. *Journal of Consulting and Clinical Psychology*. 2012;80(6):1086–96.

32. Feda DM, Roemmich JN, Roberts A, Epstein LH. Food reinforcement and delay discounting in zBMI-discordant siblings. *Appetite*. 2015;85:185–9.

33. Goldfield GS, Epstein LH. Can fruits and vegetables and activities substitute for snack foods? *Health Psychology*. 2002;21(3):299–303.

34. Epstein LH, Paluch RA, Kilanowski CK, Raynor HA. The effect of reinforcement or stimulus control to reduce sedentary behavior in the treatment of pediatric obesity. *Health Psychology*. 2004;23(4):371–80.

35. Epstein LH, Truesdale R, Wojcik A, Paluch RA, Raynor HA. Effects of deprivation on hedonics and reinforcing value of food. *Physiology & Behavior*. 2003;78(2):221–7.

36. Epstein LH, Robinson JL, Temple JL, Roemmich JN, Marusewski AL, Nadbrzuch RL. Variety influences habituation of motivated behavior for food and energy intake in children. *The American Journal of Clinical Nutrition*. 2009;89(3):746–54.

37. Temple JL, Giacomelli AM, Roemmich JN, Epstein LH. Dietary variety impairs habituation in children. *Health Psychology*. 2008;27(Suppl 1):S10–9.

38. Epstein LH, Kilanowski C, Paluch RA, Raynor H, Daniel TO. Reducing variety enhances effectiveness of family-based treatment for pediatric obesity. *Eating Behaviors*. 2015;17:140–3.

39. Epstein LH, Leddy JJ. Food reinforcement. *Appetite*. 2006;46:22–5.

40. Saelens BE, Epstein LH. Reinforcing value of food in obese and non-obese women. *Appetite*. 1996;27(1):41–50.

41. Bonato DP, Boland FJ. Delay of gratification in obese children. *Addictive Behaviors*. 1983;8(1):71–4.

42. Schlam TR, Wilson NL, Shoda Y, Mischel W, Ayduk O. Preschoolers' delay of gratification predicts their body mass 30 years later. *Journal of Pediatrics*. 2013;162(1):90–3.

43. Eigsti IM, Zayas V, Mischel W, Shoda Y, Ayduk O, Dadlani MB, et al. Predicting cognitive control from preschool to late adolescence and young adulthood. *Psychological Science*. 2006;17(6):478–84.

44. Daniel TO, Said M, Stanton CM, Epstein LH. Episodic future thinking reduces delay discounting and energy intake in children. *Eating Behaviors*. 2015;18:20–4.

45. Atance CM, O'Neill DK. Episodic future thinking. *Trends in Cognitive Sciences*. 2001;5(12):533–9.

46. Benoit RG, Gilbert SJ, Burgess PW. A neural mechanism mediating the impact of episodic prospection on farsighted decisions. *Journal of Neuroscience*. 2011;31(18):6771–9.

47. Boyer P. Evolutionary economics of mental time travel? *Trends in Cognitive Sciences*. 2008;12(6):219–24.

48. Atance CM. Future thinking in young children. *Current Directions in Psychological Science*. 2008;17(4):295–8.

11 Breast-Feeding and Infant Obesity

David A. Fields

CONTENTS

INTRODUCTION

Understanding childhood obesity is of the utmost importance today, given its precipitous, progressive, and persistent upward trajectory starting at a young age. More than 10% of 6–23-month-olds and 20% of 2–5-year-olds are either overweight or obese, with ≈70% remaining so in adulthood [1,2]. Due to the recalcitrant nature of obesity, prevention rather than treatment is key, with breast-feeding identified as a cornerstone of any prevention program. This is supported by the recommendation from a presidential task force of breast-feeding as a strategy to reduce pediatric obesity [3]. Universal breast-feeding is also supported by the Centers for Disease Control and Prevention [4], the World Health Organization [5], the American Academy of Pediatrics [6], and the American College of Obstetricians and Gynecologists [7], to name just a few. These recommendations reflect findings from seven systematic review/meta-analyses conducted using 81 studies spanning from 1970 to 2010 [5,8–13]. A review performed in 2015 of the best available evidence observed that results from all available meta-analyses indicated a reduction of 12%–24% in the prevalence of overweight/obesity in children who were breast-fed compared with those who were not breast-fed (odds ratios ranging from 0.76 to 0.88) [13]. Further, the American Academy of Pediatrics stated there is a "15%–30% reduction in adolescent and adult obesity rates if breast-feeding occurred during infancy compared with no breast-feeding" [6].

This chapter will focus solely on a single question: Is breast-feeding protective against obesity? However, it would be remiss to exclude the far-reaching benefits of breast-feeding beyond that of obesity prevention. Probative data exist showing clear associations between breast-feeding and reductions in the incidences of respiratory, allergen, gastrointestinal, and infectious-related morbidity in infancy, saying nothing of the effects of bonding and nurturing between mother and infant, and at this time it is still recommended as the preferred feeding choice of mothers [14–17]. Furthermore, a recent review reported that breast-feeding provides protection from future diabetes risk (34% reduction) while modestly improving IQ (2.2–3.5 points) [5,18,19]. This chapter will cover four broad topics that currently exist in the breast-feeding literature. The first area discussed is some of the current debate on how the literature was gathered and interpreted to come to the recommendation that breast-feeding reduces obesity. A second area will discuss the presence of nonnutritive molecules in breast milk. Building on this topic, both animal and human studies are presented that demonstrate a mechanism of action for nonnutritive molecules exerting a harmful outcome in offspring. Lastly, new and innovative study designs are discussed that advance the field forward by overcoming some of the inherent problems in conducting true randomized controlled studies in humans.

DEBATE AS TO WHETHER BREAST-FEEDING PROTECTS AGAINST OBESITY

HANDLING OF DATA AND ADEQUATE CONSIDERATION FOR PUTATIVE CONFOUNDERS

Given the biological plausibility that breast-feeding protects against pediatric obesity, along with the preponderance of the evidence and near-universal belief that breast-feeding has this effect, it would appear that the case for breast-feeding protecting against pediatric obesity risk is resolved. However, some have begun to challenge not only the recommendations but also the very evidence on which these recommendations were made [20–23]. In 2008, a critical assessment of the interpretation and handling of the data in the World Health Organization's 2007 report on "evidence of the long-term effects of breast-feeding: systematic reviews and meta-analysis" with respect to obesity was published [23]. The authors stated "while breast-feeding may have benefits beyond any putative protection against obesity, and benefits of breast-feeding most likely outweigh any harms, any statement that a strong, clear and consistent body of evidence shows that breast-feeding causally reduces the risk of overweight or obesity is unwarranted at this time" [23]. A major criticism made was in the selection or exclusion of data that may have led to an artificial inflation in the observed association between breast-feeding and reduced obesity risk. In fact, the authors brought into question the "reliability and reasonableness of the data extraction process itself" and went as far as to suggest that an independent assessment be performed.

Another issue raised by the authors is the lack of appropriate control of presumed confounders, with maternal body mass index (BMI) being especially relevant [13,20,23]. The Department of Maternal, Newborn, Child and Adolescent Health of the World Health Organization [5] reviewed the role of breast-feeding in obesity prevention, examining 71 separate studies providing 75 different estimates on the associations between breast-feeding and the risk of becoming overweight/obese. It appears that maternal BMI was collected and considered for study analyses in approximately 65% of the studies, while in the remaining studies, maternal BMI was either not collected, ambiguously obtained, or not considered at all in the analyses. The failure to consider maternal BMI and/or poor collection (i.e., retrospectively relying upon maternal recall or poor description in the methodological design) may partly explain the large range in the individual study odds ratios of 0.28 (95% CI: 0.09; 0.84) to 1.83 (95% CI: 0.53; 6.28). Failure to control for maternal BMI among breast-feeding mothers may also explain why some have concluded that there is no causal link between the duration of breast-feeding and childhood overweight/obesity, or that, at best, breast-feeding provides a modest level of protection [20–22,24]. Yet another potential confounder that is underappreciated and not commonly reported is the "length" of time that the breast-feeding took place. Oftentimes, breast-feeding is handled as a dichotomous variable, a yes or no proposition, with no regard to the length of time that the child was breast-fed. Interesting results by O'Tierney, which were part of the Helsinki Birth Cohort Study ($n = 12{,}345$), reported that infants who either breast-fed for <2 months or >8 months had the highest BMI and body fat at 60 years of age [25]. Both of the confounders presented, maternal BMI and length of breast-feeding, only highlight the difficulty and idiosyncratic complexities in categorizing a seemingly simple question, "did you breast-feed your child?"

EPIDEMIOLOGICAL EVIDENCE AGAINST BREAST-FEEDING'S BENEFICENCE

Epidemiological data have also brought into question the role of breast-feeding in reducing obesity. The Promotion of Breast-feeding Intervention Trial (PROBIT) is the largest randomized trial ever conducted with the expressed purpose of understanding the role that breast-feeding plays in reducing obesity and blood pressure [26]. The cluster-randomized trial for breast-feeding promotion was conducted in 31 Belarusian hospitals ($n = 17,046$). Given that it is unethical to randomize infants to breast-feeding or formula, the authors employed a "cluster-randomized" study design where an entire hospital/clinic was exposed to the intervention based on the Baby-Friendly Hospital Initiative, which supports and promotes breast-feeding [26]. What is important to keep in mind is that the "Baby-Friendly Initiative" is not to increase initiation of breast-feeding, but rather to support the continued practice and duration of breast-feeding in mothers who choose to initiate breast-feeding. Infants from both groups (control and experimental) were followed longitudinally with serial weight, waist/hip circumferences, and tricep/subscapular skinfolds (measures of body composition) taken over the first 6 years of life (81% were followed to their sixth birthday). The authors reported no effect on BMI or adiposity (reduction in skinfold thickness) between the groups.

PRESENCE OF NONNUTRITIVE MOLECULES IN BREAST MILK

A logical first question to ask to help understand the purported decrease in obesity risk in breast-fed infants is what evidence exists for biological plausibility? It was long thought that the primary function of breast milk was the delivery of macronutrients (protein, fat, and carbohydrates) for sustenance and immunologic primers for protection against infection and that the compositional makeup of breast milk was generally homogenous [27]. It is only now being recognized that human breast milk is a biological product generated by women with markedly varying genotypes, phenotypes, and diets, and is therefore highly variable in composition. Failure to appreciate the heterogeneity of breast milk has led to substantial gaps in our understanding, especially with regard to the effect of maternal habitus (weight and adiposity) on the composition of her breast milk, which in turn affects her infants' health. Starting in the mid-2000s, data began to emerge that showed that breast milk is composed of a myriad of appetite-regulating hormones (leptin, ghrelin, and peptide YY), cytokines (IL-6, IL-10, TNF-α), growth factors (IGF-1 and VEGF), and metabolic hormones (adiponectin and resistin) [27–29]. In all likelihood, these "analytes" are crucial players in setting early metabolism and appetite regulation, with leptin and adiponectin the most understood. In humans, breast milk leptin concentration is inversely related with weight-for-length z-scores, BMI-for-age z-scores, and delta BMI in the first month of life [30,31], while adiponectin levels are inversely related with weight-for-height and BMI in the first 2 years of life [32,33]. Animal models have demonstrated a cause and effect relationship when oral leptin supplementation is given to lactating dams, with their offspring having protection against overweight/obesity later in life [34]. What is especially important to keep in mind is the potential role that breast milk cytokines, chemokines, and metabolic hormones have on future obesity risk. We do not yet know the exact role and function of all these bioactive nonnutritive substances, though there is support for an impactful and significant role.

ASSOCIATIONS BETWEEN MATERNAL BMI AND NONNUTRITIVE MOLECULES IN BREAST MILK

A review by Andreas and colleagues on the effects of maternal BMI on bioactive nonnutritive substances (e.g., insulin, glucose, leptin, adiponectin, ghrelin, resistin, obestatin, peptide YY, and glucagon-like peptide 1) in breast milk sheds light on the importance of maternal BMI when examining associations between breast-feeding and obesity risk [35]. After taking into account the best available evidence, they found a consistent relationship between maternal BMI and breast milk leptin; however, there was no clear evidence supporting an association with breast milk adiponectin, ghrelin, insulin, peptide YY, and resistin [35]. Admittedly, most of the studies included were "proof of concept" studies, lacking rigorous study design, with inadequate sample size, poor to no standardization of sampling collection (whole milk expressions vs. fore milk vs. hind milk, time of day), and varying immunoassay methodologies (radioimmunoassay [RIA] vs. enzyme-linked immunosorbent assay [ELISA]) to determine breast milk hormone concentration levels. The review only highlights a need for more definitive well-designed studies in a field ripe for investigation. Indeed, another review investigating the biological determinants of future obesity risk and their association with mode of feeding (breast vs. formula) in infancy concluded that, "in all likelihood the mechanisms are complex and involve synergistic interactions between endocrine effects and factors that alter both inflammatory and oxidative stress in the infant" [36]. Though emergent, the role that maternal BMI has on the compositional makeup of nonnutritive molecules in breast milk is just now being appreciated, with little to nothing known of its associations with infant obesity risk.

A new and exciting component of breast milk beyond that of the molecules listed is human milk oligosaccharides (HMOs). HMOs are unconjugated glycans that serve as prebiotics and the metabolic substrate for the microbiota [37]. In a small proof of principle study, Alderete and colleagues reported at 6 months a 1 µg/mL increase in fucosyl-di sialyl lacto-N-hexaose, and lacto-N-neotetraose was associated with 0.04% higher ($p = .03$) and 0.03% lower ($p < .01$) whole body fat (by dual-energy x-ray absorptiometry) [38]. Though emergent, these findings support the hypothesis that differences in HMO composition in breast milk play a significant role in early growth and body composition.

PROPOSED MECHANISMS

ANIMAL STUDIES

Interesting data exist in both animal cross-fostering studies and a uniquely designed human study suggesting the importance of maternal BMI and/or metabolic health for healthy and appropriate breast milk composition. Both lines of study provide windows into the future that will elucidate important mechanistic pathways that are yet to be discovered. For example, these animal studies allow manipulations not ethically possible or feasible in human studies, and are often essential to understand the basic underlying mechanisms of treatments such as breast-feeding. Using a cross-fostering design, Gorski and colleagues examined the effects of the postnatal environment (i.e., breast-feeding) on offspring obesity and insulin resistance using a diet-induced obesity rat model [39]. In the obese diet–induced dams, breast milk insulin at 7 days was significantly higher (128%) compared with the diet-resistant dams, though no differences were observed in breast milk leptin. Interestingly, pups from obesity-prone dams cross-fostered to obesity-resistant dams remained obese in adulthood but improved their insulin sensitivity, while pups from obesity-resistant dams cross-fostered to obesity-prone dams had increased adiposity and decreased insulin sensitivity in adulthood. These findings are suggestive that maternal obesity affects the compositional makeup of a mother's breast milk, which in turn affects her offspring's obesity and overall metabolic health. In another cross-fostering study design using a mouse model, obese-prone dams had four times as much breast milk leptin as nonobese dams at 18 days [40]. Genetically fixed obese pups fostered to obese dams were 26% heavier than obese pups fostered to nonobese dams. Similarly, nonobese pups fostered to obese dams were 22% heavier than nonobese pups fostered to nonobese dams [40]. Taken together, these cross-fostering studies provide good evidence that breast milk composition differs by the obesity status of the mother, and pups, either obese prone or obese resistant, are significantly heavier if fostered to an obese prone mother versus a nonobese or obese-resistant dam.

HUMAN STUDIES

Several human studies have reported increased breast milk glucose and insulin concentrations from diabetic mothers compared with nondiabetic mothers [41,42], providing an opportunity to test the effects of breast milk composition on infant outcomes, namely, by comparing diabetic mothers who breast-fed with those who formula fed. As previously stated, it would be unethical to randomize human offspring to either breast-feeding or formula; however, an ingenious study design provided insight into the association between breast-feeding and infant obesity using a pseudorandomized study design [43]. Plagemann and colleagues enrolled 112 diabetic mothers ($n = 29$ who had gestational diabetes; $n = 83$ who had type 1 diabetes) prospectively and followed them for the first week of their infant's life [43]. For mothers who could not breast-feed, or stopped within the first week of life, their infant was given banked nondiabetic milk. Of note, the banked milk was from "nondiabetic" mothers (no mention was reported on maternal BMI). The findings were startling: a significantly positive correlation was observed between the volume of breast milk ingested (i.e., milk from their diabetic mother) and the risk of being overweight at 2 years of age (odds ratios 2.47; 95% CI: 1.25; 4.87). This study demonstrates that breast milk from diabetic mothers may increase the risk of obesity and diabetes later in life. Though far from conclusive, this study suggests that all breast milk is not the same and that maternal habitus/metabolic health plays a crucial role in determining the "quality" of her breast milk.

INNOVATIVE STUDY DESIGNS

Some beliefs, practices, dogmas, and ideologies are thought of so highly that they become sacrosanct, thus allowing *ipse dixit* to dominate the discussion rather than letting empirically driven, scientifically derived evidence be the prevailing driver [44]. Unfortunately, the claim that breast-feeding *causes* a reduction in obesity risk has entered the lexicon as proved by science and is factually untouchable. This persistent and impassioned belief has recently been called a myth by some and contemptuously challenged by others [13,20–22,45–47]. The proposition that "mothers who breast-feed prevent obesity in their offspring" must be based on the evidence, with more weight given to randomized controlled clinical trials than observational studies, no matter how well designed. For practical, ethical, and theoretical reasons it is impossible to have true randomization in breast-feeding studies, with few observational studies controlling for known confounders by maintaining tight controls. To date, almost all breast-feeding studies are observational in nature without controls and are purely associational in nature. This leads to a fallacy of presumption known as *cum hoc*, where it is assumed that because two events occur together (breast-feeding and less obesity), they must be causally related. Randomized controlled studies are essential for causal inference, but in the realm of breast-feeding and human obesity, are nigh impossible to carry out. The two following examples are forward thinking and advance the field forward.

Most breast-feeding studies have a multitude of methodological shortcomings that are either hard to control or impossible to eliminate. Colen and Ramey employed a unique sibling comparison using 25 years' worth of data from the National Longitudinal Survey of Youth [45]. Three models were used for analysis: Model 1 used the complete sample (between families), Model 2 included data only within siblings, and Model 3 examined discordant siblings (one sibling was breast-fed while the other sibling was formula fed). The findings were intriguing: Model 1 indicated that breast-fed children were protected not only for weight (i.e., lower) but other measured outcomes (asthma, hyperactivity, parental attachment, behavioral compliance, math and reading scores, vocabulary, intelligence, and scholastic competence). Model 2 showed similar results; however, Model 3 indicated that breast-fed siblings had, on average, only a 0.14 kg/m² smaller BMI than their formula-fed sibling. Colen et al. (2014) concluded that many of the "purported benefits attributed to breastfeeding, chiefly obesity prevention, may be primarily due to selection pressures into infant feeding practices along key demographic characteristics, such as ethnicity, socioeconomic status, education, and other yet identified confounders" [45]. This is an important consideration when understanding and interpreting the results of studies currently in the field.

More creative study designs that employ both animal and human designs are needed, such as packet randomized experiments (PREs), a framework that improves causal inference when randomization is not possible [48]. Briefly, in a PRE using an animal model (e.g., mice) of obesity, mice would be randomized to human breast milk obtained from breast-feeding mothers of varying physiological (adiposity and diabetes), sociological (education, rural vs. urban, socioeconomic), and genetic confounders that human-correlational studies (which currently dominate the literature) either cannot remove or are almost impossible to control. By randomizing mice to human milk, three sources of confounding present in human studies can be removed: (a) external/environment factors (e.g., rural vs. urban, smoking vs. none, high crime neighborhoods), (b) genetics (all mice have the same mother), and (c) maternal factors (e.g., diet, obesity status, diabetes). At this time, unique study designs that go beyond that of simple associations such as PREs are badly needed if we are to understand how maternal BMI affects human breast milk, which in turn affects her offspring. The field in general sorely needs "outside the box thinking" to resolve an important and pressing health issue.

CONCLUSIONS

This chapter focused solely on the evidence investigating the role of breast-feeding in reducing overweight/obesity risk in pediatric populations. Current evidence linking breast-feeding to reduced risk for developing obesity is inconclusive at this time. In fact, when taking into account the obesity status of the mother, data from both animal and human studies have demonstrated increased obesity in offspring nursed from either obese or diabetic mothers. Though a controversial topic, we must demand the highest scientific evidence and rigor if we are to advance the field and ultimately improve the lives of children specifically, and public health as a whole. Important questions we need to ask ourselves are where do we go from here, and what are the key issues moving forward. The most pressing issue is increasing the number of mechanistic-based studies in the science of lactation and its association with infant outcomes, while understanding the role for the maternal habitus (obesity and metabolic status). The underlying principles are important and allow for proper context (e.g., ethnicity, duration, mixed feeding) in understanding the beneficial role that breast-feeding has in obesity prevention. By understanding this role, breast-feeding can be used as a vehicle for improved health in the offspring.

ACKNOWLEDGMENTS

The author extends gratitude to Dr Richard Anderson and Dr Gregory Pavela for providing critical feedback and thoughtful input to this chapter.

REFERENCES

1. Reilly JJ. Obesity in childhood and adolescence: Evidence based clinical and public health perspectives. *Postgrad Med J.* 2006;82(969):429–37.
2. Mei Z, Ogden CL, Flegal KM, Grummer-Strawn LM. Comparison of the prevalence of shortness, underweight, and overweight among US children aged 0 to 59 months by using the CDC 2000 and the WHO 2006 growth charts. *J Pediatr.* 2008;153(5):622–8.
3. Obesity WHTFoC. *Solving the Challenge of Childhood Obesity Within a Generation.* Washington, DC: Executive office of the President of the United States, 2010.
4. CDC. Breastfeeding report card United States/2014. Atlanta, GA, 2014, p. 8.
5. Horta BL, Victora CG. *Long-Term Effects of Breastfeeding: A Systematic Review.* WHO Press, WHO, Geneva, Switzerland, 2013.
6. Section on breastfeeding: Breastfeeding and the use of human milk. *Pediatrics.* 2012;129(3):e827–41.
7. American Congress of Obstetricians and Gynecologists. ACOG Committee Opinion No. 361: Breastfeeding: Maternal and infant aspects. *Obstet Gynecol.* 2007;109(2 Pt 1):479–80.
8. Harder T, Bergmann R, Kallischnigg G, Plagemann A. Duration of breastfeeding and risk of overweight: A meta-analysis. *Am J Epidemiol.* 2005;162(5):397–403.

9. Horta B, Bahl R, Martines J, Victora C. *Evidence of the Long-Term Effects of Breastfeeding: Systematic Reviews and Meta-Analysis*. Geneva, Switzerland: WHO, Geneva, Switzerland, 2007.

10. Weng SF, Redsell SA, Swift JA, Yang M, Glazebrook CP. Systematic review and meta-analyses of risk factors for childhood overweight identifiable during infancy. *Arch Dis Child*. 2012;97(12):1019–26.

11. Owen CG, Martin RM, Whincup PH, Smith GD, Cook DG. Effect of infant feeding on the risk of obesity across the life course: A quantitative review of published evidence. *Pediatrics*. 2005;115(5):1367–77.

12. Arenz S, Ruckerl R, Koletzko B, von Kries R. Breast-feeding and childhood obesity: A systematic review. *Int J Obes Relat Metab Disord*. 2004;28(10):1247–56.

13. Woo JG, Martin LJ. Does breastfeeding protect against childhood obesity? Moving beyond observational evidence. *Curr Obes Rep*. 2015;4(2):207–16.

14. Kramer MS, Kakuma R. The optimal duration of exclusive breastfeeding: A systematic review. *Adv Exp Med Biol*. 2004;554:63–77.

15. Quigley MA, Kelly YJ, Sacker A. Breastfeeding and hospitalization for diarrheal and respiratory infection in the United Kingdom Millennium Cohort Study. *Pediatrics*. 2007;119(4):e837–42.

16. Effect of breastfeeding on infant and child mortality due to infectious diseases in less developed countries: A pooled analysis. WHO Collaborative Study Team on the Role of Breastfeeding on the Prevention of Infant Mortality. *Lancet*. 2000;355(9202):451–5.

17. Duijts L, Jaddoe VW, Hofman A, Moll HA. Prolonged and exclusive breastfeeding reduces the risk of infectious diseases in infancy. *Pediatrics*. 2010;126(1):e18–25.

18. Lucas A, Morley R. Does early nutrition in infants born before term programme later blood pressure? *BMJ*. 1994;309(6950):304–8.

19. Lucas A, Morley R, Cole TJ, Lister G, Leeson-Payne C. Breast milk and subsequent intelligence quotient in children born preterm. *Lancet*. 1992;339(8788):261–4.

20. Smithers LG, Kramer MS, Lynch JW. Effects of breastfeeding on obesity and intelligence: Causal insights from different study designs. *JAMA Pediatr*. 2015;169(8):707–8.

21. Jiang M, Foster EM. Duration of breastfeeding and childhood obesity: A generalized propensity score approach. *Health Serv Res*. 2013;48(2 Pt 1):628–51.

22. Gillman MW. Commentary: Breastfeeding and obesity—The 2011 Scorecard. *Int J Epidemiol*. 2011;40(3):681–4.

23. Cope MB, Allison DB. Critical review of the World Health Organization's (WHO) 2007 report on "evidence of the long-term effects of breastfeeding: Systematic reviews and meta-analysis" with respect to obesity. *Obes Rev*. 2008;9(6):594–605.

24. Casazza K, Fernandez JR, Allison DB. Modest protective effects of breast-feeding on obesity. *Nutr Today*. 2012;47(1):33–8.

25. O'Tierney PF, Barker DJ, Osmond C, Kajantie E, Eriksson JG. Duration of breast-feeding and adiposity in adult life. *J Nutr*. 2009;139(2):422S–5S.

26. Kramer MS, Matush L, Vanilovich I, Platt RW, Bogdanovich N, Sevkovskaya Z, et al. Effects of prolonged and exclusive breastfeeding on child height, weight, adiposity, and blood pressure at age 6.5 y: Evidence from a large randomized trial. *Am J Clin Nutr*. 2007;86(6):1717–21.

27. Ballard O, Morrow AL. Human milk composition: Nutrients and bioactive factors. *Pediatr Clin North Am*. 2013;60(1):49–74.

28. Savino F, Sorrenti M, Benetti S, Lupica MM, Liguori SA, Oggero R. Resistin and leptin in breast milk and infants in early life. *Early Hum Dev*. 2012;88(10):779–82.

29. Savino F, Liguori SA, Sorrenti M, Fissore MF, Oggero R. Breast milk hormones and regulation of glucose homeostasis. *Int J Pediatr*. 2011;2011:803985.

30. Fields DA, Demerath EW. Relationship of insulin, glucose, leptin, IL-6 and TNF-alpha in human breast milk with infant growth and body composition. *Pediatr Obes*. 2012;7(4):304–12.

31. Doneray H, Orbak Z, Yildiz L. The relationship between breast milk leptin and neonatal weight gain. *Acta Paediatr*. 2009;98(4):643–7.

32. Woo JG, Guerrero ML, Altaye M, Ruiz-Palacios GM, Martin LJ, Dubert-Ferrandon A, et al. Human milk adiponectin is associated with infant growth in two independent cohorts. *Breastfeed Med*. 2009;4(2):101–9.

33. Newburg DS, Woo JG, Morrow AL. Characteristics and potential functions of human milk adiponectin. *J Pediatr*. 2010;156(2 Suppl):S41–6.

34. Palou A, Pico C. Leptin intake during lactation prevents obesity and affects food intake and food preferences in later life. *Appetite*. 2009;52(1):249–52.

35. Andreas NJ, Hyde MJ, Gale C, Parkinson JR, Jeffries S, Holmes E, et al. Effect of maternal body mass index on hormones in breast milk: A systematic review. *PLoS One*. 2014;9(12):e115043.

36. Young BE, Johnson SL, Krebs NF. Biological determinants linking infant weight gain and child obesity: Current knowledge and future directions. *Adv Nutr.* 2012;3(5):675–86.

37. Bode L. Human milk oligosaccharides: Every baby needs a sugar mama. *Glycobiology.* 2012;22(9):1147–62.

38. Alderete TL, Autran C, Brekke BE, Knight R, Bode L, Goran MI, et al. Associations between human milk oligosaccharides and infant body composition in the first 6 mo of life. *Am J Clin Nutr.* 2015;102(6):1381–8.

39. Gorski JN, Dunn-Meynell AA, Hartman TG, Levin BE. Postnatal environment overrides genetic and prenatal factors influencing offspring obesity and insulin resistance. *Am J Physiol Regul Integr Comp Physiol.* 2006;291(3):R768–78.

40. Reifsnyder PC, Churchill G, Leiter EH. Maternal environment and genotype interact to establish diabesity in mice. *Genome Res.* 2000;10(10):1568–78.

41. Butte NF, Garza C, Burr R, Goldman AS, Kennedy K, Kitzmiller JL. Milk composition of insulin-dependent diabetic women. *J Pediatr Gastroenterol Nutr.* 1987;6(6):936–41.

42. Jovanovic-Peterson L, Fuhrmann K, Hedden K, Walker L, Peterson CM. Maternal milk and plasma glucose and insulin levels: Studies in normal and diabetic subjects. *J Am Coll Nutr.* 1989;8(2):125–31.

43. Plagemann A, Harder T, Franke K, Kohlhoff R. Long-term impact of neonatal breast-feeding on body weight and glucose tolerance in children of diabetic mothers. *Diabetes Care.* 2002;25(1):16–22.

44. Casazza K, Brown A, Astrup A, Bertz F, Baum C, Brown MB, et al. Weighing the evidence of common beliefs in obesity research. *Crit Rev Food Sci Nutr.* 2015;55(14):2014–53.

45. Colen CG, Ramey DM. Is breast truly best? Estimating the effects of breastfeeding on long-term child health and wellbeing in the United States using sibling comparisons. *Soc Sci Med.* 2014;109C:55–65.

46. Casazza K, Fontaine KR, Astrup A, Birch LL, Brown AW, Bohan Brown MM, et al. Myths, presumptions, and facts about obesity. *N Engl J Med.* 2013;368(5):446–54.

47. Cope MB, Allison DB. White hat bias: Examples of its presence in obesity research and a call for renewed commitment to faithfulness in research reporting. *Int J Obes* (Lond). 2010;34(1):84–8; discussion 3.

48. Pavela G, Wiener H, Fontaine KR, Fields DA, Voss JD, Allison DB. Packet randomized experiments for eliminating classes of confounders. *Eur J Clin Invest.* 2015;45(1):45–55.

Section III

Individual and Environmental
Factors Contributing to and/or
Associated with Childhood Obesity

12 Prenatal Risk Factors for Childhood Obesity

Suzanne Phelan and Alison K. Ventura

CONTENTS

> Biological parenting commences well before birth, even prior to conception.
>
> **Lane and Robertson [1]**

INTRODUCTION

The developmental origins of health and disease (DOHaD) is a burgeoning field of research that suggests that perturbations occurring during critical periods of early life play a significant role in shaping a person's long-term risk of obesity and negative health outcomes [2]. Although the concept of "developmental programing" most commonly refers to adverse exposures during intrauterine life, factors at the time of conception have also been implicated. As the opening quote suggests, parental health status before conception may powerfully shape child health and obesity risk. This chapter reviews prenatal exposures that may increase a child's long-term susceptibility to obesity and adverse health outcomes. We consider several potential prenatal risk factors, including poor maternal health status, complications during pregnancy (e.g., gestational diabetes, hyperglycemia), gestational weight gain (GWG; excessive or inadequate), prenatal nutrition, activity, smoking, and other potentially adverse exposures. Our review draws primarily from observational studies in humans. Other chapters review epigenetic mechanisms (Chapter 14), environmental factors (Chapters 19 and 20), and intervention research using life course prevention approaches (Chapters 32 and 33).

MATERNAL HEALTH STATUS

Several lines of research have shown that maternal obesity before and during pregnancy has an independent, adverse impact on offspring weight and health outcomes during every life stage—from birth through adulthood [3]. Such associations have been reported in several studies with effect sizes ranging from small to moderate [4]. Linear relationships are generally observed with higher maternal preconception weight related to higher offspring weight outcomes. A within-family analysis of the US population found that the risk for having a high birth weight baby, which itself is a risk factor for later obesity, increased by 1.3% for mothers who were overweight before pregnancy and 3% for mothers who were obese [5]. Greater risks have been observed for the offspring of mothers with extreme (body mass index [BMI] >50 kg/m^2) prepregnancy obesity [6]. A small number of studies have explored the relationship between maternal obesity and other offspring outcomes beyond adiposity, such as insulin sensitivity, glucose levels, lipids, and type 2 diabetes; findings generally indicated significant associations between maternal obesity and poorer offspring metabolic health [3]. Maternal prepregnancy obesity may also impact child neurological functioning. A systematic review on the topic [7] found associations between maternal obesity and several adverse child neurodevelopmental problems, including lower childhood IQ, attention-deficit/hyperactivity disorder, schizophrenia, and eating disorders, which have also been associated with child obesity; however, the review also noted several limitations in the literature.

Initially, the associations between maternal obesity and adverse offspring health outcomes were studied as evidence for a genetic underpinning of obesity risk. While shared genes partially mediate these associations, an abundance of human evidence, supported by extensive data from experimental animal studies, now suggests that intrauterine exposure to an obese intrauterine environment, *per se*, programs offspring obesity risk by influencing appetite, metabolism, and activity levels [4]. Nevertheless, the moderate size effects observed to date suggest that other early-life exposures may play a role in shaping child health outcomes.

GESTATIONAL WEIGHT GAIN

The National Academy of Science Institute of Medicine (IOM) has formulated specific recommendations based on maternal prepregnancy BMI for GWG ranges that are associated with optimal maternal-child health outcomes. However, approximately 35% of normal-weight women and 60% of obese women gain more than recommended [8]. In both normal-weight and overweight/obese women, excessive GWG is an established risk factor for obesity and obesity-related comorbidities in offspring. Meta-analyses have found that excessive GWG significantly increased the risk of offspring overweight/obesity [9,10]. One meta-analysis concluded that at least 21% of the risk for childhood overweight was related to excessive GWG [10]. Given the high prevalence of excessive GWG, many offspring, particularly in the United States, are exposed to this obesity risk factor.

Although inadequate GWG is comparably far less common in the United States (~24%), it too has been linked with future offspring weight status, but the magnitude and direction of this association remain unclear. Two, large-scale observational studies have reported significant U-shaped associations between maternal GWG and child weight outcomes [11,12] with both inadequate and excessive GWG linked with later offspring obesity risk. By contrast, two meta-analyses [9,10] concluded that inadequate GWG was associated with a small *decrease* in the risk of later childhood obesity. Studies of pregnant women during times of famine have also reported mixed effects. A series of studies examining the effects of famine in the Dutch population found small and weak positive associations between exposure to famine during pregnancy and later obesity in female (but not male) offspring [13]. By contrast, research on the effects of the Leningrad famine found no significant effects of intrauterine exposure to famine and later offspring metabolic health [14]. The extent of a nutritional "mismatch" in the intrauterine versus postnatal environment may underlie these mixed findings. Offspring exposed to inadequate GWG but adequate or excessive postnatal feeding may exhibit "catch-up growth" or a compensatory acceleration in the rate of growth that may lead to later obesity and chronic diseases [15]. However, overall, the potential adverse effects of excessive GWG appear more robust than those of inadequate GWG in predicting subsequent child obesity and metabolic risk.

PRENATAL NUTRITION

Studies of the effects of GWG commonly infer effects on "overnutrition" or "undernutrition" during pregnancy and effects on long-term child obesity, but only a few human studies have objectively measured prenatal nutrition in relation to postnatal child weight and health outcomes. One study measured maternal macronutrient intake (using a food frequency questionnaire) at 32 weeks of gestation and child adiposity (assessed using dual-energy x-ray absorptiometry [DEXA]) at 10 years of age in 5593 mother/child dyads [16]. There were no significant associations between maternal prenatal protein, fat, and carbohydrate intake and offspring adiposity or lean mass at ages 9 and 11 years. Another study of two prospective UK cohorts reported an association between low carbohydrate intake (using a food frequency questionnaire) during early pregnancy and gene methylation that was linked with higher offspring weight (DEXA measured) [17]. Other work has suggested that the ratio of carbohydrate to protein intake during pregnancy was the key risk factor for later abnormal glucose homeostasis and high blood pressure in offspring [18]. Macronutrient *components* (rather than total macronutrient content only) may more consistently relate to offspring obesity. Two studies have reported that higher maternal sugar intake during pregnancy was predictive of higher offspring weight at birth and 6 months [19], and at 5 years of age [20]. Moreover, some evidence points to a role for maternal fat intake in shaping later offspring health outcomes [20]. Overall, however, linkages between maternal prenatal dietary intake and child obesity and health have been equivocal and are not well understood. The scant research in this area limits conclusions that can be drawn. Prospective assessments with validated, repeat measures of maternal dietary intake during pregnancy are needed to move the field forward.

MATERNAL PHYSICAL ACTIVITY

The American College of Obstetricians and Gynecologists (ACOG) recommends that pregnant women engage in at least 30 min of moderate exercise each day on most, if not all, days of the week for uncomplicated pregnancies. While light and moderate leisure time and occupational physical activities have been shown to improve several maternal health outcomes, including decreasing the risk of preeclampsia, hypertension, and gestational diabetes (GDM) [21], far less is known about the potentially protective effects of maternal physical activity on child health. Sufficient evidence exists that shows that prenatal physical activity does not increase the risk of low birth weight [21]. Some observations studies have reported that prenatal physical activity reduced the occurrence of offspring neural tube malformations [22]. Evidence in animal studies has suggested potential associations between higher activity levels during gestation and improved vasomotor function in offspring. However, similar to prenatal diet, there is a clear need for research in humans, using objective, repeat measures of physical activity and objectively measured child adiposity and health outcomes.

PREGNANCY COMPLICATIONS

GDM is another widely accepted risk factor for the development of obesity and chronic disease in offspring. Several studies have shown that fetal exposure to maternal diabetes during gestation conveys a risk of several short- and long-term health problems in offspring, including obesity, type 2 diabetes, and metabolic syndrome in children, adolescents, and adults [23]. Exposure to GDM has also been linked with birth trauma, respiratory distress syndrome, and neonatal death. An analysis of data from nine studies of diverse populations showed that by age 3–16 years, the mean offspring BMI z-score was 0.28 higher for the offspring of women with diabetes compared with controls [24]. In a series of longitudinal studies of Pima Indians, most of the increased prevalence of childhood type 2 diabetes occurring over a 30-year time frame was attributable to increased exposure to maternal diabetes during pregnancy [25]. Other long-term, prospective research has shown that the adolescent offspring of mothers who had diabetes during pregnancy (regardless of type) had a significantly higher prevalence of impaired glucose tolerance (19.3% vs. 2.5%, respectively) and obesity (50% vs. 20%, respectively) than the age- and sex-matched controls [26]. Females born with obesity had an increased risk of later obesity and a doubled risk for delivering an obese infant themselves [27]. These findings suggest that prenatal exposure to diabetes could form the basis of transmission of obesity and health risks from parent to child to grandchild and beyond, creating a vicious cycle to fuel the obesity epidemic for decades to come.

Maternal gestational hypertension and preeclampsia are also significant risk factors for offspring hypertension, stroke, and cardiovascular disease, independent of maternal weight status and a range of potential confounders [28]. Using data from 6343 9-year-old participants in the Avon Longitudinal Study of Parents and Children, both preeclampsia and gestational hypertension were associated with elevated systolic and diastolic blood pressures in the 9-year-old offspring, after adjustment for parental adiposity [29]. A number of other studies have reported that offspring exposed to pre-eclampsia and gestational hypertension had an increased risk of depression and other psychiatric and psychological problems in adulthood [30].

Overall, a preponderance of evidence suggests that pregnancy complications may exert programing effects on later offspring health. In examining the effects of pregnancy complications on offspring health outcomes, studies typically "adjust" or remove the potential confounding influences of maternal obesity and excessive GWG. However, these (and other) risk factors commonly co-occur, are intertwined and, when combined, appear to exacerbate the observed adverse programing effects on child health and development [31].

MATERNAL MENTAL HEALTH

Maternal stress and depression may also play a role in programing adverse child health outcomes. In a review of nine studies, chronic maternal depression was associated with greater risk of child overweight [32], independent of a range of potential confounds. In several retrospective reports, maternal depression during pregnancy was independently associated with neonatal distress, reduced orientation and motor activity, and disrupted sleep; and longer-term effects have been observed on child neurobehavioral outcomes, including disruptive social behavior and depression [33]. Unfortunately, treatment with antidepressant medications during pregnancy also has been related to adverse long-term effects on gross motor function and language development in offspring [34].

Similarly, prenatal maternal stress and anxiety also appear to negatively impact child cognitive development, particularly if the exposure occurs early in pregnancy [35]. Moderately severe stress during pregnancy (i.e., a natural disaster) was independently associated with lower cognitive and language abilities at five and a half years of age in one Canadian study [36]. Other work has found that high levels of cortisol in mothers during the third trimester of pregnancy was negatively related to offspring cognitive skills, independent of family and postnatal factors [37]. However, most studies examining the effects of maternal mental health on offspring outcomes have only followed children through infancy. Additional long-term studies are needed with systematic follow up of women through pregnancy along with careful quantification of the degree, duration, and timing of depression, stress, and antidepressant exposures, using standardized, structured assessments of infants and children, and measurements of obesity and metabolic function.

FAMILIAL AND SOCIODEMOGRAPHIC FACTORS

Sociodemographic disparities in obesity risk are well documented, with familial-level factors, such as lower income and education levels, black race, and Hispanic ethnicity, all placing individuals at higher risk for the development of obesity. Unfortunately, sociodemographic disparities also exist for the preconception and prenatal risk factors reviewed in this chapter. The prevalence of maternal preconception obesity is higher in non-Hispanic black and Hispanic white women compared with non-Hispanic white [8]. Similarly, the risk for GDM is higher for several ethnic groups compared with non-Hispanic white mothers. Also, smoking during pregnancy is more prevalent among low-income and disadvantaged mothers. The most disadvantaged mothers are also more likely to be exposed to pesticides and toxic metals and to experience higher stress from financial challenges and life events. The reasons behind social disparities in prenatal exposures are complex and implicate a wide range of socioeconomic factors (e.g., income, education, social status) and disparities in both nutritional exposures (i.e., food availability, food security, and diet quality) and physical activity opportunities. Since socially disadvantaged populations are exposed to more risk factors, both during fetal life and after birth, developmental programing effects may serve to exacerbate health disparities from one generation to the next. Future social epidemiology research must consider whether and how the social–environmental conditions of pregnant women perpetuate social disparities in chronic disease.

NEW DIRECTIONS

This is an exciting time for research in maternal–child health and disease prevention. As reviewed earlier, the evidence in support of the DOHaD is compelling, but there are many caveats in the field requiring future research, and more work is needed to bridge the gap between animal and human studies. There are also several new avenues of inquiry on the horizon.

CHILD HEALTH OUTCOMES

Extensive research has consistently documented associations between several prenatal exposures and the risk of offspring obesity. However, far more work is needed to identify whether and how prenatal exposures impact a range of other offspring health outcomes, including insulin resistance, hypertension, dyslipidemia, adverse neurodevelopmental outcomes, and asthma.

CHILD FOOD PREFERENCES

Emergent research suggests that prenatal nutrition may be indirectly linked to offspring obesity through the influence of prenatal flavor exposures on the offspring's later food preferences [38]. Flavors of the mother's diet can be transmitted to the fetus through amniotic fluid, and the fetus has the ability to detect the flavors present in the womb, which may influence the offspring's later flavor and food preferences. In an interesting study, mothers who were randomized to drink carrot juice daily during their last trimester of pregnancy or first 6 months of lactation had infants who showed higher preferences for carrot-flavored cereal at 6 months when compared with infants whose mothers only consumed water during pregnancy and lactation [39]. Longitudinal studies that span the prenatal and postnatal periods should continue to explore how interactions between pre- and postnatal flavor and food exposures influence children's dietary patterns and obesity risk and whether long-term flavor and food preferences and, ultimately, health status can be altered by manipulating prenatal dietary exposures.

PATERNAL PRECONCEPTION HEALTH

Much research in DOHaD has focused on maternal influences on offspring outcomes. However, paternal health at the time of conception may also influence offspring development. Paternal obesity is among the strongest risk factors predicting offspring overweight [40]. Other research suggests that paternal history of smoking and/or diabetes may increase offspring susceptibility to metabolic disease. The extent to which these paternal–child health associations are due to shared genes or adverse exposures remains unclear. Data from animal models indicate that paternal obesity may negatively impair sex hormones, basic sperm function, and molecular composition, which may perturb embryo development and increase subsequent offspring disease [41]. Similar to other DOHaD research, the majority of data surrounding paternal obesity and offspring health have come from rodent models. New epidemiologic cohorts that provide repeated biological and behavioral data on fathers are needed to inform whether and how paternal health and related behaviors before and at the time of conception may influence fetal and child health.

PRECONCEPTION PERIOD

It is difficult to study the preconception period, given that approximately half of pregnancies are unplanned and that there is no readily available source of recruitment for women planning pregnancy. It is also difficult to separate preconceptual from pregnancy-specific influences on the risk of adverse health outcomes in children. As noted earlier, most women who enter pregnancy overweight remain overweight during pregnancy and may also experience excessive GWG and pregnancy complications. However, the relative impact of adverse exposures at the time of preconception versus during pregnancy remains unclear. Without prospective studies of mothers and fathers during the entire pre- to postnatal period, the optimal targets and timing for interventions remain unknown. There is a strong need for new cohort studies of families that begin before conception and follow offspring through childhood.

MICROBIOME

Fascinating research has been uncovering linkages between deviations in gut microbiota composition and the risk of obesity; specific groups of gut bacteria appear to harvest energy from food more efficiently than others and are more common in the guts of individuals with obesity versus those of normal weight status [42]. In maternal–child studies, exposures during pregnancy (e.g., maternal obesity, excessive GWG) and during the neonatal period immediately after birth (e.g., breast-feeding, vaginal delivery) appear to influence the infant microbiome and may be critical for programing child immune function and gut–brain energy-sensing systems [43]. Alterations in maternal microbiota composition during pregnancy may be transferred to infants *in utero*, impact the fetal gut, and exert significant effects on offspring immune and metabolic programing and later risk of disease [44]. As most of the work in this area has been done in animals, with limited studies during developmental periods (see Chapter 21), the time is ripe for human microbiome studies in the time surrounding pregnancy and early childhood.

EPIGENETIC MECHANISMS

The field is at the budding stages of identifying and understanding the complex epigenetic mechanisms by which preconception and intrauterine exposures impact offspring development (Chapter 14). Pathways likely differ depending on the type, timing, and duration of exposure(s) and, importantly, on the interactions with postnatal life. Further mechanistic work with humans is needed that includes a range of offspring health outcomes but also assessments of behaviors that may be amenable to intervention. Berkowtiz et al. [45] found that women who were obese before pregnancy (vs. normal weight) were more likely to have offspring who exhibited an obese eating style (large mouthfuls of food and increased caloric intake per minute during a test meal) at 4 years of age. These findings were consistent with the altered hypothalamus regulation of eating behaviors illustrated in animal models [46]. Further mechanistic work (likely through randomized controlled trials and interventions) is needed to better understand the application of findings from animal models to human systems (central nervous system [CNS], hypothalamic, metabolic) and behavior (eating, activity, smoking) and in relation to offspring health outcomes.

SUMMARY

Although much investigation has already occurred in the area of DOHaD research, the science itself is still in its infancy. It remains for researchers to tackle key questions and translate knowledge into effective interventions to reduce childhood risk of obesity and disease burden. Our review suggests several potential prenatal targets for intervention, including maternal prepregnancy over-weight, GWG, pregnancy complications, and smoking. However, long-term experimental studies in humans will be needed to determine whether and in whom altering/improving preconceptual and intrauterine environments reduces offspring risks of obesity and chronic disease. To date, prenatal intervention studies with long-term follow up of offspring weight and health outcomes are few and far between, and the optimal intervention window (before, during, and/or after pregnancy) remains unclear. The best window for intervention may not be the same for all pregnancies, ethnicities, cultures, and health-care systems.

Many of the preconceptual and pregnancy risk factors for adverse intergenerational effects correlate with socioeconomic status, race, and gender. This points to the need for societal changes rather than solely individual-level interventions. Research in health disparities and the DOHaD field provides a rationale for public health policies to improve preconceptual and pregnancy care for women and men across all levels of society. As Richardson and colleagues [47] poignantly urged, the DOHaD research findings should not be used to blame individual women. Societal-level changes are needed to support interventions that ultimately empower all women and men of childbearing age to engage in health behaviors to protect the health of future generations.

REFERENCES

1. Lane M, Robker RL, Robertson SA. Parenting from before conception. *Science*. 2014;345(6198):756–60.
2. Barker DJ. The developmental origins of chronic adult disease. *Acta Paediatr Suppl*. 2004;93(446):26–33.
3. Perng W, Gillman MW, Mantzoros CS, Oken E. A prospective study of maternal prenatal weight and offspring cardiometabolic health in midchildhood. *Ann Epidemiol*. 2014;24(11):793–800e1.
4. Oken E. Maternal and child obesity: The causal link. *Obstet Gynecol Clin North Am*. 2009;36(2):361–77, ix–x.
5. Yan J. Maternal pre-pregnancy BMI, gestational weight gain, and infant birth weight: A within-family analysis in the United States. *Econ Hum Biol*. 2015;18:1–12.
6. Marshall NE, Guild C, Cheng YW, Caughey AB, Halloran DR. Maternal superobesity and perinatal outcomes. *Am J Obstet Gynecol*. 2012;206(5):417 e1–6.
7. Van Lieshout RJ, Taylor VH, Boyle MH. Pre-pregnancy and pregnancy obesity and neurodevelopmental outcomes in offspring: A systematic review. *Obes Rev*. 2011;12(5):e548–59.
8. Chu SY, Callaghan WM, Bish CL, D'Angelo D. Gestational weight gain by body mass index among US women delivering live births, 2004–2005: Fueling future obesity. *Am J Obstet Gynecol*. 2009;200(3):271 e1–7.
9. Mamun AA, Mannan M, Doi SA. Gestational weight gain in relation to offspring obesity over the life course: A systematic review and bias-adjusted meta-analysis. *Obes Rev*. 2014;15(4):338–47.
10. Nehring I, Lehmann S, von Kries R. Gestational weight gain in accordance to the IOM/NRC criteria and the risk for childhood overweight: A meta-analysis. *Pediatr Obes*. 2013;8(3):218–24.
11. Oken E, Rifas-Shiman SL, Field AE, Frazier AL, Gillman MW. Maternal gestational weight gain and offspring weight in adolescence. *Obstet Gynecol*. 2008;112(5):999–1006.
12. Stuebe AM, Forman MR, Michels KB. Maternal recalled gestational weight gain, pre-pregnancy body mass index, and obesity in the daughter. *Int J Obes*. 2009;33(7):743–52.
13. Ravelli AC, van Der Meulen JH, Osmond C, Barker DJ, Bleker OP. Obesity at the age of 50 y in men and women exposed to famine prenatally. *Am J Clin Nutr*. 1999;70(5):811–6.
14. Stanner SA, Yudkin JS. Fetal programming and the Leningrad Siege study. *Twin Res*. 2001;4(5):287–92.
15. Kanoh M, Kaneita Y, Hara M, Harada S, Gon Y, Kanamaru H, et al. Longitudinal study of parental smoking habits and development of asthma in early childhood. *Prev Med*. 2012;54(1):94–6.
16. Brion MJ, Ness AR, Rogers I, Emmett P, Cribb V, Davey Smith G, et al. Maternal macronutrient and energy intakes in pregnancy and offspring intake at 10 y: Exploring parental comparisons and prenatal effects. *Am J Clin Nutr*. 2010;91(3):748–56.

17. Godfrey KM, Sheppard A, Gluckman PD, Lillycrop KA, Burdge GC, McLean C, et al. Epigenetic gene promoter methylation at birth is associated with child's later adiposity. *Diabetes.* 2011;60(5):1528–34.

18. Campbell DM, Hall MH, Barker DJ, Cross J, Shiell AW, Godfrey KM. Diet in pregnancy and the offspring's blood pressure 40 years later. *BJOG.* 1996;103(3):273–80.

19. Phelan S, Hart C, Phipps M, Abrams B, Schaffner A, Adams A, et al. Maternal behaviors during pregnancy impact offspring obesity risk. *Exp Diabetes Res.* 2011;2011:985139.

20. Murrin C, Shrivastava A, Kelleher CC, Lifeways Cross-generation Cohort Study Steering Group. Maternal macronutrient intake during pregnancy and 5 years postpartum and associations with child weight status aged five. *Eur J Clin Nutr.* 2013;67(6):670–9.

21. Schlussel MM, Souza EB, Reichenheim ME, Kac G. Physical activity during pregnancy and maternal–child health outcomes: A systematic literature review. *Cad Saude Publica.* 2008;24(Suppl 4):s531–44.

22. Flak AL, Yun Tark J, Tinker SC, Correa A, Cogswell ME. Major, non-chromosomal, birth defects and maternal physical activity: A systematic review. *Birth Defects Res A Clin Mol Teratol.* 2012;94(7):521–31.

23. Wendland EM, Torloni MR, Falavigna M, Trujillo J, Dode MA, Campos MA, et al. Gestational diabetes and pregnancy outcomes: A systematic review of the World Health Organization (WHO) and the International Association of Diabetes in Pregnancy Study Groups (IADPSG) diagnostic criteria. *BMC Pregnancy Childbirth.* 2012;12:23.

24. Philipps LH, Santhakumaran S, Gale C, Prior E, Logan KM, Hyde MJ, et al. The diabetic pregnancy and offspring BMI in childhood: A systematic review and meta-analysis. *Diabetologia.* 2011;54(8):1957–66.

25. Dabelea D, Hanson RL, Bennett PH, Roumain J, Knowler WC, Pettitt DJ. Increasing prevalence of Type II diabetes in American Indian children. *Diabetologia.* 1998;41(8):904–10.

26. Silverman BL, Metzger BE, Cho NH, Loeb CA. Impaired glucose tolerance in adolescent offspring of diabetic mothers: Relationship to fetal hyperinsulinism. *Diabetes Care.* 1995;18(5):611–7.

27. Ahlsson F, Gustafsson J, Tuvemo T, Lundgren M. Females born large for gestational age have a doubled risk of giving birth to large for gestational age infants. *Acta Paediatr.* 2007;96(3):358–62.

28. Kajantie E, Eriksson JG, Osmond C, Thornburg K, Barker DJ. Pre-eclampsia is associated with increased risk of stroke in the adult offspring: The Helsinki birth cohort study. *Stroke.* 2009;40(4):1176–80.

29. Geelhoed JJ, Fraser A, Tilling K, Benfield L, Davey Smith G, Sattar N, et al. Preeclampsia and gestational hypertension are associated with childhood blood pressure independently of family adiposity measures: The Avon Longitudinal Study of Parents and Children. *Circulation.* 2010;122(12):1192–9.

30. Tuovinen S, Eriksson JG, Kajantie E, Raikkonen K. Maternal hypertensive pregnancy disorders and cognitive functioning of the offspring: A systematic review. *J Am Soc Hypertens: JASH.* 2014;8(11):832–47 e1.

31. Heerman WJ, Bian A, Shintani A, Barkin SL. Interaction between maternal prepregnancy body mass index and gestational weight gain shapes infant growth. *Acad Pediatr.* 2014;14(5):463–70.

32. Lampard AM, Franckle RL, Davison KK. Maternal depression and childhood obesity: A systematic review. *Prev Med.* 2014;59:60–7.

33. Deave T, Heron J, Evans J, Emond A. The impact of maternal depression in pregnancy on early child development. *BJOG.* 2008;115(8):1043–51.

34. Suri R, Lin AS, Cohen LS, Altshuler LL. Acute and long-term behavioral outcome of infants and children exposed in utero to either maternal depression or antidepressants: A review of the literature. *J Clin Psychiatry.* 2014;75(10):e1142–52.

35. Van den Bergh BR, Mulder EJ, Mennes M, Glover V. Antenatal maternal anxiety and stress and the neurobehavioural development of the fetus and child: Links and possible mechanisms. A review. *Neurosci Biobehav Rev.* 2005;29(2):237–58.

36. Laplante DP, Brunet A, Schmitz N, Ciampi A, King S. Project Ice Storm: Prenatal maternal stress affects cognitive and linguistic functioning in 5 1/2-year-old children. *J Am Acad Child Adolesc Psychiatry.* 2008;47(9):1063–72.

37. LeWinn KZ, Stroud LR, Molnar BE, Ware JH, Koenen KC, Buka SL. Elevated maternal cortisol levels during pregnancy are associated with reduced childhood IQ. *Int J Epidemiol.* 2009;38(6):1700–10.

38. Mennella JA. The chemical senses and the development of flavor preferences in humans. In Hale TW, Hartmann PE, eds. *Textbook on Human Lactation.* Amarillo, TX: Hale Publishing, pp. 403–14, 2007.

39. Mennella JA, Jagnow CP, Beauchamp GK. Prenatal and postnatal flavor learning by human infants. *Pediatrics.* 2001;107(6):E88.

40. Heppe DH, Kiefte-de Jong JC, Durmus B, Moll HA, Raat H, Hofman A, et al. Parental, fetal, and infant risk factors for preschool overweight: The Generation R Study. *Pediatr Res.* 2013;73(1):120–7.

41. Fullston T, McPherson NO, Owens JA, Kang WX, Sandeman LY, Lane M. Paternal obesity induces metabolic and sperm disturbances in male offspring that are exacerbated by their exposure to an "obesogenic" diet. *Physiol Rep.* 2015;3(3):e12336, 1–14.

42. Diamant M, Blaak EE, de Vos WM. Do nutrient-gut-microbiota interactions play a role in human obesity, insulin resistance and type 2 diabetes? *Obes Rev.* 2011;12(4):272–81.

43. Collado MC, Isolauri E, Laitinen K, Salminen S. Effect of mother's weight on infant's microbiota acquisition, composition, and activity during early infancy: A prospective follow-up study initiated in early pregnancy. *Am J Clin Nutr.* 2010;92(5):1023–30.

44. Kalliomaki M, Collado MC, Salminen S, Isolauri E. Early differences in fecal microbiota composition in children may predict overweight. *Am J Clin Nutr.* 2008;87(3):534–8.

45. Berkowitz RI, Moore RH, Faith MS, Stallings VA, Kral TV, Stunkard AJ. Identification of an obese eating style in 4-year-old children born at high and low risk for obesity. *Obesity (Silver Spring).* 2010;18(3):505–12.

46. Chen H, Morris MJ. Differential responses of orexigenic neuropeptides to fasting in offspring of obese mothers. *Obesity (Silver Spring).* 2009;17(7):1356–62.

47. Richardson SS, Daniels CR, Gillman MW, Golden J, Kukla R, Kuzawa C, et al. Society: Don't blame the mothers. *Nature.* 2014;512(7513):131–2.

13 Genetics of Childhood Obesity

Sani M. Roy, Patrick C. Hanley, Jennifer Kelley,
Shana E. McCormack, and Struan F.A. Grant

CONTENTS

INTRODUCTION

As the worldwide prevalence of obesity increases, it is critical to elucidate the genetic basis for obesity and its associated cardiometabolic complications. The pediatric population is uniquely positioned to provide insights into the genetics of obesity, as the effect of environment on disease state is less manifest than in adults.

In this chapter, an overview is provided of the various methodologies for investigating the genetics of childhood obesity. This is followed by a description of the key genetic studies of obesity in both adults and children, as adult studies provide the foundation for genetic obesity studies in children. Finally, the known monogenic and polygenic obesity syndromes are described.

METHODS FOR STUDYING THE GENETIC COMPONENTS OF CHILDHOOD OBESITY

TWIN, ADOPTION, AND FAMILY STUDIES

It is well established that obesity has a complex and multifactorial pathogenesis, including interactions between environmental, behavioral, and genetic factors. Over the past several decades, increasing evidence has supported a substantial inherited component of human obesity risk. The first investigations linking genetics with obesity included studies in monozygotic and dizygotic twins, and in many cases occurred years prior to the identification of specific variants associated with the trait. While one of the earliest twin studies estimated a heritability of 70% for body weight and 65% for waist circumference [1], subsequent studies have produced more varied estimates, with heritability of fat mass ranging from 70% to 90% in monozygotic twins and 35%–45% in dizygotic twins [2–9]. Of note, these heritability estimates can vary greatly when additional factors including physical activity, age, and other exposures are considered. For example, higher heritability for body mass has been reported in adolescents and young adults compared with older adults [10].

In addition to twin studies, adoption and family studies have also contributed to the evidence for the heritability of obesity. During the same time period as the early twin studies, an adoption study showed that the body size of adopted children was more highly associated with that of their biological parents than their adopted parents, across multiple measures of body size and anthropometry [11]. Further, studies within different racial and/or ethnic populations have shown variation in the heritability rates of body size, with estimates of heritability of approximately 35% or less in Caucasian and Asian populations, compared with rates of 50% or more in Pima Indians and South Sea Islanders [12]. Despite the variability in study reports, the heritability of obesity is now generally accepted to be between 40% and 70%, with a typical estimate of around 50% [9,13]. Thus, approximately half of the variation of body mass within a population is attributable to genetic factors. In the case of the "common" form of diet-induced or exogenous obesity, it is also clear that inheritance is not in a predictable pattern and instead is complex, indicating the likely presence of multiple responsible genes and gene networks, many of which likely have not yet been identified.

LINKAGE STUDIES

As one of the earlier methodologies to evaluate the genes underlying disease states, linkage analysis has been very effective in identifying disease-causing genetic variants for single-gene conditions. In these studies, the genomes of multiple affected relatives are mapped using genetic markers to identify specific segments of DNA inherited more often together than would be expected by chance. The shared loci are then further analyzed to identify individual genes responsible for the disease phenotype. When applied to the evaluation of obesity, linkage studies have been successful in identifying the single-gene mutations responsible for monogenic obesity syndromes. In particular, several studies have reported that mutations in the leptin gene, identified from analysis of a region on chromosome 7q31, are responsible for severe forms of obesity, as discussed later in this chapter [14].

In contrast to the monogenic forms of obesity, the utilization of linkage analysis in common, polygenic phenotypes has proved less successful. While linkage analysis has repeatedly identified several loci associated with the so-called common forms of obesity, no genes have been identified as of yet in these regions of haplotypic sharing and there is significant variation between the results of individual studies [9,15]. This is generally due to the low power of linkage analysis to detect the effects of variation in common genes that confer only modestly increased obesity risk, as well as variations in study groups and methods. As analysis continues on larger study populations, the detection of associated loci and the possible identification of genes using linkage analysis can be refined, and can be complemented with newly available high-throughput sequencing technologies.

CANDIDATE GENE STUDIES

In candidate gene studies, potential genes are selected for association analysis based on a known or hypothesized role in a disease phenotype. Candidate genes are considered to be either functional or positional. Functional candidates are dependent on current knowledge of the disease, as they are identified through products or mechanisms that are known to be involved in the disease process. Positional candidate genes are identified through their proximity to genomic loci that have been associated with disease pathology in previous linkage or association studies as well as animal models. Large numbers of candidate genes for obesity have been published; however, many initially suggestive results demonstrated no association in additional studies [2]. As this method is based on the pathophysiological mechanisms of obesity, of which much remains unknown, there has been limited success in identifying risk genes, and the genes that have been identified appear to carry a small effect [2,15]. These studies further reveal that the genetic causes of obesity are complex and potentially involve a large amount of genes with various effect sizes. They also demonstrate the need for discovery-focused evaluations of the genetic factors associated with obesity.

GENOME-WIDE ASSOCIATION STUDIES AND META-ANALYSES

Since 2005, research into the genetic basis of human obesity has been largely driven by the development and utilization of genome-wide association studies (GWAS) and in particular the HapMap Project, which developed an extensive catalog of sequence variations along the human genome [16]. GWAS use high-throughput methodology to span a large set, often millions, of common variants (single-nucleotide polymorphisms [SNPs] or single-nucleotide variants) across the entire human genome. This method allows for an untargeted, non-hypothesis-driven approach to reveal associations between specific disease phenotypes and common variants within the genome. Several large GWAS have been conducted within the fields of human obesity and metabolism; the general approach has been to compare common variant frequencies within obesity versus normal-weight controls. This has led to the identification of robust associations between numerous genetic loci and obesity and obesity-related traits. To date, dozens of established loci have been identified for body mass index (BMI) and waist to-hip ratio [9,17–23]. A discussion of the most important of these is found in the following section of this chapter.

As GWAS are non-hypothesis-driven and have been successful in implicating genetic loci within complex, multifactorial disease processes, these robust associations are widely accepted within the research community, and are thought to offer an advantage over the linkage and candidate studies. The majority of these studies have been conducted in populations of European descent; however, recent GWAS have expanded the focus to include other ethnic populations as well as evaluating differences between sexes, pediatric populations, and longitudinal cohorts to identify potential effects by age [18,22,24–28].

Recently, meta-analyses of GWAS have become more common. Following analyses of individual GWAS datasets, statistical approaches to meta-analysis provide sufficient power to detect subtle genetic variants for common traits. By using imputation within the analyses, the number of common variants is computationally increased, which allows for a more extensive evaluation of a specific variant across the genome. In addition, meta-analyses overcome the effect of multiple testing of markers with borderline significance and thus reduce statistical noise. See subsequent sections of this chapter for more details.

MISSING HERITABILITY, RARE VARIANT–COMMON DISEASE HYPOTHESIS, AND NEXT STEPS

Despite the significant advantages that GWAS provide for our understanding of the genetic basis of obesity, there are a few particular drawbacks. The SNPs identified by GWAS are considered to be *tag SNPs*. They tag a causative variant in a particular region but are not causal themselves. Thus, the key causal factors have yet to be identified. Further, while many loci have been identified, it is estimated that GWAS results account for only 10% of the heritability of obesity. This is in contrast to the nearly 50% heritability reported in twin and family studies. The missing heritability not identified by current GWAS methods is a topic of current debate and research. One theory for the missing heritability centers on the rare variant–common disease hypothesis. GWAS methods are based on the common disease–common variant hypothesis, in which the genetic components of a complex disease are thought to be attributable to the additive effect of a moderate number of common variants, each of which explain only a small proportion of the heritability. In contrast, newer methods to study rare variants, including new microarray chips that will evaluate SNPs with minor allele frequencies as low as 0.5%, as well as larger sample sizes have emerged [29,30]. One of the most recent modalities to effectively address the missing heritability issue was reported in 2015 and utilized a new method to impute a large sample of SNP arrays. Approximately 17 million imputed variants, including common and rare alleles, were generated to evaluate the heritability of height and BMI and demonstrated that the heritability of BMI is likely to be 30%–40%, producing a smaller range of missing heritability than has previously been described [31].

In addition, several other methods of study have been identified to explain the missing heritability. Currently, copy number variants (CNVs), which are the products of large segments of genetic material that have been replicated or deleted, have been implicated in the heritability of obesity and association studies have identified such multiple loci [32]. Emerging research also focuses on the effect of epigenetic mechanisms, which include DNA methylation, histone modification, and microRNA, on the heritability of obesity. Currently, the association of DNA methylation and obesity is being studied using whole-genome sequencing. Finally, the effects of *epistasis*, or gene–gene interaction, in which variants of different genes may interact and contribute to the heritability of obesity, have been hypothesized and the methods to evaluate these interactions genome wide are under development [9,15].

RESULTS OF SPECIFIC PEDIATRIC GENETIC STUDIES

FTO Locus and Obesity Risk in Adults and Children

To date, the genetic locus most strongly associated with adult BMI using GWAS is within the fat mass– and obesity-associated (*FTO*) gene, despite only explaining less than 2% of the predicted genetic component of obesity attributable to this trait [33]. Notably, this common variant was initially identified in a GWAS of type 2 diabetes (T2D) [34]; however, it was ultimately found that the incremental increase in T2D risk attributable to the variant in *FTO* was conferred by increased BMI [18]. *FTO* was actually the second obesity locus to be identified by GWAS [18], and has been widely replicated [35]. Not all initially suggestive GWAS results demonstrate such consistency. Indeed, unlike *FTO*, the first such obesity locus identified, within insulin-induced gene 2 (*INSIG2*) [36], has not produced such consistent associations in subsequent studies [37].

Studies have also demonstrated age-dependent variations between BMI and variations harbored within *FTO*. A meta-analysis was conducted of associations between the *FTO* locus (rs9939609) and BMI in eight European cohorts of children whose ages ranged from early infancy to 13 years. An inverse relationship was found between BMI and the obesity-associated allele of *FTO* in infancy; in contrast, a positive association was noted between BMI and the obesity-associated allele of *FTO* in early childhood, corresponding to the approximate time of adiposity rebound [38]. Thus, the adult obesity–associated allele of *FTO* was related to a lower BMI during the period of infancy peak BMI and a higher BMI during the period of adiposity rebound [38]; this may be explained by variations within *FTO* altering the characteristics of the BMI trajectory. Another longitudinal study noted that the peak association between the *FTO* locus and BMI occurred by age 20 years, after which the association diminished [39]. The *FTO* risk allele has also been shown to demonstrate dynamic physiological changes during adolescence, including an association with higher BMI, fat mass index, and leptin concentrations during early puberty, followed by a nadir of these associations mid-puberty, and an eventual strengthening of these associations toward the completion of puberty [40]. These temporal associations highlight the likely complex physiology of this genetic variation with excess adiposity.

The mechanism whereby the risk allele of *FTO* is associated with obesity remains unclear, but there are some suggestions that it affects the central regulation of energy balance. *FTO* encodes 2-oxoglutarate-dependent nucleic acid demethylase, which is expressed in the appetite-regulating centers of the brain [41]. Rodent studies demonstrate that overexpression of *FTO* results in obesity [42], while a knockout of *FTO* protects against obesity [43]. Indeed, in a mechanistically focused study of 2726 Scottish children aged 4–10 years, those with the common obesity risk allele of *FTO* had significantly higher weight and BMI. In a subset analysis ($n = 97$), the risk allele was significantly associated with increased fat mass and increased energy intake but did not show associations with resting energy expenditure [44].

Notably, environmental changes over time have also been found to modify genetic risk factors. A gene-by-birth cohort interaction was identified for the rs993609 variant of the *FTO* gene within the longitudinal Framingham Heart Study, such that there was a strong linear correlation between the risk allele and BMI for individuals born after 1942, while no significant relationship existed for those born prior to 1942 [45]. This finding illustrates that some genetic variants may only contribute to obesity risk under specific adverse circumstances.

Although GWAS have yielded a large number of genomic signals, and there are a number of lines of evidence for *FTO* encoding a protein involved in the pathogenesis of obesity, these reports only represent a genomic *signal* and not necessarily, as often presumed, the localization of a culprit gene. This is because gene expression can be controlled locally or over large genomic distances; indeed, most regulatory elements do not control the nearest genes and can reside tens or hundreds of kilobases away. A paper published in *Nature* in March 2014 revealed that the signal within *FTO* was actually an embedded enhancer for the neighboring *IRX3* gene [46]; indeed a follow-up study in the *New England Journal of Medicine* in 2015 suggested that this enhancer drove the expression of two other genes, *IRX3* and *IRX5* [47]. It remains to be determined how *IRX3* and *IRX5* mechanistically mediate the risk of obesity in children specifically.

RESULTS OF GWAS AND META-ANALYSES IN ADULTS

The first GWAS meta-analysis of BMI in adults was conducted in nearly 17,000 European individuals and noted the strongest associations for adult BMI within the *FTO* locus, along with an association between BMI and a locus near the melanocortin-4 receptor [*MC4R*] gene, well known to cause severe monogenic childhood obesity [48]. Although this GWAS was initially performed in adults, the identified *MC4R* association was confirmed in both adults ($n = \sim60,000$) and children ages 7–11 years ($n = \sim6,000$) from the Avon Longitudinal Study of Parents and Children (ALSPAC). In these children, each additional copy of the risk allele was associated with a difference in BMI of 0.10–0.13 z-score units, which was approximately double the effect size noted in adults [48]. These seminal results demonstrate that GWAS could be used to determine obesity associations both in adults and in children.

The Genetic Investigation of Anthropometric Traits (GIANT) consortium was formed soon thereafter to conduct large-scale meta-analyses of multiple GWAS. The initial meta-analysis combined 15 GWAS from over 32,000 individuals of European ancestry to investigate the association between BMI and about 2.4 million SNPs that were either genotyped or imputed [49]. The SNPs from the most significantly associated loci were then further studied through *de novo* genotyping in approximately 45,000 additional individuals, along with SNP analyses in over 14,000 individuals who were genotyped in other GWAS studies. Six more genes were identified through the GIANT consortium meta-analysis that were found to be reproducibly associated with BMI, including: transmembrane protein 18 (*TMEM18*), potassium channel tetramerization domain–containing 15 (*KCTD15*), glucosamine-6-phosphate deaminase 2 (*GNPDA2*), SH2B adaptor protein 1 (*SH2B1*), mitochondrial carrier 2 (*MTCH2*), and neuronal growth regulator 1 (*NEGR1*) [49]. With regard to potential mechanistic roles for the newly identified loci, the GIANT consortium noted that *SH2B1* is involved in leptin signaling and that *SH2B1*-null mice are obese [50]. *MTCH2* is thought to function in cellular apoptosis through the encoding of a mitochondrial carrier protein [51]. *NEGR1* is thought to be involved in the outgrowth of neurons [52].

Notably, a follow-up study by the GIANT consortium of the established SNPs in a pediatric cohort (ALSPAC Study, using BMI information from age 11 years) demonstrated significant and consistent associations between BMI and variants around *TMEM18*, *KCTD15*, and *GNPDA2* [49].

In 2010, the GIANT consortium conducted another meta-analysis of BMI associations in 249,769 individuals of European ancestry. Fourteen known obesity–susceptibility loci were confirmed (nearest genes: *FTO*, *TMEM18*, *MC4R*, *GNPDA2*, *BDNF*, *NEGR1*, *SH2B1*, *ETV5*, *MTCH2*, *KCTD15*, *SEC16B*, *TFAP2B*, *FAIM2*, and *NRXN3*) and 18 new loci were identified (nearest genes: *RBJ/ADCY3/POMC*, *GPRC5B/IQCK*, *MAP2K5/LBXCOR1*, *QPCTL/GIPR*, *TNNI3K*, *SLC39A8*, *FLJ35779/HMGCR*, *LRRN6C*, *TMEM160/ZC3H4*, *FANCL*, *CADM2*, *PRKD1*, *LRP1B*, *PTBP2*, *MTIF3/GTF3A*, *ZNF608*, *RPL27A/TUB*, and *NUDT3/HMGA1*) [53].

Follow-up studies to confirm the significance of the BMI-increasing alleles included both adults and children and found a 1.016- to 1.203-fold increase in the overall odds of obesity [53]. Furthermore, for 23 of the 32 SNPs, the specific BMI-increasing allele noted in adults also increased the BMI in children and adolescents. Notably, these 32 BMI loci were found to explain only 1.45% of the interindividual variation in BMI, with each additional risk allele increasing BMI by 0.17 kg/m^2 [53]. In terms of function, the consortium considered that amid the newly found loci, mutations in *POMC* are a known rare cause of human obesity [54], and *GIPR* encodes a receptor for gastric inhibitory polypeptide [55], suggesting a potential mechanistic link between incretin secretion and the obesity phenotype.

Another GWAS meta-analysis was conducted in 2013 to investigate loci associated with BMI in individuals of African ancestry. Thirty-two of the thirty-six variants established in individuals of European ancestry were confirmed in the African sample. Furthermore, robust associations with BMI were noted at two additional loci: *GALNT10* and *MIR148A-NFE2L3*, along with a suggestive association at *KLHL32* [28]. These results indicated that BMI loci are likely shared across populations, but also underscored the need for further research to investigate ancestry-specific differences, including in children.

In 2015, the GIANT consortium conducted a GWAS and meta-analysis of BMI in over one-third of a million individuals from 125 studies derived from different ethnicities. The study found genome-wide significance for 97 BMI-associated loci, of which 56 were novel. These loci have been found to account for about 2.7% of variation in BMI [56]. The GIANT consortium then performed *fine mapping*, a form of follow-up genotyping, post-GWAS, enabling the identification of candidate genes and causal variants with a greater degree of certainty [57]. Notably, fine mapping identified a single SNP at *FTO* (rs1558902). Further studies are needed to elucidate the specific causal genes and pathways [56], including in the pediatric population.

RESULTS OF CANDIDATE GENE STUDIES, GWAS, AND META-ANALYSES IN CHILDREN AND ADOLESCENTS

The results of adult GWAS and meta-analyses have paved the way for genetic studies in the pediatric population. Candidate gene studies of 25 SNPs from 13 obesity loci previously reported in adults were performed in just over 6,000 children of European ancestry. Fifteen of the SNPs demonstrated at least nominally significant association to BMI, representing 9 of the 13 tested loci, including: *INSIG2*, *FTO*, *MC4R*, *TMEM18*, *GNPDA2*, *NEGR1*, *BDNF*, *KCTD15*, and 1q25; however, no associations were noted for *MTCH2*, *SH2B1*, 12q13, and 3q27 [58].

In 2010, 15 of 16 known adult obesity–susceptibility loci tested in children and adolescents from the European Youth Heart Study were found to have directionally consistent associations with BMI (including *NEGR1*, *SEC16B*, *LYPLAL1*, *TMEM18*, *ETV5*, *GNPDA2*, *TFAP2B*, *MSRA*, *BDNF*,

MTCH2, BCDIN3D, NRXN3, SH2B1, FTO, MC4R, and *KCTD15*) [59]. To increase statistical power, a meta-analysis was performed of 13 of the variants using previously reported data ($n = 13{,}071$ children and adolescents using cohorts from the Children's Hospital of Philadelphia and ALSPAC). All 13 variants were found to have directionally consistent associations with BMI as previously reported in adults, and 9 were found to be significant, with the greatest effect in the *TMEM18* variant. Interestingly, effect sizes for BMI were stronger in children and adolescents than in adults for the variants near *TMEM18, SEC16,* and *KCTD15* [59].

The first GWAS of pediatric and adolescent obesity was conducted in 2010 in a combined analysis of French and German cohorts ($n = 1138$ extremely obese children and 1120 normal/underweight controls). In addition to previously identified genes (*FTO, MC4R,* and *TMEM18*), two new loci were discovered within *SDCCAG8* and *TNKS/MSRA* in association with extreme obesity (BMI 97th to 99th percentile). For each loci, the odds ratios for early obesity were marginal, at approximately 1.1 per additional risk allele [60].

A larger-scale North American–Australian–European GWAS meta-analysis was performed by the Early Growth Genetics (EGG) consortium in 2012, incorporating just over 5500 cases of European ancestry (with BMI ≥95th percentile for age) and in excess of 8000 controls (with BMI <50th percentile for age) [26]. Two loci were identified that demonstrated a genome-wide significant combined *p*-value: near *OLFM4* on 13q14 and within *HOXB5* on 17q21. These signals were also tested within the GIANT meta-analysis of adult BMI [53] and also yielded directionally consistent associations.

A GWAS of BMI trajectories from ages 1 to 17 years was conducted in 2015 using repeated measures from the ALSPAC cohort ($n = \sim 8000$) and the Western Australian Pregnancy Cohort Study ($n = \sim 1500$). Replication analyses were performed for regions achieving genome-wide significance ($p < 5 \times 10^{-8}$) using the Northern Finland Birth Cohort of 1966 ($n = \sim 4000$). Genome-wide significant associations were found for three loci previously identified in GWAS of adult BMI (*FTO, MC4R,* and *ADCY3*) and for one known pediatric obesity loci (*OLFM4*) [61]. Furthermore, a novel association was found between BMI at 8 years of age and SNPs near the *FAM120AOS* gene, with effects starting around 2 years of age [61]; however, this effect was not present in the replication cohort, possibly due to potential differences in genetic profiles or generational factors between the cohorts. The function of the *FAM120AOS* gene is currently unknown, but it is near to other genes implicated in severe childhood obesity (*NINJ1*) [62], along with the development of bone and the differentiation of adipocytes (*PHF2*) [63].

KNOWN GENETIC OBESITY SYNDROMES

Current research in obesity genetics leverages next-generation high-throughput sequencing technology to use whole-exome and whole-genome sequencing approaches, along with epigenetic investigations, to further define the genetic causes of obesity. Before these techniques were available, the identification and sequencing of candidate genes in syndromic forms of obesity provided valuable genetic and molecular information in defining the neuroendocrine contribution to obesity. The most well-characterized molecular signaling pathway related to obesity is the hypothalamic leptin–melanocortin pathway [64]. The syndromic forms of obesity involving mutations in the constituents of this pathway, along with other syndromic forms of obesity, are individually rare. Despite this, they have provided valuable insight into genetic and molecular explanations for obesity.

MONOGENIC OBESITY SYNDROMES AFFECTING THE HYPOTHALAMIC LEPTIN–MELANOCORTIN PATHWAY

Congenital Leptin Deficiency

Mouse models provided the lead for a monogenic form of obesity in humans. Ingalls and colleagues described a new mutation in what they called the *obese* (*ob*) gene in 1950, when they identified mice in their laboratory that quickly grew to four times the weight of normal mice [65]. Subsequently, positional cloning of the mouse *ob* gene and its human homolog identified the *ob* locus as a highly conserved area that encoded for a secreted protein product [66]. Mouse studies further demonstrated that the *ob* gene product leptin was deficient in *ob/ob* mice, and that this secreted protein served an endocrine function in controlling fat stores in the body [67]. A later study in two severely obese children from the same consanguineous family provided the first genetic evidence that leptin was also important for energy balance in humans, and strongly suggested leptin deficiency was causative of their severe obesity [68]. Phenotypically, patients with congenital leptin deficiency have a normal birth weight, and then experience rapid weight gain in the first few months of age, causing severe obesity characterized by intense hyperphagia. Other associated abnormalities include endocrine manifestations such as hypothalamic hypothyroidism, abnormal pubertal development due to hypothalamic hypogonadism, and immunological manifestations with decreased T cell numbers and impaired function, leading to increased risk of infection [69]. Treatment with recombinant human leptin through daily subcutaneous injections has been shown to reduce body weight and fat, further confirming leptin's role in the regulation of body weight and appetite in humans [70]. Daily treatment has also been shown to alleviate the other endocrine and immunological manifestations of congenital leptin deficiency [69].

Leptin Receptor Deficiency

Patients with congenital leptin receptor deficiency are phenotypically similar to patients with congenital leptin deficiency. The prevalence of pathogenic leptin receptor gene (*LEPR*) mutations in one study in a cohort of subjects with severe, early onset obesity not associated with developmental delay was 3% [71]. Mouse models first demonstrated leptin receptor deficiency as a cause of obesity using genetic mapping and genomic analysis in the diabetes (*db*) mouse to discover *LEPR* [72]. Ensuing studies in humans showed elevated mean levels of leptin in obese subjects compared with normal-weight controls, suggesting possible insensitivity or resistance to leptin in these obese individuals [73]. Follow-up investigations not only discovered mutations in the human leptin receptor gene, but also showed that a functional leptin receptor is required for sexual maturation and the secretion of growth hormone and thyrotropin, in addition to the regulation of body weight [74].

Inactive Leptin

More recently, individuals have been identified who harbor mutations in the *leptin* gene that lead to the production of a functionally inactive protein product. Thus, these individuals have apparently high levels of circulating leptin, suggestive of resistance, but nevertheless respond to exogenously administered recombinant leptin therapy [75].

Complete Pro-Opiomelanocortin (POMC) Deficiency

The *POMC* gene is expressed in the arcuate nucleus. POMC-expressing neurons are activated by both leptin and insulin and produce peptide hormones such as alpha-melanocyte-stimulating hormone (α-MSH) that induce satiety. Patients with complete *POMC* mutations are phenotypically characterized by severe early-onset obesity, adrenal insufficiency, red hair pigmentation, and mild hypothyroidism [76,77]. The phenotypic manifestations are due to a lack of multiple POMC-derived ligands, including adrenocorticotropic hormone (ACTH), which promotes cortisol synthesis, and α-MSH, which modulates the production of skin and hair pigments.

Prohormone Convertase 1/3 Deficiency Due to Mutations in *Proprotein Convertase Subtilisin/Kexin Type 1 (PCSK1)* Gene

The *PCSK1* gene encodes a neuroendocrine-specific prohormone convertase 1/3 (PC1/3). Patients with a deficiency in PC1/3 present with early onset childhood obesity, hyperphagia, small-intestinal dysfunction, diarrhea, pituitary hypofunction including adrenal, gonadotropic, somatotropic, thyrotropic, and vasopressin insufficiency, and disordered glucose homeostasis [78–80]. PC1/3 acts on a range of substrates, including enteric hormones, proinsulin, proglucagon, and POMC, which explains how PC1/3 deficiency causes severe obesity along with other endocrine and gastrointestinal pathologies related to a deficiency in the active forms of these substrates.

Human Melanocortin-4 Receptor (*MC4R*) Deficiency

After processing by PC1/3, POMC-derived ligands α-MSH and β-MSH act on melanocortin receptors in the paraventricular nucleus to promote satiety. *MC4R* mutations can present as either dominant or recessive causes of hyperphagic obesity because this receptor plays a key role in the control of eating behaviors in humans [81]. Indeed, *MC4R* mutations were behind the first dominant form of monogenic obesity to be described, and they are also the most common form of monogenic obesity, occurring in 3%–6% of subjects with severe childhood obesity [82]. Phenotypically, patients with *MC4R* variants are hyperphagic, obese, and hyperinsulinemic. Studies have demonstrated that mutations in *MC4R* are inherited in a codominant pattern, with mutations causing a complete loss of function, producing a more severe phenotype [82].

Other Notable Genetic Mutations in the Hypothalamic Leptin–Melanocortin Pathway

With rapid advancements in sequencing techniques, several other genes have been discovered that are also associated with syndromic hyperphagic obesity and specifically related to the hypothalamus downstream of *MC4R*-containing cells in the paraventricular nucleus. A full discussion of these genes is beyond the scope of this text; however, it should be noted that in addition to the genetic syndromes already described, deficiencies in the single-minded homolog 1 (*SIM1*) gene, brain-derived neurotrophic factor (BDNF), which is encoded by the neurotrophic tyrosine kinase receptor type 2 (*NTRK2*) gene, and its associated tyrosine kinase receptor (TRKB) all cause severe monogenic hyperphagic obesity [83,84]. In addition, mutations in the *SH2B1* gene causing a deficiency in SH2B1 have been identified as a monogenic cause of obesity related to leptin signaling with a phenotype of severe obesity, insulin resistance, and behavioral abnormalities [85].

OTHER KNOWN GENETIC OBESITY SYNDROMES

Albright Hereditary Osteodystrophy (AHO)

AHO is characterized phenotypically by obesity, multihormone resistance, short stature, brachydactyly, subcutaneous ossifications, and mental deficits such as developmental delay. AHO is caused by dominantly inherited inactivating mutations of a G protein alpha subunit (G$_s$α) that couples receptors to the stimulation of adenylyl cyclase and the generation of cAMP. Maternal inheritance of this trait is referred to as pseudohypoparathyroidism type 1a (PHP1a) and paternal inheritance is classified as pseudopseudohypoparathyroidism. When the trait is inherited maternally, patients demonstrate all the characteristics of AHO plus obesity and multihormone resistance. Multihormone resistance is not seen with paternal inheritance. Obesity is a more prominent feature of PHP1a and severe obesity is a specific characteristic [86]. Parent-specific inheritance effects suggest that the imprinting of G$_s$α in central nervous system (CNS) regions and tissues acts as an important mediator of energy metabolism related to obesity [87].

Bardet–Biedl Syndrome (BBS)

BBS is a ciliopathic, genetically heterogeneous disorder inherited autosomal recessively and characterized phenotypically by the main features of obesity, retinal dystrophy, renal dysfunction, postaxial polydactyly, hypogonadism, and genitourinary malformations, with several other secondary features. Diagnosis is based on clinical features. Currently, there are 16 known genes for BBS (*BBS1–16*), which account for ~80% of BBS cases [88]. Unlike the other disorders described in this chapter, BBS can be caused by multiple genetic mutations affecting several proteins; however, the exact pathophysiologic mechanism of obesity in BBS is incompletely understood. Mouse studies have demonstrated a possible explanatory mechanism namely, leptin resistance resulting from abnormal LEPR trafficking and attenuated LEPR signaling in the hypothalamus [89]. However, this mechanism has not yet been definitively established as the cause of obesity associated with BBS.

In addition to BBS, several other disorders involving ciliary genes highlight the connection between obesity and abnormal ciliary function. Included in this class of disorders is Alström syndrome caused by mutations in the *ALMS1* gene, Carpenter syndrome caused by mutations in the *RAB23* gene, morbid obesity in humans and mice arising from homozygous mutations in the ciliary protein 19 (*CEP19*) gene, and a homozygous mutation in the *TUB* gene associated with retinal dystrophy and obesity [90,91].

Prader–Willi Syndrome (PWS)

PWS is characterized phenotypically by hyperphagic obesity (in early childhood), decreased fetal movement, hypotonia, cognitive deficits, short stature, hypogonadotropic hypogonadism, and small hands and feet. It is the most common obesity syndrome, and PWS is genetically characterized by a deficiency of one or more paternally expressed imprinted transcripts within chromosome 15q11–q13. Most cases of PWS are caused by deletion of a critical segment on the paternally inherited copy of chromosome 15q11.2–q12, while the remaining cases are caused by uniparental disomy, with the loss of the entire paternal chromosome 15 and the presence of two maternal copies [92]. The exact cause of hyperphagic obesity in PWS patients is unknown. Recently, a deletion of the HBII-85 class of small nucleolar RNAs (snoRNAs) was shown to be associated with hyperphagia, obesity, and hypogonadism in a 19-year-old patient in which previous testing for PWS was negative [93]. In this patient array, comparative genomic hybridization was used to identify a microdeletion at chromosome 15q11–q13 that encompassed the noncoding snoRNAs (including HBII-85). The findings were significant, suggesting the role of a particular family of noncoding RNAs in the regulation of energy, growth, and reproduction. Patients with PWS have also been found to have elevated levels of fasting plasma ghrelin, a gastrointestinal peptide involved in regulating appetite, though the importance of this finding to obesity in PWS remains unknown [94].

CONCLUSIONS

There has been significant progress in the development of various genetic technologies, but each strategy is associated with inherent weaknesses. Computational genetic studies of obesity have helped further unravel the heritability of obesity. Strides continue to be made using the results of large GWAS and meta-analyses, both in adults and in children. However, much work remains to be done to reveal the missing heritability of obesity, as only 10% of obesity heritability is currently explained by the results. Transethnic analyses are needed in order to investigate the effects of ancestry on genetic composition. Additionally, more functional studies are needed to translate genetic association into causation.

Furthermore, studies of specific monogenic and polygenic obesity syndromes have enriched our understanding of the complex neuroendocrine mechanisms that govern both energy intake and energy expenditure. As populations expand and unique phenotypes continue to emerge, a concerted effort is needed between clinicians and scientists alike to identify and characterize new syndromes.

Taken together, these pediatric genetic studies can inform efforts for obesity prevention and treatment starting in early childhood.

REFERENCES

1. Clark PJ. The heritability of certain anthropometric characters as ascertained from measurements of twins. *American Journal of Human Genetics*. 1956;8(1):49–54.
2. Bell CG, Walley AJ, Froguel P. The genetics of human obesity. *Nature Reviews Genetics*. 2005;6(3):221–34.
3. Farooqi IS, O'Rahilly S. New advances in the genetics of early onset obesity. *International Journal of Obesity*. 2005;29(10):1149–52.

4. Feinleib M, Garrison RJ, Fabsitz R, Christian JC, Hrubec Z, Borhani NO, et al. The NHLBI twin study of cardiovascular disease risk factors: Methodology and summary of results. *American Journal of Epidemiology.* 1977;106(4):284–5.

5. Moll PP, Burns TL, Lauer RM. The genetic and environmental sources of body mass index variability: The Muscatine Ponderosity Family Study. *The American Journal of Human Genetics.* 1991;49(6):1243–55.

6. Stunkard AJ, Foch TT, Hrubec Z. A twin study of human obesity. *JAMA.* 1986;256(1):51–4.

7. Stunkard AJ, Harris JR, Pedersen NL, McClearn GE. The body-mass index of twins who have been reared apart. *The New England Journal of Medicine.* 1990;322(21):1483–7.

8. Turula M, Kaprio J, Rissanen A, Koskenvuo M. Body weight in the Finnish Twin Cohort. *Diabetes Research and Clinical Practice.* 1990;10(Suppl. 1):S33–6.

9. Waalen J. The genetics of human obesity. *Translational Research: The Journal of Laboratory and Clinical Medicine.* 2014;164(4):293–301.

10. Pietilainen KH, Kaprio J, Rissanen A, Winter T, Rimpela A, Viken RJ, et al. Distribution and heritability of BMI in Finnish adolescents aged 16y and 17y: A study of 4884 twins and 2509 singletons. *International Journal of Obesity and Related Metabolic Disorders: Journal of the International Association for the Study of Obesity.* 1999;23(2):107–15.

11. Stunkard AJ, Sorensen TI, Hanis C, Teasdale TW, Chakraborty R, Schull WJ, et al. An adoption study of human obesity. *The New England Journal of Medicine.* 1986;314(4):193–8.

12. Knowler WC, Pettitt DJ, Saad MF, Bennett PH. Diabetes mellitus in the Pima Indians: Incidence, risk factors and pathogenesis. *Diabetes/Metabolism Reviews.* 1990;6(1):1–27.

13. Barsh GS, Farooqi IS, O'Rahilly S. Genetics of body-weight regulation. *Nature.* 2000;404(6778):644–51.

14. Farooqi IS, O'Rahilly S. Monogenic obesity in humans. *Annual Review of Medicine.* 2005;56:443–58.

15. Xia Q, Grant SF. The genetics of human obesity. *Annals of the New York Academy of Sciences.* 2013;1281:178–90.

16. International HapMap Consortium. A haplotype map of the human genome. *Nature.* 2005;437(7063):1299–320.

17. Speliotes EK, Willer CJ, Berndt SI, Monda KL, Thorleifsson G, Jackson AU, et al. Association analyses of 249,796 individuals reveal 18 new loci associated with body mass index. *Nature Genetics.* 2010;42(11):937–48.

18. Frayling TM, Timpson NJ, Weedon MN, Zeggini E, Freathy RM, Lindgren CM, et al. A common variant in the FTO gene is associated with body mass index and predisposes to childhood and adult obesity. *Science.* 2007;316(5826):889–94.

19. Loos RJ, Lindgren CM, Li S, Wheeler E, Zhao JH, Prokopenko I, et al. Common variants near MC4R are associated with fat mass, weight and risk of obesity. *Nature Genetics.* 2008;40(6):768–75.

20. Lindgren CM, Heid IM, Randall JC, Lamina C, Steinthorsdottir V, Qi L, et al. Genome-wide association scan meta-analysis identifies three loci influencing adiposity and fat distribution. *PLoS Genetics.* 2009;5(6):e1000508.

21. Thorleifsson G, Walters GB, Gudbjartsson DF, Steinthorsdottir V, Sulem P, Helgadottir A, et al. Genome-wide association yields new sequence variants at seven loci that associate with measures of obesity. *Nature Genetics.* 2009;41(1):18–24.

22. Heid IM, Jackson AU, Randall JC, Winkler TW, Qi L, Steinthorsdottir V, et al. Meta-analysis identifies 13 new loci associated with waist–hip ratio and reveals sexual dimorphism in the genetic basis of fat distribution. *Nature Genetics.* 2010;42(11):949–60.

23. Willer CJ, Speliotes EK, Loos RJ, Li S, Lindgren CM, Heid IM, et al. Six new loci associated with body mass index highlight a neuronal influence on body weight regulation. *Nature Genetics.* 2009;41(1):25–34.

24. Namjou B, Keddache M, Marsolo K, Wagner M, Lingren T, Cobb B, et al. EMR-linked GWAS study: Investigation of variation landscape of loci for body mass index in children. *Frontiers in Genetics.* 2013;4:268.

25. Graff M, Ngwa JS, Workalemahu T, Homuth G, Schipf S, Toumei A, et al. Genome-wide analysis of BMI in adolescents and young adults reveals additional insight into the effects of genetic loci over the life course. *Human Molecular Genetics.* 2013;22(17):3597–607.

26. Bradfield JP, Taal HR, Timpson NJ, Scherag A, Lecoeur C, Warrington NM, et al. A genome-wide association meta-analysis identifies new childhood obesity loci. *Nature Genetics.* 2012;44(5):526–31.

27. Wen W, Cho YS, Zheng W, Dorajoo R, Kato N, Qi L, et al. Meta-analysis identifies common variants associated with body mass index in east Asians. *Nature Genetics.* 2012;44(3):307–11.

28. Monda KL, Chen GK, Taylor KC, Palmer C, Edwards TL, Lange LA, et al. A meta-analysis identifies new loci associated with body mass index in individuals of African ancestry. *Nature Genetics.* 2013;45(6):690–6.

29. Manolio TA, Collins FS, Cox NJ, Goldstein DB, Hindorff LA, Hunter DJ, et al. Finding the missing heritability of complex diseases. *Nature*. 2009;461(7265):747–53.

30. Bogardus C. Missing heritability and GWAS utility. *Obesity*. 2009;17(2):209–10.

31. Yang J, Bakshi A, Zhu Z, Hemani G, Vinkhuyzen AA, Lee SH, et al. Genetic variance estimation with imputed variants finds negligible missing heritability for human height and body mass index. *Nature Genetics*. 2015;47(10):1114–20.

32. Glessner JT, Bradfield JP, Wang K, Takahashi N, Zhang H, Sleiman PM, et al. A genome-wide study reveals copy number variants exclusive to childhood obesity cases. *The American Journal of Human Genetics*. 2010;87(5):661–6.

33. Dina C, Meyre D, Gallina S, Durand E, Korner A, Jacobson P, et al. Variation in FTO contributes to childhood obesity and severe adult obesity. *Nature Genetics*. 2007;39(6):724–6.

34. Wellcome Trust Case Control Consortium. Genome-wide association study of 14,000 cases of seven common diseases and 3,000 shared controls. *Nature*. 2007;447(7145):661–78.

35. Hinney A, Nguyen TT, Scherag A, Friedel S, Bronner G, Muller TD, et al. Genome wide association (GWA) study for early onset extreme obesity supports the role of fat mass and obesity associated gene (FTO) variants. *PLoS One*. 2007;2(12):e1361.

36. Herbert A, Gerry NP, McQueen MB, Heid IM, Pfeufer A, Illig T, et al. A common genetic variant is associated with adult and childhood obesity. *Science*. 2006;312(5771):279–83.

37. Lyon HN, Emilsson V, Hinney A, Heid IM, Lasky-Su J, Zhu X, et al. The association of a SNP upstream of INSIG2 with body mass index is reproduced in several but not all cohorts. *PLoS Genetics*. 2007;3(4):e61.

38. Sovio U, Mook-Kanamori DO, Warrington NM, Lawrence R, Briollais L, Palmer CN, et al. Association between common variation at the FTO locus and changes in body mass index from infancy to late childhood: The complex nature of genetic association through growth and development. *PLoS Genetics*. 2011;7(2):e1001307.

39. Hardy R, Wills AK, Wong A, Elks CE, Wareham NJ, Loos RJ, et al. Life course variations in the associations between FTO and MC4R gene variants and body size. *Human Molecular Genetics*. 2010;19(3):545–52.

40. Rutters F, Nieuwenhuizen AG, Bouwman F, Mariman E, Westerterp-Plantenga MS. Associations between a single nucleotide polymorphism of the FTO Gene (rs9939609) and obesity-related characteristics over time during puberty in a Dutch children cohort. *The Journal of Clinical Endocrinology and Metabolism*. 2011;96(6):E939–42.

41. Gerken T, Girard CA, Tung YC, Webby CJ, Saudek V, Hewitson KS, et al. The obesity-associated FTO gene encodes a 2-oxoglutarate-dependent nucleic acid demethylase. *Science*. 2007;318(5855):1469–72.

42. Church C, Moir L, McMurray F, Girard C, Banks GT, Teboul L, et al. Overexpression of Fto leads to increased food intake and results in obesity. *Nature Genetics*. 2010;42(12):1086–92.

43. Fischer J, Koch L, Emmerling C, Vierkotten J, Peters T, Bruning JC, et al. Inactivation of the Fto gene protects from obesity. *Nature*. 2009;458(7240):894–8.

44. Cecil JE, Tavendale R, Watt P, Hetherington MM, Palmer CN. An obesity-associated FTO gene variant and increased energy intake in children. *The New England Journal of Medicine*. 2008;359(24):2558–66.

45. Rosenquist JN, Lehrer SF, O'Malley AJ, Zaslavsky AM, Smoller JW, Christakis NA. Cohort of birth modifies the association between FTO genotype and BMI. *Proceedings of the National Academy of Sciences of the United States of America*. 2015;112(2):354–9.

46. Smemo S, Tena JJ, Kim KH, Gamazon ER, Sakabe NJ, Gomez-Marin C, et al. Obesity-associated variants within FTO form long-range functional connections with IRX3. *Nature*. 2014;507(7492):371–5.

47. Claussnitzer M, Dankel SN, Kim KH, Quon G, Meuleman W, Haugen C, et al. FTO obesity variant circuitry and adipocyte browning in humans. *The New England Journal of Medicine*. 2015;373(10):895–907.

48. Loos RJ, Lindgren CM, Li S, Wheeler E, Zhao JH, Prokopenko I, et al. Common variants near MC4R are associated with fat mass, weight and risk of obesity. *Nature Genetics*. 2008;40(6):768–75.

49. Willer CJ, Speliotes EK, Loos RJ, Li S, Lindgren CM, Heid IM, et al. Six new loci associated with body mass index highlight a neuronal influence on body weight regulation. *Nature Genetics*. 2009;41(1):25–34.

50. Ren D, Zhou Y, Morris D, Li M, Li Z, Rui L. Neuronal SH2B1 is essential for controlling energy and glucose homeostasis. *The Journal of Clinical Investigation*. 2007;117(2):397–406.

51. Grinberg M, Schwarz M, Zaltsman Y, Eini T, Niv H, Pietrokovski S, et al. Mitochondrial carrier homolog 2 is a target of tBID in cells signaled to die by tumor necrosis factor alpha. *Molecular and Cellular Biology*. 2005;25(11):4579–90.

52. Marg A, Sirim P, Spaltmann F, Plagge A, Kauselmann G, Buck F, et al. Neurotractin, a novel neurite outgrowth-promoting Ig-like protein that interacts with CEPU-1 and LAMP. *The Journal of Cell Biology*. 1999;145(4):865–76.

53. Speliotes EK, Willer CJ, Berndt SI, Monda KL, Thorleifsson G, Jackson AU, et al. Association analyses of 249,796 individuals reveal 18 new loci associated with body mass index. *Nature Genetics*. 2010;42(11):937–48.

54. Farooqi IS, Drop S, Clements A, Keogh JM, Biernacka J, Lowenbein S, et al. Heterozygosity for a POMC-null mutation and increased obesity risk in humans. *Diabetes*. 2006;55(9):2549–53.

55. Miyawaki K, Yamada Y, Ban N, Ihara Y, Tsukiyama K, Zhou H, et al. Inhibition of gastric inhibitory polypeptide signaling prevents obesity. *Nature Medicine*. 2002;8(7):738–42.

56. Locke AE, Kahali B, Berndt SI, Justice AE, Pers TH, Day FR, et al. Genetic studies of body mass index yield new insights for obesity biology. *Nature*. 2015;518(7538):197–206.

57. Maller JB, McVean G, Byrnes J, Vukcevic D, Palin K, Su Z, et al. Bayesian refinement of association signals for 14 loci in 3 common diseases. *Nature Genetics*. 2012;44(12):1294–301.

58. Zhao J, Bradfield JP, Li M, Wang K, Zhang H, Kim CE, et al. The role of obesity-associated loci identified in genome-wide association studies in the determination of pediatric BMI. *Obesity (Silver Spring, MD)*. 2009;17(12):2254–7.

59. den Hoed M, Ekelund U, Brage S, Grontved A, Zhao JH, Sharp SJ, et al. Genetic susceptibility to obesity and related traits in childhood and adolescence: Influence of loci identified by genome-wide association studies. *Diabetes*. 2010;59(11):2980–8.

60. Scherag A, Dina C, Hinney A, Vatin V, Scherag S, Vogel CI, et al. Two new loci for body-weight regulation identified in a joint analysis of genome-wide association studies for early-onset extreme obesity in French and German study groups. *PLoS Genetics*. 2010;6(4):e1000916.

61. Warrington NM, Howe LD, Paternoster L, Kaakinen M, Herrala S, Huikari V, et al. A genome-wide association study of body mass index across early life and childhood. *International Journal of Epidemiology*. 2015;44(2):700–12.

62. Wheeler E, Huang N, Bochukova EG, Keogh JM, Lindsay S, Garg S, et al. Genome-wide SNP and CNV analysis identifies common and low-frequency variants associated with severe early-onset obesity. *Nature Genetics*. 2013;45(5):513–7.

63. Kim HJ, Park JW, Lee KH, Yoon H, Shin DH, Ju UI, et al. Plant homeodomain finger protein 2 promotes bone formation by demethylating and activating Runx2 for osteoblast differentiation. *Cell Research*. 2014;24(10):1231–49.

64. Zegers D, Van Hul W, Van Gaal LF, Beckers S. Monogenic and complex forms of obesity: Insights from genetics reveal the leptin-melanocortin signaling pathway as a common player. *Critical Reviews in Eukaryotic Gene Expression*. 2012;22(4):325–43.

65. Ingalls AM, Dickie MM, Snell GD. Obese, a new mutation in the house mouse. *Journal of Heredity*. 1950;41(12):317–8.

66. Zhang Y, Proenca R, Maffei M, Barone M, Leopold L, Friedman JM. Positional cloning of the mouse obese gene and its human homologue. *Nature*. 1994;372(6505):425–32.

67. Halaas JL, Gajiwala KS, Maffei M, Cohen SL, Chait BT, Rabinowitz D, et al. Weight-reducing effects of the plasma protein encoded by the obese gene. *Science*. 1995;269(5223):543–6.

68. Montague CT, Farooqi IS, Whitehead JP, Soos MA, Rau H, Wareham NJ, et al. Congenital leptin deficiency is associated with severe early-onset obesity in humans. *Nature*. 1997;387(6636):903–8.

69. Farooqi IS, Matarese G, Lord GM, Keogh JM, Lawrence E, Agwu C, et al. Beneficial effects of leptin on obesity, T cell hyporesponsiveness, and neuroendocrine/metabolic dysfunction of human congenital leptin deficiency. *The Journal of Clinical Investigation*. 2002;110(8):1093–103.

70. Farooqi IS, Jebb SA, Langmack G, Lawrence E, Cheetham CH, Prentice AM, et al. Effects of recombinant leptin therapy in a child with congenital leptin deficiency. *The New England Journal of Medicine*. 1999;341(12):879–84.

71. Farooqi IS, Wangensteen T, Collins S, Kimber W, Matarese G, Keogh JM, et al. Clinical and molecular genetic spectrum of congenital deficiency of the leptin receptor. *The New England Journal of Medicine*. 2007;356(3):237–47.

72. Chua SC, Jr, Chung WK, Wu-Peng XS, Zhang Y, Liu SM, Tartaglia L, et al. Phenotypes of mouse diabetes and rat fatty due to mutations in the OB (leptin) receptor. *Science*. 1996;271(5251):994–6.

73. Considine RV, Sinha MK, Heiman ML, Kriauciunas A, Stephens TW, Nyce MR, et al. Serum immunoreactive-leptin concentrations in normal-weight and obese humans. *The New England Journal of Medicine*. 1996;334(5):292–5.

74. Clement K, Vaisse C, Lahlou N, Cabrol S, Pelloux V, Cassuto D, et al. A mutation in the human leptin receptor gene causes obesity and pituitary dysfunction. *Nature*. 1998;392(6674):398–401.

75. Wabitsch M, Funcke JB, von Schnurbein J, Denzer F, Lahr G, Mazen I, et al. Severe early-onset obesity due to bioinactive leptin caused by a p.N103K mutation in the leptin gene. *The Journal of Clinical Endocrinology and Metabolism*. 2015;100(9):3227–30.

76. Krude H, Biebermann H, Luck W, Horn R, Brabant G, Gruters A. Severe early-onset obesity, adrenal insufficiency and red hair pigmentation caused by POMC mutations in humans. *Nature Genetics.* 1998;19(2):155–7.

77. Krude H, Biebermann H, Schnabel D, Tansek MZ, Theunissen P, Mullis PE, et al. Obesity due to proopiomelanocortin deficiency: Three new cases and treatment trials with thyroid hormone and ACTH4–10. *The Journal of Clinical Endocrinology and Metabolism.* 2003;88(10):4633–40.

78. Jackson RS, Creemers JW, Ohagi S, Raffin-Sanson ML, Sanders L, Montague CT, et al. Obesity and impaired prohormone processing associated with mutations in the human prohormone convertase 1 gene. *Nature Genetics.* 1997;16(3):303–6.

79. Farooqi IS, Volders K, Stanhope R, Heuschkel R, White A, Lank E, et al. Hyperphagia and early-onset obesity due to a novel homozygous missense mutation in prohormone convertase 1/3. *The Journal of Clinical Endocrinology and Metabolism.* 2007;92(9):3369–73.

80. Martin MG, Lindberg I, Solorzano-Vargas RS, Wang J, Avitzur Y, Bandsma R, et al. Congenital proprotein convertase 1/3 deficiency causes malabsorptive diarrhea and other endocrinopathies in a pediatric cohort. *Gastroenterology.* 2013;145(1):138–48.

81. Farooqi IS, Yeo GS, Keogh JM, Aminian S, Jebb SA, Butler G, et al. Dominant and recessive inheritance of morbid obesity associated with melanocortin 4 receptor deficiency. *The Journal of Clinical Investigation.* 2000;106(2):271–9.

82. Farooqi IS, Keogh JM, Yeo GS, Lank EJ, Cheetham T, O'Rahilly S. Clinical spectrum of obesity and mutations in the melanocortin 4 receptor gene. *The New England Journal of Medicine.* 2003;348(12):1085–95.

83. Michaud JL, Boucher F, Melnyk A, Gauthier F, Goshu E, Levy E, et al. Sim1 haploinsufficiency causes hyperphagia, obesity and reduction of the paraventricular nucleus of the hypothalamus. *Human Molecular Genetics.* 2001;10(14):1465–73.

84. Gray J, Yeo GS, Cox JJ, Morton J, Adlam AL, Keogh JM, et al. Hyperphagia, severe obesity, impaired cognitive function, and hyperactivity associated with functional loss of one copy of the brain-derived neurotrophic factor (BDNF) gene. *Diabetes.* 2006;55(12):3366–71.

85. Doche ME, Bochukova EG, Su HW, Pearce LR, Keogh JM, Henning E, et al. Human SH2B1 mutations are associated with maladaptive behaviors and obesity. *The Journal of Clinical Investigation.* 2012;122(12):4732–6.

86. Long DN, McGuire S, Levine MA, Weinstein LS, Germain-Lee EL. Body mass index differences in pseudohypoparathyroidism type 1a versus pseudopseudohypoparathyroidism may implicate paternal imprinting of Galpha(s) in the development of human obesity. *The Journal of Clinical Endocrinology and Metabolism.* 2007;92(3):1073–9.

87. Chen M, Berger A, Kablan A, Zhang J, Gavrilova O, Weinstein LS. Gsalpha deficiency in the paraventricular nucleus of the hypothalamus partially contributes to obesity associated with Gsalpha mutations. *Endocrinology.* 2012;153(9):4256–65.

88. Forsythe E, Beales PL. Bardet–Biedl syndrome. *European Journal of Human Genetics: EJHG.* 2013;21(1):8–13.

89. Seo S, Guo DF, Bugge K, Morgan DA, Rahmouni K, Sheffield VC. Requirement of Bardet–Biedl syndrome proteins for leptin receptor signaling. *Human Molecular Genetics.* 2009;18(7):1323–31.

90. Shalata A, Ramirez MC, Desnick RJ, Priedigkeit N, Buettner C, Lindtner C, et al. Morbid obesity resulting from inactivation of the ciliary protein CEP19 in humans and mice. *The American Journal of Human Genetics.* 2013;93(6):1061–71.

91. Borman AD, Pearce LR, Mackay DS, Nagel-Wolfrum K, Davidson AE, Henderson R, et al. A homozygous mutation in the TUB gene associated with retinal dystrophy and obesity. *Human Mutation.* 2014;35(3):289–93.

92. Angulo MA, Butler MG, Cataletto ME. Prader–Willi syndrome: A review of clinical, genetic, and endocrine findings. *Journal of Endocrinological Investigation.* 2015;38(12):1249–63.

93. de Smith AJ, Purmann C, Walters RG, Ellis RJ, Holder SE, Van Haelst MM, et al. A deletion of the HBII-85 class of small nucleolar RNAs (snoRNAs) is associated with hyperphagia, obesity and hypogonadism. *Human Molecular Genetics.* 2009;18(17):3257–65.

94. Cummings DE, Clement K, Purnell JQ, Vaisse C, Foster KE, Frayo RS, et al. Elevated plasma ghrelin levels in Prader–Willi syndrome. *Nature Medicine.* 2002;8(7):643–4.

14 Childhood Obesity
Epigenetic Factors

Keith M. Godfrey, Karen A. Lillycrop, and Robert Murray

CONTENTS

INTRODUCTION

The prevalence of obesity and associated disorders including type 2 diabetes is increasing globally at an alarming rate. While genetic variations in a number of genes have been linked to obesity (see Chapter 13), to date, single-nucleotide polymorphisms and copy number variations explain only a fraction of the risk of obesity and metabolic disease in humans [1]. However, there is now substantial evidence from both human and animal studies that the quality of the early-life environment before and after birth can affect susceptibility to obesity and associated metabolic disorders in later life [2]. Experimental studies show that the developmental environment can alter later phenotype by changing the epigenetic regulation of genes, and this chapter focuses on the evidence that perinatal influences such as maternal nutrition can alter epigenetic processes, leading to persistent phenotypic changes and an increased risk of childhood obesity.

DEVELOPMENTAL INFLUENCES ON LATER HEALTH AND DISEASE

Some of the first evidence that developmental influences play a substantial role in "programing" later health and disease came from follow-up studies of men whose mothers were exposed to famine in pregnancy during the Second World War; measurements taken in young adulthood showed that maternal famine exposure mid-pregnancy was associated with later obesity [3]. Subsequent longitudinal studies in 25,000 UK men and women related infant size at birth to later coronary heart disease and associated disorders in adulthood. People who were small or disproportionate (thin or short) at birth, or whose infant growth faltered, had high rates of coronary heart disease, raised blood pressure and cholesterol levels, and impaired glucose tolerance [4]. Large effects were particularly seen if restricted fetal and infant growth was followed by increased childhood weight gain. Replication of the initial findings in further studies worldwide has led to wide acceptance that low rates of fetal growth are associated with cardiovascular disease in later life. In the original UK studies, the relations between smaller size at birth and an increased risk of ill health and adult disease extended across the normal range of infant size in a *graded* manner, but with an increase at the highest birth weights. Maternal obesity is one of the drivers of high birth weight, and subsequent research has shown that maternal obesity is also associated with premature mortality in the off-spring from cardiovascular disease and associated disorders [5].

These observations have led to the hypothesis that obesity, coronary heart disease, type 2 diabetes, and other noncommunicable disorders (NCDs) originate through developmental plastic responses made by the fetus and infant as part of a prediction of the subsequent environment to which it anticipates that it will be exposed. Critical periods in development result in irreversible changes; if the environment in childhood and adult life differs from that predicted during fetal life and infancy, the developmental responses may increase the risk of adult disease. Evolutionary considerations and experimental findings in animals strongly support the existence of major developmental effects on health and disease in adulthood [6]. The preservation of this "programing" phenomenon across species and within the normal range of fetal growth suggests a physiological rather than a pathological basis to the developmental influences on later health. The policy implications of these concepts are now under serious consideration: the 2011 High-Level Meeting of the United Nations General Assembly on the Prevention and Control of NCDs noted that maternal and child health is inextricably linked to NCDs and their risk factors, and stressed the importance of taking a life course approach to addressing NCDs [7].

DEVELOPMENTAL INFLUENCES ON CHILD ADIPOSITY

In humans, famine exposure during pregnancy [3], maternal smoking, obesity [8], and gestational diabetes [9] are all associated with an increased risk of obesity in later life, as reviewed in Chapter 12. In the UK Southampton Women's Survey (SWS), we have demonstrated the associations of preconception, pregnancy, and early postnatal factors with childhood adiposity, determined using dual x-ray absorptiometry (DXA) at birth, and at ages 4 and 6–7 years. Using the US Institute of Medicine gestational weight gain categorization, excessive gain was associated with greater offspring fat mass at age 6–7 years [10]. Additionally, low maternal vitamin D status in pregnancy was associated with greater postnatal adiposity gain [11]. Early-life *risk factors* for greater adiposity in childhood, identified in the SWS, often coexisted, such that excess gestational weight gain and a shorter duration of breast-feeding were more common in obese mothers, and smoking during pregnancy was related to lower vitamin D status. Examining the combined impact of five early influences (maternal obesity before pregnancy, excessive gestational weight gain, smoking during pregnancy, low maternal vitamin D status, and a short duration of breast-feeding), we found strong positive associations between the number of early-life risk factors and child fat mass at both 4 and 6–7 years of age [8]. In parallel with the effects on fat mass, an increasing number of early-life risk factors was also associated with strong graded increases in the risk of being overweight or obese in childhood, according to the International Obesity Task Force definitions; when compared with children who had no perinatal risk factors, the relative risks of being overweight or obese among children who had four or five risk factors were 3.99 at four years and 4.65 at six–seven years. These findings are similar to those of an earlier US study [12], which showed that preschool children whose mothers had excess gestational weight gain and smoked during pregnancy, who were breast-fed for less than 12 months, and who slept for less than 12 hours per day in infancy had a predicted obesity prevalence of 29%, compared with 6% of children who had none of these risk factors. Importantly, these marked differences were found to persist (28% compared with 4%) when the children were aged 7–10 years [13].

DEVELOPMENTAL ADAPTATIONS AND CHILDHOOD ADIPOSITY

Our SWS studies have provided evidence that prenatal developmental adaptations play important roles in the human propensity to deposit fat [14]. Among primates, human neonates have not only the largest brains but also the highest proportion of body fat. If placental nutrient supply is limited, the fetus faces a dilemma: should resources be allocated to brain growth or to fat deposition for use as a potential postnatal energy reserve? We hypothesized that resolving this dilemma operates at the level of umbilical blood distribution entering the fetal liver. In uncomplicated third-trimester SWS pregnancies, we used ultrasound to measure blood flow perfusing the fetal liver or bypassing it via the ductus venosus to supply the brain and heart [14]. Across the range of fetal size and independent of the mother's adiposity and parity, greater liver blood flow was associated with greater offspring fat mass measured by DXA, both in the infant at birth and at age 4 years. In contrast, smaller placentas less able to meet fetal demand for essential nutrients were associated with a brain-sparing flow pattern. This led us to propose that humans have evolved a developmental strategy to prioritize nutrient allocation for prenatal fat deposition when the supply of conditionally essential nutrients requiring hepatic interconversion is limited, switching resource allocation to favor the brain if the supply of essential nutrients is limited. Facilitated placental transfer processes for glucose and other nutrients evolved in environments less affluent than those now prevalent in developed populations, and we proposed that in circumstances of maternal adiposity and nutrient excess these processes now also lead to prenatal fat deposition [14].

This proposal suggests that there may be two groups of broad developmental paths to childhood obesity. A "low" path is associated with maternal famine exposure or macronutrient deficiency, micronutrient deficiency (e.g., vitamin D insufficiency), smoking (itself associated with both toxicant exposure and low micronutrient status), and placental pathology; the infants are thin at birth but gain adiposity progressively during the infancy and preschool periods, such that they become of above-average adiposity by childhood. Conversely, a "high" path is associated with maternal obesity, excessive pregnancy weight gain, and gestational diabetes; the infants have average adiposity at birth and remain adipose during the infancy, preschool, and childhood periods.

MOLECULAR MECHANISMS LINKING DEVELOPMENTAL INFLUENCES WITH LATER OBESITY

It has been argued that the associations between fetal or infant growth and later adult disease could represent the multiple (pleiotropic) effects of genes transmitted from mother to child. The Early Growth Genetics consortium, however, showed only a small genotypic contribution to birth weight [15]. Epigenetic processes, including DNA methylation, modification of the histone proteins that package DNA, and noncoding RNAs, play a central role in regulating gene expression. DNA methylation typically involves the transfer of a methyl group to a cytosine immediately 5' to a guanine (so-called CpG dinucleotides, where p denotes the intervening phosphate group), creating 5-methylcytosine (5mC) [16]; non-CpG methylation is, however, also prevalent in embryonic stem cells [17]. Across the genome, CpG frequency is biased toward promoter regions, where they may occur in clusters termed *CpG islands*, which are mostly unmethylated. Lower-density CpG promoter sites tend to be hypermethylated. Methylation at CpG islands is typically associated with genes that require long-term repression; such genes include imprinted genes that are preferentially expressed from one parental chromosome, those located on the inactive X chromosome in female mammals, and those only requiring expression in germ and not somatic cells [18].

The traditional view has been that DNA methylation is linked to gene silencing. However, the effect of methylation on gene expression is potentially dependent on factors such as CpG density, gene product function, and site of methylation; for example, gene body methylation is not associated with gene repression [19,20]. The different epigenetic processes do not act in isolation but interact in a coordinated fashion; for example, inactive CpG island promoters are generally not methylated but are instead marked by lysine trimethylation on histone H3. Whether DNA methylation is a cause or a consequence of repressed gene expression is still under debate; some of the proposed mechanisms for methylation-associated gene silencing include disrupted transcription factor binding preventing RNA polymerase activity, the recruitment of methyl-binding proteins that in turn attract other repressor complexes, and the transcription of noncoding RNAs.

DNA methylation is a stable epigenetic mark that is transmitted through mitotic DNA replication and cell division, leading to the suggestion that epigenetic processes could be an important mechanism by which the environment alters long-term disease risk. Consistent with this suggestion, the Growing Up in Singapore Towards Healthy Outcomes (GUSTO) study has recently found that maternally mediated *in utero* environmental influences and gene–environment interactions are a more important source of variation in neonatal genome-wide methylation patterns than fixed genetic variation, as reflected by DNA sequence polymorphisms [21].

Evidence from experimental studies in animals indicates that early life is a critical period when appetite and the regulation of energy balance are programed, with lifelong consequences for the risk of excess adiposity. Variations in maternal diet have, for example, been linked to alterations in metabolism and body composition in the offspring [22]. Experimental studies show that the developmental environment induces an altered phenotype through epigenetic mechanisms, including changes in DNA methylation, histone modification, and noncoding RNAs [6]. The father's diet can also have an effect on the epigenome and phenotype of the offspring. Male mice fed a low-protein diet prior to mating showed widespread modest changes in the methylation (10%–20%) of the DNA of their offspring compared with control offspring, including a substantial increase in methylation at an intergenic CpG island 50 kilobases upstream of the PPARα gene [23]. Similarly, in rats, a paternal chronic high-fat diet led to pancreatic β-cell dysfunction in the female offspring [24]. Experimental studies of paternal environmentally induced intergenerational effects are an area of increasing research interest; for example, a recent study in marine tubeworms has shown that transgenerational adverse paternal effects can be stronger than maternal effects [25].

A classic example of maternal nutrition influencing DNA methylation in mammals is in the agouti mouse model, where coat color is influenced by the methylation status of the 5′ end of the *Agouti* gene. Differences in the mother's intake of dietary methyl donors and cofactors (including folic acid, vitamin B12, betaine, and choline) were shown to alter DNA methylation of the *Agouti* gene and induce differences in the coat color and adiposity of the offspring [26]. DNA methylation changes induced during development are highly gene and CpG specific [27], and methylation of individual CpG dinucleotides in gene promoter and intergenic regions alters gene expression. Such "tuning" has potential adaptive value and fitness advantage because it adjusts the phenotype to current circumstances and/or matches responses to the environment predicted to be experienced later [6]. When the phenotype is mismatched to the later environment—for example, from inaccurate nutritional cues from the mother or placenta, or from rapid environmental change through improved socioeconomic conditions—the risk of NCDs increases. Evidence is accruing that endocrine or nutritional interventions during early postnatal life can reverse epigenetic and phenotypic changes induced, for example, by an unbalanced maternal diet during pregnancy [28]. Elucidation of epigenetic processes may permit perinatal identification of individuals at risk of later NCDs and enable early intervention strategies to reduce such risk.

EPIGENETIC CHANGES AS A CONSEQUENCE OR CAUSE OF OBESITY

While DNA methylation states at particular loci have been associated with a range of disorders, it is generally unclear whether the methylation changes occur before disease symptoms or afterward as a consequence of the disease. A large epigenome-wide association study with replication in two independent cohorts reported that methylation levels at three CpGs in the first intron of the hypoxia inducible factor 3 alpha (*HIF3A*) locus were positively associated with adult body mass index in whole blood and adipose tissue from Caucasian subjects [29]. The finding has since been replicated by an independent group of researchers [30]. The authors of the original observation considered three possibilities that could explain the association between *HIF3A* methylation and adiposity in adults: (1) that a confounding factor (such as environment) independently affects both *HIF3A* methylation and adiposity, (2) that increased *HIF3A* methylation causes increased adiposity, and (3) that increased adiposity causes increased *HIF3A* methylation. The *HIF3A* genotype was associated with *HIF3A* methylation but not adult body mass index, and using a Mendelian randomization approach [31], Dick et al. suggested that adiposity most likely results in *HIF3A* hypermethylation [29]. However, in this context, Mendelian randomization assumes the genotype can affect the phenotype only through DNA methylation and not through other biological pathways, an assumption of unknown applicability for the *HIF3A* genotype.

Given the evidence that developmental pathways to obesity begin before birth, we used a multi-ethnic Asian mother–offspring cohort (the GUSTO cohort) to examine if *HIF3A* gene methylation levels in umbilical cord tissue are associated with birth size and adiposity [32]. Taking account of sex, ethnicity, cellular composition of umbilical cords, and interactions between ethnicity and cellular composition, the analyses showed that the link between *HIF3A* DNA methylation with weight and adiposity can be detected at birth. The association was limited to measures of adiposity (i.e., weight, BMI, and skinfolds) and not other determinants of birth size or putative proxies for gestational quality such as gestational age and birth length. Although pertaining to the same three CpGs within the *HIF3A* gene that were previously reported, these findings were derived from a different tissue (umbilical cord vs. blood and adipose), in a population-based cohort (rather than a study population of metabolic disorders and controls), and at a different stage in the life course (neonates vs. adults). The findings point away from established obesity as a cause of *HIF3A* hypermethylation [32], and suggest that prenatal factors may influence *HIF3A* methylation as well as adiposity; however, despite the extensive data collected in the GUSTO study, no responsible prenatal factor could be definitively identified. Nonetheless, as the association between *HIF3A* methylation and adiposity is detectable so early in life, *HIF3A* may be a potential biomarker of metabolic trajectory.

HUMAN STUDIES OF EPIGENETIC PROCESSES AND CHILDHOOD ADIPOSITY

While epigenetic processes operating in early development have been implicated in growth and later body composition, until recently there has been little direct evidence for the proposition in humans. Studies using candidate gene approaches have shown associations between DNA methylation in cord blood leucocytes (e.g., in the *IGF2*-imprinting control region in 24 infants) and childhood adiposity [33]. Using Sequenom MassARRAY, we measured the methylation status of 68 CpGs 5' from five candidate nonimprinted genes in umbilical cord tissue DNA from healthy neonates [34]. Methylation varied greatly at particular CpG sites. For 31 CpGs with median methylation ≥5% and a 5th to 95th percentile range ≥10%, we related methylation status to the maternal pregnancy diet and to the child's body composition at age 9 years; greater methylation of two CpGs within the retinoid X receptor alpha (*RXRA*) promoter measured in the umbilical cord was robustly associated with greater adiposity [34]. The associations reflected clinically important shifts in body composition; from the lowest to the highest quarters of the distribution of *RXRA* methylation, mean fat mass rose from 4.8 to 6.6 kg (17.3%–21.3% body fat). Regression analyses including sex and neonatal epigenetic marks explained >25% of the variance in childhood adiposity. The findings were replicated in a second independent cohort. In these human studies, associations were also observed between levels of *RXRA* methylation and mothers' carbohydrate intake [34], supportive of the concept that nutritional conditions in early pregnancy can affect a child's adiposity in later life.

As DNA methylation and gene transcription are often tissue specific, it is not possible to extrapolate how the level of methylation in the umbilical cord may affect expression in adipose or other tissues and/or whether such epigenetic alterations are causally involved in the development of fat mass. However, for a number of imprinted and nonimprinted genes, there is evidence that methylation levels are similar across a range of conceptual tissues, including buccal, brain, eye, intestine, liver, lung, muscle, and umbilical cord blood, despite the fact that these cell types arise from different germ layers [35,36]. It may be that an early environmental challenge could leave an imprint on the epigenome that is detectable across tissue types.

Another area of uncertainty arises from data showing that some DNA methylation marks can be dynamically regulated in response to postnatal environmental stimuli, raising questions about the stability of developmentally induced epigenetic marks over time. One study that examined DNA methylation stability over time in children found that the methylation levels of the genes *MAOA*, *DRD4*, and *SLC6A4* was highly dynamic between the ages of 5 and 10 years [37]. An example of dynamic regulation relates to the induction by acute physical activity of hypomethylation in the peroxisome proliferator–activated receptor gamma coactivator 1 alpha (*PGC1α*) promoter in muscle tissue [38]. In contrast, in DNA from peripheral blood cells, Clarke-Harris et al. reported year-on-year stability of the methylation levels of a different group of seven CpG sites within the *PGC1α* promoter in children 5–14 years of age [39]; this suggests that for these CpG sites methylation levels are set up in early life and their stability is maintained. Moreover, seven of the *PGC1α* promoter CpG sites analyzed at age 5–7 years were predictive of adiposity in the children at ages 9–14 [39], providing further evidence that developmentally induced methylation marks may be significant contributors to later obesity risk. The differences in the stability of the *PGC1α* methylation between the two studies may reflect differences in the location of the CpGs or tissue-specific differences between blood and muscle (*PGC1α* has a muscle-specific transcript). Whether the changes in methylation in response to exercise occur on top of a developmentally induced methylation change is also not known.

EPIGENETICS IN SEVERE CHILDHOOD OBESITY

Much of the research to date has examined the role of epigenetic processes in potentially mediating variations in child adiposity across the range in general population samples of children. To examine whether severe childhood obesity is associated with differential DNA methylation, we studied DNA methylation profiles in whole blood from 78 obese children (mean BMI z-score: 2.6) and 71 age- and sex-matched controls (mean BMI z-score: 0.1) [40]. Using the Infinium HumanMethylation450 BeadChip array, comparison of the methylation profiles between obese and control subjects revealed 129 differentially methylated CpG (DMCpG) loci associated with 80 unique genes that had a greater than 10% difference in methylation. Undertaking pathway analysis of these DMCpG loci, the top pathways enriched included developmental processes, immune system regulation, regulation of cell signaling, and small GTPase-mediated signal transduction. The associations between the methylation of selected DMCpGs within the *FYN*, *PIWIL4*, and *TAOK3* genes and childhood obesity were then validated using sodium bisulfite pyrosequencing in individual subjects. Three CpG loci within *FYN* were hypermethylated in obese individuals, while obesity was associated with lower methylation of CpG loci within *PIWIL4* and *TAOK3*. Using logistic regression models, a 1% increase in methylation in *TAOK3* multiplicatively decreased the odds of being obese by 0.91, and a 1% increase in *FYN* methylation multiplicatively increased the odds of being obese by 1.03 [40]. The findings provide further evidence that childhood obesity is associated with specific DNA methylation changes.

CONCLUSION

Research has demonstrated that during prenatal development, responses to a range of environmental stimuli are likely to "program" the risk of obesity and associated metabolic disorders. Subsequent environmental exposures during infancy, childhood, and adult life may modify or condition this later risk of obesity. This life course approach is central to the concept of the "developmental origins of health and disease." Development, growth, and metabolism are influenced by a combination of genetic, epigenetic, and environmental factors. Experimental studies indicate that environmental factors in early life, including nutrition, stress, endocrine disruption, and pollution, induce altered body composition in ways that are influenced or mediated by epigenetic mechanisms. These mechanisms include DNA methylation, covalent modifications of histones, and noncoding RNAs, and increasing evidence implicates similar mechanisms in the developmental programing of childhood obesity. This evidence suggests that efforts to improve the nutrition of young women before and during pregnancy will be central to future strategies to achieve the primary prevention of childhood obesity [41].

REFERENCES

1. Locke AE, Kahali B, Berndt SI, et al. Genetic studies of body mass index yield new insights for obesity biology. *Nature* 2015;518:197–206.
2. Godfrey KM, Inskip HM, Hanson MA. The long-term effects of prenatal development on growth and metabolism. *Sem Repro Med* 2011;29: 257–265.
3. Ravelli GP, Stein ZA, Susser MW. Obesity in young men after famine exposure *in utero* and early infancy. *N Engl J Med* 1976;295:349–353.
4. Barker DJ, Winter PD, Osmond C, Margetts B, Simmonds SJ. Weight in infancy and death from ischaemic heart disease. *Lancet* 1989;8663:577–580.
5. Lee KK, Raja EA, Lee AJ, Bhattacharya S, Bhattacharya S, Norman JE, Reynolds RM. Maternal obesity during pregnancy associates with premature mortality and major cardiovascular events in later life. *Hypertension* 2015;66:938–944.
6. Hanson MA, Godfrey KM, Lillycrop KA, Burdge GC, Gluckman P. Developmental plasticity and developmental origins of non-communicable disease: Theoretical considerations and epigenetic mechanisms. *Prog Biophys Mol Biol* 2011;106: 272–280.
7. WHO. *Global Action Plan for the Prevention and Control of Non-communicable Diseases 2013–2020.* Geneva, Switzerland: WHO, 2013.
8. Robinson SM, Crozier SR, Harvey NC, et al. Modifiable early-life risk factors for childhood adiposity and overweight: An analysis of their combined impact and potential for prevention. *Am J Clin Nutr* 2015;101:368–375.
9. Pettitt DJ, Bennett PH, Saad MF, et al. Abnormal glucose tolerance during pregnancy in Pima Indian women: Long-term effects on offspring. *Diabetes* 1991;40(Suppl. 2): 126–130.
10. Crozier SR, Inskip HM, Godfrey KM, Cooper C, Harvey NC, Cole ZA, Robinson SM, SWS Study Group. Weight gain in pregnancy and childhood body composition: Findings from the Southampton Women's Survey. *Am J Clin Nutr* 2010;91:1745–1751.
11. Crozier SR, Harvey NC, Inskip HM, Godfrey KM, Cooper C, Robinson SM, SWS Study Group. Maternal vitamin D status in pregnancy is associated with adiposity in the offspring: Findings from the Southampton Women's Survey. *Am J Clin Nutr* 2012;96:57–63.
12. Gillman MW, Rifas-Shiman SL, Kleinman K, Oken E, Rich-Edwards JW, Taveras EM. Developmental origins of childhood overweight: Potential public health impact. *Obesity (Silver Spring)* 2008;16: 1651–1656.
13. Gillman MW, Ludwig DS. How early should obesity prevention start? *N Engl J Med* 2013;369:2173–2175.
14. Godfrey KM, Haugen G, Kiserud T, Inskip HM, Cooper C, Harvey NCW, Crozier SR, Robinson SM, Davies L, SWS Study Group, Hanson MA. Fetal liver blood flow distribution: Role in human developmental strategy to prioritize fat deposition versus brain development. *PLoS One* 2012;7:e41759.
15. Horikoshi M, Yaghootkar H, Mook-Kanamori DO, et al. Novel loci associated with birth weight reveal genetic links between intrauterine growth and adult height and metabolism. *Nat Genet* 2013;45:76–82.
16. Godfrey KM, Lillycrop KA, Burdge GC, Gluckman PD, Hanson MA. Epigenetic mechanisms and the mismatch concept of the developmental origins of health and disease. *Pediatr Res* 2007;61:5R–10R.
17. Ramsahoye BH, Biniszkiewicz D, Lyko F, Clark V, Bird AP, Jaenisch R. Non-CpG methylation is prevalent in embryonic stem cells and may be mediated by DNA methyltransferase 3a. *Proc Nat Acad Sci* 2000;97:5237–5242.
18. Jones PA. Functions of DNA methylation: Islands, start sites, gene bodies and beyond. *Nat Rev Genet* 2012;13:484–492.
19. Weber M, Hellmann I, Stadler MB, et al. Distribution, silencing potential and evolutionary impact of promoter DNA methylation in the human genome. *Nat Genet* 2007;39:457–466.
20. Messerschmidt DM, Knowles BB, Solter D. DNA methylation dynamics during epigenetic reprogramming in the germline and preimplantation embryos. *Genes Dev* 2014;28:812–828.
21. Teh AL, Pan H, Chen L, et al. The effect of genotype and in utero environment on interindividual variation in neonate DNA methylomes. *Genome Res* 2014;24:1064–1074.
22. Godfrey KM, Costello PM, Lillycrop KA. The developmental environment, epigenetic biomarkers and long-term health. *J Dev Origins Health Dis* 2015;6:399–406.

23. Carone BR, Fauquier L, Habib N, et al. Paternally induced transgenerational environmental reprogramming of metabolic gene expression in mammals. *Cell* 2010;143:1084–1096.

24. Ng S-F, Lin RCY, Laybutt DR, Barres R, Owens JA, Morris MJ. Chronic high-fat diet in fathers programs β-cell dysfunction in female rat offspring. *Nature* 2010;467:963–966.

25. Guillaume AS, Monro K, Marshall DJ. Transgenerational plasticity and environmental stress: Do paternal effects act as a conduit or a buffer? *Funct Ecol* 2015;10.1111/1365-2435.12604.

26. Waterland RA, Jirtle RL. Transposable elements: Targets for early nutritional effects on epigenetic gene regulation. *Mol Cell Biol* 2003;23:5293–5300.

27. Lillycrop KA, Phillips ES, Torrens C, Hanson MA, Jackson AA, Burdge GC. Feeding pregnant rats a protein-restricted diet persistently alters the methylation of specific cytosines in the hepatic PPARα promoter of the offspring. *Br J Nutr* 2008;100:278–282.

28. Hoile SP, Lillycrop KA, Grenfell LR, Hanson MA, Burdge GC. Increasing the folic acid content of maternal or post-weaning diets induces differential changes in phosphoenolpyruvate carboxykinase mRNA expression and promoter methylation in rats. *Br J Nutr* 2012;108:852–857.

29. Dick KJ, Nelson CP, Tsaprouni L, Sandling JK, Aissi D, Wahl S, et al. DNA methylation and body-mass index: A genome-wide analysis. *Lancet* 2014;383:1990–1998.

30. Agha G, Houseman EA, Kelsey KT, Eaton CB, Buka SL, Loucks EB. Adiposity is associated with DNA methylation profile in adipose tissue. *Int J Epidemiol* 2015;44:1277–1287.

31. Murphy TM, Mill J. Epigenetics in health and disease: Heralding the EWAS era. *Lancet* 2014;383:1952–1954.

32. Pan H, Lin X, Wu Y, et al., GUSTO study group. *HIF3A* association with adiposity: The story begins before birth. *Epigenomics* 2015;7:937–950.

33. Perkins E, Murphy SK, Murtha AP, Schildkraut J, Jirtle RL, Demark-Wahnefried W, Forman MR, Kurtzberg J, Overcash F, Huang Z, Hoyo C. Insulin-like growth factor 2/H19 methylation at birth and risk of overweight and obesity in children. *J Pediatr* 2012;161:31–39.

34. Godfrey KM, Sheppard A, Gluckman PD, et al. Epigenetic gene promoter methylation at birth is associated with child's later adiposity. *Diabetes* 2011;60:1528–1534.

35. Murphy SK, Huang Z, Hoyo C. Differentially methylated regions of imprinted genes in prenatal, perinatal and postnatal human tissues. *PLoS One* 2012;7:e40924.

36. Talens RP, Boomsma DI, Tobi EW, et al. Variation, patterns, and temporal stability of DNA methylation: Considerations for epigenetic epidemiology. *FASEB J* 2010;24:3135–3144.

37. Wong CCY, Caspi A, Williams B, et al. A longitudinal study of epigenetic variation in twins. *Epigenetics* 2010;5:516–526.

38. Barres R, Yan J, Egan B, et al. Acute exercise remodels promoter methylation in human skeletal muscle. *Cell Metab* 2012;15:405–411.

39. Clarke-Harris R, Wilkin TJ, Hosking J, et al. PGC1α promoter methylation in blood at 5–7 years predicts adiposity from 9 to 14 years (EarlyBird 50). *Diabetes* 2014;63:2528–2537.

40. Huang RC, Garratt ES, Pan H, Wu Y, Davis EA, Barton SJ, Burdge GC, Godfrey KM, Holbrook JH, Lillycrop KA. Genome-wide methylation analysis identifies differentially methylated CpG loci associated with severe obesity in childhood. *Epigenetics* 2015;10:995–1005.

41. Hanson M, Godfrey K, Poston L, Bustreo F, Stephenson J. Preconception health. In Davies SC, ed. Annual Report of the Chief Medical Officer, 2014: The Health of the 51%; Women. London: Department of Health, 2015, pp. 53–66.

15 Parent- and Family-Level Factors Associated with Childhood Obesity

Kyung E. Rhee and Kerri N. Boutelle

CONTENTS

INTRODUCTION

Many factors have been associated with the development of childhood obesity. The socioecological model [1] suggests that the closest level of influence to the child besides individual-level factors such as biology, epigenetics, and genetics, is the microsystem that involves interpersonal relationships with parents and family. Parents are responsible for the home environment and control what foods are available, provide opportunities for physical activity, model important eating and activity behaviors, set limits and behavioral expectations, create a socioemotional environment that shapes the child's socialization and growth, and influence the overall family functioning in the home. As such, parents are critical to the overall growth and development of the child, as well as to the development of obesity and obesity-related behaviors. Their participation is also essential to the success of the child's efforts in weight control interventions [2,3]. The goal of this chapter is to highlight the parent- and family-level factors that influence the development of childhood obesity and obesity-related behaviors through a number of different mechanisms.

There are a few caveats that are necessary to consider while evaluating the influence of parent- and family-level factors on the development of childhood obesity. First, it is important to recognize that parents and children can influence each other's behaviors, reflecting a bidirectional relationship [4]. As shown in Figure 15.1, specific parenting practices and other broader parent- and family-level factors can influence the child, but may also be shaped by the child's own behaviors and weight status. However, much of the work in this area is cross-sectional and does not take into account the bidirectional nature of the parent–child relationship. Additionally, the role and influence of parents

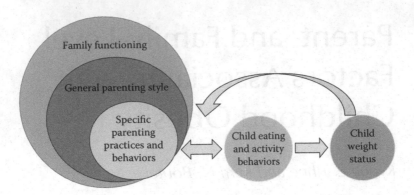

FIGURE 15.1   Parent and family influences on child behaviors and weight. (Modified from Rhee et al. *International Journal of Behavioral Nutrition and Physical Activity*. 2015;12[1]:49.)

and family need to be considered in the context of child development, where many of the influences may be stronger when children are younger and more dependent on their parents and weaken as the child transitions into adolescence and adulthood. As a result, much of the work reviewed in this chapter will focus on preschool and grade school children, on whom the influence of parents may be more pronounced.

Using Figure 15.1 as a framework for the relationship between parent and child behaviors, we will first address specific parenting practices and behaviors that can affect child eating, activity, and sedentary behaviors and ultimately weight status. We will then review the effect of general parenting style, a broader level of parenting that can set the tone for child development and socialization, on child outcomes. In particular, we will examine how general parenting styles can influence or moderate the effect of specific parenting practices on child eating and activity behaviors. Finally, we will address family functioning and how the overall functioning of the family as a unit can influence the development of childhood obesity and obesity-related behaviors.

SPECIFIC PARENTING PRACTICES AND BEHAVIORS

Parenting practices are considered to change based on the context, or in this case, the child's and parent's traits and behaviors. Specific parenting practices are the most proximal parent-level factor to the outcome of interest (childhood obesity) [5] and can directly address the child's eating behaviors, physical activity behaviors, and sedentary behaviors that ultimately affect weight status. Some of the more commonly studied parenting practices and behaviors are described in the following sections.

ENCOURAGING CHILDREN TO EAT PAST SATIETY

One of the most commonly studied feeding practices includes encouraging children to eat beyond satiety (i.e., to "clean their plate") [6]. This practice can have a direct effect on the child's energy balance. Parents often encourage their child to clean his or her plate because they are concerned about the quality and quantity of the child's intake or because they were taught to clean their own plate. This is particularly salient during the toddler and preschool years, when children's growth trajectories naturally slow down and dietary consumption decreases proportionally. However, encouraging children to "clean their plate" may lead to overeating and a loss of attention to internal satiety and hunger cues that help a child to naturally self-regulate his or her caloric intake [7]. Similarly, directly prompting, encouraging, or reminding a child to eat (e.g., "take another bite," "finish your peas") has been associated with higher child weight, faster rates of eating, and longer durations of eating [8–10]. Overweight mothers in particular may prompt their child to eat more often [10], further increasing their child's risk of obesity. As a result, it may be beneficial to allow some children, particularly young children who are developing eating habits and are not yet overweight, to respond to internal cues of hunger and satiety and self-regulate their caloric intake, rather than prompt them to clean their plate [11].

USING FOOD AS A REWARD AND FOR EMOTION REGULATION

It is natural for family members to use food as a reward, as it is a primary reinforcer and can almost always motivate children. Some parents will use this feeding behavior to encourage children to finish their plate or eat an undesired food, such as vegetables. Other parents use food as a reward for participating in an uncomfortable event (e.g., visiting the dentist) or for celebrations (e.g., getting good grades or winning a competition). However, this behavior can have some undesired consequences, such as lower satiety responsiveness and greater caloric intake [6]. Using food as a reward can also increase the value of the reward food (typically dessert) and decrease the value of the required food (often vegetables) [12,13], which ultimately undermines the intention of the parent to get the child to eat the required food. By offering food when the child is sad, bored, or stressed, particularly high–energy density sweet or salty foods, parents may also alter the child's ability to respond to internal cues of satiety and be more responsive to emotional cues that trigger a person to eat [14].

RESTRICTING ACCESS AND OVERTLY CONTROLLING A CHILD'S INTAKE

Restricting a child from a desired high–energy density food (e.g., potato chips) may increase the child's desire for that food. However, restricting access to these foods may also prevent weight gain and promote disordered eating behaviors or cognitions. The literature regarding controlling feeding behaviors and restriction reflects this quandary. A number of studies suggest that restricting a child's intake is associated with greater caloric intake when the child has free access to the restricted food and weight gain [15–17]. However, not all studies show a relationship between restriction and weight gain [18,19]. Recent studies suggest that restriction may be a response to a child's weight status or disinhibited eating behaviors [20,21]. Because of the concern that parents have regarding their child's weight, they could be using restriction to limit the child's intake of excess calories. Restriction may also be beneficial in limiting a child's intake if he or she is an impulsive eater or is highly stimulated by external food cues. Therefore, the use of restriction may have some benefits depending on the individual child and his or her responsivity to food in the environment.

EXPOSURE AND AVAILABILITY OF FOODS

Studies have shown that frequent exposure to an unfamiliar food can result in increased consumption, liking, and preference for that food [22,23]. Exposing children to healthy foods over time and making them available in the home has been associated with greater consumption of these foods [24]. Furthermore, increasing the accessibility of these foods (e.g., by precutting fruits and vegetables, putting them on a lower shelf in the refrigerator, or putting them on the counter top in plain sight) has also been shown to increase their consumption [25]. On the other hand, covertly limiting the availability of unhealthy snack foods by not buying them and bringing them into the house will decrease the likelihood that children will eat these foods; if these foods are not available in the home, children cannot eat them and must choose another healthier option. Several studies have demonstrated that decreased availability of these foods in the home leads to decreased snack intake [26,27], and it appears that in teenagers, healthy food availability is more strongly correlated with fruit and vegetable intake than restriction of unhealthy foods [28].

PORTION SIZE

Research shows that children as young as 2 years old and adults will often respond to external food cues and consume more calories when given larger portion sizes [29–31]. Interestingly, in one study of preschool children, those who were allowed to serve themselves and determine their own portion size ate 24% less of the entrée than when someone else provided them with a large portion on their plate [30]. While this technique may be effective in young children who are not overweight and are not stimulated by food, it may not be effective in older children who are overweight or highly responsive to food stimuli. These factors have yet to be explored. Nevertheless, the size of a portion can influence a child's caloric intake, and if left unchecked, can lead to excess weight gain.

MODELING

According to social cognitive theory [32], individuals learn behaviors by observing the behaviors of others. Initial research shows that modeling healthy eating and activity behaviors can result in healthier habits among children [33]. Children who have parents who eat fruits and vegetables [34,35] and have low dietary fat intake [36] are more likely to report similar behaviors themselves. Several researchers have also demonstrated that preschool children will more quickly accept and consume a novel food when an adult is eating something similar [37] or a teacher makes an enthusiastic comment about the targeted food [38]. Unfortunately, parents or adults who model negative behaviors can have the same effect on a child, as is seen with the development of emotional eating, snacking, and body dissatisfaction [33]. The power of modeling is demonstrated in weight control programs where parents are the primary agent of change [39,40]. Research also suggests that parent weight change is one of the best predictors of child weight change in a behavioral weight loss program [3].

Parent modeling of physical activity behavior has also been thought to influence child and adolescent physical activity behavior [41,42]. However, several reviews suggest that parent physical activity in and of itself may not be significantly related to child and adolescent physical activity [43–45], and a more recent meta-analysis suggests that there might only be a small effect of parent modeling of physical activity on child physical activity [46]. Instead, the type of support that parents provide may be a stronger moderator of child physical activity (see the following section, "Access to and Support for Physical Activity Opportunities") [46].

With regard to sedentary activity, research shows that children watch more television when their parents watch television frequently [47–49] and when there are few rules regarding the amount of time that they are allowed to watch television [48–50]. Setting up guidelines and boundaries as to when and how much television can be viewed may help to decrease this activity and the associated caloric intake that happens when watching television [51]. Given the potential influence of parent modeling, parents who actively engage their children in other healthy activities may be able to shape these behaviors at an early age and work toward developing healthy habits.

ACCESS TO AND SUPPORT FOR PHYSICAL ACTIVITY OPPORTUNITIES

Parents who enroll their child in sports and increase the availability of physically active opportunities often have children who are more physically active [52]. Parents can also influence their child's participation in physical activity by providing the appropriate support for this behavior. Parental support comes in a variety of forms, including informational (i.e., providing physical activity advice), emotional (i.e., letting the child know that the parent cares about his or her physical activity by watching the child's games), appraisal (i.e., direct prompts or verbal encouragement), and instrumental support (i.e., providing transportation to recreational facilities). Several studies have demonstrated that parental instrumental support is associated with higher physical activity among girls and boys [53]. Other types of parental support, particularly emotional and positive appraisal or encouragement, have also been associated with increased child physical activity behavior [43,54]. This type of support may lead to increased child self-efficacy and confidence to engage in physical activity, which has also been a positive correlate to physical activity in children and adolescents [45]. Thus, increasing access to and support for physical activity behaviors may be useful in tipping the energy balance toward a lower, healthier weight status.

TELEVISION ACCESS

Research consistently shows that children watch more television when they have televisions in their bedrooms [47,50]. This is associated with increased calorie consumption [55,56] and has been attributed to mindless eating while the child's attention is focused on the screen rather than what he or she is putting in his or her mouth [57]. In one of the only longitudinal studies evaluating correlates of television viewing, the number of meals eaten while watching television was significantly associated with the amount of time children at age 6 and 12 years were watching television [58]. The amount of time spent watching television was also associated with overweight status at both 6 and 12 years of age. Efforts to reduce screen time have demonstrated a decrease in caloric intake [51] and may be an effective way to decrease weight [59].

GENERAL PARENTING STYLE

General parenting style is often thought of as a higher-order construct [60] that embodies the overall socialization goals parents have for their child and provides the social and emotional context for child rearing [61]. As such, it provides the backdrop or emotional context in which children interpret the specific parenting practices that parents use. Parenting style, then, represents *how* a parent delivers an intervention, while specific parenting practices, such as restriction, describe *what* a parent does. There are four classic parenting styles that are each defined by varying levels of emotional involvement, warmth, and support as well as demands for self-control, discipline, and maturity [62,63]. The *authoritative* parenting style is characterized by high levels of warmth, support, and involvement, as well as discipline and demands for self-control, and is often considered the optimal parenting style. Several cross-sectional studies have found an association between the authoritative parenting style and lower body mass index (BMI) in children and adolescents [64,65]. On the other hand, more *authoritarian* parenting styles that show little warmth and affection but use high levels of behavioral control defined by psychological control (characterized by the use of coercion, guilt induction, shame, love withdrawal, and possessiveness) have been associated with increased BMI z-scores [66]. Our own longitudinal study found that children of authoritarian parents (high demandingness, low responsiveness) had almost a fivefold increase in odds of being overweight [67]. At this time, an intervention that targeted general parenting behaviors for families with children with behavioral problems found a decreased rate of obesity three to five years later, despite not having targeted any weight-related eating and activity behaviors during the intervention [68].

The authoritative parenting style has also been associated with greater consumption of fruits and vegetables [69–71], more frequent physical activity behavior in children [69,72], and greater weight loss during treatment [73]. However, general parenting style is more often thought to moderate the effect of specific parenting practices, such as feeding practices, on child eating and activity behaviors or weight [74,75]. In one study, van der Horst and colleagues found that parents who limited their child's consumption of sugar-sweetened beverages in the context of an authoritative parenting style had children who drank fewer calories than children whose parents used an authoritarian parenting style [74]. Therefore, a higher-order general parenting style may be important to consider when examining the impact of specific parenting practices and behaviors on child outcomes. Our work suggests that it is the *emotional responsiveness* parents display that is particularly associated with decreased child weight status [67]. Parental displays of warmth and sensitivity may work via their effects on increasing the child's ability to regulate negative emotions, work cooperatively with the parents, and have greater psychosocial functioning [76]. This emotional connection and responsivity may create a supportive environment in which the child can develop the confidence to explore behaviors and test boundaries while becoming an independent being. Consequently, children may be able to develop greater self-regulation across several domains, including eating and physical activity. Nevertheless, creating an environment with some behavioral expectations and boundaries may also be needed to guide children in the development of healthy eating and activity behaviors.

As such, specific parenting practices delivered within the context of an authoritative parenting style may result in optimal outcomes for the child.

In contrast to research on parenting style and eating, cross-sectional evidence regarding general parenting and physical activity report inconsistent results. Some studies suggest that more permissive approaches are associated with greater child engagement in moderate-to-vigorous physical activity [53], while other studies suggest that an authoritative parenting style is associated with increased physical activity in the child [77]. Interestingly, findings from longitudinal studies indicate that authoritative parenting is a positive predictor of physical activity [72,78], but the same relationship was not significant in others [79]. Because of the relatively few studies conducted in this area and the variability in outcomes, additional research in this area using consistent definitions of parenting style and longitudinal designs need to be conducted.

Studies regarding sedentary behavior and parenting are much fewer. The majority of the studies focus on television viewing. In two longitudinal studies, it appears that authoritative parenting is inversely related to sedentary behavior [72,78]. However, as with physical activity outcomes, further research needs to be conducted in this area.

FAMILY FUNCTIONING

In addition to parenting style, family functioning is another higher-order construct that can influence child development and childhood obesity risk. Family functioning refers to the structural/organizational properties and the interpersonal interactions of the family group, such as how they problem solve, communicate, adopt roles, adapt to each other, display warmth and closeness, and demonstrate behavior control [80]. Overall, poor family communication [81] and lower family functioning [82,83] were associated with higher BMI in youth. In a few studies using videotape assessments of family meals, positive qualities during mealtime (e.g., group enjoyment, higher relationship quality and interpersonal involvement, and warmth/nurture) were associated with reduced prevalence of child overweight/obesity, while negative qualities (e.g., hostility, being indulgent and permissive, and inconsistent discipline) were associated with a higher prevalence of child overweight/obesity [18,84]. Interestingly, it appears that mothers of overweight/obese children may use more maladaptive behavioral control strategies, particularly a permissive feeding style, which may contribute to their child's obesity risk.

With regard to eating behaviors, higher family functioning is associated with greater fruit and vegetable intake, family meals, and breakfast consumption [85–87]. Positive communication about the food and reinforcement for eating appropriately was associated with these more positive family functions [84]. However, in families where there is a discordant-weight sibling pair, mothers showed more interpersonal involvement with the lower-weight child, more maladaptive feeding control behaviors (authoritarian) with younger children with low restraint during eating and overweight, and permissive feeding control behaviors with older children with low restraint and overweight [88]. Thus, parents seem to respond to the characteristics of the child, and overall family functioning may be altered as a result.

With regard to activity levels in children, most studies show a positive association between higher family functioning and physical activity [87,89,90]. Recent research also suggests that the gender of the child and parent may be a moderator of this relationship [87]. Overall, the creation of more positive interactions and family functioning in the home setting appears to support positive health behaviors in children. As seen with some of the research around eating behaviors, the degree to which child characteristics or traits contribute to how the family functions remains to be seen.

SUMMARY

In summary, there are a number of parent- and family-level factors that play a role in the development or maintenance of childhood obesity. Specific parenting practices such as prompting the child to eat or turn off the television can directly influence the eating and activity behaviors of children. Other behaviors such as providing a healthy food environment, access to physical activity opportunities, and modeling of healthy behaviors also influence the child's behaviors. Furthermore, higher-order constructs of parenting style and family functioning may act to moderate the specific parenting practices and behavioral strategies that parents use and make them more palatable for children, ultimately reducing obesity risk. From this body of work, we can see that parents can potentially have great influence on their child's development and health. However, we must realize that parents often respond to child behaviors, temperament, and body size [20,21,91,92], and while certain parent behaviors (e.g., restricting food) may have a positive outcome for some children, they may result in greater food intake in others (e.g., those with low inhibitory control and high food responsivity) [93,94]. Additional factors such as parent and child gender, parent weight status, and child age may also moderate the relationship between parenting behaviors and child outcomes [95–97]. For example, fathers may have greater influence over child physical activity behaviors than dietary behaviors [95], but mothers appear to provide more logistic support for physical activity than fathers [52,98]. With regard to eating behaviors, there are greater correlations between same-sex parents and children [99,100], but paternal control behaviors may have a stronger effect on the child's BMI status [64,65]. Furthermore, overweight parents may have greater concern for their child's weight status and utilize more monitoring and controlling parenting practices to help decrease the risk of obesity in their child [101]. Overall, parents can greatly influence their child's health and development. However, this relationship is not unidirectional, and interacts with many child, family, and environmental factors. Further research in this complex interaction is needed to develop recommendations for parents and providers as they work to decrease the risk of obesity for their child.

Specific parenting practices and behaviors can directly affect child eating and physical activity behaviors and ultimately child weight status. These practices are the most proximal parent-level factor to the outcome of interest, but are often implemented within the context of general parenting style and family functioning. These broader constructs can moderate the effect of the specific parenting practices and are therefore important to consider when examining factors affecting childhood obesity risk.

REFERENCES

1. Bronfenbrenner U. *The Ecology of Human Development: Experiments by Nature and Design.* Cambridge, MA: Harvard University Press, 1979, pp. xv, 330.
2. Golan M, Crow S. Parents are key players in the prevention and treatment of weight-related problems. *Nutr Rev.* 2004;62(1):39–50.
3. Boutelle KN, Cafri G, Crow SJ. Parent-only treatment for childhood obesity: A randomized controlled trial. *Obesity (Silver Spring).* 2011;19(3):574–80.
4. Costanzo P, Woody E. Domain-specific parenting styles and their impact on the child's development of particular deviance: The example of obesity proneness. *J Soc Clin Psychol.* 1985;3:425–45.
5. De Bourdeaudhuij I, Te Velde SJ, Maes L, Perez-Rodrigo C, de Almeida MD, Brug J. General parenting styles are not strongly associated with fruit and vegetable intake and social-environmental correlates among 11-year-old children in four countries in Europe. *Public Health Nutr.* 2009;12(2):259–66.
6. Birch LL, McPhee L, Shoba B, Steinberg L, Krehbiel R. "Clean up your plate": Effects of child feeding practices on the conditioning of meal size. *Learn Motiv.* 1987;18:301–17.
7. Remy E, Issanchou S, Chabanet C, Boggio V, Nicklaus S. Impact of adiposity, age, sex and maternal feeding practices on eating in the absence of hunger and caloric compensation in preschool children. *Int J Obes (Lond).* 2015;39(6):925–30.
8. Drucker RR, Hammer LD, Agras WS, Bryson S. Can mothers influence their child's eating behavior? *J Dev Behav Pediatr.* 1999;20(2):88–92.
9. Klesges RC, Coates TJ, Brown G, Sturgeon-Tillisch J, Moldenhauer-Klesges LM, Holzer B, et al. Parental influences on children's eating behavior and relative weight. *J Appl Behav Anal.* 1983;16(4):371–8.
10. Lumeng JC, Burke LM. Maternal prompts to eat, child compliance, and mother and child weight status. *J Pediatr.* 2006;149(3):330–5.

11. Birch LL, Deysher M. Caloric compensation and sensory specific satiety: Evidence for self-regulation of food intake by young children. *Appetite*. 1986;7:323–31.
12. Birch LL, Birch D, Marlin DW, Kramer L. Effects of instrumental consumption on children's food preference. *Appetite*. 1982;3(2):125–34.
13. Newman J, Taylor A. Effect of a means-end contingency on young children's food preferences. *J Exp Child Psychol*. 1992;53(2):200–16.
14. Blissett J, Haycraft E, Farrow C. Inducing preschool children's emotional eating: Relations with parental feeding practices. *Am J Clin Nutr*. 2010;92(2):359–65.
15. Fisher JO, Birch LL. Restricting access to foods and children's eating. *Appetite*. 1999;32(3):405–19.
16. Birch LL, Fisher JO, Davison KK. Learning to overeat: Maternal use of restrictive feeding practices promotes girls' eating in the absence of hunger. *Am J Clin Nutr*. 2003;78(2):215–20.
17. Anzman SL, Birch LL. Low inhibitory control and restrictive feeding practices predict weight outcomes. *J Pediatr*. 2009;155(5):651–6.
18. Moens E, Braet C, Soetens B. Observation of family functioning at mealtime: A comparison between families of children with and without overweight. *J Pediatr Psychol*. 2007;32(1):52–63.
19. Keller KL, Pietrobelli A, Johnson SL, Faith MS. Maternal restriction of children's eating and encouragements to eat as the "non-shared environment": A pilot study using the child feeding questionnaire. *Int J Obes (Lond)*. 2006;30(11):1670–5.
20. Rhee KE, Coleman SM, Appugliese DP, Kaciroti NA, Corwyn RF, Davidson NS, et al. Maternal feeding practices become more controlling after and not before excessive rates of weight gain. *Obesity (Silver Spring)*. 2009;17(9):1724–9.
21. Webber L, Cooke L, Hill C, Wardle J. Associations between children's appetitive traits and maternal feeding practices. *J Am Diet Assoc*. 2010;110(11):1718–22.
22. Wardle J, Herrera ML, Cooke L, Gibson EL. Modifying children's food preferences: The effects of exposure and reward on acceptance of an unfamiliar vegetable. *Eur J Clin Nutr*. 2003;57(2):341–8.
23. Wardle J, Cooke LJ, Gibson EL, Sapochnik M, Sheiham A, Lawson M. Increasing children's acceptance of vegetables: A randomized trial of parent-led exposure. *Appetite*. 2003;40(2):155–62.
24. Reinaerts E, de Nooijer J, Candel M, de Vries N. Explaining school children's fruit and vegetable consumption: The contributions of availability, accessibility, exposure, parental consumption and habit in addition to psychosocial factors. *Appetite*. 2007;48(2):248–58.
25. Baranowski T, Cullen KW, Baranowski J. Psychosocial correlates of dietary intake: Advancing dietary intervention. *Annu Rev Nutr*. 1999;19:17–40.
26. Rodenburg G, Kremers SP, Oenema A, van de Mheen D. Associations of parental feeding styles with child snacking behaviour and weight in the context of general parenting. *Public Health Nutr*. 2014;17(5):960–69.
27. Sleddens EF, Kremers SP, Stafleu A, Dagnelie PC, De Vries NK, Thijs C. Food parenting practices and child dietary behavior: Prospective relations and the moderating role of general parenting. *Appetite*. 2014;79:42–50.
28. Loth KA, MacLehose RF, Larson N, Berge JM, Neumark-Sztainer D. Food availability, modeling and restriction: How are these different aspects of the family eating environment related to adolescent dietary intake? *Appetite*. 2016;96:80–6.
29. Fisher JO. Effects of age on children's intake of large and self-selected food portions. *Obesity (Silver Spring)*. 2007;15(2):403–12.
30. Orlet Fisher J, Rolls BJ, Birch LL. Children's bite size and intake of an entree are greater with large portions than with age-appropriate or self-selected portions. *Am J Clin Nutr*. 2003;77(5):1164–70.
31. Rolls BJ, Morris EL, Roe LS. Portion size of food affects energy intake in normal-weight and overweight men and women. *Am J Clin Nutr*. 2002;76(6):1207–13.
32. Bandura A. *Social Learning Theory*. Englewood Cliffs, NJ: Prentice Hall, 1977.
33. Brown R, Ogden J. Children's eating attitudes and behaviour: A study of the modelling and control theories of parental influence. *Health Educ Res*. 2004;19(3):261–71.
34. Rodenburg G, Oenema A, Kremers SP, van de Mheen D. Parental and child fruit consumption in the context of general parenting, parental education and ethnic background. *Appetite*. 2012;58(1):364–72.
35. Fisher JO, Mitchell DC, Smiciklas-Wright H, Birch LL. Parental influences on young girls' fruit and vegetable, micronutrient, and fat intakes. *J Am Diet Assoc*. 2002;102(1):58–64.
36. Tibbs T, Haire-Joshu D, Schechtman KB, Brownson RC, Nanney MS, Houston C, et al. The relationship between parental modeling, eating patterns, and dietary intake among African-American parents. *J Am Diet Assoc*. 2001;101(5):535–41.

37. Addessi E, Galloway AT, Visalberghi E, Birch LL. Specific social influences on the acceptance of novel foods in 2–5-year-old children. *Appetite*. 2005;45(3):264–71.

38. Hendy HM, Raudenbush B. Effectiveness of teacher modeling to encourage food acceptance in preschool children. *Appetite*. 2000;34(1):61–76.

39. Golan M, Crow S. Targeting parents exclusively in the treatment of childhood obesity: Long-term results. *Obes Res*. 2004;12(2):357–61.

40. Golan M, Weizman A, Apter A, Fainaru M. Parents as the exclusive agents of change in the treatment of childhood obesity. *Am J Clin Nutr*. 1998;67(6):1130–5.

41. Sallis JF, Patterson TL, Buono MJ, Atkins CJ, Nader PR. Aggregation of physical activity habits in Mexican-American and Anglo families. *J Behav Med*. 1988;11(1):31–41.

42. Sallis JF, Patterson TL, McKenzie TL, Nader PR. Family variables and physical activity in preschool children. *J Dev Behav Pediatr*. 1988;9(2):57–61.

43. Gustafson SL, Rhodes RE. Parental correlates of physical activity in children and early adolescents. *Sports Med*. 2006;36(1):79–97.

44. Sleddens EF, Gerards SM, Thijs C, de Vries NK, Kremers SP. General parenting, childhood overweight and obesity-inducing behaviors: A review. *Int J Pediatr Obes*. 2011;6(2–2):e12–27.

45. Bauman AE, Reis RS, Sallis JF, Wells JC, Loos RJ, Martin BW, et al. Correlates of physical activity: Why are some people physically active and others not? *Lancet*. 2012;380(9838):258–71.

46. Yao CA, Rhodes RE. Parental correlates in child and adolescent physical activity: A meta-analysis. *Int J Behav Nutr Phys Act*. 2015;12:10.

47. Davison KK, Francis LA, Birch LL. Links between parents' and girls' television viewing behaviors: A longitudinal examination. *J Pediatr*. 2005;147(4):436–42.

48. Barradas DT, Fulton JE, Blanck HM, Huhman M. Parental influences on youth television viewing. *J Pediatr*. 2007;151(4):369–73.e4.

49. Salmon J, Timperio A, Telford A, Carver A, Crawford D. Association of family environment with children's television viewing and with low level of physical activity. *Obes Res*. 2005;13(11):1939–51.

50. Springer AE, Kelder SH, Barroso CS, Drenner KL, Shegog R, Ranjit N, et al. Parental influences on television watching among children living on the Texas–Mexico border. *Prev Med*. 2010;51(2):112–7.

51. Epstein LH, Roemmich JN, Robinson JL, Paluch RA, Winiewicz DD, Fuerch JH, et al. A randomized trial of the effects of reducing television viewing and computer use on body mass index in young children. *Arch Pediatr Adolesc Med*. 2008;162(3):239–45.

52. Davison KK, Cutting TM, Birch LL. Parents' activity-related parenting practices predict girls' physical activity. *Med Sci Sports Exerc*. 2003;35(9):1589–95.

53. Jago R, Davison KK, Brockman R, Page AS, Thompson JL, Fox KR. Parenting styles, parenting practices, and physical activity in 10- to 11-year olds. *Prev Med*. 2011;52(1):44–7.

54. Loprinzi PD, Trost SG. Parental influences on physical activity behavior in preschool children. *Prev Med*. 2010;50(3):129–33.

55. Matheson DM, Killen JD, Wang Y, Varady A, Robinson TN. Children's food consumption during television viewing. *Am J Clin Nutr*. 2004;79(6):1088–94.

56. Matheson DM, Wang Y, Klesges LM, Beech BM, Kraemer HC, Robinson TN. African-American girls' dietary intake while watching television. *Obes Res*. 2004;12(Suppl.):32S–7S.

57. Robinson TN. Reducing children's television viewing to prevent obesity: A randomized controlled trial. *JAMA*. 1999;282(16):1561–7.

58. Saelens BE, Sallis JF, Nader PR, Broyles SL, Berry CC, Taras HL. Home environmental influences on children's television watching from early to middle childhood. *J Dev Behav Pediatr*. 2002;23(3):127–32.

59. Robinson TN. Television viewing and childhood obesity. *Pediatr Clin North Am*. 2001;48(4):1017–25.

60. Rhee K. Childhood overweight and the relationship between parent behaviors, parenting style, and family functioning. *Ann Am Acad Pol Soc Sci*. 2008;615:12–37.

61. Darling N, Steinberg L. Parenting style as context: An integrative model. *Psychol Bull*. 1993;113(3):487–96.

62. Baumrind D. Current patterns of parental authority. *Dev Psychol Mono*. 1971;4:101–3.

63. Maccoby E, Martin J. Socialization in the context of the family: Parent–child interaction. In Hetherington E, ed. *Handbook of Child Psychology: Socialization, Personality and Social Development*, 4 edn. New York: Wiley, 1983, pp. 1–101.

64. Berge JM, Wall M, Bauer KW, Neumark-Sztainer D. Parenting characteristics in the home environment and adolescent overweight: A latent class analysis. *Obesity (Silver Spring)*. 2010;18(4):818–25.

65. Wake M, Nicholson JM, Hardy P, Smith K. Preschooler obesity and parenting styles of mothers and fathers: Australian national population study. *Pediatrics*. 2007;120(6):e1520–7.

66. Rodenburg G, Kremers SP, Oenema A, van de Mheen D. Psychological control by parents is associated with a higher child weight. *Int J Pediatr Obes.* 2011;6(5–6):442–9.
67. Rhee KE, Lumeng JC, Appugliese DP, Kaciroti N, Bradley RH. Parenting styles and overweight status in first grade. *Pediatrics.* 2006;117(6):2047–54.
68. Brotman LM, Dawson-McClure S, Huang KY, Theise R, Kamboukos D, Wang J, et al. Early childhood family intervention and long-term obesity prevention among high-risk minority youth. *Pediatrics.* 2012;129(3):e621–8.
69. Kremers SP, Brug J, de Vries H, Engels RC. Parenting style and adolescent fruit consumption. *Appetite.* 2003;41(1):43–50.
70. Pearson N, Atkin AJ, Biddle SJ, Gorely T, Edwardson C. Parenting styles, family structure and adolescent dietary behaviour. *Public Health Nutr.* 2010;13(8):1245–53.
71. Lytle LA, Varnell S, Murray DM, Story M, Perry C, Birnbaum AS, et al. Predicting adolescents' intake of fruits and vegetables. *J Nutr Educ Behav.* 2003;35(4):170–5.
72. Schmitz KH, Lytle LA, Phillips GA, Murray DM, Birnbaum AS, Kubik MY. Psychosocial correlates of physical activity and sedentary leisure habits in young adolescents: The Teens Eating for Energy and Nutrition at School study. *Prev Med.* 2002;34(2):266–78.
73. Stein RI, Epstein LH, Raynor HA, Kilanowski CK, Paluch RA. The influence of parenting change on pediatric weight control. *Obes Res.* 2005;13(10):1749–55.
74. van der Horst K, Kremers S, Ferreira I, Singh A, Oenema A, Brug J. Perceived parenting style and practices and the consumption of sugar-sweetened beverages by adolescents. *Health Educ Res.* 2007;22(2):295–304.
75. Hennessy E, Hughes SO, Goldberg JP, Hyatt RR, Economos CD. Parent behavior and child weight status among a diverse group of underserved rural families. *Appetite.* 2010;54(2):369–77.
76. Steinberg L, Lamborn S, Darling N, Mounts N, Dornbusch S. Over-time changes in adjustment and competence among adolescents from authoritative, authoritarian, indulgent, and neglectful families. *Child Dev.* 1994;65:754–70.
77. Arredondo EM, Elder JP, Ayala GX, Campbell N, Baquero B, Duerksen S. Is parenting style related to children's healthy eating and physical activity in Latino families? *Health Educ Res.* 2006;21(6):862–71.
78. Berge JM, Wall M, Loth K, Neumark-Sztainer D. Parenting style as a predictor of adolescent weight and weight-related behaviors. *J Adolesc Health.* 2010;46(4):331–8.
79. Saunders J, Hume C, Timperio A, Salmon J. Cross-sectional and longitudinal associations between parenting style and adolescent girls' physical activity. *Int J Behav Nutr Phys Act.* 2012;9:141.
80. Epstein NB, Bishop DS, Levin S. The McMaster Model of family functioning. *J Marriage Fam Counsel.* 1978;4:19–31.
81. Chen JL, Kennedy C. Factors associated with obesity in Chinese-American children. *Pediatr Nurs.* 2005;31(2):110–5.
82. Zeller MH, Reiter-Purtill J, Modi AC, Gutzwiller J, Vannatta K, Davies WH. Controlled study of critical parent and family factors in the obesigenic environment. *Obesity (Silver Spring).* 2007;15(1):126–36.
83. Wen LM, Simpson JM, Baur LA, Rissel C, Flood VM. Family functioning and obesity risk behaviors: Implications for early obesity intervention. *Obesity (Silver Spring).* 2011;19(6):1252–8.
84. Berge JM, Rowley S, Trofholz A, Hanson C, Rueter M, MacLehose RF, et al. Childhood obesity and interpersonal dynamics during family meals. *Pediatrics.* 2014;134(5):923–32.
85. Berge JM, Jin SW, Hannan P, Neumark-Sztainer D. Structural and interpersonal characteristics of family meals: Associations with adolescent body mass index and dietary patterns. *J Acad Nutr Diet.* 2013;113(6):816–22.
86. Berge JM, Wall M, Larson N, Forsyth A, Bauer KW, Neumark-Sztainer D. Youth dietary intake and weight status: Healthful neighborhood food environments enhance the protective role of supportive family home environments. *Health Place.* 2014;26:69–77.
87. Berge JM, Wall M, Larson N, Loth KA, Neumark-Sztainer D. Family functioning: Associations with weight status, eating behaviors, and physical activity in adolescents. *J Adolesc Health.* 2013;52(3):351–7.
88. Moens E, Braet C, Vandewalle J. Observation of parental functioning at mealtime using a sibling design. *Appetite.* 2013;68:132–8.
89. Mellin AE, Neumark-Sztainer D, Story M, Ireland M, Resnick MD. Unhealthy behaviors and psychosocial difficulties among overweight adolescents: The potential impact of familial factors. *J Adolesc Health.* 2002;31(2):145–53.
90. Ornelas IJ, Perreira KM, Ayala GX. Parental influences on adolescent physical activity: A longitudinal study. *Int J Behav Nutr Phys Act.* 2007;4:3.

91. Hughes SO, Shewchuk RM, Baskin ML, Nicklas TA, Qu H. Indulgent feeding style and children's weight status in preschool. *J Dev Behav Pediatr.* 2008;29(5):403–10.
92. Carnell S, Benson L, Driggin E, Kolbe L. Parent feeding behavior and child appetite: Associations depend on feeding style. *Int J Eat Disord.* 2014;47(7):705–9.
93. Rollins BY, Loken E, Savage JS, Birch LL. Effects of restriction on children's intake differ by child temperament, food reinforcement, and parent's chronic use of restriction. *Appetite.* 2014;73:31–9.
94. Rollins BY, Loken E, Savage JS, Birch LL. Maternal controlling feeding practices and girls' inhibitory control interact to predict changes in BMI and eating in the absence of hunger from 5 to 7 y. *Am J Clin Nutr.* 2014;99(2):249–57.
95. Lloyd AB, Lubans DR, Plotnikoff RC, Collins CE, Morgan PJ. Maternal and paternal parenting practices and their influence on children's adiposity, screen-time, diet and physical activity. *Appetite.* 2014;79:149–57.
96. Gevers DW, van Assema P, Sleddens EF, de Vries NK, Kremers SP. Associations between general parenting, restrictive snacking rules, and adolescent's snack intake: The roles of fathers and mothers and interparental congruence. *Appetite.* 2015;87:184–91.
97. Larsen JK, Hermans RC, Sleddens EF, Engels RC, Fisher JO, Kremers SP. How parental dietary behavior and food parenting practices affect children's dietary behavior: Interacting sources of influence? *Appetite.* 2015;89:246–57.
98. Edwardson CL, Gorely T. Activity-related parenting practices and children's objectively measured physical activity. *Pediatr Exerc Sci.* 2010;22(1):105–13.
99. de Lauzon-Guillain B, Romon M, Musher-Eizenman D, Heude B, Basdevant A, Charles MA. Cognitive restraint, uncontrolled eating and emotional eating: Correlations between parent and adolescent. *Matern Child Nutr.* 2009;5(2):171–8.
100. Blissett J, Meyer C, Haycraft E. Maternal and paternal controlling feeding practices with male and female children. *Appetite.* 2006;47(2):212–9.
101. Francis LA, Hofer SM, Birch LL. Predictors of maternal child-feeding style: Maternal and child characteristics. *Appetite.* 2001;37(3):231–43.

16 Social Networks and Childhood Obesity

Kayla de la Haye and Sarah-Jeanne Salvy

CONTENTS

INTRODUCTION

High rates of childhood obesity have been attributed to a complex system of individual, social, and environmental factors, as reviewed in other chapters. The vital role of social networks in the propagation of obesity in children and adults has been highlighted in recent studies, and is emerging as an important component of this social-ecological system to understand and intervene on. Some of this research suggests that obesity spreads within social networks as a result of interpersonal "contagion" [1–3]. However, the social contagion hypothesis is just one potential mechanism driving associations between social networks and childhood obesity. Advances in *social network analysis* (SNA) and applied social network research are helping to refine our understanding of the broader set of social factors and processes at play in the development and maintenance of childhood obesity. This chapter briefly introduces the key concepts in SNA, before summarizing research findings that identify mechanisms linking social networks to childhood obesity, and then discussing directions for future research and implications for childhood obesity interventions. *Network interventions*, which typically alter or leverage social network structures (e.g., by targeting influential individuals or naturally occurring social groups), show great promise to more effectively promote and sustain diverse health behaviors [4–6]. Interventions that leverage social networks to prevent and treat childhood obesity are in their infancy, but are likely to be bolstered by considerable interest in this approach [7–9].

SOCIAL NETWORK THEORY AND METHODS

SNA is a set of theories and methodological tools that seek to understand social systems by studying the patterns of relationships among social entities (i.e., people or organizations). These relationships (referred to as *ties*) between social entities (referred to as *actors*) can represent any affiliation of interest: close friendship, acquaintance, marriage, group comembership, monetary transactions, online or offline communication, and so on. Social network research often focuses on understanding (1) the processes that *predict network ties* and generate complex social network structures, and (2) the individual and group processes/outcomes that *are influenced by* social networks. Social network methods provide tools for the measurement and analysis of social relations, including techniques to describe specific network structures (i.e., particular patterns or configurations of ties) that enable a more formal understanding of the key features of our social environments [10,11]. Social network theorists emphasize the role of social connections as a source of influence, support, and resources that influence actors, as well actors' positions in the global network, whereby individuals' attitudes, perceptions, and behaviors are influenced by where they are situated in the larger social system [12]. For example, SNA can be used to understand whether a social network is densely or sparsely connected, and to identify actors that occupy central, potentially influential positions in a network. Additionally, social networks can be evaluated from two perspectives: *personal social network measures* capture information on the social actors and relationships that surround a focal individual, while *complete social network measures* evaluate information on all actors and relationships within a bounded social group, such as a school, a family, or a community [13].

In the context of obesity research, SNA makes it possible to assess how patterns of relationships are related to, and potentially impact, actors' health behaviors and outcomes. Akin to traditional statistical approaches, the analysis of social network data can be descriptive or inferential. Table 16.1

TABLE 16.1
Summary of Descriptive Network Measures

Measure	Description	Applied Example in a Friendship Network
In-degree	The sum of directed ties that are received by an actor.	The number of friendship nominations a child receives from their peers.
Out-degree	The sum of directed ties that an actor sends to other people in the network.	The number of friends that a child nominates from a set of peers.
Geodesic	The shortest path (i.e., sequence of ties) that connects two actors in a network.	The "degrees of separation" between two children.
Centrality	The extent to which an actor is central to the network. This is often evaluated based on an actor's in-degree and the extent to which they are connected to other high-degree actors.	The extent to which a child is popular (is nominated as a friend by many peers) and is friends with other popular children.
Size	The number of actors in a network.	The number of children in a school friendship network.
Density	A measure of the actual number of ties as a proportion of total possible ties in the network.	The proportion of observed friendship ties among children, relative to the number of ties there would be if all children in the network were friends.
Reciprocity	The proportion of directed ties in the network that are reciprocated.	The extent to which children nominate friends who have nominated them as a friend.
Degree distribution	The distribution of in-degrees or out-degrees across all actors in the network.	The variability in the number of friendship nominations that children receive and make.
Transitivity	The proportion of two-path relations (where ties exist between i and j, and j and k) that form triads (where ties exist between i and j, j and k, and i and k).	When the friends of a child's friends become the child's friends as well.
Cliques	Subgroups of densely connected nodes, identified based on degree (i.e., high density) or reachability (i.e., short geodesics).	When smaller groups of peers in a network share many friendships among each other, but have few friendships to peers outside of their densely connected friendship group.
Homophily	Tendency for actors who share a tie to have a similar actor attribute.	Children who are friends tend to have similar BMIs, more so than children who are not friends.

summarizes important descriptive measures that are often of interest to applied social network researchers. SNA also goes beyond the description of network structures and provides statistical methods to test research hypotheses—for example, to test whether actors who share a network tie are similar in weight status, or to test whether the characteristics of actors' social connections significantly impact their weight outcomes. Because the network perspective assumes that individuals and relationships in a network are interdependent, traditional statistical models that assume data are *independent* are often not appropriate. Therefore, probabilistic network models have been developed that account for dependencies inherent in network data. These include dependencies between actors who share a tie, as well as more complex dependencies based on broader social structures that are important network building blocks [14]. For example, actors are often more likely to have a social connection, such as friendship, if they share a common friend (a process referred to as *transitivity*).

Statistical models for social networks are available for cross-sectional data (e.g., exponential random graph models) and longitudinal data (e.g., temporal exponential random graph models; stochastic actor-based [SAB] models) [15,16]. The relatively recent advancements in models for longitudinal social network data have provided a sophisticated and statistically sound approach for teasing apart micromechanisms of social selection, social influence, and confounding processes [17]. Specifically, it allows us to isolate factors that predict friendship choices from among a set of potential friends, while simultaneously testing for network and confounding effects that predict changes in individual attributes (e.g., health beliefs, behaviors, or outcomes). As we outline in the subsequent sections, this is important to accurately test the social diffusion hypothesis for obesity.

SOCIAL NETWORKS AND CHILDHOOD OBESITY

Social networks have been found to exert influence on various health behaviors and outcomes in children and adults [6,18], including obesity [1,3]. Broadly, social networks are important milieus to consider in health because they provide models for healthy or unhealthy behaviors, are sources or barriers of support, information, and resources, and can ultimately promote or impede healthy behavior change and behavior maintenance. Access to support in ones' social network can also reduce stress and increase self-efficacy, which in turn may reduce barriers to adopting healthy behaviors and achieving better health outcomes.

The adoption of a social network framework has been a natural progression for researchers interested in social influences on obesity because of the convincing evidence that social connections, such as family [19,20] and peers [21], influence behaviors and beliefs related to childhood obesity. SNA and social network theories provide a framework that goes beyond the study of social influence from an individual or dyadic (interpersonal) perspective, enabling a broader examination of how the emergent properties of social systems and their structures relate to childhood obesity. Although social network studies of childhood obesity to date are sparse and have focused predominantly on peer social networks in late childhood and adolescence, when many children are already overweight or obese, there is compelling evidence that social networks and childhood obesity dynamically influence one another. These processes are likely to be consequential for the development and diffusion of childhood obesity in diverse settings and populations.

Peer Social Networks

The prevention and treatment of childhood obesity has typically focused on the role of families. However, children's social and physical environments expand throughout development, with peer and school contexts playing an increasingly important role. To date, the influence of these social contexts on childhood obesity has been understudied [21,22], but social network studies are providing new and valuable insights into peer effects on childhood obesity.

Studies of adolescents' peer social networks provide evidence that obesity and related health behaviors are not distributed in networks randomly; rather, these attributes are associated with social network structures in important ways. One key finding is that friends are similar in weight status and weight-related behaviors [23], and that friends' weight similarities increase over time [24,25]. These findings have prompted claims that excess weight is "socially contagious" among peers, causing the social diffusion of obesity in social networks, and have stimulated interest in network-based obesity interventions that leverage social diffusion [5,8,26,27].

Although friend similarities in weight status may occur due to social influence, whereby youth with overweight friends are at a greater risk of gaining excess weight [2,24], it may also be explained by one or more of the following processes: (1) the *selection of friends* who are similar in weight status because of weight-based stigma [25,28–30] or a preference to befriend peers who have similar attributes that are correlated with obesity (e.g., gender, ethnicity) [31]; and (2) *shared environments*, such as school or neighborhood settings, that impact the risk of overweight. Research providing support for these various mechanisms is outlined here.

Social Selection

One mechanism that can lead to body mass index (BMI) similarities among friends is social selection or *homophily*: specifically, the tendency for friendships to form among peers who are similar in weight status (see Figure 16.1). Overweight youth have limited opportunities to form friendships because of weight-based stigma [25,28,30,32]. Social network studies have found that as a result of this stigma, overweight youth are likely to befriend other marginalized, overweight peers, resulting in the clustering of overweight youth in peer networks [3,25,29,30,33]. Additionally, friend similarities in weight status are likely to arise because youths prefer to affiliate with peers who have similar attributes and behaviors that are often correlated with or predict overweight. Specifically, youth have been found to befriend peers who engage in similar physical activities and sports [34,35], and additionally show strong preferences to affiliate with peers who are similar in gender, socioeconomic status, and race/ethnicity [31], preferences that are likely to contribute to correlations in weight status among friends and the clustering of obesity in peer networks.

Social Influence

Among adults, the likelihood of becoming obese increases with social connections (particularly friendship) to obese individuals [1]. Related findings have been reported among adolescents:

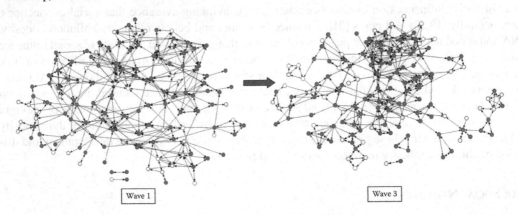

Wave 1   Wave 3

FIGURE 16.1 Evolution of an adolescent friendship network and weight status. Nodes are adolescents, directed ties represent close friendship nominations, and node color is based on weight status (black = nonoverweight, white = overweight or obese). In this network, increasing similarity in weight status among friends (i.e., nodes in the network that share a friendship tie) is largely explained by friendship selection, and specifically the marginalization of overweight youth by their nonoverweight peers.

adolescents' BMIs were found to be similar to the BMIs of their close friends, and these similarities increased over time [2,3,24,36–39]. These findings may reflect direct *social influence*, whereby friends' weight statuses influence changes in adolescent weight status. Importantly, a few of these studies have utilized longitudinal models for social network dynamics to test for network effects on weight status, while also controlling for the effects of weight status (and other related attributes) on social selection. Their findings provide some evidence that peer networks and obesity coevolve in a mutually dependent way. One study found evidence of weight-based friendship selection in an Australian school social network but not of peer influence on weight status over 18 months [29]. Other researchers used network data from two schools in the US-based Add Health cohort, and found evidence that both social selection and social influence predicted similarity in BMI [3,35]. Because these studies looked at only one or two schools, and because of the different study populations, it is not possible to draw firm conclusions about the different results.

Social psychology and health behavior theories point to several mechanisms that may explain social network influence on weight status [21], whereby friends' behaviors or characteristics influence adolescents' behaviors and/or beliefs about obesity-related behaviors. First, adolescents' diets and activities are likely to be influenced by the diets and activities of their friends. Research based on youths' perceptions of their peers' behaviors, and exploring social influence among pairs or small groups, has documented diverse and pervasive peer effects on physical activity [40] and diet [41–43]. Various mechanisms have been found to underpin these peer effects, including normative influence, behavior imitation, and motivations for peer approval [21]. These peer effects are likely to be especially prominent among older children and adolescents, at a time when half of their consumption of low-nutrient, energy-dense foods occurs out of the home [44], lunches and snacks are often eaten with friends [45], and leisure time and opportunities for physical activity are increasingly based in peer and school contexts.

Social network research also provides support that *interpersonal social influence* on obesity-related behaviors among friends gives rise to *peer network effects* on obesity-related behaviors (diet, physical activity), processes that may underpin the observed social contagion of obesity. This research has found that obesity-related behaviors, such as energy-dense food intake, physical activity, and physical inactivity (i.e., screen time), tend to be similar among friends, and thus cluster in friendship groups and larger peer networks [23,46,47]. And longitudinal social network studies have found that similarities among friends in physical activity [3,34,47] and consumption of energy-dense foods [48] were also explained by social influence, evidenced by the fact that adolescents' behaviors were predicted by their friends' behaviors, controlling for similarities when the friendships were formed. Interestingly, the influence of friends' behaviors on adolescent behaviors was not found to be mediated via a range of social-cognitive mechanisms proposed by many health behavior theories. Specifically, the effect of friends' behaviors on adolescent behaviors over time was not explained by a process whereby friends' behaviors influenced adolescent descriptive peer norms, attitudes, or intentions. These findings suggest that it may be modeling processes and implicit cues, more so than normative influences, that underpin the influence of friends on these weight-related behaviors in naturalistic social networks. Alternately, adolescents' adoption of their friends' behaviors may be driven by impression management and goals to fit into their peer group, rather than their own beliefs about weight, eating, or physical activity. Further research is needed to better understand the mechanisms driving these social network effects.

A second process that might underpin the social contagion of obesity is the influence of friends' weight statuses on youths' weight norms, which may impact their weight monitoring and indirectly affect their diet and physical activity. Youth with overweight friends are also more likely to underestimate their own weight and develop inaccurate perceptions of appropriate weight status [49]. These mechanisms could normalize obesity and reinforce obesogenic behaviors among friends, resulting in the spread of obesity [50,51]. Simulation studies with adults suggest that this is a plausible mechanism explaining the diffusion of obesity in adult populations [50].

Confounding Influence

A third mechanism of note in explaining similarities in weight status among socially connected individuals is the tendency for friends to experience *shared environmental risk factors* for excess weight. This could lead to parallel changes in BMI, processes called *confounding influences* or *exogenous contextual effects* [52]. Adolescent friendships play out to a large extent in school, neighborhood, and community settings: environments that are linked to obesity risk. Indeed, Cohen-Cole and Fletcher's analysis of the Add Health data suggests that peer network effects on BMI were actually better explained by shared school environments, because these friendships clustered in schools, and school characteristics and physical environments differed in the extent to which they promoted obesity [36].

Summary

In sum, the research outlined thus far suggests that the clustering and diffusion of obesity through adolescent peer networks is likely to be driven by social selection, social influence (on weight-related behaviors and weight norms), *and* confounding factors. However, no study to date has tested all of these mechanisms simultaneously to adequately evaluate the social contagion hypothesis. Additional research is needed that utilizes longitudinal social network data, and that includes multiple social networks nested in different settings and environments, to accurately test for the effects of weight-based social selection and social influence while accounting for the extent to which children who share social connections are exposed to the same environmental risk factors for obesity. Additional research is also needed on younger children, to understand differences in these network dynamics over children's developmental stages. These findings can inform effective school and health policy, and contribute to the development of multilevel interventions that successfully impede or harness social network processes for obesity prevention in youth.

FAMILY SOCIAL NETWORKS

The importance of family social systems in influencing and addressing childhood obesity is clear, and is covered in detail in Chapter 15. Much of this work has focused on parent–child dyads in isolation of broader family social networks, and has been limited in its focus on a narrow dimension of parent–child relationships, typically parents' influence on their children. Family social networks extend beyond these parent–child dyads; they encompass characteristics of the relationships and interactions among family members, and emergent patterns of these interactions, and thus capture much broader features of the family social environment that are also important milieus that impact childhood obesity and related behaviors.

Children and family members are likely to influence one another's eating behaviors, activities, and obesity risks recursively, rather like a cascading chain of actions and reactions. Evidence that these more complex dependencies within family systems are relevant to childhood obesity include findings that multiple types of family members, including children and multigenerational family members, tend to engage in similar health behaviors in the areas of food choice [53], eating behavior [54], and physical activity [55,56]. And family-level support for healthy behaviors such as healthful eating has been associated with better behavioral outcomes in children [53].

However, few studies have actually mapped the multiplexity of relationships within families to understand how the characteristics of these family social networks (rather than parent or family-group characteristics) impact childhood obesity risk. A handful of studies have found evidence that particular patterns of relationships that entail health-related communication and encouragement among family members are linked to individual engagement in healthy behaviors and coengagement in healthy behaviors among parents and children (e.g., physical activity) [57,58]. These findings suggest that additional research utilizing SNA to understand family influences on childhood obesity has the potential to identify family processes that could be harnessed to reduce childhood obesity risk.

CHILDHOOD OBESITY AND SOCIAL NETWORKS AS COMPLEX SYSTEMS

The research reviewed here indicates that childhood obesity, social networks, and broader setting and environmental factors need to be considered jointly, as they operate as a social-ecological system that may give rise to similarities in weight status among social connections and lead to the diffusion of childhood obesity [59]. Further research is needed that examines the coevolution of childhood obesity and social networks within diverse family and peer settings, and that models this social-ecological environment as a complex, evolving, and interdependent system. A systems-oriented approach is necessary to identify *emergent properties* that impact the risk of childhood overweight, which are not evident when testing the effects of isolated components of this system. This is critical in light of evidence that networks don't just impact childhood obesity, but that this is a system with bidirectional influences and likely feedback loops.

For example, a well-specified systems dynamics model of childhood obesity and peer networks within school and neighborhood settings (Figure 16.2) would enable a formal integration of processes that lead to friend similarities in BMI and the clustering of obesity in social networks, such as social selection (Figure 16.2A), social influence (Figure 16.2B), and shared environments (Figure 16.2D). This multilevel, systems-focused perspective would allow us to identify processes across this system that promote obesity in youth, and assess the relative impact of individual factors, social influence and diffusion, and environments on youth overweight, which are important to designing targeted strategies to reduce obesity in youth.

CONCLUSIONS

The literature reviewed here provides compelling evidence of the effects of social networks on childhood obesity, and valuable insights into diverse and complex social network processes. As with research that has identified features of physical environments that may be obesogenic, children's

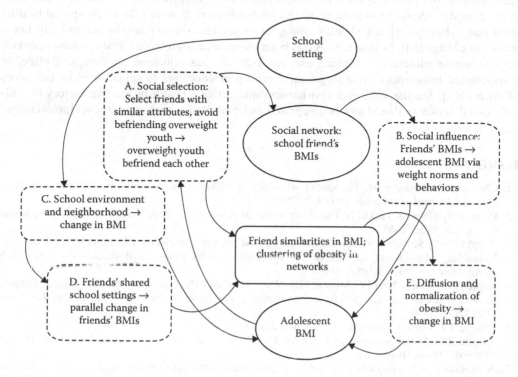

FIGURE 16.2 A model of childhood obesity and peer network system dynamics.

social environments and social networks, and the cues, norms, values, and opportunities entrenched within these contexts, can also be obesogenic or protective.

However, despite these promising findings and the prominence of conceptual and theoretical complex-system models for obesity [59], empirical research identifying social system dynamics that propagate or protect against childhood obesity is lacking. This is in part because the models for social network dynamics that provide the most sophisticated means for addressing these questions were developed fairly recently, and because the longitudinal complete social network data (i.e., data on the patterns of relationships among *all* individuals in a bounded population, such as all students in a school) required to adequately model social selection and influence have not been widely available. Another important gap is the limited research on the role of peer networks among younger children, and the changing impact of different relationships (e.g., family, peers, close friends, or romantic partners) on children's behaviors and weight status across developmental stages. Additionally, important moderators of these processes, such as race and ethnicity, may play an important role in peer network–obesity dynamics but have received little consideration. For example, because rates of overweight and obesity differ markedly by race/ethnicity, with the highest rates in the United States found among Latino and African American youth [60], and because youth show strong preferences to befriend peers of the same race/ethnic background, there is likely stronger clustering of overweight in peer groups composed predominantly of Latino and African American youth. This may impact weight norms and weight-based stigma [61], and ultimately differences in peer network and obesity dynamics.

A comprehensive understanding of the links between social networks and childhood obesity can inform future obesity prevention efforts. Social networks can be leveraged for various stages of obesity initiatives, and those that holistically target relevant and important features of children's social contexts to harness and activate social networks that support healthy behavioral change have the potential to improve their reach, effectiveness, adoption, implementation, and maintenance [4,62,63]. Broader efforts to develop *network-mediated interventions* that address or activate network processes for health promotion show great promise [5,6]. For example, SNA has been used to identify and train network *opinion leaders* to more effectively spread healthy norms and behaviors [5] and identify strategies to activate support within networks to boost behavioral change [64]. In youth, SNA has been used successfully to understand how peer networks influence adolescent substance use, research that has informed the design of effective network-based interventions that target influential peer educators to spread healthy behaviors and norms [65]. Similar strategies that harness and activate health-promoting factors in children's social networks should now be integrated and evaluated as part of multilevel interventions on childhood obesity.

REFERENCES

1. Christakis NA, Fowler JH. The spread of obesity in a large social network over 32 years. *The New England Journal of Medicine.* 2007;357:370–9.
2. Renna F, Grafova IB, Thakur N. The effect of friends on adolescent body weight. *Economics & Human Biology.* 2008;6:377–87.
3. Simpkins SD, Schaefer DR, Price CD, Vest AE. Adolescent friendships, BMI, and physical activity: Untangling selection and influence through longitudinal social network analysis. *Journal of Research on Adolescence.* 2013;23(3):537–49.
4. Burke JG, Lich KH, Neal JW, Meissner HI, Yonas M, Mabry PL. Enhancing dissemination and implementation research using systems science methods. *International Journal of Behavioral Medicine.* 2015;22(3):283–91.
5. Valente TW. Network interventions. *Science.* 2012;337:49–53.
6. Valente TW. *Social Networks and Health: Models, Methods, and Applications.* New York: Oxford University Press, 2010.
7. de la Haye K. RE: "Are network-based interventions a useful antiobesity strategy?" *American Journal of Epidemiology.* 2013;178(5):837–8.

8. El-Sayed AM, Seemann L, Scarborough P, Galea S. Are network-based interventions a useful anti-obesity strategy? An application of simulation models for causal inference in epidemiology. *American Journal of Epidemiology*. 2013;178(2):287–95.

9. Zhang J, Tong L, Lamberson PJ, Durazo-Arvizu RA, Luke A, Shoham DA. Leveraging social influence to address overweight and obesity using agent-based models: The role of adolescent social networks. *Social Science & Medicine*. 2015;125:203–13.

10. Robins G. *Doing Social Network Research: Network-Based Research Design for Social Scientists*. Los Angeles, CA: SAGE, 2015, p. 300.

11. Wasserman S, Faust K. *Social Network Analysis: Methods and Applications*. Cambridge, MA: Cambridge University Press, 1994.

12. Friedkin NE. *A Structural Theory of Social Influence*. New York: Cambridge University Press, 1998.

13. Carrington PJ, Scott J, Wasserman S. *Models and Methods in Social Network Analysis*. New York: Cambridge University Press, 2005.

14. Robins G, Pattison P. Interdependencies and social processes: Dependence graphs and generalized dependence structures. In Carrington PJ, Scott J, Wasserman S, eds. *Models and Methods in Social Network Analysis*. New York: Cambridge University Press, 2005, pp. 192–214.

15. Snijders TAB, van de Bunt GG, Steglich CEG. Introduction to stochastic actor-based models for network dynamics. *Social Networks*. 2010;32:44–60.

16. Lusher D, Koskinen J, Robins G. *Exponential Random Graph Models for Social Networks: Theory, Methods, and Applications*. New York: Cambridge University Press, 2012, p. 361.

17. Veenstra R, Dijkstra JK, Steglich C, Van Zalk M. Network–behavior dynamics. *Journal of Research on Adolescence*. 2013;23:399–412.

18. Smith KP, Christakis NA. Social networks and health. *Annual Review of Sociology*. 2008;34:405–29.

19. Birch LL, Davison KK. Family environmental factors influencing the developing behavioral controls of food intake and childhood overweight. *Pediatric Clinics of North America*. 2001;48:893–907.

20. Patrick H, Nicklas TA. A review of family and social determinants of children's eating patterns and diet quality. *Journal of the American College of Nutrition*. 2005;24:83–92.

21. Salvy S-J, de la Haye K, Bowker JC, Hermans RCJ. Influence of peers and friends on children's and adolescents' eating and activity behaviors. *Physiology & Behavior*. 2012;106:369–78.

22. Badaly D. Peer similarity and influence for weight-related outcomes in adolescence: A meta-analytic review. *Clinical Psychology Review*. 2013;33(8):1218–36.

23. de la Haye K, Robins G, Mohr P, Wilson C. Obesity-related behaviors in adolescent friendship networks. *Social Networks*. 2010;32:161–7.

24. Fowler JH, Christakis NA. Estimating peer effects on health in social networks: A response to Cohen-Cole and Fletcher; and Trogdon, Nonnemaker, and Pais. *Journal of Health Economics*. 2008;27:1400–5.

25. Valente TW, Fujimoto K, Chou C-P, Spruijt-Metz D. Adolescent affiliations and adiposity: A social network analysis of friendships and obesity. *Journal of Adolescent Health*. 2009;45:202–4.

26. de la Haye K, Green HD, Kennedy DP, Pollard MS, Tucker JS. Selection and influence mechanisms associated with marijuana initiation and use in adolescent friendship networks. *Journal of Research on Adolescence*. 2013;23:474–86.

27. Gesell SB, Bess KD, Barkin SL. Understanding the social networks that form within the context of an obesity prevention intervention. *Journal of Obesity*. 2012;2012:10.

28. Crosnoe R, Frank K, Muener AS. Gender, body size and social relations in American high schools. *Social Forces*. 2008;86:1189–216.

29. de la Haye K, Robins G, Mohr P, Wilson C. Homophily and contagion as explanations for weight similarities among adolescent friends. *Journal of Adolescent Health*. 2011;49:421–7.

30. Strauss RS, Pollack HA. Social marginalization of overweight children. *Archives of Pediatrics & Adolescent Medicine*. 2003;157:746–52.

31. Moody J. Race, school integration, and friendship segregation in America. *American Journal of Sociology*. 2001;107:679–716.

32. Tang-Péronard JL, Heitmann BL. Stigmatization of obese children and adolescents, the importance of gender. *Obesity Reviews*. 2008;9:522–34.

33. Schaefer DR, Simpkins SD. Using social network analysis to clarify the role of obesity in selection of adolescent friends. *American Journal of Public Health*. 2014;104:1223–29.

34. de la Haye K, Robins G, Mohr P, Wilson C. How physical activity shapes, and is shaped by, adolescent friendships. *Social Science & Medicine*. 2011;73:719–28.

35. Shoham DA, Tong L, Lamberson PJ, Auchincloss AH, Zhang J, Dugas L, et al. An actor-based model of social network influence on adolescent body size, screen time, and playing sports. *PLoS ONE*. 2012;7:29.

36. Cohen-Cole E, Fletcher JM. Is obesity contagious? Social networks vs. environmental factors in the obesity epidemic. *Journal of Health Economics.* 2008;27:1382–7.

37. Halliday TJ, Kwak S. Weight gain in adolescents and their peers. *Economics & Human Biology.* 2009;7:181–90.

38. Shoham DA, Hammond R, Rahmandad H, Wang Y, Hovmand P. Modeling social norms and social influence in obesity. *Current Epidemiology Reports.* 2015;2(1):71–9.

39. Trogdon JG, Nonnemaker J, Pais J. Peer effects in adolescent overweight. *Journal of Health Economics.* 2008;27:1388–99.

40. Voorhees CC, Murray D, Welk G, Birnbaum A, Ribisi KM, Johnson CC, et al. The role of peer social network factors and physical activity in adolescent girls. *American Journal of Health Behavior.* 2005;29:183–90.

41. Hermans RCJ, Lichtwarck-Aschoff A, Bevelander KE, Herman CP, Larsen JK, Engels RCME. Mimicry of food intake: The dynamic interplay between eating companions. *PLoS ONE.* 2012;7:e31027.

42. Salvy SJ, Coelho JS, Kieffer E, Epstein LH. Effects of social contexts on overweight and normal-weight children's food intake. *Physiology & Behavior.* 2007;92(5):840–6.

43. Salvy S-J, Howard M, Read M, Mele E. The presence of friends increases food intake in youth. *American Journal of Clinical Nutrition.* 2009;90:282–7.

44. Briefel RR, Wilson A, Gleason PM. Consumption of low-nutrient, energy-dense foods and beverages at school, home, and other locations among school lunch participants and nonparticipants. *Journal of the American Dietetic Association.* 2009;109:S79–90.

45. Feunekes GIJ, de Graaf C, Meyboom S, van Staveren WA. Food choice and fat intake of adolescents and adults: Associations of intakes within social networks. *Preventive Medicine.* 1998;27:645–56.

46. Fletcher A, Bonell C, Sorhaindo A. You are what your friends eat: Systematic review of social network analyses of young people's eating behaviours and bodyweight. *Journal of Epidemiology and Community Health.* 2011;65:548–55.

47. Macdonald-Wallis K, Jago R, Sterne JAC. Social network analysis of childhood and youth physical activity: A systematic review. *American Journal of Preventive Medicine.* 2012;43:636–42.

48. de la Haye K, Robins G, Mohr P, Wilson C. Adolescents' intake of junk food: Processes and mechanisms driving consumption similarities among friends. *Journal of Research on Adolescence.* 2013;23:524–36.

49. Maximova K, McGrath JJ, Barnett T, Loughlin JO, Paradis G, Lamber M. Do you see what I see? Weight status misperception and exposure to obesity among children and adolescents. *International Journal of Obesity.* 2008;32:1008–15.

50. Hammond RA, Ornstein JT. A model of social influence on body mass index. *Annals of the New York Academy of Sciences.* 2014;1331(1):34–42.

51. Burke MA, Heiland F. Social dynamics of obesity. *Economic Inquiry.* 2007;45:571–91.

52. Manski CF. Identification of endogenous social effects: The reflection problem. *The Review of Economic Studies.* 1993;60:531–42.

53. Ayala GX, Baquero B, Arredondo EM, Campbell N, Larios S, Elder JP. Association between family variables and Mexican American children's dietary behaviors. *Journal of Nutrition Education and Behavior.* 2007;39:62–9.

54. Munsch S, Hasenboehler K, Michael T, Meyer AH, Roth B, Biedert E, et al. Restrained eating in overweight children: Does eating style run in families? *International Journal of Pediatric Obesity.* 2007;2:97–103.

55. Sallis JF, Patterson TL, Buono MJ, Atkins CJ, Nader PR. Aggregation of physical activity habits in Mexican-American and Anglo families. *Journal of Behavioral Medicine.* 1988;11:31–41.

56. Simonen RL, Pérusse L, Rankinen T, Rice T, Rao DC, Bouchard C. Familial aggregation of physical activity levels in the Quebec family study. *Medicine & Science in Sports & Exercise.* 2002;34:1137–42.

57. de Heer HD, de la Haye K, Skapinsky KF, Goergen AF, Wilkinson AV, Koehly LM. Let's move together a randomized trial of the impact of family health history on encouragement and co-engagement in physical activity of Mexican-origin parents and their children. *Health Education and Behavior.* doi: 1090198116644703.

58. Haye K de la, Heer HD de, Wilkinson AV, Koehly LM. Predictors of parent–child relationships that support physical activity in Mexican-American families. *Journal of Behavioral Medicine.* 2012;37(2):234–44.

59. Huang TT, Drewnosksi A, Kumanyika S, Glass TA. A systems-oriented multilevel framework for addressing obesity in the 21st century. *Preventing Chronic Disease.* 2009;6:A82.

60. Ogden CL, Carroll MD, Kit BK, Flegal KM. Prevalence of childhood and adult obesity in the United States, 2011–2012. *JAMA.* 2014;311(8):806–14.

61. Lanza HI, Echols L, Graham S. Deviating from the norm: Body mass index (BMI) differences and psychosocial adjustment among early adolescent girls. *Journal of Pediatric Psychology.* 2013;38:376–86.
62. Gest S, Osgood D, Feinberg M, Bierman K, Moody J. Strengthening prevention program theories and evaluations: Contributions from social network analysis. *Prevention Science.* 2011;12(4):349–60.
63. Shin H-S, Valente TW, Riggs NR, Huh J, Spruijt-Metz D, Chou C-P, et al. The interaction of social networks and child obesity prevention program effects: The pathways trial. *Obesity.* 2014;22(6):1520–6.
64. Ashida S, Hadley DW, Goergen AF, Skapinsky KF, Devlin HC, Koehly LM. The importance of older family members in providing social resources and promoting cancer screening in families with a hereditary cancer syndrome. *The Gerontologist.* 2011;51:833–42.
65. Campbell R, Starkey F, Holliday J, Audrey S, Bloor M, Parry-Langdon N, et al. An informal school-based peer-led intervention for smoking prevention in adolescence (ASSIST): A cluster randomised trial. *Lancet.* 2008;371:1595–602.

17 Role of the Built Environment in Childhood Obesity

Deborah A. Cohen

CONTENTS

INTRODUCTION

The *built environment* refers to physical and social living conditions—the human-made space in which people live, work, and recreate on a day-to-day basis [1]. The built environment is the most important determinant of health. It underlies population-level obesity for both children and adults, because contextual factors influence people to consume more calories than they burn. This chapter will provide specific evidence as to how modern physical and social environments have driven too many children to become overweight or obese.

ENERGY BALANCE

Energy balance is the difference between energy intake and energy expenditure. In order to support increases in height and developmental maturation, growing children need energy and nutrients beyond what would be required for maintaining a steady state. When children consume and absorb nutrients beyond what is needed for growth, the extra calories are stored as fat. Energy expenditure can reduce the amount of calories that might be available for storage, but too little physical activity (PA) is never the primary cause of obesity. PA is, nevertheless, necessary for normal growth and development, particularly to enable youths to build strong bones and muscles. Today, children and adults are being set up for overconsumption because of the multiple ways in which food is promoted.

Secondarily, most people need fewer calories than in the past because of active utilitarian transport and the decreasing need for physical labor.

ENERGY INTAKE (DIET)

Other chapters in this book review a wide variety of factors that contribute to dietary intake in children. Among them is the likelihood that many children consume excess calories simply because they are served too much food [2,3]. Most children and adults lack the capacity to tell whether they have eaten too much simply by paying attention to their appetite or feelings of fullness [4]. Total energy intake among US children and adolescents rose considerably from 1989 to 2004, and subsequently declined through 2010. Part of the increase in caloric consumption is also explained by increases in the number of daily eating occasions [5]. Overall, eating patterns indicate that children (like adults) consume too many discretionary calories. Seven sources were consistently major contributors across all time points: sugar-sweetened beverages (SSBs), pizza, full-fat milk, grain-based desserts, breads, pasta dishes, and savory snacks. Intakes of full-fat milk, meats and processed meat products, ready-to-eat cereals, burgers, fried potatoes, fruit juice, and vegetables decreased between 1989 and 2010, whereas intakes of nonfat milk, poultry, sweet snacks and candies, and tortilla- and corn-based dishes increased linearly over the 21-year period [6]. The discretionary foods consumed are a reflection of the aggressive marketing of these products in stores and on television, as well as their low cost and convenience. Food is relatively inexpensive in the United States, with the percentage of total income spent on food decreasing from 13.9% in 1970 to 9.6% in 2012 [7] and the percentage of food dollars spent away from home increasing from 25.9% to 43% over the same time period [8]. With more dollars to spend, food has taken on a strong element of entertainment (dubbed *eatertainment*), with advertisers promoting "fun" foods for children [9].

CHILDREN AND MARKETING

Multiple studies have examined how exposure to food advertising is associated with greater food consumption. Harris et al. conducted a study showing that children watching a TV show with food commercials consumed 45% more of a goldfish cracker snack than children watching the same TV show with no food commercials [10]. Halford et al. also conducted multiple studies showing that children watching food advertisements consume more and obese children are more likely than non-obese children to recognize food advertising [11,12].

Other studies have examined the impact of cartoon characters on children's requests for food. One study that examined the impact of branding on taste preferences found that among young children aged 3–5, burgers wrapped in McDonald's-branded packaging were rated as tasting better than the same burgers wrapped in a different packaging [13]. Similar findings have been shown in multiple experiments with adults, where the brand names are intentionally mislabeled [14], indicating that food (and beverage) preferences are anything but rational.

Marketing to children often promotes the least healthy foods in the most aggressive ways, showing, for example, food with high levels of sugar to have extraordinary powers [15]. The use of mixed messages and unrealistic associations are confusing and misleading [15]. A study of the use of athletes to promote food indicated that the majority of endorsements were for energy-dense and nutrient-poor foods and for beverages with added sugar [16,17].

Efforts to persuade the food industry to voluntarily refrain from targeting children has resulted in decreases in offering toys as incentives for restaurant meals and modest expenditure declines in targeting younger children (from $2.1 billion in 2006 to $1.8 billion in 2009), but marketing dollars may have shifted to older children [18]. Although the dollars spent on television advertising declined, the number of commercials broadcast was still 12–16 per day for low-nutrient foods. Large amounts of marketing dollars are being shifted to new media, such as social media and web advertising [18].

PLACE-BASED EXPOSURES TO EXCESS CALORIES

In 2009–10, the sources of the low-nutrient foods that children consumed excessively were relatively equally divided among schools (32%), stores (33%), and fast-food restaurants (35%) [19]. The following is a discussion of factors associated with increased consumption in these settings.

FOOD IN SCHOOLS

The intent of new federal school meal guidelines is to ensure access to balanced, healthy meals and to reduce exposure to low-nutrient foods, and particularly to reduce the levels of high-fat milk and pizza consumed in schools [20]. The new federal standards for school meals are currently being evaluated. One study indicated that the consumption of fruits and vegetables in school cafeterias is increasing [21]. Another showed improvements in overweight and obesity trends in California schools after policies were implemented to limit competitive foods and beverages in public schools [22].

While lunches offered by schools have improved, the food that children bring from home is still considered suboptimal. In a study of bag lunches in Houston, researchers found lunches brought from home contained more sodium and fewer servings of fruits, vegetables, whole grains, and fluid milk, compared with the National School Lunch Program (NSLP) guidelines. About 90% of lunches from home contained desserts, snack chips, and sweetened beverages, which are not permitted in reimbursable school meals [23]. Clearly, many families are unaware of what constitutes healthy balanced meals.

FOOD IN CONVENIENCE STORES/SUPERMARKETS

Retail food outlets use multiple strategies to pressure families to buy more than they need as well as to make impulse purchases. At big-box stores, foods are sold in bulk and families take home large quantities. While the intent may be to save money with large-volume purchases, people end up eating more. The consumption of stockpiled convenience foods tend to be greater than nonstockpiled foods, especially when they are visually salient [24].

One study examining the impact of salient junk food in supermarkets showed that the "pester power" effect was extremely high. Seventy-three percent of parents reported a food request from their child during the supermarket visit. Most child-requested food items were unhealthy foods (88%), with chocolate/confectionery being the most common food category requested (40%). Most parents (70%) purchased at least one food item requested during the shopping trip [25]. The availability of low-nutrient snack foods, candies, chips, and sodas has expanded to multiple nonfood outlets such as book stores, hardware stores, and car washes, and vending sodas/candies at cash registers. This makes it difficult for people to avoid low-nutrient foods.

FOOD IN RESTAURANTS

In 2010, the Boards of Supervisors in both San Francisco and Santa Clara County adopted legislation requiring that meals that include free incentive items such as toys meet certain nutritional standards, including limits on calories and sodium [26]. The San Francisco standards additionally require a minimum number of servings of fruits and vegetables. These ordinances set a national precedent in establishing an explicit regulatory standard for meals sold in the private sector but made the achievement of these standards conditional on free incentives. The response of some chain restaurants, including Burger King and McDonald's, has been to simply charge for the toy rather than reformulate their meals; however, other restaurants are seeking to achieve the meal standards. Requiring the achievement of nutritional standards for all marketed children's meals, regardless of the presence of an incentive, may have been a more effective policy to achieve the public health goal.

The National Restaurant Association developed the Kids LiveWell program to create nutritional standards for children's meals. Several chains have adopted these and more restaurants are making efforts to improve the quality of children's meals. Disney was a leader in this, offering healthier side options in children's meals in their theme parks. Most recently, Dairy Queen, McDonald's, Wendy's, Burger King, Subway, Chipotle, Arby's, and Panera have taken soda off their children's menus. This trend signifies broader recognition of the need to reduce children's intake of SSBs. Because the trend to eat away from home has been steadily increasing, a move toward standards for healthier restaurant meals should be considered a positive trend.

Food at Home and Destinations Including Friends' Houses

Many studies have also examined predictors of what and how often children eat while at home. It was found that when kids had a TV in the bedroom, they had a higher probability of viewing more television. In turn, a TV in the bedroom was linked to three times the odds of a high waist circumference, high cardiometabolic risk, and elevated triglycerides [27]. Other studies have shown that watching TV is associated with snacking [28,29]. In a study following adolescent girls who wore global positioning system (GPS) monitors and kept a diary of where they went and what they ate at various destinations, it was found that at 50% of all places that girls visited food was served. Of all the places visited, including stores and restaurants, girls were most likely to get foods high in solid oils, fats, and added sugars (SOFAS) when they visited friends' houses [30]. Such studies indicate how deeply integrated low-nutrient foods have become in daily life.

Summary of Food Exposures

By making the availability of low-nutrient foods ubiquitous, such that youth encounter and are served these foods at multiple destinations, the environment nudges people to consume too much food. Schools are beginning to address this exposure to too much low-nutrient food through standards. Standards are beginning to play a role in restaurants, but have yet to be considered in other retail food outlets. Advertising makes these low-nutrient foods more desirable, but efforts to constrain marketing on a voluntary basis have been disappointing. Other approaches to advertising, such as counteradvertising, will need to be considered.

ENERGY EXPENDITURE (PHYSICAL ACTIVITY)

Children expend energy throughout the day, but are more active outdoors than indoors, partially due to constraints on space but also because they are purposefully being asked to stay sedentary and limit their movement in indoor settings [31]. Opportunities for moderate-to-vigorous physical activity (MVPA) are thus found during (1) utilitarian transport, (2) school-based PA programs and curricula, (3) community settings such as parks and other open spaces, and (4) organized extracurricular activities in and outside of school.

Utilitarian Transport

There are declining trends in active transport to school in part due to safety concerns (increasing traffic, fear of kidnapping and other crimes), but also because schools have been sited far from local communities, particularly middle and high schools, where more children are typically served than in elementary schools. Efforts to address this trend include programs such as the Walking School Bus, and Safe Routes to Schools. One evaluation in New York City found that Safe Routes to Schools programs reduced pedestrian injuries and was cost-effective [32].

SCHOOL-BASED PHYSICAL ACTIVITY

Many curricula have been developed to help youth be more active in school, especially during designated physical education (PE) classes. The standard goal is for youth to engage in MVPA at least 50% of the time during a PE class. However, achieving this goal is often elusive, despite the rigorous training of instructors. Many studies of PE classes indicate that youth are active less than 50% of the time because of teaching techniques that result in many students watching and waiting. Solutions may be as simple as having more equipment (a ball for each student) or promoting exercise and sports that allow all the students to be active [33,34]. Studies have tried to promote more vigorous physical activity during PE, and the most positive effects have been among boys [35]. Supervision during recess and the presence of outdoor equipment was strongly associated with PA during recess in middle schools [36]. One study in elementary school settings found that simply painting playgrounds using multicolored paints resulted in increased minutes of PA, with the largest effects seen among children who initially were the most sedentary [37].

After-School Programs

Opportunities for increasing PA can be provided after school, yet several studies that have tried to promote these activities have had difficulty in recruiting and sustaining participation [38,39]. Barriers to participation in after-school sports and PA programs include transportation, lack of funding, and the increased emphasis on academic achievement. In addition, a study of the accessibility of schoolyards and school facilities on weekends indicates that in many localities a large proportion of schools lock their gates. An analysis of the data showed a correlation between girls' body mass index (BMI) and weekend schoolyard accessibility, such that girls who lived in neighborhoods with more locked schoolyards had higher BMI [40].

In many school districts there are no requirements for daily PE. The reduction in time allocated to school PE has been attributed to increasing academic requirements. One way to maintain PE and meet new increased academic standards would be to lengthen the school day. Indeed, some districts are already doing this. However, whether this will translate into more PA for youth is still unknown. Some studies have suggested that there is a set point for PA among youth, and that if they exercise more in school, they will compensate by exercising less after school [41]. Other studies have not found this, and have shown that absolute PA levels can be increased among school-age youth [42].

School-Based Competitive Sports

Although many schools have competitive sports programs, they may exclude those who are not sufficiently talented to make the team. With limited funding, many schools do not offer intramural sports opportunities for those youth. The problem of insufficient opportunities is exacerbated in large schools, since more students are competing for the same number of limited slots. Descriptive studies of after-school PA programs show that large schools may offer more programs, but typically have lower rates of participation, considering the size of the student body [43]. In addition, schools that serve lower-income populations tend to have fewer after school–based opportunities for PA [44].

COMMUNITY SETTINGS FOR PHYSICAL ACTIVITY (STREETS, SIDEWALKS, PARKS)

In urban areas, many cities have been increasing the number of parks, so people are all within 10 minutes' walk of one. Yet a recent national study on parks indicated that they are designed to serve children more than adults. For example, 89% of neighborhood parks have playground equipment, but fewer than one-third have facilities such as tennis courts or walking paths [45]. More than 50% of park users were children and teens, while these age groups comprise less than 27% of the population [45]. Many park systems also sponsor a wide variety of leagues and activities for children, but very few for adults or seniors. Large gender disparities also exist in park use. Among children under 13, 60% of park users are boys, and among teens aged 13–19, 65% of park users are boys [45]. This likely reflects a greater emphasis on team sports for boys than for girls. There are also disparities between parks in socioeconomic status. While gender distribution is similar across income levels, parks in low-income neighborhoods have fewer programed activities.

Over the past few decades, investments in local parks have declined [46] and park systems often limit their oversight to maintenance rather than programing and event planning. Increasingly, it is up to private groups to manage and provide PA programing for youth and others in the community.

STREET NETWORKS, STREET CONNECTIVITY, AND SPRAWL

Many studies that have examined street design in relationship to PA among adults show that adults walk more in neighborhoods with more intersections and which are more densely populated [47,48]. Frank et al. developed an index of walkable neighborhoods strongly based on land use and found that a difference of one standard deviation in walkability could increase PA by more than 8% [47]. The association between street connectivity with children's PA appears to be mixed. For example, in one study no association with street design was found [49], in another more PA was seen only with boys [50], and in another the association with PA in youth was opposite that of adults (more PA in streets with lower connectivity for children, less for adults) [51].

CONCLUSION

Without addressing the conditions in which people live, it will be very difficult, if not impossible, to end the epidemic of childhood obesity. Given that food is the major source of obesity, food outlets are where interventions hold the greatest promise in moderating intake. Supermarkets and restaurants need standards to guide them to offer foods in ways that will not increase the risk of obesity and chronic diseases among both youth and adults. Standards and oversight could protect consumers from being served too much and from being exposed to settings that limit their ability to make thoughtful choices in their own best interests. Investments in spaces and programing for active recreation will be necessary to counter the pull of electronic media and encourage children to spend more time outdoors, where they will be most likely to engage in PA.

REFERENCES

1. Frumkin H, Frank L, Jackson RJ. *Urban Sprawl and Public Health: Designing, Planning, and Building for Healthy Communities.* Washington, DC: Island Press, 2004.
2. Orlet Fisher J, Rolls BJ, Birch LL. Children's bite size and intake of an entree are greater with large portions than with age-appropriate or self-selected portions. *Am J Clin Nutr.* 2003;77(5):1164–70.
3. Birch LL, Savage JS, Fisher JO. Right sizing prevention: Food portion size effects on children's eating and weight. *Appetite.* 2015;88:11–6.
4. Popkin BM, Duffey KJ. Does hunger and satiety drive eating anymore? Increasing eating occasions and decreasing time between eating occasions in the United States. *Am J Clin Nutr.* 2010;91(5):1342–7.
5. Duffey KJ, Popkin BM. Causes of increased energy intake among children in the U.S., 1977–2010. *Am J Prev Med.* 2013;44(2):e1–8.
6. Slining MM, Mathias KC, Popkin BM. Trends in food and beverage sources among US children and adolescents: 1989–2010. *J Acad Nutr Diet.* 2013;113(12):1683–94.
7. ERS. Food expenditures. http://www.ers.usda.gov/data-products/food-expenditures.aspx. June 17, 2015.
8. Blackford K, Jancey J, Lee AH, James AP, Howat P, Hills AP, et al. A randomised controlled trial of a physical activity and nutrition program targeting middle-aged adults at risk of metabolic syndrome in a disadvantaged rural community. *BMC Public Health.* 2015;15:284.
9. CSPI. Pestering parents: How food companies market obesity to children. https://cspinet.org/new/pdf/pages_from_pestering_parents_final_pt_1.pdf. Washington, DC: CSPI, 2003.
10. Harris JL, Bargh JA, Brownell KD. Priming effects of television food advertising on eating behavior. *Health Psychol.* 2009;28(4):404–13.

11. Halford JC, Boyland EJ, Hughes G, Oliveira LP, Dovey TM. Beyond-brand effect of television (TV) food advertisements/commercials on caloric intake and food choice of 5–7-year-old children. *Appetite.* 2007;49(1):263–7.

12. Halford JC, Boyland EJ, Hughes GM, Stacey L, McKean S, Dovey TM. Beyond-brand effect of television food advertisements on food choice in children: The effects of weight status. *Public Health Nutr.* 2008;11(9):897–904.

13. Robinson TN, Borzekowski DLG, Matheson DM, Kraemer HC. Effects of fast food branding on young children's taste preferences. *Arch Pediatr Adolesc Med.* 2007;161(8):792–7.

14. Alison R, Uhl K. Influence of beer brand identification on taste perception. *J Mark Res.* 1964;1:36–9.

15. LoDolce ME, Harris JL, Schwartz MB. Sugar as part of a balanced breakfast? What cereal advertisements teach children about healthy eating. *J Health Commun.* 2013;18(11):1293–309.

16. Bragg MA, Yanamadala S, Roberto CA, Harris JL, Brownell KD. Athlete endorsements in food marketing. *Pediatrics.* 2013;132(5):805–10.

17. Bragg MA, Liu PJ, Roberto CA, Sarda V, Harris JL, Brownell KD. The use of sports references in marketing of food and beverage products in supermarkets. *Public Health Nutr.* 2013;16(4):738–42.

18. Powell LM, Harris JL, Fox T. Food marketing expenditures aimed at youth: Putting the numbers in context. *Am J Prev Med.* 2013;45(4):453–61.

19. Poti JM, Slining MM, Popkin BM. Where are kids getting their empty calories? Stores, schools, and fast-food restaurants each played an important role in empty calorie intake among US children during 2009–2010. *J Acad Nutr Diet.* 2014;114(6):908–17.

20. IOM. *School Meals: Building Blocks for Healthy Children.* Washington, DC: National Academies Press, 2009.

21. Cohen JF, Richardson S, Parker E, Catalano PJ, Rimm EB. Impact of the new U.S. Department of Agriculture school meal standards on food selection, consumption, and waste. *Am J Prev Med.* 2014;46(4):388–94.

22. Sanchez-Vaznaugh EV, Sanchez BN, Crawford PB, Egerter S. Association between competitive food and beverage policies in elementary schools and childhood overweight/obesity trends: Differences by neighborhood socioeconomic resources. *JAMA Pediatr.* 2015;169(5):e150781.

23. Caruso ML, Cullen KW. Quality and cost of student lunches brought from home. *JAMA Pediatr.* 2015;169(1):86–90.

24. Wansink B. Environmental factors that increase the food intake and consumption volume of unknowing consumers. *Annu Rev Nutr.* 2004;24:455–79.

25. Campbell S, James EL, Stacey FG, Bowman J, Chapman K, Kelly B. A mixed-method examination of food marketing directed towards children in Australian supermarkets. *Health Promot Int.* 2014;29(2):267–77.

26. Otten JJ, Hekler EB, Krukowski RA, Buman MP, Saelens BE, Gardner CD, et al. Food marketing to children through toys: Response of restaurants to the first U.S. toy ordinance. *Am J Prev Med.* 2012;42(1):56–60.

27. Staiano AE, Harrington DM, Broyles ST, Gupta AK, Katzmarzyk PT. Television, adiposity, and cardiometabolic risk in children and adolescents. *Am J Prev Med.* 2013;44(1):40–7.

28. Anderson GH, Khodabandeh S, Patel B, Luhovyy BL, Bellissimo N, Mollard RC. Mealtime exposure to food advertisements while watching television increases food intake in overweight and obese girls but has a paradoxical effect in boys. *Appl Physiol Nutr Metab.* 2015;40(2):162–7.

29. Montoye AH, Pfeiffer KA, Alaimo K, Betz HH, Paek HJ, Carlson JJ, et al. Junk food consumption and screen time: Association with childhood adiposity. *Am J Health Behav.* 2013;37(3):395–403.

30. Cohen DA, Ghosh-Dastidar B, Beckman R, Lytle L, Elder J, Pereira MA, et al. Adolescent girls' most common source of junk food away from home. *Health Place.* 2012;18(5):963–70.

31. McKenzie TL, Sallis JF, Nader PR, Patterson TL, Elder JP, Berry CC, et al. BEACHES: An observational system for assessing children's eating and physical activity behaviors and associated events. *J Appl Behav Anal.* 1991;24(1):141–51.

32. Muennig PA, Epstein M, Li G, DiMaggio C. The cost-effectiveness of New York City's Safe Routes to School program. *Am J Public Health.* 2014;104(7):1294–9.

33. McKenzie TL, Sallis JF, Nader PR. SOFIT: System for observing fitness instruction time. *J Teach Phys Educ.* 1991;11:195–205.

34. McKenzie TL, Catellier DJ, Conway T, Lytle LA, Grieser M, Webber LA, et al. Girls' activity levels and lesson contexts in middle school PE: TAAG baseline. *Med Sci Sports Exerc.* 2006;38(7):1229–35.

35. Sallis JF, McKenzie TL, Alcaraz JE, Kolody B, Faucette N, Hovell MF. The effects of a 2-year physical education program (SPARK) on physical activity and fitness in elementary school students: Sports, Play and Active Recreation for Kids. *Am J Public Health.* 1997;87(8):1328–34.

36. Sallis JF, Conway TL, Prochaska JJ, McKenzie TL, Marshall SJ, Brown M. The association of school environments with youth physical activity. *Am J Public Health.* 2001;91(4):618–20.

37. Stratton G, Mullan E. The effect of multicolor playground markings on children's physical activity level during recess. *Prev Med.* 2005;41(5–6):828–33.

38. Pate RR, Saunders RP, Ward DS, Felton G, Trost SG, Dowda M. Evaluation of a community-based intervention to promote physical activity in youth: Lessons from Active Winners. *Am J Health Promot.* 2003;17(3):171–82.

39. *Urban After-School Programs: Evaluations and Recommendations.* ERIC/CUE Digest 140 (071 Information Analyses: ERIC IAPs, report no.: EDO-UD-98-0). New York: ERIC Clearinghouse on Urban Education, 1998.

40. Scott MM, Cohen DA, Evenson KR, Elder J, Catellier D, Ashwood JA, et al. Weekend schoolyard accessibility, physical activity, and obesity: 3. The Trial of Activity in Adolescent Girls (TAAG) study. *Prev Med.* 2007;44(5):398–403. doi:10.1016/j.ypmed.2006.12.010.

41. Wilkin TJ, Mallam KM, Metcalf BS, Jeffery AN, Voss LD. Variation in physical activity lies with the child, not his environment: Evidence for an "activitystat" in young children (EarlyBird 16). *Int J Obes.* 2006;30(7):1050–5.

42. van Sluijs EM, McMinn AM, Griffin SJ. Effectiveness of interventions to promote physical activity in children and adolescents: Systematic review of controlled trials. *Br J Sports Med.* 2008;42(8):653–7.

43. McNeal RB, Jr. Participation in high school extracurricular activities: Investigating school effects. *Soc Sci Q.* 1999;80(2):291–309.

44. Cohen DA, Taylor S, Zonta M, Vestal KD, Schuster M. Availability of high school extra-curricular sports programs. *J Sch Health.* 2007;77:80–6.

45. Cohen DA, Han B, Nagel C, Harnik P, McKenzie T, Evenson KR, et al. The first national study of neighborhood parks: Implications for physical activity. *AJPM.* 2016, doi:http://dx.doi.org/10.1016/j.amepre.2016.03.021.

46. NRPA. Economic Update Survey Report. https://www.nrpa.org/uploadedFiles/nrpa.org/Publications_and_Research/Research/Projects/Economic%20Update%20Survey%20Report%20Spring%202010.pdf. June 28, 2010.

47. Frank LD, Schmid TL, Sallis JF, Chapman J, Saelens BE. Linking objectively measured physical activity with objectively measured urban form: Findings from SMARTRAQ. *Am J Prev Med.* 2005;28(2) (Suppl. 2):117–25.

48. Frank LD, Andresen MA, Schmid TL. Obesity relationships with community design, physical activity, and time spent in cars. *Am J Prev Med.* 2004;27(2):87–96.

49. Cohen D, Ashwood S, Scott M, Overton A, Evenson KR, Voorhees CC, et al. Proximity to school and physical activity among middle school girls: The trial of activity for adolescent girls study. *J Phys Act Health.* 2006;3(Suppl. 1):S129–38.

50. Roemmich JN, Epstein LH, Raja S, Yin L. The neighborhood and home environments: Disparate relationships with physical activity and sedentary behaviors in youth. *Ann Behav Med.* 2007;33(1):29–38.

51. Norman GJ, Nutter SK, Ryan S, Sallis JF, Calfas KJ, Patrick K. Community design and access to recreational facilities as correlates of adolescent physical activity and body mass index. *J Phys Act Health.* 2006;3(Suppl. 1):S118–28.

18 The Influence of Stress on Obesity Development in Children

Sydney G. O'Connor, Eleanor T. Shonkoff, and Genevieve Fridlund Dunton

CONTENTS

INTRODUCTION

This chapter explores the extent to which stress influences the development of obesity in pediatric populations. Our focus is on the types of stressors and stress, both objectively and subjectively measured, which have been associated with adverse weight outcomes in children and youth. We also discuss two broad pathways, behavioral and biological, through which stress may operate on the genesis and maintenance of obesity. This chapter concludes with an overview of the limitations of the current literature, as well as recommendations for future research in the area to address these gaps.

DEFINING STRESS

Stress can be defined as an imbalance between the demands placed on an individual and the resources that he or she has to manage them [1]. Stressors are external factors (e.g., events, experiences, circumstances) that may threaten safety, security, and well-being. In contrast, psychological stress is described as a reaction that occurs when the demands of stressors outweigh one's ability to cope with those demands, which can eventually lead to poor health [2]. Both stressors and psychological stress are difficult to measure. Stressors are often characterized by *objective* external events, whereas psychological stress consists of an individual's *subjective* internal appraisal of, or reaction to, external stressors. Whether exposure to external stressors leads to psychological stress may vary depending on individual characteristics, resources, and coping abilities. Exposure to excessive stressors and psychological stress in early life, whether objective or perceived, can have a profound impact on many developmental processes, including increased biological reactivity to stress or altered behavioral patterns that can lead to heightened obesity risk over time [3,4].

PREVALENCE OF STRESS IN CHILDREN AND YOUTH

External Stressors

Exposure to stressful circumstances is common among US children. Poverty, low parental education, minority status, and being raised outside of a two-parent family are highly prevalent. More than 50% of all US children are estimated to experience at least one of these four stressors, and worse child health outcomes are associated with experiencing a greater number of these stressors [5]. Furthermore, as much as 50% of US youth are exposed to community violence [6], another circumstance that can be viewed as a stressor.

Psychological Stress

Despite an abundance of information on the prevalence of perceived stress among adults, stress prevalence in pediatric populations is less understood. Available data illuminate perceived stress as a salient issue in the lives of youth. In 2009, the American Psychological Association (APA) expanded their annual Stress in America survey to include 1206 youth aged 8–17. Overall, children self-reported experiencing stress to a greater extent than their parents reported for them; 14% of youth aged 8–12 and 28% of teens aged 13–17 reported worrying "a lot or a great deal," while only 2%–5% of parents reported that their child experienced "extreme stress." The most commonly reported sources of stress in the sample included the desire to do well in school (44%) and concern for family finances (30%) [7].

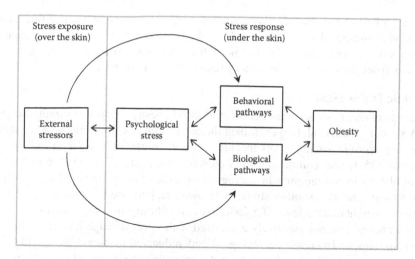

FIGURE 18.1 Conceptual model of stress and obesity.

CONCEPTUAL MODEL OF CHILDHOOD STRESS AND OBESITY RISK

Although there is growing evidence for the contributing role of stress in the onset and perpetuation of obesity in children [3], the underlying mechanisms are not well understood. In this chapter, we propose a conceptual model linking stress and obesity in youth to delineate and explore potential pathways leading from stressful exposures to stress responses, and obesogenic processes. This model is summarized in Figure 18.1.

Our conceptual model provides a general organizational framework to understand these potential mechanisms. The model differentiates between (1) external "over the skin" exposures to objective stressors and (2) internal "under the skin" responses to stressors, including subjective perceptions and psychophysiological indicators (e.g., cortisol and heart rate reactivity) of psychological stress. The model also proposes two major pathways, behavioral and biological, through which exposure to stressors and psychological stress may lead to obesity in children.

To illustrate, an external stressor might consist of a child experiencing physical abuse, whereas psychological stress can be illustrated as the child's subjective evaluation of the extent to which abuse is perceived as stressful, the latter of which may vary from child to child. Stressful exposures and heightened perceptions of stress can lead to behavioral consequences, such as decreased physical activity [8], and alterations in biological response, such as the accumulation of abdominal adipose tissue [9]. Over time, it is hypothesized that repeated stress exposures and responses can contribute to the development of obesity in youth [3,10,11].

EXPOSURE TO STRESSORS AND CHILD OBESITY RISK

The following sections describe major external stressors that have been found to be related to child obesity risk. A socioecological approach [12,13] is used, distinguishing between external stressors at the community/neighborhood, family, and individual levels.

COMMUNITY/NEIGHBORHOOD-LEVEL STRESSORS

Crime and Violence

Exposure of youth to community violence is as high as 50% within some US inner-city populations, and can range from witnessing stabbing to death by gunshot [6]. A review by Midei et al. [14] of six separate studies of interpersonal violence in the community and youth obesity risk found a positive association in half of the studies. In those studies finding an association, residing in an unsafe neighborhood was associated with greater odds of obesity in children. This review found that studies examining younger children tended to find null results, suggesting that obesogenic processes related to stress from community violence may take longer to manifest.

Socioeconomic Status (SES)

One of the most consistent stressors associated with child obesity risk is community/neighborhood-level SES. A study by Shih et al. [15] examined the correlation of community-level economic hardship, a summary score of six indicators including education and income, with the rate of obesity in youth. Across 135 distinct communities in Los Angeles County, they found more than twice the prevalence of obesity in communities in the highest quartile of economic hardship, compared with those in the lowest quartile. Another study by Grow et al. [16] used spatial analyses to examine the link between neighborhood-level SES indicators and obesity in census tract data from a large US city. Child obesity risk was positively associated with lower average household income, lower home ownership rates, and a greater percentage of undereducated women at the neighborhood level. A continuing challenge in this area, however, is disentangling the stress-related effects of living in a low SES neighborhood from other features (e.g., low walkability, limited access to grocery stores) that may contribute to child obesity.

FAMILY-LEVEL STRESSORS

Racial/Ethnic Minority Status

Evidence suggests that children of racial and ethnic minorities are at an increased risk of overweight and obesity. Although the mechanism for this stress obesity outcome is not clear, increased risk could be because children of racial and ethnic minorities are exposed to racial discrimination as well as other stressors such as financial and food insecurity, and neighborhood safety threats [3]. Research also suggests that racial/ethnic minority youth may experience stress from low SES differently than white children. A review by Dixon et al. [17] found that SES and obesity were positively associated among white children, but there was no clear relationship between SES and weight within black and Mexican American youth.

Negative Family Events

The term *family stressor* is used to describe stressful circumstances that originate within the family system. A study by Garasky et al. [18] examined a large nationally representative sample to determine the impact of six distinct family-level stressors, including financial strain, mental and physical health problems, conflict and disruption, housing or health insurance struggles, and lack of cognitive and emotional support in the home, on children's obesity risk. They found that the types of family stressors associated with child obesity risk varied by child age. Children 5–11 years of age from households characterized by a dearth of cognitive stimulation and emotional support were at greater risk of overweight and obesity, whereas children 6–12 years of age living in households characterized by greater physical and mental health issues and financial difficulties were at greater risk of overweight and obesity.

Parental Stress

Parental perceived stress has been implicated as an independent external stressor associated with child obesity risk [3]. Using a cross-sectional design, Parks et al. [19] found that parents reporting stress from a greater number of sources (e.g., financial strain, physical health problems, poverty) in a stressor index were more likely to have obese children. This same study also collected measures of parent self-reported perceived stress (using a general stress question); although they found no relationship between the number of stressors experienced and child dietary behaviors, there was a positive association between parent perceived stress and frequency of child fast-food consumption, suggesting that parental perceived stress but not the number of stressors experienced may lead to obesogenic parenting behaviors.

INDIVIDUAL-LEVEL STRESSORS

Victimization/Bullying

Youth who are bullied may be at increased risk for overweight and obesity. Midei et al. [14] conducted a literature review examining the link between exposure to bullying and obesity risk in children, finding general agreement that victimization by bullying confers greater risk of obesity in youth both cross-sectionally and longitudinally. In a longitudinal study of 1200 youth aged 12–13 years at baseline and followed for 4 years, Adams and Bukowski [20] found that bullying at the onset of the study predicted increases in body mass index (BMI) among initially obese females. This relationship was inverted for initially obese males, such that victimization at study onset predicted a decrease in BMI over time. There was no relationship between victimization and change in BMI in nonobese youth. Additionally, a meta-analysis by van Geel et al. [21] of 16 internationally representative studies and 28 independent effect sizes found a significantly greater likelihood of obese youth to be bullied, regardless of gender.

Maltreatment

Physical, sexual, or emotional maltreatment has been demonstrated to impact child obesity risk. A 2013 meta-analysis of 41 studies revealed that exposure to maltreatment in childhood is associated with increased odds of becoming obese over the lifespan, as measured through a variety of populations and study designs [22]. Although this meta-analysis also included studies assessing obesity outcomes in adults, several studies focused exclusively on child and adolescent weight outcomes, supporting the link between exposure to maltreatment and increased obesity risk during youth. A review by Midei et al. [14] examining 36 unique studies of weight outcomes in individuals who experienced interpersonal violence before the age of 18 similarly reported increased odds of overweight and obesity in individuals who experienced physical or sexual abuse in their youth.

RESPONSE TO STRESS AND CHILD OBESITY RISK

PSYCHOLOGICAL STRESS

Children's psychological responses to stress, including their appraisals of the severity of stress and psychophysiological stress reactions, are thought to play a contributing role in obesity risk [3], with some variation depending on the age of the child, as summarized in the following sections.

Preschool-Age Children (Ages 0–6 Years)

A limited number of studies have examined how psychological responses to stress in preschool-age children are related to obesity risk. Psychological responses to chronic stress, indicated by blunted cortisol and salivary alpha-amylase responses, have been associated with higher obesity in low-income preschool-age children [23,24].

School-Age Children (Ages 6–10 Years)

Among school-age youth, some evidence indicates that psychological stress is higher among obese youth, but findings are mixed. Using an experimental paradigm, Roemmich et al. [25] found that youth with greater reactivity to stress, assessed by perceived stress ratings and heart rate reactivity in reaction to a laboratory stressor, had a higher-percentage body fat among adolescents of average BMI percentile.

Preadolescents (Ages 10–12 Years)

A larger body of research has investigated these relationships in preadolescents, with most cross-sectional studies finding that psychological stress is associated with higher rates of obesity. One study of 10–12-year-olds measured how participants would expect to feel in response to hypothetical stressful situations. In this group, psychological stress was positively correlated with adiposity (BMI and waist circumference), but did not predict BMI status above the effects of depression and was only marginally predictive of waist circumference, accounting for the effects of depression [26]. A large, longitudinal study following children from age 7 to 11 years, which assessed stress and BMI once each year, found that perceived stress at any time point did not predict change in obesity (measured by BMI and waist circumference) for any of the subsequent years. However, children who had consistently higher perceived stress across the 3 years had higher obesity compared with those with moderate and low stress over that time period [27].

Adolescents (Ages 13–20 Years)

Evidence is mixed for the association between psychological stress and obesity among adolescents. A small, cross-sectional study of Middle Eastern adolescents aged 14–17 years found that higher perceived stress was correlated with higher odds of overweight and obesity [28]. In a cross-sectional study by De Vrient et al. [29], a measure of how stressful certain situations, such as home life or peer pressure, are perceived to be was assessed in youth aged 12.5–17.5 years. In girls, higher perceived stress was associated with overall and central adiposity (measured by BMI z-score, six skinfold measures, and body fat analysis), adjusting for overall dietary quality and moderate-to-vigorous physical activity. Other cross-sectional studies have shown contradictory results, with levels of perceived stress not differing between overweight/obese and healthy weight teenagers [30]. Another longitudinal study of adolescents (aged 12–18 years) examined whether stress at baseline predicted obesity 6–8 years later, finding no association [31]. Some studies suggest that race and ethnicity may be moderating factors, including a large, longitudinal study of girls, which found a faster rate of increase in BMI from 10–19 years for girls who experienced high versus low chronic stress, with stronger effects for black girls [32].

Behavioral Pathways Linking Stress and Obesity Risk

Stress may promote the onset and perpetuation of obesity in youth, through its effect on children's eating and activity behavior [18,33].

Stress and Eating

Different types of stress are related to increased food intake or decreased healthy food consumption in youth. In one study of school-age children, stressful life events were linked to lower fruit and vegetable intake. However, gender was an important moderator, and after controlling for emotional eating, the link between stress and dietary intake was significant only for girls [34]. Experimental evidence suggests that social stressors, such as social ostracism, can lead overweight youth to be more motivated to work for palatable, high-calorie snack foods and to consume more of these foods [35]. Another study found that among children who were highly reactive to stress, restrained eaters consumed more calories and ate for longer after a social stressor than when they were not exposed to the stressor [36]. In a longitudinal study of fourth-grade youth, perceived stress predicted subsequent higher intake of high-calorie snack foods, mediated by emotion-driven eating [37]. Other evidence suggests contradictory evidence, and one study found that emotional distress was not correlated with unhealthy eating in a sample of school-age children [38]. Overall, findings suggest that stress may be associated with poorer dietary patterns, but evidence for effects on dietary intake are mixed and may only occur for girls. The effects of stress on dietary intake may be greater for youth who are obese, highly reactive to stress, or highly restrained eaters.

Stress and Physical Activity

Youth may be less likely to engage in physical activity following exposure to a stressor, though results are mixed. Using an experimental paradigm, Roemmich et al. [8] found that youth who were exposed to a social stressor chose to perform less leisure physical activity than those who were not exposed. Further, youth who were highly reactive to stress, as measured by heart rate reactivity, performed less physical activity than those who were less reactive. However, results may vary depending on the age of the child. One study found that negative emotions increased physical activity in children under 8 years of age but decreased physical activity in older children [34]. Physical activity may also serve as a buffer against the negative effects of being exposed to stressors [3]. Cross-sectional research indicates that adolescents who report more frequent physical activity have lower psychological stress [39,40]. However, not all studies find that physical activity is linked to lower psychological stress among adolescents [41], and more research on youth samples is needed [3].

Interactions between Stress, Eating, Physical Activity, and Obesity

Physical activity may also moderate the effects of stress on eating behavior and obesity. Experimentally, physical activity has been shown to buffer against stress-induced compensatory eating [42]. In this study, both normal weight and overweight/obese children did not engage in compensatory eating after physical activity following a social stressor. Compared with children in the sedentary behavior condition, children who engaged in physical activity burned more calories but did not increase caloric intake, leading to a more favorable energy balance. In a cross-sectional study of older youth and young adults (aged 12–24 years), physical activity buffered the effect of stress on adiposity, such that for physically active youth there was a weaker positive relationship between stress and adiposity (measured by BMI, waist circumference, and skinfold) [43]. In a similar vein, one longitudinal study found that higher stress led to lower adiposity for children who had low sedentary behavior or high moderate-to-vigorous physical activity [44].

BIOLOGICAL PATHWAYS LINKING STRESS AND OBESITY RISK

Stress may also indirectly influence obesity risk in children through biological pathways that are independent of changes in eating and physical activity behavior [18,25,45]. Prolonged chronic activation of the metabolic, cardiovascular, inflammatory, and endocrine systems in response to stress has been linked to the onset and progression of obesity [10,33,45]. The experience of stress activates the hypothalamic–pituitary–adrenal (HPA) axis, leading to the release of glucocorticoids into the bloodstream. One glucocorticoid of particular importance is cortisol, produced by the adrenal cortex, which has been implicated for its role in metabolic processes [33]. Excess cortisol may lead to visceral fat formation over time [10,33]. Although the exact mechanisms are not well understood, it is thought that cortisol and other glucocorticoids are involved in the process of adipogenesis and may increase the expression of numerous genes involved in fat deposition [46]. Emerging evidence also suggests that disrupted circadian adrenal rhythms within the stress system can lead to disrupted diurnal rhythms within the adipose deposition system, triggering obesogenesis [47]. Furthermore, stress may trigger inflammatory responses such as the release of interleukin-1 beta (IL-1β) signaling within subcutaneous adipose tissue, which may lead to the development of visceral obesity. Repeated stress-induced release of IL-1β in the subcutaneous adipose tissue may impair its ability to uptake energy substrates, which may cause them to be disproportionately deposited in visceral adipose tissue, leading to obesity progression [48]. Through these biological pathways, chronic hyperactivation of the stress system may lead to the development of adiposity and ultimately increase the risk of obesity [45]. However, the exact nature of these mechanisms in children is not well understood.

RECIPROCAL EFFECTS AND BIDIRECTIONALITY

A small line of research suggests that there may be a reciprocal relationship between stress and obesity in children, such that being obese can serve as a stressor itself or lead to increased stress reactivity [11,25]. For example, one experimental study found that, compared with normal weight peers, obese youth aged 12–18 years showed increased stress reactivity to a social stressor, indicated by cortisol response [49]. In another experimental study among 9-year-old youth, children with higher BMI percentile, percentage body fat, and central adiposity experienced higher levels of perceived stress, as well as greater heart rate reactivity, after a social stressor than youth with lower BMI, body fat, and abdominal girth [25]. A longitudinal study of children aged 5–12 years found that adiposity at baseline led to increased stress over time, and this association was stronger for children with elevated morning cortisol levels and who consumed the greatest amount of sweet foods [44].

RESEARCH CHALLENGES

CHALLENGES IN OBESITY OUTCOME MEASUREMENT

Research in this area typically uses BMI percentile as the primary indicator of obesity in children. However, BMI does not differentiate between fat and lean body mass in terms of how they contribute to body weight. Given the potential role of stress in the accumulation of adipose tissue, other measures such as waist circumference, skinfolds, and percentage of body fat (e.g., via duel-energy x-ray absorptiometry [DXA] or bioelectrical impedance analysis [BIA]) should be incorporated in future studies of stress and obesity risk in youth.

CHALLENGES IN STRESS MEASUREMENT

Most studies rely on instruments that neglect to collect information on the length or intensity of stressor experience [3]. Additionally, measures of stress experienced by children often rely on parent reports, adding yet another potential layer of inaccuracy [3]. Furthermore, few studies collect both self-reported measures of stress and biomarkers of stress psychophysiology (e.g., cortisol), which, combined, may yield a more complete picture of the experience of psychological stress in children.

RESEARCH GAPS AND RECOMMENDATIONS FOR FUTURE RESEARCH

LONGITUDINAL STUDIES AND NATURAL EXPERIMENTS

Most studies examining the association between stress and obesity risk during childhood are cross-sectional in nature. This type of study design makes it difficult to disentangle directionality—whether stress leads to obesity or obesity causes stress or both. Longitudinal studies with measures of stress and obesity across multiple time points as well as natural experiments (i.e., examining changes in stress and obesity risk before and after stressful events such as natural disasters or school shootings) are needed to establish directionality.

RESEARCH DURING EARLY CHILDHOOD

Research on how prenatal and early-life exposure to negative events and stressful circumstances may establish unhealthy weight trajectories during the first few years of life is lacking [50]. Prenatal and early-life stressors may play a role in the etiology of early childhood obesity through maternal and infant food consumption, basal metabolism, and adipose deposition.

REAL-TIME DATA CAPTURE

Studies of stress, physical activity, and eating in children typically assess these exposures and behaviors on an infrequent basis (e.g., once, semiannually, or annually). Although this measurement approach can capture *interindividual* (i.e., between-person) differences or change over longer periods of time, the effects of day-to-day (i.e., *intraindividual*) variation in key exposures and responses are unknown. Also, studies often rely on retrospective reports of perceived stress, which may be vulnerable to recall biases. These methodological limitations can be addressed through real-time data capture, repeated measures designs that can capture daily covariation between stress exposures and experiences, and energy balance behaviors.

RESEARCH EXAMINING MEDIATING MECHANISMS (BEHAVIORAL AND BIOLOGICAL RESPONSES)

Due to the cross-sectional nature of work in this area, few studies examine mediating mechanisms and the behavioral and biological pathways leading from stress to obesity progression in children. Future research is needed to uncover intermediary factors to target in prevention and treatment programs to reduce and buffer the effects of stress on child obesity.

RESEARCH ON RISK AND PROTECTIVE FACTORS

Research on moderating mechanisms and effect modifiers is needed to identify risk and protective factors to identify families whose children are at the greatest risk of obesity progression, and strategies to effectively buffer these effects. These risk and protective factors may include parenting styles, household rules, and weight-related parenting practices [12], among other factors.

SUMMARY AND CONCLUSIONS

Overall, a sizable body of evidence implicates the potential role of psychological stress on the etiology of childhood obesity. Exposure to external stressors such as poverty, victimization/bullying, and maltreatment may be particularly salient experiences during childhood that increase obesity risk. Variations in children's individual perceptions of, and reactions to, stress are important factors to consider in addition to objective measures of exposures to potential stressors. Whereas growing evidence has shown that psychological stress may influence children's eating and physical activity behaviors, fewer studies have examined how stress can directly alter biological processes (e.g., metabolism, inflammation, fat deposition) that can lead to obesity in children.

The conceptual model illustrates the mechanisms through which stress may impact child obesity outcomes. The model differentiates between (1) external "over the skin" exposures to objective stressors and (2) internal "under the skin" responses to stressors, including subjective perceptions and psychophysiological indicators (e.g., cortisol and heart rate reactivity) of psychological stress, and proposes two major pathways, behavioral and biological, through which exposure to stressors and psychological stress may lead to obesity in children.

REFERENCES

1. Lazarus RS, Folkman S. *Stress, Appraisal, and Coping.* New York: Springer, 1984, pp. xiii, 445.
2. Palmer S. Occupational stress. *Health Saf Pract.* 1989;7:16–18.
3. Wilson SM, Sato AF. Stress and paediatric obesity: What we know and where to go. *Stress Health.* 2014;30(2):91–102.
4. Lupien SJ, McEwen BS, Gunnar MR, Heim C. Effects of stress throughout the lifespan on the brain, behaviour and cognition. *Nat Rev Neurosci.* 2009;10(6):434–45.
5. Bauman LJ, Silver EJ, Stein REK. Cumulative social disadvantage and child health. *Pediatrics.* 2006;117(4):1321–8.
6. Buka SL, Stichick TL, Birdthistle I, Earls FJ. Exposure to violence: Prevalence, risks. *Am J Orthopsychiatr.* 2001;71(3):298–310.
7. The American Psychological Association. *Stress in America: Paying with Our Health.* 2009. Released 2015. Available from: http://www.apa.org/news/press/releases/stress/2014/stress-report.pdf.

8. Roemmich JN, Gurgol CM, Epstein LH. Influence of an interpersonal laboratory stressor on youths' choice to be physically active. *Obes Res.* 2003;11(9):1080–7.

9. Pervanidou P, Chrousos GP. Stress and obesity/metabolic syndrome in childhood and adolescence. *Int J Pediatr Obes.* 2011;6(Suppl.1):21–8.

10. Chrousos GP. Pediatric stress: Hormonal mediators and human development. *Horm Res.* 2003;1583:161–79.

11. Kyrou I, Chrousos GP, Tsigos C. Stress, visceral obesity, and metabolic complications. *Ann NY Acad Sci.* 2006;1083:77–110.

12. Davidson K, Birch L. Childhood overweight: A contextual model and recommendations for future research. *Obes Rev.* 2001;2(3):159–171.

13. Ohri-Vachaspati P, DeLia D, DeWeese RS, Crespo NC, Todd M, Yedidia MJ. The relative contribution of layers of the social ecological model to childhood obesity. *Public Health Nutr.* 2015;18(11):2055–66.

14. Midei AJ, Matthews KA. Interpersonal violence in childhood as a risk factor for obesity: A systematic review of the literature and proposed pathways. *Obes Rev.* 2011;12(501):159–72.

15. Shih M, Dumke KA, Goran MI, Simon PA. The association between community-level economic hardship and childhood obesity prevalence in Los Angeles. *Pediatr Obes.* 2013;8(6):411–7.

16. Greves Grow HM, Cook AJ, Arterburn DE, Saelens BE, Drewnowski A, Lozano P. Child obesity associated with social disadvantage of children's neighborhoods. *Soc Sci Med.* 2010;71(3):584–91.

17. Dixon B, Peña M, Taveras EM. Lifecourse approach to racial/ethnic disparities in childhood obesity 1–3. *Adv Nutr.* 2012;3:73–82.

18. Garasky S, Stewart SD, Gundersen C, Lohman BJ, Eisenmann JC. Family stressors and child obesity. *Soc Sci Res.* 2009;38(4):755–66.

19. Parks EP, Kumanyika S, Moore RH, Stettler N, Wrotniak BH, Kazak A. Influence of stress in parents on child obesity and related behaviors. *Pediatrics.* 2012;130(5):e1096–104.

20. Adams RE, Bukowski WM. Peer victimization as a predictor of depression and body mass index in obese and non-obese adolescents. *J Child Psychol Psychiatry.* 2008;49(8):858–66.

21. van Geel M, Vedder P, Tanilon J. Are overweight and obese youth more often bullied by their peers? A meta-analysis on the relation between weight status and bullying. *Int J Obes (Lond).* 2014;38:1263–7.

22. Danese A, Tan M. Childhood maltreatment and obesity: Systematic review and meta-analysis. *Mol Psychiatry.* 2014;19(5):544–54.

23. Miller AL, Clifford C, Sturza J, Rosenblum K, Vazquez DM, Kaciroti N, et al. Blunted cortisol response to stress is associated with higher body mass index in low-income preschool-aged children. *Psychoneuroendocrinology.* 2013;38(11):2611–7.

24. Miller AL, Sturza J, Rosenblum K, Vazquez DM, Kaciroti N, Lumeng JC. Salivary alpha amylase diurnal pattern and stress response are associated with body mass index in low-income preschool-aged children. *Psychoneuroendocrinology.* 2015;53:40–8.

25. Roemmich JN, Smith JR, Epstein LH, Lambiase M. Stress reactivity and adiposity of youth. *Obesity (Silver Spring).* 2007;15(9):2303–10.

26. Lam T. The effects of psychological stress, depressive symptoms, and cortisol on body mass and central adiposity in 10- to 12-year-old children. PhD dissertation, University of Alabama at Birmingham, 2012.

27. van Jaarsveld CHM, Fidler JA, Steptoe A, Boniface D, Wardle J. Perceived stress and weight gain in adolescence: A longitudinal analysis. *Obesity (Silver Spring).* 2009;17(12):2155–61.

28. Hamaideh SH, Al-Khateeb RY, Al-Rawashdeh AB. Overweight and obesity and their correlates among Jordanian adolescents. *J Nurs Scholarsh.* 2010;42(4):387–94.

29. De Vriendt T, Clays E, Maes L, De Bourdeaudhuij I, Vicente-Rodriguez G, Moreno LA, et al. European adolescents' level of perceived stress and its relationship with body adiposity: The HELENA Study. *Eur J Public Health.* 2012;22(4):519–24.

30. Martyn-Nemeth PA, Penckofer S. Psychological vulnerability among overweight/obese minority adolescents. *J Sch Nurs.* 2012;28(4):291–301.

31. Carter JS, Dellucci T, Turek C, Mir S. Predicting depressive symptoms and weight from adolescence to adulthood: Stressors and the role of protective factors. *J Youth Adolesc.* 2015;44(11):2122–40.

32. Tomiyama AJ, Puterman E, Epel ES, Rehkopf DH, Laraia BA. Chronic psychological stress and racial disparities in body mass index change between black and white girls aged 10–19. *Ann Behav Med.* 2013;45(1):3–12.

33. De Vriendt T, Moreno LA, De Henauw S. Chronic stress and obesity in adolescents: Scientific evidence and methodological issues for epidemiological research. *Nutr Metab Cardiovasc Dis.* 2009;19(7):511–9.

34. Michels N, Sioen I, Boone L, Braet C, Vanaelst B, Huybrechts I. Longitudinal association between child stress and lifestyle. *Health Psychol.* 2015;34(1):40–50.

35. Salvy SJ, Bowker JC, Nitecki LA, Kluczynski MA, Germeroth LJ, Roemmich JN. Effects of ostracism and social connection-related activities on adolescents' motivation to eat and energy intake. *J Pediatr Psychol*. 2012;37(1):23–32.
36. Balantekin KN, Roemmich JN. Children's coping after psychological stress: Choices among food, physical activity, and television. *Appetite*. 2012;59(2):298–304.
37. Tate EB, Spruijt-Metz D, Pickering TA, Pentz MA. Two facets of stress and indirect effects on child diet through emotion-driven eating. *Eat Behav*. 2015;18:84–90.
38. van Kooten M, de Ridder D, Vollebergh W, van Dorsselaer S. What's so special about eating? Examining unhealthy diet of adolescents in the context of other health-related behaviours and emotional distress. *Appetite*. 2007;48(3):325–32.
39. Moljord IEO, Moksnes UK, Eriksen L, Espnes GA. Stress and happiness among adolescents with varying frequency of physical activity. *Percept Mot Skills*. 2011;113(2):631–46.
40. Norris R, Carroll D, Cochrane R. The effects of physical activity and exercise training on psychological stress and well-being in an adolescent population. *J Psychosom Res*. 1992;36(1):55–65.
41. Allison KR, Adlaf EM, Irving HM, Hatch JL, Smith TF, Dwyer JJM, et al. Relationship of vigorous physical activity to psychologic distress among adolescents. *J Adolesc Health*. 2005;37(2):164–6.
42. Horsch A, Wobmann M, Kriemler S, Munsch S, Borloz S, Balz A, et al. Impact of physical activity on energy balance, food intake and choice in normal weight and obese children in the setting of acute social stress: A randomized controlled trial. *BMC Pediatr*. 2015;15(1):1–10.
43. Yin Z, Davis CL, Moore JB, Treiber FA. Physical activity buffers the effects of chronic stress on adiposity in youth. *Ann Behav Med*. 2005;29(1):29–36.
44. Michels N, Sioen I, Boone L, Clays E, Vanaelst B, Huybrechts I, et al. Cross-lagged associations between children's stress and adiposity. *Psychosom Med*. 2015;77(1):50–8.
45. Pervanidou P, Chrousos GP. Metabolic consequences of stress during childhood and adolescence. *Metabolism*. 2012;61(5):611–9.
46. Lee MJ, Pramyothin P, Karastergiou K, Fried SK. Deconstructing the roles of glucocorticoids in adipose tissue biology and the development of central obesity. *Biochim Biophys Acta*. 2014;1842(3):473–81.
47. Kolbe I, Dumbell R, Oster H. Circadian clocks and the interaction between stress axis and adipose function. *Int J Endocrinol*. 2015;2015:693204.
48. Speaker KJ, Fleshner M. Interleukin-1 beta: A potential link between stress and the development of visceral obesity. *BMC Physiol*. 2012;12(1):8.
49. Verdejo-Garcia A, Moreno-Padilla M, Garcia-Rios MC, Lopez-Torrecillas F, Delgado-Rico E, Schmidt-Rio-Valle J, et al. Social stress increases cortisol and hampers attention in adolescents with excess weight. *PLoS One*. 2015;10(4):e0123565.
50. Tate EB, Wood W, Liao Y, Dunton GF. Do stressed mothers have heavier children? A meta-analysis on the relationship between maternal stress and child body mass index. *Obes Rev*. 2015;16(5):351–61.

19 Early Toxicant Exposures and the Development of Obesity in Childhood

Yun Liu and Karen E. Peterson

CONTENTS

INTRODUCTION

Worldwide increases in child obesity have been attributed to changes in diet, a sedentary lifestyle, and genetic predisposition, as reviewed in other chapters, but these risk factors do not fully account for the pace and pattern of recent secular trends [1,2]. The health consequences of obesity across the life course [3–6] coupled with challenges and costs of management [7,8] underscore the importance of disentangling the origins of pediatric obesity. The environment to which humans are exposed has changed, due to the exponential growth in the production and use of synthetic chemicals since the late nineteenth century [9]. In 2002, researchers offered ecologic evidence relating elevated production of endocrine-disrupting chemicals (EDCs) to US obesity trends and highlighted paradoxical weight gains at low levels of exposure to these ubiquitous compounds [2]. The mechanisms underlying the association of EDCs, collectively termed *obesogens* [10], with the developmental programing of obesity are described in Chapter 20.

This chapter considers evidence from human studies on the impacts of early-life exposure to persistent organic pollutants (POPs), short-lived compounds, and heavy metals on measures of off-spring fat mass and distribution. While cross-sectional studies have suggested that some EDCs are associated with obesity [11,12], accumulating evidence from longitudinal studies suggests that the timing of exposure and the direction of effects varies by sex across sensitive periods of development [13]. We restricted our review to human, nonexperimental studies with a prospective longitudinal design that examined the associations of perinatal toxicant exposures (*in utero*, breast milk) or those measured in children under 2 years with obesity-related outcomes from birth to young adulthood. For POPs and nonpersistent compounds, we summarize evidence from epidemiologic studies published over a 5-year period from 2011 to 2015 [14], given the availability of three extensive reviews of earlier studies [15–17]. For heavy metals, we discuss all human research available to date evaluating the effect of early exposure on the development of child obesity. Different lengths of follow-up across studies can provide insights on toxicant effects across sensitive periods for obesity development [18].

PERSISTENT ORGANIC POLLUTANTS AND OBESITY

POPs have been widely used as pesticides, solvents, pharmaceuticals, or industrial chemicals [19], raising global concern due to their potential for long-range transport, capacity to persist in the environment, ability to bioaccumulate in ecosystems, and their negative effects on human health [20]. Humans are exposed to these persistent substances primarily through dietary ingestion, inhalation, or dermal exposure [21]. Although POPs are presently banned or restricted by the Stockholm Convention, these toxicants can bioaccumulate within the food chain and are still detectable in human tissues around the world [16]. Polychlorinated biphenyl (PCBs), organochlorine pesticides, perfluorinated compounds (PFCs), and polybrominated diphenyl ethers (PBDEs) were found in 99%–100% of pregnant women [22], and POPs have been detected in cord blood, placenta, amniotic fluid, and breast milk [23–25]. Therefore, it is possible that perinatal POPs exposure may start *in utero*, passing through the placenta, and continue after delivery through breast-feeding. POPs are categorized into dioxins/dioxin-like substances or non-dioxin-like substances, as determined by their capacity to bind the aryl hydrocarbon receptor (AhR) [26]. Dioxins and dioxin-like compounds such as coplanar PCBs can promote adipogenesis by increasing peroxisome proliferator–activated receptor (PPAR) expression [27] and by disturbing initiation of estrogen receptors to encourage the progress of obesity [28]. In contrast, the underlying mechanism is not fully understood for non-dioxin-like compounds such as noncoplanar PCBs, organochlorine pesticides, hexachlorobenzene (HCB), hexachlorocyclohexane (HCH), PFCs, and PBDEs. Previous studies suggest that dichlorodiphenyltrichloroethane (DDT) and p,p′-dichlorodiphenyldichloroethylene (p,p′-DDE) can exert toxicity through antiandrogenic, estrogenic, and antiestrogenic effects [16]. HCB may lead to disrupted gluconeogenic reactions. Perfluroalkyls (PFOAs) and tributyltin (TBT) can affect fat storage, adipocyte differentiation, and insulin sensitivity via interfering with PPAR expression [16]. Polycyclic aromatic hydrocarbons (PAHs), which are a group of persistent chemicals generated in the course of incomplete combustion processes of organic materials, are suspected to act as endocrine disruptors and were recently suggested to be obesogens [29–31]. An animal study reported that benzo[a]pyrene, a high-molecular-weight PAH, directly inhibits the release of free fatty acids by adipocytes and leads to weight gain by accumulating fat mass [32].

Prior to 2011, numerous experimental reports and a limited number of epidemiological studies in humans linked perinatal exposure to synthetic chemicals to obesity in later life. Earlier prospective human studies documented an association between elevated levels of DDT or its main metabolite DDE [33] during pregnancy and obesity in their offspring [15]. The few cohort studies that examined the obesogenic effects of other organochlorine pesticides such as HCB and HCH provided inconsistent conclusions [15]. Far fewer researchers have examined the obesogenicity of other POPs, including PFCs, PBDEs, organotins, or PAHs. We identified 19 papers published between 2011 and 2015 that examined the relationship between obesity and perinatal exposure to POPs, including PCBs, DDE, DDT, HCB, HCH, PFOAs, PFOS, PBDEs, TBT, and PAHs. Most reports considered the influence of POPs, for example, PCBs (9 studies), and DDE (12 studies), while fewer investigated the impact of other compounds.

POLYCHLORINATED BIPHENYLS

Most of the nine prospective studies evaluating the impact of early PCB exposures failed to support the hypothesis that these synthetic chemicals predicted infant or child obesity prior to adolescence (Table 19.1). In the Spanish Infancia y Medio Ambiente (INMA)-Sabadell birth cohort, serum PCB levels during the first trimester were not associated with rapid weight gain in the first 6 months of life or overweight at 14 months, although this study was limited by sample size ($n = 518$) [34].

TABLE 19.1

Prospective Studies of Associations between Early-Life Exposure to Toxicants and Childhood Obesity and Related Outcomes

Study Setting n = mother–child pairs (Child Sex)	Exposure	Child Age at Follow-Up	Outcome[a]	Ref.
		Persistent Chemicals		
PCBs				
The Netherlands (Zwolle) n = 61 (♂♀)	Cord plasma (ng/L or ng/mL)	12 months	NS BMI	36
Spain (Sabadell) n = 518 (♂♀)	1st trimester serum (ng/g lipid)	6, 14 months	NS WAZ birth to 6 months, NS BMIz 14 months	34
Spain (Sabadell, Valencia and Gipuzkoa) n = 1285 (♂♀)	1st trimester serum (ng/g lipid)	6, 14 months	NS WAZ 6–14 months, NS overweight 14 months	35
Europe (pooled 7 birth cohorts) n = 1864 (♂♀)	Cord blood and postnatal exposure estimated with a validated pharmacokinetic model	Birth and 24 months	Postnatal PCBs: – WAZ β = –0.10 (95% CI: –0.19, –0.01)	41
Spain (Island of Menorca) n = 344 (♂♀)	Cord blood (ng/mL)	6.5 years	+ [T3 (>0.9 ng/mL) vs. T1 (<0.6 ng/mL)] Overweight RR = 1.70 (95% CI: 1.09, 2.64)	25
Denmark (Faroe Islands) n = 561 (♂♀)	Maternal serum and breast milk (µg/g)	5 and 7 years	+ in ♀, NS in ♂: BMI (kg/m^2) 7 years β = 1.13 (95% CI: 0.33, 1.93) WC (cm) 7 years β = 0.60 (95% CI: 0.05, 1.16) BMI change from 5 to 7 years β = 0.70 (95% CI: 0.26, 1.14) with overweight mothers	40
United States n = 1915 (♂♀)	3rd trimester serum (µg/L)	7 years	NS overweight and obesity	38
Greenland, Poland (Warsaw), and Ukraine (Kharkiv); n = 1109 (♂♀)	Second- and third-trimester serum and estimated postnatal (ng/g lipid)	5–9 years	NS BMI	37
Belgium (Flanders); n = 114 (♂♀)	Cord blood (ng/g fat)	7–9 years	+ in ♀, NS in ♂: WC β = 0.014 (p = .033)	39
DDE/DDT				
Mexico (Morelos); n = 253 (♂♀)	First-, second-, and third-trimester serum (ng/mL)	Birth to 12 months	DDE: NS WAZ, NS BMIz	44
The Netherlands (Zwolle); n = 61 (♂♀)	Cord plasma (ng/L or ng/mL)	12 months	DDE: NS BMI	36
Spain (Sabadell); n = 518 (♂♀)	First-trimester serum (ng/g lipid)	6 and 14 months	DDE: + WAZ birth to 6 months RR = 2.42 (95% CI: 1.25, 4.67) BMIz at 14 months RR = 1.22 (95% CI: 0.96, 1.55)	34
Spain (Sabadell, Valencia, and Gipuzkoa) n = 1285 (♂♀)	1st trimester serum (ng/g lipid)	6, 14 months	DDE: + WAZ 6–14 months RR = 1.13 (95% CI: 1.01, 1.26) Overweight 14 months RR = 1.15 (95% CI: 1.03, 1.28)	35
Europe (pooled 7 birth cohorts) n = 1864 (♂♀)	Cord blood and postnatal exposure estimated with a validated pharmacokinetic model	Birth and 24 months	Prenatal DDE: + WAZ β = 0.12 (95% CI: 0.03, 0.22)	41

(Continued)

TABLE 19.1 (CONTINUED)
Prospective Studies of Associations between Early-Life Exposure to Toxicants and Childhood Obesity and Related Outcomes

Study Setting n = mother–child pairs (Child Sex)	Exposure	Child Age at Follow-Up	Outcome[a]	Ref.
Spain (Island of Menorca); n = 344 (♂♀)	Cord blood (ng/mL)	6.5 years	DDE: + [T2 (0.7–1.5 ng/mL) vs. T1 (<0.7 ng/mL)] Overweight RR = 1.67 (95% CI: 1.10, 2.55) DDT: + in ♂, NS in ♀: [T2 (0.06–0.18 ng/mL) vs. T1 (<0.06 ng/mL)] Overweight RR = 1.96 (95% CI: 1.06, 3.62)	25
Denmark (Faroe Islands); n = 561 (♂♀)	Maternal serum and breast milk (µg/g)	5 and 7 years	DDE: + in ♀, NS in ♂: WC 7 years β = 0.93 (95% CI: 0.36, 1.51) BMI change 5–7 years β = 0.46 (95% CI: 0.12, 0.80) with overweight mothers	40
United States; n = 1915 (♂♀)	Third-trimester serum (µg/L)	7 years	DDE, DDT: NS overweight and obesity	38
United States (Salinas Valley); n = 270 (♂♀)	Second-trimester serum (ng/g lipid)	7 years	DDE, DDT: + obesity trend with age (2, 3.5, 5, 7 years) NS at 7 years	43
Greenland, Poland (Warsaw), and Ukraine (Kharkiv); n = 1109 (♂♀)	Second- and third-trimester serum and estimated postnatal (ng/g lipid)	5–9 years	DDE: NS BMI	37
Belgium (Flanders); n = 114 (♂♀)	Cord blood (ng/g fat)	7–9 years	DDE: + in ♀, NS in ♂: WC (cm) β = 0.013 (p = .021) WHR β = 0.015 (p = .004)	39
United States (Salinas Valley); n = 261 (♂♀)	Second-trimester serum (ng/g lipid)	9 years	DDT: + in ♂, NS in ♀: Overweight and obesity OR = 2.51 (95% CI: 1.00, 6.28) WC OR = 2.05 (95% CI: 1.10, 3.82) DDE: NS ♀♂	42
HCB/HCH				
Spain (Sabadell); n = 518 (♂♀)	First-trimester serum (ng/g lipid)	6 and 14 months	HCB, HCH: NS WAZ birth to 6 months, NS BMIz 14 months	34
Spain (Sabadell, Valencia, and Gipuzkoa); n = 1285 (♂♀)	First-trimester serum (ng/g lipid)	6 and 14 months	HCB: + WAZ 6–14 months RR = 1.13 (95% CI: 1.00, 1.29) Overweight 14 months RR = 1.19 (95% CI: 1.05, 1.34)	35
United States; n = 1915 (♂♀)	Third-trimester serum (µg/L)	7 years	HCH: NS overweight and obesity	38
Belgium (Flanders); n = 114 (♂♀)	Cord blood (ng/g fat)	7–9 years	HCB: NS ♀♂	39
Other POPs				
The Netherlands (Zwolle); n = 61 (♂♀)	Cord plasma (ng/L or ng/mL)	12 months	PFOS, PFOA: NS BMI	36
Great Britain (Avon); n = 320 (♀)	Pregnancy serum (10–28 weeks) (ng/mL)	20 months	PFOS: + [T3 (>23.0 ng/mL) vs. T1 (<16.6 ng/mL)] Weight (g) β = 579.82 (95% CI: 301.40, 858.25) PFOA: NS	45
Denmark; n = 811 (♂♀)	First- and second-trimester plasma (ng/mL)	7 years	PFOS, PFOA: NS BMI, WC, overweight	47
Greenland and Ukraine (Kharkiv); n = 1022 (♂♀)	Second-trimester serum (ng/mL)	5–9 years	PFOA, PFOS: NS overweight	48

TABLE 19.1 (CONTINUED)
Prospective Studies of Associations between Early-Life Exposure to Toxicants and Childhood Obesity and Related Outcomes

Study Setting n = mother–child pairs (Child Sex)	Exposure	Child Age at Follow-Up	Outcome[a]	Ref.
Denmark (Aarhus); $n = 665$ (♀♂)	Third-trimester serum (µg/L)	20 years	PFOA in ♀, NS in ♂: [Q4 (4.8–19.8 µg/L) vs. Q1 (0.1–2.8 µg/L)] + BMI (kg/m²) $\beta = 1.6$ (95% CI: 0.6, 2.6) + WC (cm) $\beta = 4.3$ (95% CI: 1.4, 7.3) + Overweight RR = 3.1 (95% CI: 1.4, 6.9) + Insulin (mmol/L) $\beta = 4.5$ (95% CI: 1.8, 7.2) + Leptin (ng/L) $\beta = 4.8$ (95% CI: 0.5, 9.4) – Adiponectin (µg/L) $\beta = -2.3$ (95% CI: –4.5, –0.2)	46
United States (Salinas Valley); $n = 224$ (♂♀)	Second- and third-trimester serum (ng/g lipid)	7 years	Maternal PBDEs in ♀, NS in ♂: – BMIz $\beta = -0.41$ (95% CI: –0.87, –0.05)	49
Finland (Turku); $n = 110$ (♂)	Placenta (ng/g)	Birth, 3, and 18 months	TBT: + weight gain (kg/week) 0–3 months $\beta = 0.024$ (95% CI: 0.003, 0.044) NS at other time points	50
United States (New York); $n = 324$ (♂♀)	Third-trimester personal air (ng/m³)	5 and 7 years	PAHs: + [T3 (≥3.08 ng/m³) vs. T1 (<1.73 ng/m³)] BMIz 5 years $\beta = 0.39$ (95% CI: 0.08, 0.70) Obesity 5 years RR = 1.79 (95% CI: 1.09, 2.96) BMIz 7 years $\beta = 0.30$ (95% CI: 0.01, 0.59) Percentage of body fat 7 years $\beta = 1.93$ (95% CI: 0.33, 3.54) Obesity 7 years RR = 2.26 (95% CI: 1.28, 4.00)	30

Nonpersistent Chemicals

BPA

Study Setting n = mother–child pairs (Child Sex)	Exposure	Child Age at Follow-Up	Outcome[a]	Ref.
Spain (Sabadell); $n = 402$ (♂♀)	First- and third-trimester urine (µg/g creatinine)	6, 14 months, and 4 years	+ WCz 4 years $\beta = 0.28$ (95% CI: 0.01, 0.57) NS: change in WAZ, overweight	58
United States (Salinas Valley); $n = 311$ (♂♀)	First- and second-trimester urine (µg/L)	9 years	– in ♀, NS in ♂: BMIz $\beta = -0.47$ (95% CI: –0.87, –0.07) Body fat (%) $\beta = -4.36$ (95% CI: –8.37, –0.34) Overweight and obesity OR = 0.38 (95% CI: 0.16, 0.91)	57
United States (Salinas Valley); $n = 188$ (♂♀)	First-, second-, and third-trimester urine (µg/g creatinine)	9 years	BPA during late pregnancy (first and second): + Leptin (ng/mL) in ♂ $\beta = 0.06$ (95% CI: 0.01, 0.11) BPA during early pregnancy (second and third): + Adiponectin (µg/mL) in ♀ $\beta = 3.71$ (95% CI: 0.38, 7.04)	33

Phthalates

Study Setting n = mother–child pairs (Child Sex)	Exposure	Child Age at Follow-Up	Outcome[a]	Ref.
The Netherlands (Zwolle); $n = 61$ (♂♀)	Cord plasma (ng/L or ng/mL)	12 months	High MEOHP: – in ♂, NS in ♀ BMI (kg/m²) $p = .029$	36
Spain (Sabadell); $n = 391$ (♂♀)	First- and third-trimester urine (µg/g creatinine)	Birth and 6 months; 1, 4, and 7 years	High-molecular weight phthalate metabolites: – in ♂, NS in ♀ WAZ 0–6 months $\beta = -0.41$ (95% CI: –0.75, –0.06) BMI (kg/m²) 4 years $\beta = -0.38$ (95% CI: –0.76, –0.01) BMI 7 years $\beta = -0.40$ (95% CI: –0.78, –0.02)	60
United States (New York); $n = 326$ (♂♀)	Third-trimester urine (µg/g creatinine)	5 and 7 years	Non-DEHP: – in ♂, NS in ♀ BMIz $\beta = -0.30$ (95% CI: –0.50, –0.10) Body fat (%) $\beta = -1.62$ (95% CI: –2.91, –0.34) WC $\beta = -2.02$ (95% CI: –3.71, –0.32)	61

(Continued)

TABLE 19.1 (CONTINUED)
Prospective Studies of Associations between Early-Life Exposure to Toxicants and Childhood Obesity and Related Outcomes

Study Setting n = mother–child pairs (Child Sex)	Exposure	Child Age at Follow-Up	Outcome[a]	Ref.
		Heavy Metals		
Lead				
Mexico (Mexico City); n = 329 (♂♀)	One month postpartum maternal bone (μg of lead/g of mineral bone) and infant blood (μg/dL)	Birth to 1 month	Maternal lead: – attained weight (g) 1 month β = –3.69 (95% CI: –7.21, –0.16) Infancy lead: – weight gain (g) from birth to 1 month β = –15.1 (95% CI: –28.3, –1.8)	66
United States (New York); n = 211 (♂♀)	Second-trimester and postnatal 6-month blood (μg/dL)	6 and 12 months	Second-trimester lead: Higher (≥3 μg/dL) vs. lower lead (<3 μg/dL) WAZ 6 months β = –0.771 (p = .03) UAZ 12 months β = –1.063 (p = .02) Infancy lead: NS	67
South Korea; n = 247 (♂♀)	Early pregnancy (first and second trimester) and late-pregnancy (delivery) blood (μg/dL)	Birth, 6, 12, and 24 months	Late-pregnancy lead: WAZ 12 months β = –0.31 (95% CI: –0.59, –0.04) WAZ 24 months β = –0.41 (95% CI: –0.71, –0.11) Early-pregnancy lead: NS	68
Mexico (Mexico City); n = 171 (♂♀)	One month postpartum maternal bone (μg/g), average infancy (between birth and 24 months), and average early-childhood blood (30 and 48 months)(μg/dL)	2 years	NS BMI	69
Mexico (Mexico City); n = 1000 (♂♀)	One month postpartum maternal bone (μg/g)	Birth to 5 years	– in ♀, NS in ♂: weight (g) 0 to 5 years β = –130.9 (95% CI: –227.4, –34.4)	63
Bangladesh (Matlab); n = 1505 (♂♀)	First- and third-trimester urine (μg/L)	Birth to 5 years	NS weight	64
Yugoslavia (Kosovo); n = 309 (♂♀)	Pregnancy maternal blood (9–28 weeks) (μg/dL)	Birth to 10 years	NS BMI	70
Mexico (Mexico City); n = 647 (♂♀)	Maternal bone (μg/g) and early-childhood blood (μg/dL)	7–15 years	Maternal bone lead in ♀, NS in ♂: – BMI (kg/m²) β = –0.0368 (p = .01) Early-childhood lead: NS ♂♀	71
Cadmium				
Taiwan; n = 402 (♂♀)	Cord blood (μg/L)	Birth to 3 years	– Weight (kg) 0–3 years β (×100) = –1.81 (95% CI [×100]: –3.01, –0.61)	72
Bangladesh (Matlab); n = 1505 (♂♀)	First- and third-trimester urine (μg/L)	Birth to 5 years	NS weight	64
Belgium (Flanders); n = 114 (♂♀)	Cord blood (μg/L)	7 to 8 years	– in ♀, NS in ♂: Weight (kg) β (ln-transformed)= 0.937 (95% CI: 0.900, 0.979) BMIz β = –0.749 (95% CI: –1.261, –0.237) WC (cm) β (ln-transformed) = 0.973 (95% CI: 0.953, 0.997) Sum of four skin folds (mm) β (ln-transformed) = 0.728 (95% CI: 0.587, 0.900)	39

TABLE 19.1 (CONTINUED)

Prospective Studies of Associations between Early-Life Exposure to Toxicants and Childhood Obesity and Related Outcomes

Study Setting n = mother–child pairs (Child Sex)	Exposure	Child Age at Follow-Up	Outcome[a]	Ref.
Other Metals				
Bangladesh (Matlab); n = 2087 (♂♀)	First- and third-trimester and postnatal 18-month urine (µg/L)	Birth to 2 years	Postnatal arsenic: – in ♀, NS in ♂ [Q4 (46–96 µg/L) vs. Q1 (2.4–16 µg/L)] Weight (kg) 18 months $\beta = -0.34$ (95% CI: -0.52, -0.15) Weight (kg) 21 months $\beta = -0.27$ (95% CI: -0.47, -0.075) Weight (kg) 24 months $\beta = -0.22$ (95% CI: -0.42, -0.014) Gestational arsenic: NS in ♂♀	73
Bangladesh (Matlab); n = 1505 (♂♀)	First- and third-trimester urine (µg/L)	Birth to 5 years	Arsenic: NS weight	64
South Korea; n = 164 (♂♀)	Early pregnancy (first and second), late pregnancy (third trimester), and cord blood (µg/L)	Birth to 2 years	Late-pregnancy mercury: – Attained weight (kg) until 2 years $\beta = -0.186$ ($p = .05$) Cord blood mercury: – Attained weight (kg) until 2 years $\beta = -0.359$ ($p = .01$) Early-pregnancy mercury: NS	74

Abbreviations: BMI, body mass index; BMIz, BMI z-score for age and sex; WCz, waist circumference z-score; NS, nonsignificant statistical test of association; overweight defined as BMI ≥85th and <95th percentile for age and sex; obesity defined as children BMI ≥95th percentile for age and sex based on reference growth curves used by primary authors; OR, odds ratio; Q, quartile; RR, relative risk; T, tertile; WAZ, weight-for-age z-score for age and sex; WC, waist circumference in cm; WHR, waist-to-hip ratio; UAZ, upper-arm circumference-for-age z-score for age and sex; PCBs, polychlorinated biphenyls; DDE, dichlorodiphenyldichloroethylene; DDT, dichlorodiphenyltrichloroethane; HCB, hexachlorobenzene; HCH, hexachlorocyclohexane; TBT, tributyltin; PFOA, perfluorooctanoic acid; PFOS, perfluorooctane sulfate; PBDEs, polybrominated diphenyl ethers; BPA, bisphenol A; MEOHP, mono-2-ethyl-5-oxohexyl phthalate; PAHs, polycyclic aromatic hydrocarbons.

a   Change in outcome per 1-unit change in the exposure unless otherwise specified.

An expansion of the original INMA-Sabadell cohort to a larger study population ($n = 1285$) confirmed earlier findings that PCBs were unrelated to infant growth in this cohort [35]. A Dutch study among pregnant mothers from Zwolle, the Netherlands, also found no association between PCB 153 measured in cord blood and infant growth [36]. Two studies found no evidence that PCBs affect weight status in school-age children. A prospective cohort study [37] of maternal–child pairs from Greenland, Poland, and Ukraine found no clear associations between PCB exposure during pregnancy and children's body mass index (BMI) at 5–9 years. This study was consistent with earlier findings [38] from the US Collaborative Perinatal Project (CPP) showing that high levels of total PCB exposures during the third trimester were not linked to overweight or obesity in children aged 7 years. Notably, PCB exposure levels were relatively high in the CPP population, since blood samples were collected before these toxic substances were phased out in the United States.

Counter to the preceding studies that failed to demonstrate a relationship between PCBs and obesity-related outcomes in infancy or at school entry, four prospective studies showed that prenatal PCB exposure may have different impacts on child growth by age and sex (Table 19.1). A pooled analysis of seven European birth cohorts [39], the largest study to date examining the obesogenic effects of POPs, found a negative association between postnatal exposure to PCBs and weight from birth to 24 months. In mid-childhood, however, positive associations of perinatal PCB exposures with fat mass and distribution were documented in girls but not boys in three observational studies. In a Flemish cohort [40], PCB levels in cord blood were positively correlated with waist circumference (WC), an indirect measure of central fat distribution in girls aged 7–9 years, but cord blood PCB levels were unrelated to BMI in children in the sample. Maternal PCB levels in pregnancy of Faroese women similarly were related to higher WC in female children aged 7 years, but only those who had overweight mothers [41]. Additionally, these authors found a significant association between prenatal PCBs and a change of BMI in girls from 5 to 7 years of age as well as BMI at 7 years [41]. In the INMA-Sabadell cohort, the concentration of PCBs in cord blood positively predicted BMI and overweight in Spanish children aged 6.5 years, an association that appeared to be stronger in girls than in boys, in contrast to nonsignificant findings at earlier ages [25].

ORGANOCHLORINE PESTICIDES

Of the 12 recent prospective studies of maternal exposure to DDE or DDT we reviewed, eight documented a statistically significant, positive association with child obesity–related outcomes across different developmental periods (Table 19.1). Among maternal–child dyads in the Spanish INMA-Sabadell cohort, *in utero* DDE exposure was related to rapid growth in the first 6 months of life and overweight at age 14 months [34,35]. In the same cohort, DDE concentrations in cord blood also were related to an increased risk of overweight at 6.5 years of age, but DDT was significantly associated with overweight only in boys, not girls [25]. Across seven pooled European birth cohorts, DDE levels in cord blood were associated with greater weight change from birth to 24 months of age, although this effect was not seen in infants with postnatal exposure via breast milk [39]. Studies conducted in Faroese and in Flemish children reported significant positive associations between prenatal DDE and BMI change from 5 to 7 years of age [41] and obesity-related outcomes at 7 years [40] in girls but not in boys, respectively. In contrast, reports from the Center for the Health Assessment of Mothers and Children of Salinas (CHAMACOS) study found that prenatal DDT concentrations in second-trimester serum were related to increased WC, overweight, and obesity at 9 years of age only in boys [42]. However, these authors also documented a significant trend of increased odds of obesity across ages 2, 3.5, 5, and 7 years in boys and girls combined [43].

Despite a preponderance of evidence linking persistent organochlorine pesticides to offspring weight gain and status in US and European settings, four recent studies found no association of developmental exposure to DDE with infant or child obesity (Table 19.1). A study among 253 women in Morelos State, Mexico, suggested that maternal exposure to DDE during pregnancy may not affect infant growth [44]. Similarly, three prospective studies found no clear association between maternal exposure to DDE or DDT and growth in the first year of life among children in the Netherlands [36], or with BMI in Greenlandic, Polish, and Ukrainian children aged 5–9 years [37], or 7-year-old children in the United States. [38].

Few human studies have examined early-life exposures to HCB and HCH (Table 19.1). Of four epidemiological studies considering these perinatal exposures, three found no significant association between prenatal HCB and infant growth at 6 and 14 months [34], obesity in children aged 7 years [38], or obesity in children aged 7–9 years [40], respectively. No association with HCH was found in these three studies. Only one study reported HCB was positively associated with rapid growth and overweight in Spanish infants in the INMA-Sabadell cohort [35].

OTHER POPS

Other new POPs on the Stockholm Convention list, including PFOA, PFOS, PBDEs, TBT, and PAHs, have attracted attention because their potential to promote obesity has been suggested by several animal studies. We identified five human studies published since 2011 that evaluated the effects of PFOA and PFOS on offspring obesity (Table 19.1). British girls at 20 months of age with prenatal PFOS exposure in the upper tertile were 580 g heavier compared with those in the lower tertile, but no differences in weight were found with PFOA [45]. In contrast, a Danish cohort study [46] of 665 pregnant women found that *in utero* exposure to PFOA was significantly associated with BMI, WC, and overweight among female offspring followed to early adulthood, as well as levels of insulin, adiponectin, and leptin, but no association was observed for PFOS [46]. One prospective study observed a null association of prenatal PFOA/PFOS with infant BMI at 12 months [36], and two reports found no association with overweight in school-age children [47,48]. In the single human study of developmental exposure to PBDEs and risk of obesity in the Salinas Valley, California, maternal PBDE serum levels during pregnancy were significantly related to decreased BMI in 7-year-old girls [49]. Despite the relatively extensive number of experimental studies of TBT described in Chapter 11 (Blumberg), we identified only one study exploring the possible obesogenic effect of TBT in humans. A Finnish cohort study reported that TBT levels in placental tissue were associated with the weight gain of male infants during the first 3 months of life, but no associations were observed at 3 or 18 months [50]. One study found that personal airborne PAHs during the third trimester were positively associated with BMI z-score and risk of obesity at 5 years and with BMI z-score, percentage of fat mass, and risk of obesity at 7 years of age among a sample of African American and Dominican children residing in New York City [30].

Short-Lived Ubiquitous Pollutants and Obesity

In addition to persistent environmental chemicals, nonpersistent compounds such as bisphenol A (BPA) and phthalates have been related to human health. BPA has been used in a wide range of consumer products including can linings, packaging materials, and children's toys. The major route of exposure is through the consumption of foods and beverages that have been contaminated with BPA [51]. Detectable levels of BPA in blood have been found in human fetuses [52]. BPA is considered an EDC that can regulate insulin and leptin production by exerting estrogenic activity, acting as agonist and antagonist of PPARγ [16]. Experimental data suggest that prenatal BPA promotes weight gain in offspring, but this association has not been extensively studied in humans using longitudinal studies. Similarly, phthalates [53] such as diethylhexyl phthalate (DEHP), oxidative DEHP, and metabolite mono-(2-ethyl-5-oxohexyl) phthalate (MEOHP) are used in hundreds of consumer products, including plastics, cosmetics, and personal care products. Measurable levels of phthalate metabolites haven been reported in the urine of pregnant women, in amniotic fluids, and in cord blood [53–55]. Growing experimental evidence has shown that phthalates are thyroid hormone and androgen antagonists and may affect adipogenesis, lipid accumulation, and insulin resistance by regulating activation of PPARγ [56].

Nonpersistent compounds such as phthalates and BPA have been related to pediatric obesity in experimental studies, but human data are insufficient to support such a relationship [16]. The three prospective studies published between 2011 and 2015 that examined the effects of urinary BPA levels during pregnancy on postnatal growth and obesity reported inconsistent results. In the Spanish population participating in the INMA-Sabadell study, prenatal BPA was weakly associated with increased WC in 4-year-old children but not at earlier ages [57]. In the CHAMACOS cohort, maternal urinary BPA concentrations during pregnancy were inversely associated with BMI, percentage of body fat, and obesity in 9-year-old Mexican American girls, but these effects were not yet evident at 5 years [58]. In the same population, BPA exposure during late pregnancy was related to increased leptin in boys, whereas BPA in early pregnancy was associated with increased adiponectin in girls at 9 years of age [33]. Although the mechanistic pathways for sex-specific effects seen in these studies are not fully understood, one potential explanation is that BPA may affect estrogen activity by interrupting original binding at nuclear estrogen receptors. The synthesis and function of estrogen as well as the distribution of estrogen receptors vary in males and females [59]. Previous studies of associations between prenatal phthalate exposure and obesity among children are limited to a few cross-sectional reports. A recent prospective study in a small Danish sample ($n = 61$) reported that higher MEOHP in cord blood was related to lower BMI in male offspring from birth to 11 months [36].

Similar results were seen in a prospective study of high-molecular-weight phthalate metabolites and postnatal growth in the Spanish INMA-Sabadell birth cohort; pregnancy urinary levels were associated with reduced weight gain in the first 6 months of life and lower BMI at 4–7 years in boys [60]. In addition, one study conducted in New York City among 326 African American and Dominican mothers revealed a significant inverse association of third-trimester phthalates with BMI z-score, percentage of body fat, and WC in boys at 5 and 7 years old [61].

HEAVY METALS AND OBESITY

Other than synthetic industrial substances, heavy metals have also been proposed to exert obesogenic effects [2,16]. Although the underlying mechanism remains uncertain, heavy metals such as lead, cadmium, arsenic, and mercury have been found to exhibit endocrine-disrupting features in animal studies [62]. For example, lead may disrupt endocrine functions through its impact on estrogen metabolism, which leads to altered insulin-like growth factor 1 (IGF-1) levels and subsequent body growth [63]. Since the level of estrogen varies by sex, the effects of lead on child growth may have been more pronounced in girls than in boys. Similarly, cadmium, arsenic, and mercury have also been indicated to exert endocrine-disrupting properties and affect children's growth in a sex-dependent manner [62,64]. Evidence in both animal and human studies supports the hypothesis that cadmium and mercury interrupt steroidogenesis in the placenta and affect estradiol functions [62,65]. With regard to arsenic, it has been suggested to disrupt insulin signaling and glucose uptake by tissues, resulting in impaired growth [62,64].

Most studies of early exposure to heavy metals in relation to obesity have focused on the toxic effects of endocrine-disrupting metals on birth outcomes, whereas research to determine the persistence of these effects into childhood is limited and current evidence is inconsistent. Among these four toxicants, the influence of lead on child obesity has been the most extensively studied. We identified eight longitudinal studies that evaluated the toxicity of lead exposure during early life on anthropometry in children (Table 19.1). In the Early-Life Exposure in Mexico to Environmental Toxicants (ELEMENT) birth cohort, maternal bone lead at 1 month postpartum, a measure of cumulative *in utero* exposure, was significantly and negatively associated with attained weight at 1 month of life, and infant blood lead with weight gain from birth to 1 month of age [66]. A longitudinal study performed in Albany, New York [67], also revealed an inverse association of higher blood lead levels (≥ 3 µg/dL) during pregnancy with postnatal weight-for-age z-scores at 6 months and upper-arm circumference-for-age z-scores at 12 months, whereas postnatal exposure to lead at 6 months was not significantly related to infant growth. Another investigation confirmed that blood lead level at delivery but not early pregnancy (first and second trimester) negatively predicted infant weight from 12 to 24 months among participants from the Mothers and Children's Environmental Health (MOCEH) birth cohort in South Korea, and this influence was more pronounced in pregnant women with lower levels of calcium intake (<541 mg/d) [68]. To examine the persistence of these effects into preschool years, a follow-up study of 522 boys and 477 girls in the Mexico City ELEMENT cohorts found that maternal bone lead at 1 month postpartum was related to a reduced weight trajectory among female participants from birth to 5 years of age [63]. However, these authors did not observe associations of prenatal or early postnatal lead exposure with BMI at 48 months of age using the same cohort [69]. In contrast, a prospective cohort study of 1505 mother–offspring pairs living in rural Bangladesh provided evidence that pregnancy urinary lead levels were not significantly associated with child weight at age 5 [64]. Two studies considered the effects of early lead exposure on obesity-related outcomes in school-age children. A cohort study in 309 mother–offspring pairs from Kosovo, Yugoslavia, reported that gestational lead exposure was not correlated with children's BMI up to 10 years of age [70]. However, another study using the ELEMENT cohort provided evidence that maternal patella lead but not early childhood blood lead was associated with reduced BMI in 267 Mexican girls at 7–15 years of age but not in 290 boys [71].

Three prospective studies that examined the influence of early-life cadmium on child growth and obesity-related outcomes reported equivocal results. A prospective Taiwanese study reported that cadmium cord blood concentrations were negatively associated with children's weight up to 3 years of age [72]. In the Flemish population, prenatal cadmium exposure was found to be associated with reduced weight, WC, BMI z-score, and skinfolds only in girls aged 7–8 years [40]. In contrast, a study in the Matlab cohort in rural Bangladesh indicated a null association of maternal cadmium level in urine during the first and third trimesters with body weight in 5-year-old children [64,73]. Arsenic and mercury are the least documented toxic metals in terms of obesogenic effects. In the Matlab cohort, postnatal exposure to arsenic at 18 months negatively predicted child weight from 1.5 to 2 years of age in girls but not boys, whereas this effect was not observed with *in utero* arsenic exposure [73]. Maternal arsenic also was unrelated to body weight in these Bangladeshi children in the first 5 years of life [64]. A study in the South Korean MOCEH birth cohort revealed an inverse relationship between maternal blood mercury concentrations during late pregnancy and cord blood with attained weight over the first 24 months of life, whereas no significant association was found for early pregnancy exposure [74].

CONCLUSIONS

The 35 studies discussed in this chapter reveal inconsistent conclusions about the obesogenic effects of early-life exposure to environmental toxicants that may be attributable to differences in the study population, chemical congeners, levels of exposure, time windows for outcomes, and measured and unmeasured confounders. Most longitudinal human studies on the effects of early-life exposure to synthetic chemicals on overweight or obesity in childhood have focused on the prenatal period, whereas few have examined exposure via breast-feeding or early childhood or a combination. Rapid growth, overweight, and obesity among children were primarily assessed using indirect measures of adiposity such as weight gain, BMI, and WC, whereas direct measures were less commonly employed—for example, skinfolds, bioimpedance, dual-energy x-ray absorptiometry, or adipokines. Most current epidemiological data consider the influence of these chemicals on overweight and obesity during infancy and early childhood up to 9 years of age, but few studies examine the persistence of obesity in adolescence and adulthood due to the challenges of long-term follow-up. Of the reports we reviewed, the majority focused on understanding the toxic effects of DDE, PCBs, and lead, while investigations of other environmental toxicants were scarce, particularly for PBDEs, organotin compounds, PAHs, and nonpersistent chemicals, as well as other heavy metals. Overall, we found continued support for the predominantly positive effect of maternal DDE on increased risk of child obesity and less consistent associations for other substances. Several studies were limited by relatively small-to-modest sample sizes, whereas those with large sample sizes were constrained by heterogeneity across pooled populations, which could contribute to imprecision. Some longitudinal investigations also reported a substantial loss of participants during the follow-up time, which could bias findings across different developmental periods. Many authors modeled relationships with categorical measures of exposure, which may reduce statistical power, although categorical measures could reveal nonlinear or nonmonotonic relationships that could be explored in studies with larger sample sizes [14]. Among the strengths of the 35 papers reviewed here was that they all utilized a prospective, longitudinal design that can enhance causal inference. A few studies used advanced modeling for estimating postnatal exposure and measured levels of adipokines and skinfolds to assess adiposity.

Further research in larger study populations and various settings worldwide is needed to confirm the observed associations, especially for less-studied chemicals, and to evaluate potential underlying mechanisms. Studies with longer follow-up time to ascertain the persistence of compounds' effects into later ages and developmental periods, including the transition to young adulthood, should be considered a priority for future investigations. Research with complete information about both maternal prenatal and postnatal exposure and that utilizes direct measures of adiposity is recommended. Considering that many studies report inconsistent results regarding differential effects on boys and girls, the systematic evaluation of interaction by sex is needed. Other factors that appear to serve as effect modifiers of chemical exposures, such as maternal weight status and intake of fat, minerals such as calcium and zinc, and other micronutrients that affect their bioavailability, also require confirmation in larger studies. In addition, birth weight deserves special attention as it shows divergent functions in different analyses as a confounder or as an intermediate variable. Lastly, studies of mixtures of chemicals should be taken into consideration, given that humans have detectable levels of various obesogenic compounds and toxicants may have opposing effects on obesity-related outcomes in male and female offspring at different ages.

In conclusion, studies on the risk of obesity in relation to environmental toxicant exposures during early life provide suggestive evidence for some but not all chemicals, and many uncertainties require further exploration. With prospective study designs, large sample sizes, improved exposure assessments, direct measures of obesity, and advanced statistical analyses, data generated from these studies can contribute to a strong evidence base for recommendations and strategies to prevent pediatric obesity and its long-term sequelae.

ACKNOWLEDGMENTS

This work was supported in part by 1P01ES022844–01/RD-83543601 and the National Institute of Public Health of Mexico.

REFERENCES

1. Grun F, Blumberg B. Environmental obesogens: Organotins and endocrine disruption via nuclear receptor signaling. *Endocrinology.* 2006;147(Suppl. 6):S50–5.
2. Baillie-Hamilton PF. Chemical toxins: A hypothesis to explain the global obesity epidemic. *J Altern Complement Med.* 2002;8(2):185–92.
3. Freedman DS, Mei Z, Srinivasan SR, Berenson GS, Dietz WH. Cardiovascular risk factors and excess adiposity among overweight children and adolescents: The Bogalusa Heart Study. *J Pediatr.* 2007;150(1):12–7 e2.
4. Li C, Ford ES, Zhao G, Mokdad AH. Prevalence of pre-diabetes and its association with clustering of cardiometabolic risk factors and hyperinsulinemia among U.S. adolescents: National Health and Nutrition Examination Survey 2005–2006. *Diabetes Care.* 2009;32(2):342–7.
5. Maffeis C, Tato L. Long-term effects of childhood obesity on morbidity and mortality. *Horm Res.* 2001;55 Suppl 1:42–5.
6. Singh AS, Mulder C, Twisk JW, van Mechelen W, Chinapaw MJ. Tracking of childhood overweight into adulthood: A systematic review of the literature. *Obes Rev.* 2008;9(5):474–88.
7. Cawley J, Meyerhoefer C. The medical care costs of obesity: An instrumental variables approach. *J Health Econ.* 2012;31(1):219–30.
8. Wang Y, Beydoun MA, Liang L, Caballero B, Kumanyika SK. Will all Americans become overweight or obese? Estimating the progression and cost of the US obesity epidemic. *Obesity.* 2008;16(10):2323–30.
9. Landrigan PJ, Goldman LR. Children's vulnerability to toxic chemicals: A challenge and opportunity to strengthen health and environmental policy. *Health Aff.* 2011;30(5):842–50.
10. Grun F, Blumberg B. Endocrine disrupters as obesogens. *Mol Cell Endocrinol.* 2009;304(1–2):19–29.
11. Trasande L, Attina TM, Blustein J. Association between urinary bisphenol A concentration and obesity prevalence in children and adolescents. *JAMA.* 2012;308(11):1113–21.
12. Eng DS, Lee JM, Gebremariam A, Meeker JD, Peterson K, Padmanabhan V. Bisphenol A and chronic disease risk factors in US children. *Pediatrics.* 2013;132(3):e637–45.
13. Veiga-Lopez A, Kannan K, Liao C, Ye W, Domino SE, Padmanabhan V. Gender-specific effects on gestational length and birth weight by early pregnancy BPA exposure. *J Clin Endocrinol Metab.* 2015;100(11):E1394–403.
14. Liu Y, Peterson KE. Maternal exposure to synthetic chemicals and obesity in the offspring: Recent findings. *Curr Environ Health Rep.* 2015;2:339–47.
15. La Merrill M, Birnbaum LS. Childhood obesity and environmental chemicals. *Mt Sinai J Med.* 2011;78(1):22–48.

16. Grant KL, Carpenter DO, Sly LJ, Sly PD. Environmental contributions to obesity and type 2 diabetes. *J Environ Immunol Toxicol*. 2014;1(2):80–91.
17. Tang-Peronard JL, Andersen HR, Jensen TK, Heitmann BL. Endocrine-disrupting chemicals and obesity development in humans: A review. *Obes Rev*. 2011;12(8):622–36.
18. Dietz WH. Overweight in childhood and adolescence. *N Engl J Med*. 2004;350(9):855–7.
19. Vested A, Giwercman A, Bonde JP, Toft G. Persistent organic pollutants and male reproductive health. *Asian J Androl*. 2014;16(1):71–80.
20. Yu GW, Laseter J, Mylander C. Persistent organic pollutants in serum and several different fat compartments in humans. *J Environ Public Health*. 2011;2011:417980.
21. Li QQ, Loganath A, Chong YS, Tan J, Obbard JP. Persistent organic pollutants and adverse health effects in humans. *J Toxicol Environ Health A*. 2006;69(21):1987–2005.
22. Woodruff TJ, Zota AR, Schwartz JM. Environmental chemicals in pregnant women in the United States: NHANES 2003–2004. *Environ Health Perspect*. 2011;119(6):878–85.
23. Foster W, Chan S, Platt L, Hughes C. Detection of endocrine disrupting chemicals in samples of second trimester human amniotic fluid. *J Clin Endocrinol Metab*. 2000;85(8):2954–7.
24. Longnecker MP, Rogan WJ, Lucier G. The human health effects of DDT (dichlorodiphenyltrichloroethane) and PCBS (polychlorinated biphenyls) and an overview of organochlorines in public health. *Annu Rev Public Health*. 1997;18:211–44.
25. Valvi D, Mendez MA, Martinez D, Grimalt JO, Torrent M, Sunyer J, et al. Prenatal concentrations of polychlorinated biphenyls, DDE, and DDT and overweight in children: A prospective birth cohort study. *Environ Health Perspect*. 2012;120(3):451–7.
26. Ahlborg UG, Brouwer A, Fingerhut MA, Jacobson JL, Jacobson SW, Kennedy SW, et al. Impact of polychlorinated dibenzo-p-dioxins, dibenzofurans, and biphenyls on human and environmental health, with special emphasis on application of the toxic equivalency factor concept. *Eur J Pharmacol*. 1992;228(4):179–99.
27. Casals-Casas C, Feige JN, Desvergne B. Interference of pollutants with PPARs: Endocrine disruption meets metabolism. *Int J Obes*. 2008;32(Suppl. 6):S53–61.
28. Cooke PS, Naaz A. Role of estrogens in adipocyte development and function. *Exp Biol Med*. 2004;229(11):1127–35.
29. Santodonato J. Review of the estrogenic and antiestrogenic activity of polycyclic aromatic hydrocarbons: Relationship to carcinogenicity. *Chemosphere*. 1997;34(4):835–48.
30. Rundle A, Hoepner L, Hassoun A, Oberfield S, Freyer G, Holmes D, et al. Association of childhood obesity with maternal exposure to ambient air polycyclic aromatic hydrocarbons during pregnancy. *Am J Epidemiol*. 2012;175(11):1163–72.
31. Kim HW, Kam S, Lee DH. Synergistic interaction between polycyclic aromatic hydrocarbons and environmental tobacco smoke on the risk of obesity in children and adolescents: The U.S. National Health and Nutrition Examination Survey 2003–2008. *Environ Res*. 2014;135:354–60.
32. Irigaray P, Ogier V, Jacquenet S, Notet V, Sibille P, Mejean L, et al. Benzo[a]pyrene impairs beta-adrenergic stimulation of adipose tissue lipolysis and causes weight gain in mice. A novel molecular mechanism of toxicity for a common food pollutant. *FEBS J*. 2006;273(7):1362–72.
33. Volberg V, Harley K, Calafat AM, Dave V, McFadden J, Eskenazi B, et al. Maternal bisphenol a exposure during pregnancy and its association with adipokines in Mexican-American children. *Environ Mol Mutagen*. 2013;54(8):621–8.
34. Mendez MA, Garcia-Esteban R, Guxens M, Vrijheid M, Kogevinas M, Goni F, et al. Prenatal organochlorine compound exposure, rapid weight gain, and overweight in infancy. *Environ Health Perspect*. 2011;119(2):272–8.
35. Valvi D, Mendez MA, Garcia-Esteban R, Ballester F, Ibarluzea J, Goni F, et al. Prenatal exposure to persistent organic pollutants and rapid weight gain and overweight in infancy. *Obesity*. 2014;22(2):488–96.
36. de Cock M, de Boer MR, Lamoree M, Legler J, van de Bor M. First year growth in relation to prenatal exposure to endocrine disruptors: A Dutch prospective cohort study. *Int J Environ Res Public Health*. 2014;11(7):7001–21.
37. Hoyer BB, Ramlau-Hansen CH, Henriksen TB, Pedersen HS, Goralczyk K, Zviezdai V, et al. Body mass index in young school-age children in relation to organochlorine compounds in early life: A prospective study. *Int J Obes*. 2014;38(7):919–25.
38. Cupul-Uicab LA, Klebanoff MA, Brock JW, Longnecker MP. Prenatal exposure to persistent organochlorines and childhood obesity in the US collaborative perinatal project. *Environ Health Perspect*. 2013;121(9):1103–9.

39. Iszatt N, Stigum H, Verner MA, White RA, Govarts E, Palkovicova Murinova L, et al. Prenatal and postnatal exposure to persistent organic pollutants and infant growth: A pooled analysis of seven european birth cohorts. *Environ Health Perspect.* 2015;123:730–736.

40. Delvaux I, Van Cauwenberghe J, Den Hond E, Schoeters G, Govarts E, Nelen V, et al. Prenatal exposure to environmental contaminants and body composition at age 7–9 years. *Environ Res.* 2014;132:24–32.

41. Tang-Peronard JL, Heitmann BL, Andersen HR, Steuerwald U, Grandjean P, Weihe P, et al. Association between prenatal polychlorinated biphenyl exposure and obesity development at ages 5 and 7 y: A prospective cohort study of 656 children from the Faroe Islands. *Am J Clin Nutr.* 2014;99(1):5–13.

42. Warner M, Wesselink A, Harley KG, Bradman A, Kogut K, Eskenazi B. Prenatal exposure to dichlorodiphenyltrichloroethane and obesity at 9 years of age in the CHAMACOS study cohort. *Am J Epidemiol.* 2014;179(11):1312–22.

43. Warner M, Aguilar Schall R, Harley KG, Bradman A, Barr D, Eskenazi B. *In utero* DDT and DDE exposure and obesity status of 7-year-old Mexican-American children in the CHAMACOS cohort. *Environ Health Perspect.* 2013;121(5):631–6.

44. Garced S, Torres-Sanchez L, Cebrian ME, Claudio L, Lopez-Carrillo L. Prenatal dichlorodiphenyldichloroethylene (DDE) exposure and child growth during the first year of life. *Environ Res.* 2012;113:58–62.

45. Maisonet M, Terrell ML, McGeehin MA, Christensen KY, Holmes A, Calafat AM, et al. Maternal concentrations of polyfluoroalkyl compounds during pregnancy and fetal and postnatal growth in British girls. *Environ Health Perspect.* 2012;120(10):1432–7.

46. Halldorsson TI, Rytter D, Haug LS, Bech BH, Danielsen I, Becher G, et al. Prenatal exposure to perfluorooctanoate and risk of overweight at 20 years of age: A prospective cohort study. *Environ Health Perspect.* 2012;120(5):668–73.

47. Andersen CS, Fei C, Gamborg M, Nohr EA, Sorensen TI, Olsen J. Prenatal exposures to perfluorinated chemicals and anthropometry at 7 years of age. *Am J Epidemiol.* 2013;178(6):921–7.

48. Hoyer BB, Ramlau-Hansen CH, Vrijheid M, Valvi D, Pedersen HS, Zviezdai V, et al. Anthropometry in 5- to 9-year-old Greenlandic and Ukrainian children in relation to prenatal exposure to perfluorinated alkyl substances. *Environ Health Perspect.* 2015;123(8):841–6.

49. Erkin-Cakmak A, Harley KG, Chevrier J, Bradman A, Kogut K, Huen K, et al. *In utero* and childhood polybrominated diphenyl ether exposures and body mass at age 7 years: The CHAMACOS study. *Environ Health Perspect.* 2015;123(6):636–42.

50. Rantakokko P, Main KM, Wohlfart-Veje C, Kiviranta H, Airaksinen R, Vartiainen T, et al. Association of placenta organotin concentrations with growth and ponderal index in 110 newborn boys from Finland during the first 18 months of life: A cohort study. *Environ Health.* 2014;13(1):45.

51. Carwile JL, Michels KB. Urinary bisphenol A and obesity: NHANES 2003–2006. *Environ Res.* 2011;111(6):825–30.

52. Vom Saal FS, Nagel SC, Coe BL, Angle BM, Taylor JA. The estrogenic endocrine disrupting chemical bisphenol A (BPA) and obesity. *Mol Cell Endocrinol.* 2012;354(1–2):74–84.

53. Yan X, Calafat A, Lashley S, Smulian J, Ananth C, Barr D, et al. Phthalates biomarker identification and exposure estimates in a population of pregnant women. *Hum Ecol Risk Assess.* 2009;15(3):565–78.

54. Cantonwine DE, Cordero JF, Rivera-Gonzalez LO, Anzalota Del Toro LV, Ferguson KK, Mukherjee B, et al. Urinary phthalate metabolite concentrations among pregnant women in Northern Puerto Rico: Distribution, temporal variability, and predictors. *Environ Int.* 2014;62:1–11.

55. Jensen MS, Norgaard-Pedersen B, Toft G, Hougaard DM, Bonde JP, Cohen A, et al. Phthalates and perfluorooctanesulfonic acid in human amniotic fluid: Temporal trends and timing of amniocentesis in pregnancy. *Environ Health Perspct.* 2012;120(6):897–903.

56. Hao C, Cheng X, Xia H, Ma X. The endocrine disruptor mono-(2-ethylhexyl) phthalate promotes adipocyte differentiation and induces obesity in mice. *Biosci Rep.* 2012;32(6):619–29.

57. Valvi D, Casas M, Mendez MA, Ballesteros-Gomez A, Luque N, Rubio S, et al. Prenatal bisphenol a urine concentrations and early rapid growth and overweight risk in the offspring. *Epidemiology.* 2013;24(6):791–9.

58. Harley KG, Aguilar Schall R, Chevrier J, Tyler K, Aguirre H, Bradman A, et al. Prenatal and postnatal bisphenol A exposure and body mass index in childhood in the CHAMACOS cohort. *Environ Health Perspect.* 2013;121(4):514–20.

59. Gillies GE, McArthur S. Estrogen actions in the brain and the basis for differential action in men and women: A case for sex-specific medicines. *Pharmacol Rev.* 2010;62(2):155–98.

60. Valvi D, Casas M, Romaguera D, Monfort N, Ventura R, Martinez D, et al. Prenatal Phthalate exposure and childhood growth and blood pressure: Evidence from the Spanish INMA-Sabadell birth cohort study. *Environ Health Perspect.* 2015;123:1022–1029.

61. Maresca MM, Hoepner LA, Hassoun A, Oberfield SE, Mooney SJ, Calafat AM, et al. Prenatal exposure to phthalates and childhood body size in an urban cohort. *Environ Health Perspect.* 2016;124(4):514–20.

62. Georgescu B, Georgescu C, Dărăban S, Bouaru A, Paşcalău S. Heavy metals acting as endocrine disrupters. *J Anim Sci Biotechnol.* 2011;44(2):89–93.

63. Afeiche M, Peterson KE, Sanchez BN, Cantonwine D, Lamadrid-Figueroa H, Schnaas L, et al. Prenatal lead exposure and weight of 0- to 5-year-old children in Mexico city. *Environ Health Perspect.* 2011;119(10):1436–41.

64. Gardner RM, Kippler M, Tofail F, Bottai M, Hamadani J, Grander M, et al. Environmental exposure to metals and children's growth to age 5 years: A prospective cohort study. *Am J Epidemiol.* 2013;177(12):1356–67.

65. Henson MC, Chedrese PJ. Endocrine disruption by cadmium, a common environmental toxicant with paradoxical effects on reproduction. *Exp Biol Med.* 2004;229(5):383–92.

66. Sanin LH, Gonzalez-Cossio T, Romieu I, Peterson KE, Ruiz S, Palazuelos E, et al. Effect of maternal lead burden on infant weight and weight gain at one month of age among breastfed infants. *Pediatrics.* 2001;107(5):1016–23.

67. Schell LM, Denham M, Stark AD, Parsons PJ, Schulte EE. Growth of infants' length, weight, head and arm circumferences in relation to low levels of blood lead measured serially. *Am J Hum Biol.* 2009;21(2):180–7.

68. Hong YC, Kulkarni SS, Lim YH, Kim E, Ha M, Park H, et al. Postnatal growth following prenatal lead exposure and calcium intake. *Pediatrics.* 2014;134(6):1151–9.

69. Afeiche M, Peterson KE, Sánchez BN, Schnaas L, Cantonwine D, Ettinger AS, et al. Windows of lead exposure sensitivity, attained height, and body mass index at 48 months. *J Pediatr.* 2012;160(6):1044–9.

70. Lamb MR, Janevic T, Liu X, Cooper T, Kline J, Factor-Litvak P. Environmental lead exposure, maternal thyroid function, and childhood growth. *Environ Res.* 2008;106(2):195–202.

71. Peterson KE WK, Sánchez BN, Afeiche M, Ettinger A, et al. Influence of *in utero* and childhood lead exposure on body mass index and waist circumference at ages 7–15 years. The International Society for Environmental Epidemiology, Barcelona, Spain, September 2011.

72. Lin CM, Doyle P, Wang D, Hwang YH, Chen PC. Does prenatal cadmium exposure affect fetal and child growth? *Occup Environ Med.* 2011;68(9):641–6.

73. Saha KK, Engstrom A, Hamadani JD, Tofail F, Rasmussen KM, Vahter M. Pre- and postnatal arsenic exposure and body size to 2 years of age: A cohort study in rural Bangladesh. *Environ Health Perspect.* 2012;120(8):1208–14.

74. Kim BM, Lee BE, Hong YC, Park H, Ha M, Kim YJ, et al. Mercury levels in maternal and cord blood and attained weight through the 24 months of life. *Sci Total Environ.* 2011;410–411:26–33

20 Impact of Environmental Obesogens

Focus on Mechanisms Linking to Childhood Obesity

Bassem M. Shoucri and Bruce Blumberg

CONTENTS

THE OBESITY EPIDEMIC: BEYOND DIET AND EXERCISE

Although the prevailing paradigm of obesity remains one of energy intake versus energy expenditure, the abrupt rise in global childhood obesity rates has led researchers to explore alternative contributors. While genetics undoubtedly bestow some obesity risk, the handful of genetic loci associated with obesity in human studies account for <2% of variance in body weight [1], as reviewed in Chapter 13. This observation is not surprising given the abrupt time line of the obesity epidemic. Beyond excess caloric intake and sedentarism, well-studied environmental risk factors for obesity include stress, smoking, sleep patterns, and the microbiome, as reviewed in other chapters in this book. In this chapter, we will discuss mounting evidence implicating developmental exposure to xenobiotic compounds as a hitherto underinvestigated contributor to the global obesity epidemic [2]. This chapter complements Chapter 19, with a focus on understanding the potential mechanisms that might link obesogens to obesity development.

ENVIRONMENTAL CHEMICALS AND OBESITY

A study setting out to examine the potential effects of the environment on obesity observed over 20,000 animals, representing 12 distinct populations and 8 different species, living in proximity to industrialized societies [3]. These animals included pets (cats and dogs), laboratory animals (mice, rats, and primates) that were fed controlled diets, and feral rats. Notably, nearly every one of these populations showed positive trends in both weight gain and odds of obesity over the past several decades. The chance of these populations all concomitantly exhibiting the same trend in obesity was calculated as approximately 1 in 10 million [3]. These data strongly suggest that an environmental insult, independent of diet and exercise, is responsible for the parallel trend in obesity in humans and animals.

The use of synthetic chemicals in commerce has grown exponentially since the 1940s, numbering in the tens of thousands today [4]. Of particular concern is a subset of nearly 3000 chemicals, termed *endocrine disrupting chemicals* (EDCs), that interfere with any aspect of hormone action [5,6]. The "endocrine" label can be misleading as EDCs can perturb the action of any chemical messenger, endocrine or otherwise (autocrine, paracrine, neurotransmitter). EDCs can alter hormone synthesis and transport, or they can interfere with the cell signaling and receptor systems that regulate hormone response in target tissues. Since hormones play critical roles in development and metabolism, investigators suspect that EDCs might interfere with hormonal systems to promote weight gain and ultimately obesity [7].

THE OBESOGEN HYPOTHESIS

In 2006, our group proposed the obesogen hypothesis, which asserts that there are EDCs in the environment that confer obesity risk on exposed individuals, principally those exposed during critical windows of development [8]. These "obesogens" promote adiposity through a variety of mechanisms that include

- Disturbing normal fat development, thereby increasing the number of fat cells
- Encouraging the storage of energy within fat cells, increasing fat cell size
- Altering metabolic set points programed during development
- Interfering with neurologic and hormonal control of hedonic reward and appetite

A number of obesogens have been identified in humans and animals and the list continues to lengthen. Obesogens identified in animal studies include estrogenic chemicals (such as diethylstilbestrol [DES] [9], genistein [10], Bisphenol A [BPA] [11], and nonylphenol [12]); organotins, such as tributyltin (TBT) [13]; organochlorine pesticides (including polychlorinated biphenyls [PCBs] [14], dichlorodiphenyltrichloroethane [DDT] [15], triflumizole [16], and tolylfluanid [17]); organophosphates (such as chlorpyrifos [18] and diazinon [19]); brominated [20] and nonbrominated flame-retardants [21] and a number of other chemicals including nicotine [22], benzo[a]pyrene [23], phthalates [24]; and perfluorooctanoic acid (PFOA) [25]. In humans, urinary phthalates are associated with waist circumference and insulin resistance in adults [26] and in children and adolescents [27,28]. Likewise, multiple studies of US [29–31] and Chinese [32] children associate urine BPA levels with obesity prevalence. Urinary phenol pesticides are correlated with obesity in adolescents [33]. Serum levels of several persistent organic pollutants (POPs), including dichlorodiphenyldichloroethylene (DDE, a metabolite of DDT), PCBs, hexachlorobenzene (HCB), and β-hexachlorocyclohexane (β-HCH), are associated with BMI in adults [34]. Prenatal exposure to PCBs [35], DDE [36], and HCB [37] are associated with obesity later in life. Chapter 19 provides a detailed overview of the findings from human cohort studies that have examined the effects of these obesogens on obesity development.

In addition to these environmental exposures, there is a wide range of obesogenic pharmaceuticals for which weight gain is an established side effect. These include first- and second-generation antipsychotics [38], selective serotonin-reuptake inhibitors (SSRIs) [39], systemic glucocorticoids [40], and the antidiabetic thiazolidinediones (rosi-, pio-, and troglitazone) [41]. If clinicians have already accepted weight gain as an established side effect of these medications, then it is not unreasonable to infer that exposure to physiologically relevant doses of nonpharmaceutical xenobiotic compounds (such as EDCs) could have the same effect.

DEVELOPMENTAL OBESOGEN EXPOSURE

Applying the developmental origins of health and disease (DOHaD) model to the obesogen hypothesis requires monitoring of early-life EDC exposure during sensitive developmental windows together with subsequent observation of obesity and metabolic disease throughout life. Given the relatively recent establishment of the DOHaD and EDC fields, such studies are limited in number and by low sample size and lack of long-term follow-up. The strongest epidemiological evidence of an environmental obesogen programing obesity risk *in utero* is maternal smoking. It is well established that the children of smoking mothers are born small-for-gestational-age; however, these children experience catch-up growth in the first year of life and eventually outpace their peers. Tens of epidemiological studies have all shown an increased overweight/obesity risk in children whose mothers smoked during pregnancy [42].

A number of studies have evaluated perinatal exposure to POPs, which have long half-lives and persist in the environment despite significant regulation and outright bans on many (reviewed in Chapter 19). Taken together, these studies indicate that POPs may affect intrauterine and postnatal growth to increase risk of obesity later in childhood [43–46]. The continued follow up of ongoing cohorts will be informative in addition to new, well-designed prospective studies of precise exposure windows that track obesity and metabolic health into adulthood. It must also be accepted that human studies will always be limited by overall numbers together with confounding and interacting variables. Therefore, these should be supplemented with cell culture and animal studies that can provide a controlled environment to carry out exposures and study them mechanistically.

DEVELOPMENT OF FAT

One facet of the obesogen hypothesis that has received ample attention is the notion that EDCs can promote the excessive development of fat tissue. Adipocytes appear during the second trimester of pregnancy and proliferate through childhood and adolescence before leveling off at approximately 10% renewal per year in adulthood [47]. This phenomenon is independent of BMI, as weight gain/loss in adults is predominantly attributed to changes in cell size rather than cell number [47]. Visceral fat, which is linked to insulin resistance, may be the exception to this rule. In humans, visceral depot size is determined by cell number [48], and adult mice fed a high-fat diet generate new fat cells in visceral depots [49]. Therefore, adipogenic stimuli (such as an obesogen) during gestation and early life establish the number of fat cells in an individual, while fat mass in adults is regulated both by cell number and cell size in a depot-specific manner.

Adipocytes originate from the mesodermal lineage via the mesenchymal stem cell (MSC or multipotent stromal cell), a multipotent cell capable of forming bone, muscle, cartilage, tendon, fat, and other tissues. MSCs and their lineage-restricted derivatives can be found in the perivascular niche of any vascularized organ, including adipose tissue [50]. Transformation of an MSC into a mature adipocyte requires initial commitment to the adipose lineage, followed by terminal differentiation into a functioning fat cell [51]. Adipose lineage commitment requires the concerted action of multiple signaling cascades regulated by adipogenic transcription factors that induce the expression of the peroxisome proliferator–activated receptor gamma (PPARγ), the "master regulator" of adipogenesis [52]. PPARγ, a member of the nuclear receptor family, is a ligand-activated, DNA-binding transcription factor that dimerizes with the retinoid X receptor (RXR) to bind and regulate genomic targets that promote adipose differentiation [53]. Both MSCs and mouse 3T3-L1 cells (a committed preadipocyte cell line) have become valuable *in vitro* tools for screening candidate obesogens and characterizing their mechanisms of action.

TRIBUTYLTIN: A MODEL OBESOGEN

We and others first showed that the TBT binds and activates both PPARγ and its heterodimeric partner, RXR, to promote adipogenesis and alter lipid homeostasis [13,54]. Human and mouse MSCs, as well as mouse 3T3–L1 preadipocytes exposed to environmentally relevant levels (nanomolar) of TBT, or the pharmaceutical PPARγ agonist rosiglitazone, were shunted toward the adipocyte lineage via a PPARγ-dependent pathway [55,56]. Mice exposed to TBT, *in utero,* showed lipid accumulation in adipose depots, livers, and testes, and have MSCs biased toward the adipose lineage and away from the bone lineage [13,56,57]. Treatment of adult mice or rats with TBT resulted in obesity and fatty liver [58,59], as well as disrupted thyroid function [60].

Beyond concerns over organotin exposure, there is an expanding group of obesogens to which humans are exposed that also activate PPARγ. These include phthalates [61]; triflumizole [16]; flava-nones [62,63]; bixin [64]; dioctyl sodium sulfosuccinate (DOSS), a component of the oil dispersant COREXIT [65]; and several flame-retardants including the polybrominated diphenyl ether (PBDE) BDE-47 [66], tetrabromo- and tetrachloro-BPA (TBBPA, TCBPA) [67], and triphenyl phosphate (TPP), a component of the flame-retardant Firemaster® 550 (FM550) [68].

Phthalates are widely used as plasticizers and solubilizing agents and are commonly found in personal-care products, medications, and medical equipment. Phthalates and their metabolites can be detected in the urine of nearly all humans [69], including infants [70]. These chemicals promote adipose differentiation of 3T3-L1 cells [71] and they stimulate adipogenesis and suppress osteogen-esis in mouse MSCs [72]. Several *in vivo* studies show that prenatal phthalate exposure promotes obesity in adult mice [24,73]. In addition to activation of PPARγ, phthalates may program obesity risk through their effects on PPARα or PPARδ, thyroid metabolism, or gestational growth [74]. Urinary phthalates are associated with obesity and insulin resistance in children, adolescents, and adults [26–28,75]. Studies of prenatal phthalate exposure that examine obesity as a primary out-come are sparse, though one study of African American and Dominican mothers in New York showed a negative correlation between third trimester urine phthalates and BMI of the offspring at 5 and 7 years [76].

For a half century, brominated chemicals, such as PBDEs and hexabromocyclododecane (HBCD), have been used as flame-retardants in a variety of products [77]. Due to safety concerns, several PBDEs were phased out of U.S. production in 2005, though these chemicals linger in prod-ucts and migrate into house dust, a major source of human exposure [77]. BDE-47 induces adipo-genesis in 3T3-L1 cells [78], in part due to a weak activation of PPARγ [66]. A recent screen of flame-retardants and their metabolites revealed that 3-hydroxy-BDE-47 activates PPARγ with the same potency as the pharmaceutical rosiglitazone [79]. TBBPA and TCBPA have not been phased out and are still widely used. Recently, these halogenated bisphenols were identified as PPARγ agonists that stimulate differentiation of 3T3-L1 preadipocytes [67,79]. The phase out of PBDEs increased demand for alternative flame-retardants such as the organophosphate-based FM550. Perinatal FM550 exposure results in varied phenotypes in rat offspring including obesity, advanced puberty, cardiac hypertrophy, and anxiety [21]. In a subsequent study, FM550 was shown to be a PPARγ activator along with TPP, a triaryl phosphate that comprises 10%–20% of FM550 [68]. FM550 and TPP were further shown to increase adipogenesis and inhibit osteogenic differentiation of mouse MSCs [80].

PFOA is a persistent fluorochemical with hundreds of industrial applications that is found in the serum of most humans living in the United States [81]. PFOA purportedly activates PPARγ [82], though this assertion is controversial [83], and PFOA does not induce adipogenesis in 3T3-L1 pre-adipocytes [78]. However, *in utero* exposure to low-dose PFOA results in increased body weight and elevated serum insulin and leptin in postpubertal female mice [25]. These animal data were mir-rored in a prospective study of 665 Danish pregnant mothers whose gestational PFOA exposure was associated with the BMI of female, but not male, offspring at 20 years of age [84]. Another Danish cohort showed no such associations [85].

Taken together, these results indicate a continued need to screen for industrial chemicals that can activate PPARγ, since there is sufficient evidence in cells, animals, and humans to believe these compounds will act as obesogens, *in vivo*.

ESTROGENIC OBESOGENS

Estrogens are protective against obesity and cardiovascular disease in adults, as is well demonstrated by the onset of abdominal obesity and dyslipidemia following the loss of estrogen at menopause. Emerging research, however, implicates early-life exposure to low-dose estrogens to be obesogenic. Prenatal exposure to the estrogenic EDCs, DES, genistein, and BPA results in obese adult animals [86], and urine BPA is associated with obesity prevalence in children [29,30,32]. DDT and its metabolite DDE are estrogenic and antiandrogenic, respectively, and have been implicated as obesogens in humans and animals [15,36].

DES is a synthetic estrogen that was widely prescribed to pregnant women in the midtwentieth century to prevent miscarriage. Though mothers were unaffected, among the millions of children born to DES-treated mothers, there was a well-documented increase in several rare pathologies of the reproductive tract. Data from the National Cancer Institute's DES Follow-Up Study showed a modest increase in obesity risk among females prenatally exposed to DES, and this risk was higher in those exposed to lower doses [87]. Mice exposed to low doses of DES prenatally become obese later in life, while high-dose exposure resulted in decreased birth weight followed by catch-up growth and subsequent obesity [88]. Similar results were observed in mice exposed postnatally, during the first 5 days of life [86,89]. Importantly, these results were recapitulated with other estrogens (2- and 4-hydroxyestradiol), suggesting an estrogen-dependent mechanism [9].

Of all the data on estrogenic EDCs, data implicating BPA as a potent obesogen are most concerning. BPA, used in polycarbonate plastics and epoxy resins, is produced in millions of tons annually and can be detected in most humans [11,69]. BPA is a potent activator of the estrogen receptor (ER) in the nucleus and also at the cell membrane where it induces rapid cell signaling events [90]. BPA promotes differentiation of 3T3-L1 preadipocytes [91] and human preadipocytes via an ER-dependent mechanism [92]. Low-dose prenatal BPA exposure in animals results in increased body weight in adult life [93]. Perinatal BPA exposure results in increased visceral fat depot size in females at weaning, as well as adipocyte hypertrophy and increased expression of adipogenic and lipogenic genes [94]. Both Trasande et al. and Bhandari et al. have shown a correlation between urinary BPA and obesity prevalence in US children from the National Health and Nutrition Examination Survey (NHANES) [27,29], results echoed in a Chinese cohort [32]. Despite these extensive data (and data implicating BPA in numerous other pathologies), regulatory agencies do not believe levels of BPA exposure are sufficient to result in adverse outcomes, and production of the high-volume chemical continues.

OTHER OBESOGENS AND THEIR MECHANISMS OF ACTION

Much attention has been paid to the ability of obesogens to act as hormone mimics that can bind nuclear receptors. Numerous EDCs have been shown to bind PPARγ and ER, though other nuclear receptors are known to be obesogen targets. BPA, whose obesogenic effects are largely attributed to its ability to bind and activate ER, is also an activator of the steroid and xenobiotic receptor (SXR) [95], the glucocorticoid receptor (GR) [96], and an antagonist of the androgen receptor (AR) [97]. Likewise, phthalates activate all three PPAR receptors (α, δ, γ) [71,98] as well as SXR [98]. The obesogenic effects of PCB 77 were shown to be dependent on the activation of the aryl hydrocarbon receptor (AhR) both *in vitro* and *in vivo* [14]. Tolylfluanid, a fungicide commonly used in Europe, promotes adipose differentiation of 3T3-L1 cells through activation of the GR [99], and mice fed a diet supplemented with tolylfluanid gain more weight and fat mass than controls [17]. Hence, obesogens can act through several members of the nuclear receptor family, at times simultaneously, to promote obesity.

Not all obesogens are nuclear receptor ligands, and obesogens that do activate nuclear receptors may also act through alternative pathways. For example, TBT, BPA, and phthalates, all of which activate nuclear receptors, also inhibit the enzyme 11β-hydroxysteroid dehydrogenase, a critical regulator of active/inactive intracellular glucocorticoid levels [100]. TBT is further known to inhibit aromatase [101] and isocitrate dehydrogenase [102]. Prenatal exposure to nicotine results in obesity and metabolic complications [22,103], presumably through its action on nicotinic acetylcholine receptors (nAChRs), plasma membrane–associated ion channels present in the brain, hypothalamus, adrenal medulla, and other organs [104]. The pharmaceutical obesogen lithium, which has diverse mechanisms of action, promotes weight gain through increased appetite, hypothyroidism, and even a combination of thirst and improved mood that leads to the consumption of high-calorie beverages [105]. Therefore, obesogens can act through varied nuclear receptor–independent mechanisms to promote weight gain.

EPIGENETICS AND THE ENVIRONMENT

A central tenet of the DOHaD hypothesis is the notion of "developmental plasticity," whereby the developing fetus adapts to environmental stimuli, permanently altering phenotypic expression [106]. While these adaptations may benefit the fetus in the short term, they may confer disease risk later in life within a different environmental context [107]. The definitive example of this concept is the "thrifty phenotype" seen in the offspring of malnourished mothers. These children are programed to survive in a food-scarce environment, but when faced with caloric excess in adult life these adaptations increase the risk for cardiometabolic diseases [108]. Crucially, the genotype of these individuals remains unchanged, though environmental inputs during development have permanently altered their phenotype. That is, there are changes in gene expression during development without any alteration of DNA sequence. Of the mechanisms thought to be responsible for such a phenomenon, epigenetics is the most widely accepted, and its role in childhood obesity is discussed in detail in Chapter 14.

Epigenetics is the study of heritable changes in phenotype that are not the result of altered DNA sequence, but rather environmentally influenced modifications of the genome. These modifications include methylation and/or hydroxymethylation of DNA at cytosine residues of 5' to guanine (CpG sites), chemical modifications of the histone proteins that package DNA into chromatin, and expression of noncoding RNAs. Epigenetic marks can alter chromatin accessibility by encouraging or disrupting transcription factor/cofactor binding to regulatory elements and recruiting silencing complexes to the genome. In mammalian development there are two major epigenetic reprograming events during which there is a genome-wide erasure of DNA methylation marks and subsequent remethylation [109]. The first reprograming occurs in the preimplantation embryo and the second in the developing primordial germ cells. This process plays a critical role in regulating the potency of developing cell populations from pluripotency through lineage commitment and eventual terminal differentiation [110].

There is ample evidence that environmental inputs during development can alter the epigenetic landscape to alter gene expression, development, and phenotype [111,112]. A classic model of this phenomenon is the viable yellow agouti (A^{vy}) mouse described in Chapter 14. Studies in wild-type animals have explored the effects of maternal and paternal nutrition on the epigenetic landscape and phenotype of the offspring [113]. The progeny of rat dams fed a low-protein diet had livers with promoter hypomethylation and increased expression of PPARα (Ppara) and the GR (NR3C1) [114], later attributed to a reduction in DNA methyltransferase 1 (DNMT1) expression [115]. Maternal protein restriction in mice resulted in fetal livers with promoter hypermethylation and underexpression of the liver X receptor alpha gene (LXR-alpha) in addition to several of its target genes [116]. Maternal high-fat diet altered the feeding behavior of the offspring via altered methylation and expression of genes in the dopamine and opioid pathways within areas of the brain associated with reward [117]. Interestingly, a paternal high-fat diet resulted in glucose intolerance and pancreatic β-cell dysfunction in female offspring, as well as hypomethylation and upregulation of a member of the JAK-STAT signaling pathway in pancreatic islets [118]. This study suggests that the phenotype seen in female offspring is due to high fat diet–induced epigenetic modifications of the paternal germ line. Recent work furthered this notion using a fly model, where as little as 2 days of paternal dietary intervention prior to mating resulted in obese progeny [119]. The authors went on to show this phenotype was passed through the male germ line via modifications of histone marks passed on from sperm to developing embryos [119].

Humans exposed to famine early, but not late, in gestation have a slight hypomethylation of the maternally imprinted insulin-like growth factor 2 gene (IGF2), as compared with their unexposed, same-gender siblings at 60 years of age [120]. Strikingly, the degree of methylation of a single CpG residue associated with the RXA alpha (RXRA) gene in an umbilical cord at birth predicts adiposity of the offspring at 9 years of age [121]. An ensuing study showed that hypermethylation of 4 CpGs in a differentially methylated region (DMR) upstream of RXRA was inversely associated with bone mineral density of offspring at 4 years [122]. Finally, recent data show that obesity is associated with altered small noncoding RNA expression and DNA methylation of sperm, though further studies are needed to assess whether and how these alterations of the germ line are manifested in offspring [123].

EPIGENETICS AND EDCS

Substantial research shows that developmental exposure to EDCs alters the epigenome. Maternal exposure of agouti (A^{vy}) mice to BPA [124] or the phytoestrogen genistein [125] results in hypo- or hyperretrotransposon methylation, respectively, and a corresponding obese or lean phenotype in the offspring. Wild-type mice exposed to DES [126] or BPA [127] in utero have increased uterine expression and altered methylation of the Homeobox A10 gene (HOXA10), which plays critical roles in uterine development and the maintenance of mature endometrium. Rats treated postnatally with PCBs have diminished global liver DNA methylation and decreased hepatic expression of DNA methyltransferases (DNMTs) [128]. Prenatal PCB exposure in rats induces liver expression of histone-modifying enzymes that subsequently reduce the transcriptional activating histone marks H3K4me3 and H4K16ac [129]. Perinatal BPA exposure results in hepatocellular damage in adult male rats and decreased hepatic expression of the β-oxidative gene carnitine palmitoyltransferase 1a (CPT1a) at birth, attributed to altered DNA methylation, transcription factor binding, and histone modification of CPT1a [130]. Hence, perinatal exposure to EDCs can permanently alter the development and function of varied tissues at least in part through stable alterations of the epigenome.

Adipogenesis is also regulated by epigenetic mechanisms that respond to environmental influences [131,132]. 3T3-L1 preadipocytes treated with a panel of EDCs, including TBT and BPA, experienced global changes in DNA methylation during adipose differentiation [78]. Bone marrow MSCs from mice treated with dexamethasone favor an adipose fate over bone due to reduced promoter methylation of the proadipogenic gene CCAAT/enhancer binding protein alpha (CEBPA) [133]. Mice prenatally exposed to TBT have MSCs biased toward the adipose lineage and a hypomethylated promoter region of the PPARγ target gene, fatty acid binding protein 4 (FABP4) [56]. Postnatal genistein exposure resulted in increased fat mass in female rats and diminished adipose expression and hypermethylation of wingless-type MMTV integration site 10B (WNT-10B), a regulator of adipose lineage commitment [134]. Finally, prenatal exposure to polycyclic aromatic hydrocarbon (PAH) increased weight and fat mass of the offspring and adipose expression of PPARγ, which correlated with promoter methylation of a single CpG site [135]. The ability of EDCs to epigenetically reprogram the MSC compartment to favor the fat lineage is an emerging and exciting area of research.

ENVIRONMENTAL EXPOSURES CAN HAVE TRANSGENERATIONAL CONSEQUENCES

Of great concern is accumulating evidence linking developmental EDC exposure to disease risk not only in offspring, but also in multiple generations of unexposed descendants. Skinner and colleagues showed that high-dose exposure of pregnant F0 rats to the fungicide vinclozolin caused reproductive abnormalities in male rats through four generations (F1–F4) [136]. While the F1 fetus and F2 primordial germ cells were exposed to vinclozolin *in utero*, the F3 and F4 generations received no direct exposure and hence their phenotype is considered transgenerational. This study went on to show that the F3 and F4 phenotype was due to heritable epigenetic alterations of the male germ line [136]. Similar adverse effects on male reproductive health were demonstrated in F1–F3 male descendants of rodents exposed to BPA [137] and phthalates [138]. Our group first showed that developmental EDC exposure could result in a transgenerational obesity phenotype [57]. The F1, F2, and F3 progeny of F0 mothers exposed to environmentally relevant doses of TBT display increased adipose depot weights, hepatic steatosis, and MSCs reprogramed to favor the adipocyte lineage [57]. There is a small, but growing list of environmental chemicals that induce a heritable, transgenerational obesity phenotype, including a mixture of plastics-derived EDCs (BPA and phthalates) [139], a hydrocarbon mixture (jet fuel, JP-8) [140], and DDT [141].

How exactly these developmental exposures propagate disease phenotypes to unexposed generations remains an open question. Some assert that an altered intrauterine environment is sufficient to propagate a phenotype through multiple generations, independent of epigenetic changes to the germ line [142]. This assertion is contradicted by evidence of transgenerational phenotypes following paternal exposures and studies showing phenotypes beyond the F2 generation [143]. DNA methylation marks are stable through mitosis and meiosis; hence, altered epigenetic reprograming of the germ line is a key mechanism through which EDCs are proposed to cause transgenerational phenotypes [112]. DNA methylation remains the most studied epigenetic factor responsible for EDC-induced transgenerational phenomena. However, DNA hydroxymethylation, histone modifications, and a variety of noncoding RNAs have all been implicated in epigenetic inheritance [144]. That developmental EDC exposure may contribute to the vast and abrupt rise in global obesity through several generations raises the stakes of identifying obesogens, studying their mechanisms of action, and ultimately reducing human exposure.

ECONOMIC BURDEN OF EDCS

A series of studies set out to estimate the economic burden of EDC exposure in the European Union [44,145]. The total cost of EDC exposure in health-care expenditures and lost productivity were conservatively estimated to be $209 billion annually, with the true cost likely being many times higher [145]. The cost of obesity and diabetes due to EDC exposure was in the range of $20–30 billion annually [44]. It should be noted that this analysis only assessed three EDCs (DDE, phthalates, and BPA) that were backed by the strongest animal studies and longitudinal epidemiological studies in humans with measurements of prenatal exposure. EDCs, for which animal data are strong but human studies are sparse, cross-sectional and/or inconclusive (e.g., PFOA and TBT) were not included. Moreover, this study did not take into account the harrowing possibility that EDCs are programing transgenerational disease susceptibility into multiple generations of humans. Hence, the actual societal burden of EDC exposure is likely to be many fold higher than the conservative estimate.

CONCLUSIONS

The tremendous cost of obesity warrants full consideration of all risk factors that may contribute to the disease. While physicians continue to prescribe diet and exercise as a panacea for obesity, the collective weight of the US population continues to rise, even at the bottom of the BMI distribution [146]. Current clinical management of obesity and its comorbidities remains fixated on disease prevention in adults whose health is already deteriorating. Lifestyle interventions are rarely successful, yet physicians continue to attribute these failures to genetics or even to a lack of will and determination. We have presented strong evidence that environmental exposures (EDCs, in particular) in the womb and during early development can program our obesity risk for the rest of our adult lives and possibly the lives of future generations. With this in mind, it would be appropriate to shift our focus away from adults that are already in poor health and toward young adults that are planning to have children, pregnant mothers, infants, and children. On the side of industry, there are some efforts to design chemicals that lack bioactivity [147]. However, these efforts cannot counter the vast production of EDCs worldwide and governments must take action to regulate these chemicals or incentivize industry to screen for bioactivity prior to their introduction into the manufacturing process.

ACKNOWLEDGMENTS

This research was supported by the National Institutes of Health (1R01ES023316 to BB and 5T32GM008620 supporting BMS) and the American Heart Association (15PRE25090030 to BMS).

REFERENCES

1. Loos RJ. Recent progress in the genetics of common obesity. *British Journal of Clinical Pharmacology.* 2009;68(6):811–29.
2. Janesick A, Blumberg B. Endocrine disrupting chemicals and the developmental programming of adipogenesis and obesity. *Birth Defects Research Part C, Embryo Today: Reviews.* 2011;93(1):34–50.
3. Klimentidis YC, Beasley TM, Lin HY, Murati G, Glass GE, Guyton M, et al. Canaries in the coal mine: A cross-species analysis of the plurality of obesity epidemics. *Proceedings Biological Sciences/The Royal Society.* 2011;278(1712):1626–32.
4. Meeker JD. Exposure to environmental endocrine disruptors and child development. *Archives of Pediatrics & Adolescent Medicine.* 2012;166(10):952–8.
5. Diamanti-Kandarakis E, Bourguignon JP, Giudice LC, Hauser R, Prins GS, Soto AM, et al. Endocrine-disrupting chemicals: An Endocrine Society scientific statement. *Endocrine Reviews.* 2009;30(4):293–342.
6. Zoeller RT, Brown TR, Doan LL, Gore AC, Skakkebaek NE, Soto AM, et al. Endocrine-disrupting chemicals and public health protection: A statement of principles from The Endocrine Society. *Endocrinology.* 2012;153(9):4097–110.
7. Heindel JJ. Endocrine disruptors and the obesity epidemic. *Toxicological Sciences: An Official Journal of the Society of Toxicology.* 2003;76(2):247–9.
8. Grun F, Blumberg B. Environmental obesogens: Organotins and endocrine disruption via nuclear receptor signaling. *Endocrinology.* 2006;147(6 Suppl):S50–5.
9. Newbold RR, Padilla-Banks E, Snyder RJ, Jefferson WN. Developmental exposure to estrogenic compounds and obesity. *Birth Defects Research Part A, Clinical and Molecular Teratology.* 2005;73(7):478–80.
10. Penza M, Montani C, Romani A, Vignolini P, Pampaloni B, Tanini A, et al. Genistein affects adipose tissue deposition in a dose-dependent and gender-specific manner. *Endocrinology.* 2006;147(12):5740–51.
11. Vom Saal FS, Nagel SC, Coe BL, Angle BM, Taylor JA. The estrogenic endocrine disrupting chemical bisphenol A (BPA) and obesity. *Molecular and Cellular Endocrinology.* 2012;354(1–2):74–84.
12. Hao CJ, Cheng XJ, Xia HF, Ma X. The endocrine disruptor 4-nonylphenol promotes adipocyte differentiation and induces obesity in mice. *Cellular Physiology and Biochemistry: International Journal of Experimental Cellular Physiology, Biochemistry, and Pharmacology.* 2012;30(2):382–94.
13. Grun F, Watanabe H, Zamanian Z, Maeda L, Arima K, Cubacha R, et al. Endocrine-disrupting organotin compounds are potent inducers of adipogenesis in vertebrates. *Molecular Endocrinology.* 2006;20(9):2141–55.
14. Arsenescu V, Arsenescu RI, King V, Swanson H, Cassis LA. Polychlorinated biphenyl-77 induces adipocyte differentiation and proinflammatory adipokines and promotes obesity and atherosclerosis. *Environmental Health Perspectives.* 2008;116(6):761–8.

15. La Merrill M, Karey E, Moshier E, Lindtner C, La Frano MR, Newman JW, et al. Perinatal exposure of mice to the pesticide DDT impairs energy expenditure and metabolism in adult female offspring. *PloS One*. 2014;9(7):e103337.

16. Li X, Pham HT, Janesick AS, Blumberg B. Triflumizole is an obesogen in mice that acts through per-oxisome proliferator activated receptor gamma (PPARgamma). *Environmental Health Perspectives*. 2012;120(12):1720–6.

17. Regnier SM, Kirkley AG, Ye H, El-Hashani E, Zhang X, Neel BA, et al. Dietary exposure to the endocrine disruptor tolylfluanid promotes global metabolic dysfunction in male mice. *Endocrinology*. 2015;156(3):896–910.

18. Meggs WJ, Brewer KL. Weight gain associated with chronic exposure to chlorpyrifos in rats. *Journal of Medical Toxicology: Official Journal of the American College of Medical Toxicology*. 2007;3(3):89–93.

19. Roegge CS, Timofeeva OA, Seidler FJ, Slotkin TA, Levin ED. Developmental diazinon neurotoxicity in rats: Later effects on emotional response. *Brain Research Bulletin*. 2008;75(1):166–72.

20. Suvorov A, Battista MC, Takser L. Perinatal exposure to low-dose 2,2′,4,4′-tetrabromodiphenyl ether affects growth in rat offspring: What is the role of IGF-1? *Toxicology*. 2009;260(1–3):126–31.

21. Patisaul HB, Roberts SC, Mabrey N, McCaffrey KA, Gear RB, Braun J, et al. Accumulation and endo-crine disrupting effects of the flame retardant mixture Firemaster(R) 550 in rats: An exploratory assess-ment. *Journal of Biochemical and Molecular Toxicology*. 2013;27(2):124–36.

22. Gao YJ, Holloway AC, Zeng ZH, Lim GE, Petrik JJ, Foster WG, et al. Prenatal exposure to nico-tine causes postnatal obesity and altered perivascular adipose tissue function. *Obesity Research*. 2005;13(4):687–92.

23. Ortiz L, Nakamura B, Li X, Blumberg B, Luderer U. *In utero* exposure to benzo[a]pyrene increases adi-posity and causes hepatic steatosis in female mice, and glutathione deficiency is protective. *Toxicology Letters*. 2013;223(2):260–7.

24. Schmidt JS, Schaedlich K, Fiandanese N, Pocar P, Fischer B. Effects of di(2-ethylhexyl) phthalate (DEHP) on female fertility and adipogenesis in C3H/N mice. *Environmental Health Perspectives*. 2012;120(8):1123–9.

25. Hines EP, White SS, Stanko JP, Gibbs-Flournoy EA, Lau C, Fenton SE. Phenotypic dichotomy follow-ing developmental exposure to perfluorooctanoic acid (PFOA) in female CD-1 mice: Low doses induce elevated serum leptin and insulin, and overweight in mid-life. *Molecular and Cellular Endocrinology*. 2009;304(1–2):97–105.

26. Stahlhut RW, van Wijngaarden E, Dye TD, Cook S, Swan SH. Concentrations of urinary phthalate metabolites are associated with increased waist circumference and insulin resistance in adult U.S. males. *Environmental Health Perspectives*. 2007;115(6):876–82.

27. Trasande L, Spanier AJ, Sathyanarayana S, Attina TM, Blustein J. Urinary phthalates and increased insulin resistance in adolescents. *Pediatrics*. 2013;132(3):e646–55.

28. Buser MC, Murray HE, Scinicariello F. Age and sex differences in childhood and adulthood obesity association with phthalates: Analyses of NHANES 2007–2010. *International Journal of Hygiene and Environmental Health*. 2014;217(6):687–94.

29. Bhandari R, Xiao J, Shankar A. Urinary bisphenol A and obesity in U.S. children. *American Journal of Epidemiology*. 2013;177(11):1263–70.

30. Trasande L, Attina TM, Blustein J. Association between urinary bisphenol A concentration and obesity prevalence in children and adolescents. *JAMA: The Journal of the American Medical Association*. 2012;308(11):1113–21.

31. Harley KG, Aguilar Schall R, Chevrier J, Tyler K, Aguirre H, Bradman A, et al. Prenatal and postnatal bisphenol A exposure and body mass index in childhood in the CHAMACOS cohort. *Environmental Health Perspectives*. 2013;121(4):514–20.

32. Li DK, Miao M, Zhou Z, Wu C, Shi H, Liu X, et al. Urine bisphenol-a level in relation to obesity and overweight in school-age children. *PloS One*. 2013;8(6):e65399.

33. Buser MC, Murray HE, Scinicariello F. Association of urinary phenols with increased body weight measures and obesity in children and adolescents. *The Journal of Pediatrics*. 2014;165(4):744–9.

34. Tang-Peronard JL, Andersen HR, Jensen TK, Heitmann BL. Endocrine-disrupting chemicals and obesity development in humans: A review. *Obesity Reviews: An Official Journal of the International Association for the Study of Obesity*. 2011;12(8):622–36.

35. Verhulst SL, Nelen V, Hond ED, Koppen G, Beunckens C, Vael C, et al. Intrauterine exposure to environmental pollutants and body mass index during the first 3 years of life. *Environmental Health Perspectives*. 2009;117(1):122–6.

36. Valvi D, Mendez MA, Martinez D, Grimalt JO, Torrent M, Sunyer J, et al. Prenatal concentrations of polychlorinated biphenyls, DDE, and DDT and overweight in children: A prospective birth cohort study. *Environmental Health Perspectives.* 2012;120(3):451–7.

37. Smink A, Ribas-Fito N, Garcia R, Torrent M, Mendez MA, Grimalt JO, et al. Exposure to hexachlorobenzene during pregnancy increases the risk of overweight in children aged 6 years. *Acta Paediatrica.* 2008;97(10):1465–9.

38. Rummel-Kluge C, Komossa K, Schwarz S, Hunger H, Schmid F, Lobos CA, et al. Head-to-head comparisons of metabolic side effects of second generation antipsychotics in the treatment of schizophrenia: A systematic review and meta-analysis. *Schizophrenia Research.* 2010;123(2–3):225–33.

39. Blumenthal SR, Castro VM, Clements CC, Rosenfield HR, Murphy SN, Fava M, et al. An electronic health records study of long-term weight gain following antidepressant use. *JAMA Psychiatry.* 2014;71(8):889–96.

40. Huscher D, Thiele K, Gromnica-Ihle E, Hein G, Demary W, Dreher R, et al. Dose-related patterns of glucocorticoid-induced side effects. *Annals of the Rheumatic Diseases.* 2009;68(7):1119–24.

41. Nesto RW, Bell D, Bonow RO, Fonseca V, Grundy SM, Horton ES, et al. Thiazolidinedione use, fluid retention, and congestive heart failure: A consensus statement from the American Heart Association and American Diabetes Association. *Circulation.* 2003;108(23):2941–8.

42. Thayer KA, Heindel JJ, Bucher JR, Gallo MA. Role of environmental chemicals in diabetes and obesity: A National Toxicology Program workshop review. *Environmental Health Perspectives.* 2012;120(6):779–89.

43. Vafeiadi M, Georgiou V, Chalkiadaki G, Rantakokko P, Kiviranta H, Karachaliou M, et al. Association of prenatal exposure to persistent organic pollutants with obesity and cardiometabolic traits in early childhood: The rhea mother-child cohort (Crete, Greece). *Environmental Health Perspectives.* 2015;123(10):1015–21.

44. Legler J, Fletcher T, Govarts E, Porta M, Blumberg B, Heindel JJ, et al. Obesity, diabetes, and associated costs of exposure to endocrine-disrupting chemicals in the European union. *The Journal of Clinical Endocrinology and Metabolism.* 2015;100(4):1278–88.

45. Iszatt N, Stigum H, Verner MA, White RA, Govarts E, Palkovicova Murinova L, et al. Prenatal and postnatal exposure to persistent organic pollutants and infant growth: A pooled analysis of seven European birth cohorts. *Environmental Health Perspectives.* 2015;123(7):730–6.

46. Cupul-Uicab LA, Klebanoff MA, Brock JW, Longnecker MP. Prenatal exposure to persistent organochlorines and childhood obesity in the US collaborative perinatal project. *Environmental Health Perspectives.* 2013;121(9):1103–9.

47. Spalding KL, Arner E, Westermark PO, Bernard S, Buchholz BA, Bergmann O, et al. Dynamics of fat cell turnover in humans. *Nature.* 2008;453(7196):783–7.

48. Arner P, Andersson DP, Thorne A, Wiren M, Hoffstedt J, Naslund E, et al. Variations in the size of the major omentum are primarily determined by fat cell number. *The Journal of Clinical Endocrinology and Metabolism.* 2013;98(5):E897–901.

49. Jeffery E, Church CD, Holtrup B, Colman L, Rodeheffer MS. Rapid depot-specific activation of adipocyte precursor cells at the onset of obesity. *Nature Cell Biology.* 2015;17(4):376–85.

50. Crisan M, Yap S, Casteilla L, Chen CW, Corselli M, Park TS, et al. A perivascular origin for mesenchymal stem cells in multiple human organs. *Cell Stem Cell.* 2008;3(3):301–13.

51. Rosen ED, Spiegelman BM. What we talk about when we talk about fat. *Cell.* 2014;156(1–2):20–44.

52. Cristancho AG, Lazar MA. Forming functional fat: A growing understanding of adipocyte differentiation. *Nature Reviews Molecular Cell Biology.* 2011;12(11):722–34.

53. Tontonoz P, Spiegelman BM. Fat and beyond: The diverse biology of PPARgamma. *Annual Review of Biochemistry.* 2008;77:289–312.

54. Kanayama T, Kobayashi N, Mamiya S, Nakanishi T, Nishikawa J. Organotin compounds promote adipocyte differentiation as agonists of the peroxisome proliferator-activated receptor gamma/retinoid X receptor pathway. *Molecular Pharmacology.* 2005;67(3):766–74.

55. Li X, Ycaza J, Blumberg B. The environmental obesogen tributyltin chloride acts via peroxisome proliferator activated receptor gamma to induce adipogenesis in murine 3T3–L1 preadipocytes. *The Journal of Steroid Biochemistry and Molecular Biology.* 2011;127(1–2):9–15.

56. Kirchner S, Kieu T, Chow C, Casey S, Blumberg B. Prenatal exposure to the environmental obesogen tributyltin predisposes multipotent stem cells to become adipocytes. *Molecular Endocrinology.* 2010;24(3):526–39.

57. Chamorro-Garcia R, Sahu M, Abbey RJ, Laude J, Pham N, Blumberg B. Transgenerational inheritance of increased fat depot size, stem cell reprogramming, and hepatic steatosis elicited by prenatal exposure to the obesogen tributyltin in mice. *Environmental Health Perspectives.* 2013;121(3):359–66.

58. Bertuloso BD, Podratz PL, Merlo E, de Araujo JF, Lima LC, de Miguel EC, et al. Tributyltin chloride leads to adiposity and impairs metabolic functions in the rat liver and pancreas. *Toxicology Letters.* 2015;235(1):45–59.
59. Zuo Z, Chen S, Wu T, Zhang J, Su Y, Chen Y, et al. Tributyltin causes obesity and hepatic steatosis in male mice. *Environmental Toxicology.* 2011;26(1):79–85.
60. Sharan S, Nikhil K, Roy P. Disruption of thyroid hormone functions by low dose exposure of tributyltin: An *in vitro* and *in vivo* approach. *General and Comparative Endocrinology.* 2014;206:155–65.
61. Feige JN, Gelman L, Rossi D, Zoete V, Metivier R, Tudor C, et al. The endocrine disruptor monoethyl-hexyl-phthalate is a selective peroxisome proliferator-activated receptor gamma modulator that promotes adipogenesis. *The Journal of Biological Chemistry.* 2007;282(26):19152–66.
62. Saito T, Abe D, Sekiya K. Flavanone exhibits PPARgamma ligand activity and enhances differentiation of 3T3–L1 adipocytes. *Biochemical and Biophysical Research Communications.* 2009;380(2):281–5.
63. Christensen KB, Petersen RK, Kristiansen K, Christensen LP. Identification of bioactive compounds from flowers of black elder (*Sambucus nigra* L.) that activate the human peroxisome proliferator-activated receptor (PPAR) gamma. *Phytotherapy Research: PTR.* 2010;24 Suppl 2:S129–32.
64. Takahashi N, Goto T, Taimatsu A, Egawa K, Katoh S, Kusudo T, et al. Bixin regulates mRNA expression involved in adipogenesis and enhances insulin sensitivity in 3T3–L1 adipocytes through PPARgamma activation. *Biochemical and Biophysical Research Communications.* 2009;390(4):1372–6.
65. Temkin AM, Bowers RR, Magaletta ME, Holshouser S, Maggi A, Ciana P, et al. Effects of crude oil/dispersant mixture and dispersant components on PPARgamma activity and: Identification of dioctyl sodium sulfosuccinate (DOSS; CAS #577–11-7) as a probable obesogen. *Environmental Health Perspectives.* 2016;124(1):112–9.
66. Kamstra JH, Hruba E, Blumberg B, Janesick A, Mandrup S, Hamers T, et al. Transcriptional and epigenetic mechanisms underlying enhanced *in vitro* adipocyte differentiation by the brominated flame retardant BDE-47. *Environmental Science & Technology.* 2014;48(7):4110–9.
67. Riu A, Grimaldi M, le Maire A, Bey G, Phillips K, Boulahtouf A, et al. Peroxisome proliferator-activated receptor gamma is a target for halogenated analogs of bisphenol A. *Environmental Health Perspectives.* 2011;119(9):1227–32.
68. Belcher SM, Cookman CJ, Patisaul HB, Stapleton HM. *In vitro* assessment of human nuclear hormone receptor activity and cytotoxicity of the flame retardant mixture FM 550 and its triarylphosphate and brominated components. *Toxicology Letters.* 2014;228(2):93–102.
69. Crinnion WJ. The CDC fourth national report on human exposure to environmental chemicals: What it tells us about our toxic burden and how it assist environmental medicine physicians. *Alternative Medicine Review: A Journal of Clinical Therapeutic.* 2010;15(2):101–9.
70. Sathyanarayana S, Karr CJ, Lozano P, Brown E, Calafat AM, Liu F, et al. Baby care products: Possible sources of infant phthalate exposure. *Pediatrics.* 2008;121(2):e260–8.
71. Hurst CH, Waxman DJ. Activation of PPARalpha and PPARgamma by environmental phthalate monoesters. *Toxicological Sciences: An Official Journal of the Society of Toxicology.* 2003;74(2):297–308.
72. Watt J, Schlezinger JJ. Structurally-diverse, PPARgamma-activating environmental toxicants induce adipogenesis and suppress osteogenesis in bone marrow mesenchymal stromal cells. *Toxicology.* 2015;331:66–77.
73. Hao C, Cheng X, Xia H, Ma X. The endocrine disruptor mono-(2-ethylhexyl) phthalate promotes adipocyte differentiation and induces obesity in mice. *Bioscience Reports.* 2012;32(6):619–29.
74. Kim SH, Park MJ. Phthalate exposure and childhood obesity. *Annals of Pediatric Endocrinology & Metabolism.* 2014;19(2):69–75.
75. Hatch EE, Nelson JW, Qureshi MM, Weinberg J, Moore LL, Singer M, et al. Association of urinary phthalate metabolite concentrations with body mass index and waist circumference: A cross-sectional study of NHANES data, 1999–2002. *Environmental Health: A Global Access Science Source.* 2008;7:27.
76. Maresca MM, Hoepner LA, Hassoun A, Oberfield SE, Mooney SJ, Calafat AM, et al. Prenatal exposure to phthalates and childhood body size in an urban cohort. *Environmental Health Perspectives.* 2016;124(4):514–20.
77. Shaw SD, Harris JH, Berger ML, Subedi B, Kannan K. Brominated flame retardants and their replacements in food packaging and household products: Uses, human exposure, and health effects. In: Snedeker MS, ed. *Molecular and Integrative Toxicology.* London: Springer, pp. 61–93, 2014.
78. Bastos Sales L, Kamstra JH, Cenijn PH, van Rijt LS, Hamers T, Legler J. Effects of endocrine disrupting chemicals on *in vitro* global DNA methylation and adipocyte differentiation. *Toxicology In Vitro: An International Journal Published in Association with BIBRA.* 2013;27(6):1634–43.

79. Fang M, Webster TF, Ferguson PL, Stapleton HM. Characterizing the peroxisome proliferator-activated receptor (PPARgamma) ligand binding potential of several major flame retardants, their metabolites, and chemical mixtures in house dust. *Environmental Health Perspectives*. 2015;123(2):166–72.

80. Pillai HK, Fang M, Beglov D, Kozakov D, Vajda S, Stapleton HM, et al. Ligand binding and activation of PPARgamma by Firemaster(R) 550: Effects on adipogenesis and osteogenesis *in vitro*. *Environmental Health Perspectives*. 2014;122(11):1225–32.

81. Kato K, Wong LY, Jia LT, Kuklenyik Z, Calafat AM. Trends in exposure to polyfluoroalkyl chemicals in the U.S. population: 1999–2008. *Environmental Science & Technology*. 2011;45(19):8037–45.

82. Vanden Heuvel JP, Thompson JT, Frame SR, Gillies PJ. Differential activation of nuclear receptors by perfluorinated fatty acid analogs and natural fatty acids: A comparison of human, mouse, and rat peroxisome proliferator-activated receptor-alpha, -beta, and -gamma, liver X receptor-beta, and retinoid X receptor-alpha. *Toxicological Sciences: An Official Journal of the Society of Toxicology*. 2006;92(2):476–89.

83. Takacs ML, Abbott BD. Activation of mouse and human peroxisome proliferator-activated receptors (alpha, beta/delta, gamma) by perfluorooctanoic acid and perfluorooctane sulfonate. *Toxicological Sciences: An Official Journal of the Society of Toxicology*. 2007;95(1):108–17.

84. Halldorsson TI, Rytter D, Haug LS, Bech BH, Danielsen I, Becher G, et al. Prenatal exposure to perfluorooctanoate and risk of overweight at 20 years of age: A prospective cohort study. *Environmental Health Perspectives*. 2012;120(5):668–73.

85. Andersen CS, Fei C, Gamborg M, Nohr EA, Sorensen TI, Olsen J. Prenatal exposures to perfluorinated chemicals and anthropometry at 7 years of age. *American Journal of Epidemiology*. 2013;178(6):921–7.

86. Newbold RR, Padilla-Banks E, Jefferson WN. Environmental estrogens and obesity. *Molecular and Cellular Endocrinology*. 2009;304(1–2):84–9.

87. Hatch EE, Troisi R, Palmer JR, Wise LA, Titus L, Strohsnitter WC, et al. Prenatal diethylstilbestrol exposure and risk of obesity in adult women. *Journal of Developmental Origins of Health and Disease*. 2015;6(3):201–7.

88. Hurst CH, Waxman DJ. Environmental phthalate monoesters activate pregnane X receptor-mediated transcription. *Toxicology and Applied Pharmacology*. 2004;199(3):266–74.

89. Newbold RR, Padilla-Banks E, Jefferson WN, Heindel JJ. Effects of endocrine disruptors on obesity. *International Journal of Andrology*. 2008;31(2):201–8.

90. Watson CS, Jeng YJ, Kochukov MY. Nongenomic signaling pathways of estrogen toxicity. *Toxicological Sciences: An Official Journal of the Society of Toxicology*. 2010;115(1):1–11.

91. Masuno H, Kidani T, Sekiya K, Sakayama K, Shiosaka T, Yamamoto H, et al. Bisphenol A in combination with insulin can accelerate the conversion of 3T3-L1 fibroblasts to adipocytes. *Journal of Lipid Research*. 2002;43(5):676–84.

92. Zong G, Grandjean P, Wu H, Sun Q. Circulating persistent organic pollutants and body fat distribution: Evidence from NHANES 1999–2004. *Obesity*. 2015;23(9):1903–10.

93. Howdeshell KL, Hotchkiss AK, Thayer KA, Vandenbergh JG, vom Saal FS. Exposure to bisphenol A advances puberty. *Nature*. 1999;401(6755):763–4.

94. Somm E, Schwitzgebel VM, Toulotte A, Cederroth CR, Combescure C, Nef S, et al. Perinatal exposure to bisphenol a alters early adipogenesis in the rat. *Environmental Health Perspectives*. 2009;117(10):1549–55.

95. Sui Y, Ai N, Park SH, Rios-Pilier J, Perkins JT, Welsh WJ, et al. Bisphenol A and its analogues activate human pregnane X receptor. *Environmental Health Perspectives*. 2012;120(3):399–405.

96. Sargis RM, Johnson DN, Choudhury RA, Brady MJ. Environmental endocrine disruptors promote adipogenesis in the 3T3-L1 cell line through glucocorticoid receptor activation. *Obesity*. 2010;18(7):1283–8.

97. Teng C, Goodwin B, Shockley K, Xia M, Huang R, Norris J, et al. Bisphenol A affects androgen receptor function via multiple mechanisms. *Chemico-Biological Interactions*. 2013;203(3):556–64.

98. Lampen A, Zimnik S, Nau H. Teratogenic phthalate esters and metabolites activate the nuclear receptors PPARs and induce differentiation of F9 cells. *Toxicology and Applied Pharmacology*. 2003;188(1):14–23.

99. Neel BA, Brady MJ, Sargis RM. The endocrine disrupting chemical tolylfluanid alters adipocyte metabolism via glucocorticoid receptor activation. *Molecular Endocrinology*. 2013;27(3):394–406.

100. Vitku J, Starka L, Bicikova M, Hill M, Heracek J, Sosvorova L, et al. Endocrine disruptors and other inhibitors of 11beta-hydroxysteroid dehydrogenase 1 and 2: Tissue-specific consequences of enzyme inhibition. *The Journal of Steroid Biochemistry and Molecular Biology*. 2016;155:207–16.

101. Heidrich DD, Steckelbroeck S, Klingmuller D. Inhibition of human cytochrome P450 aromatase activity by butyltins. *Steroids*. 2001;66(10):763–9.

102. Yamada S, Kotake Y, Demizu Y, Kurihara M, Sekino Y, Kanda Y. NAD-dependent isocitrate dehydrogenase as a novel target of tributyltin in human embryonic carcinoma cells. *Scientific Reports.* 2014;4:5952.

103. Somm E, Schwitzgebel VM, Vauthay DM, Camm EJ, Chen CY, Giacobino JP, et al. Prenatal nicotine exposure alters early pancreatic islet and adipose tissue development with consequences on the control of body weight and glucose metabolism later in life. *Endocrinology.* 2008;149(12):6289–99.

104. Tweed JO, Hsia SH, Lutfy K, Friedman TC. The endocrine effects of nicotine and cigarette smoke. *Trends in Endocrinology and Metabolism: TEM.* 2012;23(7):334–42.

105. Torrent C, Amann B, Sanchez-Moreno J, Colom F, Reinares M, Comes M, et al. Weight gain in bipolar disorder: Pharmacological treatment as a contributing factor. *Acta Psychiatrica Scandinavica.* 2008;118(1):4–18.

106. Hanson MA, Gluckman PD. Early developmental conditioning of later health and disease: Physiology or pathophysiology? *Physiological Reviews.* 2014;94(4):1027–76.

107. Bateson P, Barker D, Clutton-Brock T, Deb D, D'Udine B, Foley RA, et al. Developmental plasticity and human health. *Nature.* 2004;430(6998):419–21.

108. Hales CN, Barker DJ. The thrifty phenotype hypothesis. *British Medical Bulletin.* 2001;60:5–20.

109. Seisenberger S, Peat JR, Reik W. Conceptual links between DNA methylation reprogramming in the early embryo and primordial germ cells. *Current Opinion in Cell Biology.* 2013;25(3):281–8.

110. Hemberger M, Dean W, Reik W. Epigenetic dynamics of stem cells and cell lineage commitment: Digging Waddington's canal. *Nature Reviews Molecular Cell Biology.* 2009;10(8):526–37.

111. Feil R, Fraga MF. Epigenetics and the environment: Emerging patterns and implications. *Nature Reviews Genetics.* 2011;13(2):97–109.

112. Jirtle RL, Skinner MK. Environmental epigenomics and disease susceptibility. *Nature Reviews Genetics.* 2007;8(4):253–62.

113. Seki Y, Williams L, Vuguin PM, Charron MJ. Minireview: Epigenetic programming of diabetes and obesity: Animal models. *Endocrinology.* 2012;153(3):1031–8.

114. Lillycrop KA, Phillips ES, Jackson AA, Hanson MA, Burdge GC. Dietary protein restriction of pregnant rats induces and folic acid supplementation prevents epigenetic modification of hepatic gene expression in the offspring. *The Journal of Nutrition.* 2005;135(6):1382–6.

115. Lillycrop KA, Slater-Jefferies JL, Hanson MA, Godfrey KM, Jackson AA, Burdge GC. Induction of altered epigenetic regulation of the hepatic glucocorticoid receptor in the offspring of rats fed a protein-restricted diet during pregnancy suggests that reduced DNA methyltransferase-1 expression is involved in impaired DNA methylation and changes in histone modifications. *The British Journal of Nutrition.* 2007;97(6):1064–73.

116. van Straten EM, Bloks VW, Huijkman NC, Baller JF, van Meer H, Lutjohann D, et al. The liver X-receptor gene promoter is hypermethylated in a mouse model of prenatal protein restriction. *American Journal of Physiology Regulatory, Integrative and Comparative Physiology.* 2010;298(2):R275–82.

117. Vucetic Z, Kimmel J, Totoki K, Hollenbeck E, Reyes TM. Maternal high-fat diet alters methylation and gene expression of dopamine and opioid-related genes. *Endocrinology.* 2010;151(10):4756–64.

118. Ng SF, Lin RC, Laybutt DR, Barres R, Owens JA, Morris MJ. Chronic high-fat diet in fathers programs beta-cell dysfunction in female rat offspring. *Nature.* 2010;467(7318):963–6.

119. Ost A, Lempradl A, Casas E, Weigert M, Tiko T, Deniz M, et al. Paternal diet defines offspring chromatin state and intergenerational obesity. *Cell.* 2014;159(6):1352–64.

120. Heijmans BT, Tobi EW, Stein AD, Putter H, Blauw GJ, Susser ES, et al. Persistent epigenetic differences associated with prenatal exposure to famine in humans. *Proceedings of the National Academy of Sciences of the United States of America.* 2008;105(44):17046–9.

121. Godfrey KM, Sheppard A, Gluckman PD, Lillycrop KA, Burdge GC, McLean C, et al. Epigenetic gene promoter methylation at birth is associated with child's later adiposity. *Diabetes.* 2011;60(5):1528–34.

122. Harvey NC, Sheppard A, Godfrey KM, McLean C, Garratt E, Ntani G, et al. Childhood bone mineral content is associated with methylation status of the *RXRA* promoter at birth. *Journal of Bone and Mineral Research: The Official Journal of the American Society for Bone and Mineral Research.* 2014;29(3):600–7.

123. Donkin I, Versteyhe S, Ingerslev LR, Qian K, Mechta M, Nordkap L, et al. Obesity and bariatric surgery drive epigenetic variation of spermatozoa in humans. *Cell Metabolism.* 2016;23(2):369–78.

124. Dolinoy DC, Huang D, Jirtle RL. Maternal nutrient supplementation counteracts bisphenol A-induced DNA hypomethylation in early development. *Proceedings of the National Academy of Sciences of the United States of America.* 2007;104(32):13056–61.

125. Dolinoy DC, Weidman JR, Waterland RA, Jirtle RL. Maternal genistein alters coat color and protects Avy mouse offspring from obesity by modifying the fetal epigenome. *Environmental Health Perspectives*. 2006;114(4):567–72.

126. Bromer JG, Wu J, Zhou Y, Taylor HS. Hypermethylation of homeobox A10 by in utero diethylstilbestrol exposure: An epigenetic mechanism for altered developmental programming. *Endocrinology*. 2009;150(7):3376–82.

127. Bromer JG, Zhou Y, Taylor MB, Doherty L, Taylor HS. Bisphenol-A exposure in utero leads to epigenetic alterations in the developmental programming of uterine estrogen response. *FASEB Journal: Official Publication of the Federation of American Societies for Experimental Biology*. 2010;24(7):2273–80.

128. Desaulniers D, Xiao GH, Lian H, Feng YL, Zhu J, Nakai J, et al. Effects of mixtures of polychlorinated biphenyls, methylmercury, and organochlorine pesticides on hepatic DNA methylation in prepubertal female Sprague-Dawley rats. *International Journal of Toxicology*. 2009;28(4):294–307.

129. Casati L, Sendra R, Colciago A, Negri-Cesi P, Berdasco M, Esteller M, et al. Polychlorinated biphenyls affect histone modification pattern in early development of rats: A role for androgen receptor-dependent modulation? *Epigenomics*. 2012;4(1):101–12.

130. Strakovsky RS, Wang H, Engeseth NJ, Flaws JA, Helferich WG, Pan YX, et al. Developmental bisphenol A (BPA) exposure leads to sex-specific modification of hepatic gene expression and epigenome at birth that may exacerbate high-fat diet-induced hepatic steatosis. *Toxicology and Applied Pharmacology*. 2015;284(2):101–12.

131. Ost A, Pospisilik JA. Epigenetic modulation of metabolic decisions. *Current Opinion in Cell Biology*. 2015;33:88–94.

132. Stel J, Legler J. The role of epigenetics in the latent effects of early life exposure to obesogenic endocrine disrupting chemicals. *Endocrinology*. 2015;156(10):3466–72.

133. Li J, Zhang N, Huang X, Xu J, Fernandes JC, Dai K, et al. Dexamethasone shifts bone marrow stromal cells from osteoblasts to adipocytes by C/EBPalpha promoter methylation. *Cell Death & Disease*. 2013;4:e832.

134. Strakovsky RS, Lezmi S, Flaws JA, Schantz SL, Pan YX, Helferich WG. Genistein exposure during the early postnatal period favors the development of obesity in female, but not male rats. *Toxicological Sciences: An Official Journal of the Society of Toxicology*. 2014;138(1):161–74.

135. Yan Z, Zhang H, Maher C, Arteaga-Solis E, Champagne FA, Wu L, et al. Prenatal polycyclic aromatic hydrocarbon, adiposity, peroxisome proliferator-activated receptor (PPAR) gamma methylation in offspring, grand-offspring mice. *PloS One*. 2014;9(10):e110706.

136. Anway MD, Cupp AS, Uzumcu M, Skinner MK. Epigenetic transgenerational actions of endocrine disruptors and male fertility. *Science*. 2005;308(5727):1466–9.

137. Salian S, Doshi T, Vanage G. Perinatal exposure of rats to Bisphenol A affects the fertility of male offspring. *Life Sciences*. 2009;85(21–22):742–52.

138. Doyle TJ, Bowman JL, Windell VL, McLean DJ, Kim KH. Transgenerational effects of di-(2-ethylhexyl) phthalate on testicular germ cell associations and spermatogonial stem cells in mice. *Biology of Reproduction*. 2013;88(5):112.

139. Manikkam M, Tracey R, Guerrero-Bosagna C, Skinner MK. Plastics derived endocrine disruptors (BPA, DEHP and DBP) induce epigenetic transgenerational inheritance of obesity, reproductive disease and sperm epimutations. *PloS One*. 2013;8(1):e55387.

140. Tracey R, Manikkam M, Guerrero-Bosagna C, Skinner MK. Hydrocarbons (jet fuel JP-8) induce epigenetic transgenerational inheritance of obesity, reproductive disease and sperm epimutations. *Reproductive Toxicology*. 2013;36:104–16.

141. Skinner MK, Manikkam M, Tracey R, Guerrero-Bosagna C, Haque M, Nilsson EE. Ancestral dichloro-diphenyltrichloroethane (DDT) exposure promotes epigenetic transgenerational inheritance of obesity. *BMC Medicine*. 2013;11:228.

142. Aiken CE, Ozanne SE. Transgenerational developmental programming. *Human Reproduction Update*. 2014;20(1):63–75.

143. Lane M, Robker RL, Robertson SA. Parenting from before conception. *Science*. 2014;345(6198):756–60.

144. Xin F, Susiarjo M, Bartolomei MS. Multigenerational and transgenerational effects of endocrine disrupting chemicals: A role for altered epigenetic regulation? *Seminars in Cell & Developmental Biology*. 2015;43:66–75.

145. Trasande L, Zoeller RT, Hass U, Kortenkamp A, Grandjean P, Myers JP, et al. Estimating burden and disease costs of exposure to endocrine-disrupting chemicals in the European union. *The Journal of Clinical Endocrinology and Metabolism*. 2015;100(4):1245–55.

146. Yang L, Colditz GA. Prevalence of overweight and obesity in the United States, 2007–2012. *JAMA Internal Medicine.* 2015;175(8):1412–3.

147. Schug TT, Abagyan R, Blumberg B, Collins TJ, Crews D, DeFur PL, et al. Designing endocrine disruption out of the next generation of chemicals. *Green Chemistry: An International Journal and Green Chemistry Resource: GC.* 2013;15(1):181–98.

21 Potential Role of the Microbiome in the Development of Childhood Obesity

Christopher Mulligan and Jacob E. Friedman

CONTENTS

INTRODUCTION

The human body is covered with trillions of bacteria collectively known as the *human microbiome*, which is separated into five distinct regions; oral, nasal, skin, vaginal, and gut. Each region contains its own unique abundance and diversity of microbes. The gut contains the most abundant microbiome community, consisting of approximately 100 trillion microbes, outnumbering the cells of the human body 10 to 1 and containing more than 1000 different bacterial species and 10 times the genes of the human genome. The four main phyla of bacteria that populate the human gut are Firmicutes, Bacteroidetes, Actinobacteria, and Proteobacteria with the two primary phyla being Firmicutes and Bacteroidetes. The human gut microbiome is established during infancy and contains a diverse and dynamic community of microbes that serves numerous important functions. These include the metabolism of otherwise indigestible polysaccharides that impact energy harvest and storage, the modulation of the host immune system, and protection from pathogens through gut barrier defense. Given the critical functions of the gut microbiota in the human body, any deviation in microbial composition that leads to impairments of these functions can drastically compromise host health. Alteration of the early infant gut microbiome has been correlated with the development of childhood obesity and autoimmune conditions, including asthma, allergies, and, more recently, type 1 diabetes. This is likely due to complex interactions between the mode of delivery, antibiotic use, maternal diet, components of breast-feeding, and a network of regulatory events involving both the innate and adaptive immune systems within the infant host. The main approach to studying changes in the composition of the intestinal microbiota in relation to obesity has relied primarily on the phylogenetic characterization of the microbiota of diseased individuals in comparison with apparently healthy individuals. More recently, strong evidence supporting a role for commensal bacteria on mammalian host metabolism has accumulated based on the biochemical and physiological characteristics of germ-free (GF) mice following their colonization with human microbes from obese adults. However, there are substantial interindividual and intraindividual variations in the composition of the intestinal microbiota that occur during the first 2–3 years of life, making it

235

difficult to establish precise cause–effect relationships between human health and the presence and relative abundance of specific microbial communities [1].

POSSIBLE MECHANISMS BY WHICH THE GUT MICROBIOME CONTRIBUTES TO OBESITY

As a result of studies in GF mice, the gut microbiome has been implicated as a contributing factor to the development of obesity. This concept was first described by Hooper et al. [3], who noticed that GF mice (mice free of all microorganisms) had 40% less total body fat than mice with a normal gut microbiota, even though they consumed 30% more calories than the normal mice [2]. They also showed that when GF mice were conventionalized with gut microbiota harvested from a normal mouse, it resulted in a 60% increase in body fat within 2 weeks, despite a significantly lower food intake. These early studies suggested a role for the gut microbiome in energy harvest and metabolism. This was perhaps not surprising given that the distal human intestine harbors trillions of microbes that allow us to extract calories from otherwise indigestible dietary polysaccharides. For example, Hooper et al. [3] showed that the colonization of GF mice with *Bacteroides thetaiotaomicron*, a common anaerobic human commensal bacteria, induced the expression of sodium/glucose transporter-1 (SGLT1) in the small intestine, resulting in a doubling of glucose absorption from the intestine.

Studies in both humans and animals investigating the role of the microbiome in the development of obesity have found that an obesity-associated microbiome has an increased capacity to harvest energy from the diet [4,5]. The obesity-associated microbiome has been shown to be enriched with genes coding for enzymes that use otherwise indigestible carbohydrates to produce the short-chain fatty acids (SCFA): acetate, propionate, and butyrate [5]. In humans, 95% of synthesized SCFA are absorbed by the colon and used by the host for energy, or serve as signaling molecules. Butyrate is the preferred source of energy for colonic epithelial cells. Acetate and propionate are transported in the portal circulation to the liver where they contribute to lipogenesis and gluconeogenesis, respectively. Furthermore, acetate is the principal SCFA found in the blood, where it can be used as an important energy source for peripheral tissues.

In addition to its role in extracting energy from the diet, the gut microbiome has been shown to contribute to the regulation of energy metabolism and storage. SCFAs have been found to not only be important energy substrates, but also effective signaling molecules, influencing energy intake and metabolism [6]. SCFAs, primarily acetate and propionate, are ligands for the G protein–coupled receptors, GPR41 and GPR43, which are broadly expressed in the gut and adipose tissue, where they have been shown to promote adipogenesis through the uptake of fatty acids and glucose, and the inhibition of lipolysis [7,8]. Furthermore, the colonization of GF mice has been shown to impact enzymes involved in fatty acid metabolism. Backhed et al. [2] found that inoculation of GF mice led to the suppression of fasting-induced adipocyte factor (FIAF), also known as *angiopoietin-like 4*, a circulating inhibitor of lipoprotein lipase (LPL), resulting in increased cellular uptake of fatty acids and adipocyte triglyceride accumulation. It was also observed by Backhed et al. [9] that adenosine monophosphate (AMP)-activated protein kinase (AMPK), an enzyme that functions as a fuel gauge and monitors cellular energy status, is significantly lower in conventionalized mice compared with GF mice, resulting in reduced fatty acid oxidation. While it is clear from these studies that just having a gut microbiome can increase energy harvest and storage capacity, it is unknown whether these factors contribute to the development of obesity. The microbiome may be linked to behaviors in humans, such as appetite, inflammation, or adipocyte metabolism, which can be revealed when transplanted into GF mice. However, more work needs to be done in children before they become obese, by examining the molecular biomarkers when transplanted into GF mice, including an exploration of their functional influence on adiposity and behavioral traits.

Obesity is associated with an increase in gut permeability, which allows for an increase in bacteria and bacterial components to enter the circulation and lead systemic inflammation. Alterations in microbial composition may lead to alterations in gut barrier function resulting in translocation of endotoxic compounds such as lipopolysaccharides (LPS), a component of gram-negative intestinal bacteria and a natural ligand for toll-like receptors (TLRs). Binding of LPS to TLRs triggers the release of cytokines and an associated inflammatory response. Cani et al. [10] found that infusion of LPS for 4 weeks in mice led to an increase in weight gain, similar to that seen in mice following diet-induced obesity (DIO) as a result of a high-fat diet (HFD), providing a causative role for gut microbiota and inflammation in the development of obesity.

Over the years, investigations of the microbial composition of lean and overweight/obese adults [11], children [12], and infants have resulted in the discovery of associations of particular bacteria with obesity. Ley et al. [13] analyzed the microbial composition of the gut in leptin-deficient ob/ob mice, an established model of obesity, and their lean counterpart, to determine if distinct variations existed. They reported that ob/ob mice had a reduced abundance of Bacteroidetes and concomitantly higher proportions of Firmicutes relative to their lean counterparts. This particular shift was confirmed in a mouse model of DIO by Turnbaugh et al. [14] and was also reported in obese humans by Ley et al. [11]. Whether these particular bacterial compositions are causative or correlative of weight gain continues to be investigated. Previous investigations in both mice and humans by Turnbaugh et al. [4] and Ridaura et al. [5], respectively, transplanted the microbiome from obese and lean donors to GF mice and found that colonization of an obese donor microbiome led to a greater increase in fat mass compared with their lean counterpart. The increase in fat mass was found to be as a result of an increased energy harvest from the diet suggesting a causative role of the microbiome in the development of obesity. Furthermore, evidence from a study by Hildebrandt et al. [15] found that shifts in microbiota composition occurred prior to the development of obesity. Additional data from Santacruz et al. [16] found that microbiome characteristics can influence potential weight loss outcomes.

It is clear from the aforementioned research that the microbiome is altered in obese individuals and there is evidence suggesting that those alterations may precede the development of obesity. When and how these alterations occur is still a matter of debate. While changes in the adult microbiome can occur through long-term dietary changes and antibiotic use, the adult microbiome is considered relatively stable. The most unstable period for the microbiome is in the first 2–3 years of life when the initial colonization and development is taking place. It is also during this time that the microbiome is most vulnerable to disruptions that could be maintained throughout life. Given the animal and human data suggesting a link between microbial composition and obesity, a disruption in normal acquisition of the microbiome may be an early contributing factor to the development of obesity. Understanding how early-life events impact the development of the microbiome may help establish points of intervention to reduce the risk of developing obesity.

EVENTS THAT IMPACT EARLY DEVELOPMENT OF THE MICROBIOME

The initial colonization of the human microbiome primarily occurs at birth and continues to increase in diversity and abundance in response to various environmental exposures until reaching a relatively stable, fully developed microbiome at approximately 2 years of age. Emerging evidence suggests that the development of the infant microbiome follows a distinct pattern of colonization punctuated by new environmental exposures such as breast-feeding and introduction to solid foods [17]. Facultative anaerobic bacteria including Staphylococcus, Streptococcus, Escherichia coli, and Enterobacteria are thought to be the initial colonizers of the gut where they consume oxygen and create an environment for obligate anaerobes [18,19]. Later, these are replaced by facultative anaerobes that dominate the gastrointestinal tract, primarily Actinobacteria and Firmicutes [20]. Deviations from this colonization pattern have been found to contribute to disease such as asthma and allergies. An emerging area of inquiry in the field of childhood obesity is determining the impact of variability in the initial and subsequent colonization of the microbiome on weight gain. Although there is a lack of direct causative evidence supporting the link between gut bacterial composition and the development of childhood obesity, there are a few studies to date that provide indirect evidence by associating microbial composition with childhood weight gain [21–24]. Additionally, there are a number of factors that have been associated with increased risk of developing childhood obesity that also have been found to contribute to variability in initial bacterial colonization and subsequent development, including maternal health status, mode of delivery, infant diet, and antibiotic use.

Four primary factors contribute to variability in the development of the infant microbiome. The first factor influencing the infant microbiome is the mother's microbiome. Given the vertical transmission of the microbiome from the mother to the infant, any maternal health status that confers changes to the mother's microbiome will likely directly impact the initial colonization of the infant microbiome. Mother's weight status, dietary intake, and antibiotic use have all been shown to impact the composition of the mother's gut microbiome. Santacruz et al. [25] showed that overweight pregnant women had reduced numbers of *Bifidobacterium* and *Bacteroides* and increased numbers of *Staphylococcus*, Enterobacteriaceae, and *Escherichia coli* compared with normal-weight pregnant women. The contention that maternal weight status impacts infant microbiome composition was supported in a study by Collado et al. [26] They found that fecal *Bacteroides* and *Staphylococcus* concentrations were significantly higher in infants of overweight mothers during the first 6 months. Furthermore, higher maternal weights and BMIs were associated with higher concentrations of *Bacteroides*, *Clostridium*, and *Staphylococcus*, and lower concentrations of the *Bifidobacterium* group. Additionally, infants born to normal-weight mothers and mothers with normal weight gains during pregnancy had lower *Akkermansia muciniphila*, *Staphylococcus*, and *Clostridium difficile* [26]. In addition to maternal weight status, diabetes, and the intake of a HFD in nonhuman primates has also been shown to impact maternal and infant microbiome composition beyond weaning, even when the offspring were switched to a healthy diet, implicating early colonization may have persistent effects [27–29].

The second factor contributing to the infant's microbiome composition is the mode of birth delivery. Infants born by vaginal delivery are colonized by microbes resident in the birth canal and the mother's own gastrointestinal tract, whereas infants born by cesarean section (C-section) are initially colonized by skin flora [23,30,31]. The microbial composition of the vagina is substantially different from the microbial composition of the skin. Dominguez-Bello et al. [30] found, in samples taken less than 24 h after delivery, that vaginally delivered infants acquired bacterial communities resembling their own mother's vaginal microbiota, dominated by *Lactobacillus*, *Prevotella*, or *Sneathia* spp., and C-section infants harbored bacterial communities similar to those found on the skin's surface, dominated by *Staphylococcus*, *Corynebacterium*, and *Propionibacterium* spp., and they had a deficiency of anaerobes with lower numbers of *Bacteroides* and *Bifidobacterium*.

The third factor influencing the infant microbiome composition is the infant diet. Immediately after birth, the primary source of nutrition for the infant is maternal breast milk or infant formula, which will contribute to the next stage of bacterial colonization in the gut. Breast milk contains hundreds of species of bacteria and also contains prebiotic human milk oligosaccharides (HMOs), which are sugar polymers that bypass small intestinal degradation to serve as metabolic substrates for bacteria in the colon, particularly bifidobacteria, and help shape the infant microbiome [32]. The combination of probiotics in the form of bacteria and prebiotics in the form of HMOs provides breast milk infants with a stable and relatively uniform gut microbiome compared with formula-fed babies. Formula-fed infants are not exposed to the same nutrients that breast-fed infants are and so develop an entirely different microbiome [33]. Compared with breast-fed infants, the diversity and abundance of the genus *Bifidobacterium* was decreased in formula-fed infants [34]. Furthermore, Kalliomaki et al. [21] reported that bifidobacterial numbers in fecal samples during infancy were higher in children remaining normal weight compared with children becoming overweight. Finally, the introduction of solid foods during the development of the microbiome can have significant influences on bacterial colonization [35]. The introduction of solid foods requires a shift in microbiome function to meet the metabolic demand of changing nutrients. This could lead to substantial individual differences in colonization based on the type of food introduced.

A fourth factor that impacts the colonization of the microbiome is early exposure to antibiotics. Antibiotics have been shown to alter the normal assembly of the infant microbiome. Antibiotics can decrease the colonization of certain microbes while allowing others to flourish. Dardas et al. [36] found that antibiotics given within the first 30 days after birth resulted in a reduction in the dominant Firmicutes and Bacteroidetes phyla and an increase in the Proteobacteria and Actinobacteria. Multiple studies have reported that antibiotics can have long-lasting effects on gut microbiome composition. It was found in these studies that microbiome composition either took weeks to recover to preexposure levels or failed to fully recover after 6 months [37]. Antibiotics have been used for years in farm animals to accelerate weight gain. This has been shown to be the result of shifting digestion toward enhanced energy harvest [38]. Furthermore, early-life exposure to antibiotics has been shown to be associated with increased body mass and adiposity in children [39,40]. Although these studies provide evidence that antibiotics promote weight gain in humans, whether this effect is dependent on a specific antibiotic type or the amount of exposure has been insufficiently explored.

IMPACT OF EARLY COLONIZERS ON INFANT HEALTH

It is currently unclear whether early disruption in infant microbiome colonization contributes to the development of childhood obesity. It has, however, been extensively reported that early disruption in microbiome colonization can impact the development of the infant immune system. Groundbreaking studies in nonhuman primates have shown that a maternal HFD reduced the diversity of offspring intestinal microbiota in juvenile animals at 1 year of age [16], even after switching to a healthy diet at the time of weaning. This persistent effect of early-life diet suggests that maternal diet exposure during gestation and breast-feeding can pattern the composition of the microbial community, with long-lasting effects. However, studies assessing the duration of microbial disruption in these offspring are lacking.

CONCLUSION

The human gut contains a diverse and dynamic community of microbes that serve numerous important functions for the host, including metabolism of otherwise indigestible polysaccharides impacting energy harvest and storage, modulation of the host immune system, and providing protection from pathogens through gut barrier defense. Although there is substantial evidence that the microbiome itself can contribute to increased energy harvest and fat accumulation, it is still unclear whether composition shifts in the microbiome have significant impacts on these functions. The shifts in gut microbiome composition reported in obesity have been shown to increase capacity to harvest energy, but whether these changes are a cause or a consequence of obesity requires further study. A few studies have reported differences in infant microbiome composition that are associated with childhood obesity but again these differences are yet to be causatively linked to weight status. Colonization of the infant microbiome can be influenced by a wide variety of environmental exposures and has already been implicated in a number of diseases associated with its function. Ultimately, to prove causation, large, longitudinal, prospective studies are needed that serially evaluate the gut microbiome from infancy into adulthood. Future studies will hopefully shed light on which bacteria are necessary and at what abundance for proper metabolic function. The introduction of these bacteria early in development may prove to be an extremely useful tool in preventing the development of childhood obesity.

REFERENCES

1. Carding S, Verbeke K, Vipond DT, Corfe BM, Owen LJ. Dysbiosis of the gut microbiota in disease. *Microb Ecol Health Dis.* 2015;26:26191.
2. Backhed F, Ding H, Wang T, Hooper LV, Koh GY, Nagy A, et al. The gut microbiota as an environmental factor that regulates fat storage. *Proc Natl Acad Sci U S A.* 2004;101(44):15718–23.

3. Hooper LV, Wong MH, Thelin A, Hansson L, Falk PG, Gordon JI. Molecular analysis of commensal host-microbial relationships in the intestine. *Science*. 2001;291(5505):881–4.
4. Turnbaugh PJ, Ley RE, Mahowald MA, Magrini V, Mardis ER, Gordon JI. An obesity-associated gut microbiome with increased capacity for energy harvest. *Nature*. 2006;444(7122):1027–31.
5. Ridaura VK, Faith JJ, Rey FE, Cheng J, Duncan AE, Kau AL, et al. Gut microbiota from twins discordant for obesity modulate metabolism in mice. *Science*. 2013;341(6150):1241214.
6. Conterno L, Fava F, Viola R, Tuohy KM. Obesity and the gut microbiota: Does up-regulating colonic fermentation protect against obesity and metabolic disease? *Genes Nutr*. 2011;6(3):241–60.
7. Hong YH, Nishimura Y, Hishikawa D, Tsuzuki H, Miyahara H, Gotoh C, et al. Acetate and propionate short chain fatty acids stimulate adipogenesis via GPCR43. *Endocrinology*. 2005;146(12):5092–9.
8. Ge H, Li X, Weiszmann J, Wang P, Baribault H, Chen JL, et al. Activation of G protein-coupled receptor 43 in adipocytes leads to inhibition of lipolysis and suppression of plasma free fatty acids. *Endocrinology*. 2008;149(9):4519–26.
9. Backhed F, Manchester JK, Semenkovich CF, Gordon JI. Mechanisms underlying the resistance to diet-induced obesity in germ-free mice. *Proc Natl Acad Sci U S A*. 2007;104(3):979–84.
10. Cani PD, Amar J, Iglesias MA, Poggi M, Knauf C, Bastelica D, et al. Metabolic endotoxemia initiates obesity and insulin resistance. *Diabetes*. 2007;56(7):1761–72.
11. Ley RE, Turnbaugh PJ, Klein S, Gordon JI. Microbial ecology: Human gut microbes associated with obesity. *Nature*. 2006;444(7122):1022–3.
12. Karlsson CL, Onnerfalt J, Xu J, Molin G, Ahrne S, Thorngren-Jerneck K. The microbiota of the gut in preschool children with normal and excessive body weight. *Obesity (Silver Spring)*. 2012;20(11):2257–61.
13. Ley RE, Backhed F, Turnbaugh P, Lozupone CA, Knight RD, Gordon JI. Obesity alters gut microbial ecology. *Proc Natl Acad Sci U S A*. 2005;102(31):11070–5.
14. Turnbaugh PJ, Backhed F, Fulton L, Gordon JI. Diet-induced obesity is linked to marked but reversible alterations in the mouse distal gut microbiome. *Cell Host Microbe*. 2008;3(4):213–23.
15. Hildebrandt MA, Hoffmann C, Sherrill-Mix SA, Keilbaugh SA, Hamady M, Chen YY, et al. High-fat diet determines the composition of the murine gut microbiome independently of obesity. *Gastroenterology*. 2009;137(5):1716–24.e1–2.
16. Santacruz A, Marcos A, Warnberg J, Marti A, Martin-Matillas M, Campoy C, et al. Interplay between weight loss and gut microbiota composition in overweight adolescents. *Obesity (Silver Spring)*. 2009;17(10):1906–15.
17. Koenig JE, Spor A, Scalfone N, Fricker AD, Stombaugh J, Knight R, et al. Succession of microbial consortia in the developing infant gut microbiome. *Proc Natl Acad Sci U S A*. 2011;108 Suppl 1:4578–85.
18. Palmer C, Bik EM, DiGiulio DB, Relman DA, Brown PO. Development of the human infant intestinal microbiota. *PLoS Biol*. 2007;5(7):e177.
19. Jost T, Lacroix C, Braegger CP, Chassard C. New insights in gut microbiota establishment in healthy breast fed neonates. *PLoS One*. 2012;7(8):e44595.
20. Turroni F, Peano C, Pass DA, Foroni E, Severgnini M, Claesson MJ, et al. Diversity of bifidobacteria within the infant gut microbiota. *PLoS One*. 2012;7(5):e36957.
21. Kalliomaki M, Collado MC, Salminen S, Isolauri E. Early differences in fecal microbiota composition in children may predict overweight. *Am J Clin Nutr*. 2008;87(3):534–8.
22. Scheepers LE, Penders J, Mbakwa CA, Thijs C, Mommers M, Arts IC. The intestinal microbiota composition and weight development in children: The KOALA Birth Cohort Study. *Int J Obes (Lond)*. 2015;39(1):16–25.
23. Dogra S, Sakwinska O, Soh SE, Ngom-Bru C, Bruck WM, Berger B, et al. Dynamics of infant gut microbiota are influenced by delivery mode and gestational duration and are associated with subsequent adiposity. *MBio*. 2015;6(1):e02419-14.
24. Vael C, Verhulst SL, Nelen V, Goossens H, Desager KN. Intestinal microflora and body mass index during the first three years of life: An observational study. *Gut Pathog*. 2011;3(1):8.
25. Santacruz A, Collado MC, Garcia-Valdes L, Segura MT, Martin-Lagos JA, Anjos T, et al. Gut microbiota composition is associated with body weight, weight gain and biochemical parameters in pregnant women. *Br J Nutr*. 2010;104(1):83–92.
26. Collado MC, Isolauri E, Laitinen K, Salminen S. Effect of mother's weight on infant's microbiota acquisition, composition, and activity during early infancy: A prospective follow-up study initiated in early pregnancy. *Am J Clin Nutr*. 2010;92(5):1023–30.
27. Ma J, Prince AL, Bader D, Hu M, Ganu R, Baquero K, et al. High-fat maternal diet during pregnancy persistently alters the offspring microbiome in a primate model. *Nat Commun*. 2014;5:3889.

28. Larsen N, Vogensen FK, van den Berg FW, Nielsen DS, Andreasen AS, Pedersen BK, et al. Gut microbiota in human adults with type 2 diabetes differs from non-diabetic adults. *PLoS One.* 2010;5(2):e9085.

29. Hu J, Nomura Y, Bashir A, Fernandez-Hernandez H, Itzkowitz S, Pei Z, et al. Diversified microbiota of meconium is affected by maternal diabetes status. *PLoS One.* 2013;8(11):e78257.

30. Dominguez-Bello MG, Costello EK, Contreras M, Magris M, Hidalgo G, Fierer N, et al. Delivery mode shapes the acquisition and structure of the initial microbiota across multiple body habitats in newborns. *Proc Natl Acad Sci U S A.* 2010;107(26):11971–5.

31. van Nimwegen FA, Penders J, Stobberingh EE, Postma DS, Koppelman GH, Kerkhof M, et al. Mode and place of delivery, gastrointestinal microbiota, and their influence on asthma and atopy. *J Allergy Clin Immunol.* 2011;128(5):948–55.e1–3.

32. Chichlowski M, German JB, Lebrilla CB, Mills DA. The influence of milk oligosaccharides on microbiota of infants: Opportunities for formulas. *Annu Rev Food Sci Technol.* 2011;2:331–51.

33. Azad MB, Konya T, Maughan H, Guttman DS, Field CJ, Chari RS, et al. Gut microbiota of healthy Canadian infants: Profiles by mode of delivery and infant diet at 4 months. *CMAJ.* 2013;185(5):385–94.

34. Roger LC, Costabile A, Holland DT, Hoyles L, McCartney AL. Examination of faecal Bifidobacterium populations in breast- and formula-fed infants during the first 18 months of life. *Microbiology.* 2010;156(Pt 11):3329–41.

35. Backhed F, Roswall J, Peng Y, Feng Q, Jia H, Kovatcheva-Datchary P, et al. Dynamics and stabilization of the human gut microbiome during the first year of life. *Cell Host Microbe.* 2015;17(6):852.

36. Dardas M, Gill SR, Grier A, Pryhuber GS, Gill AL, Lee YH, et al. The impact of postnatal antibiotics on the preterm intestinal microbiome. *Pediatr Res.* 2014;76(2):150–8.

37. Dethlefsen L, Huse S, Sogin ML, Relman DA. The pervasive effects of an antibiotic on the human gut microbiota, as revealed by deep 16S rRNA sequencing. *PLoS Biol.* 2008;6(11):e280.

38. Looft T, Johnson TA, Allen HK, Bayles DO, Alt DP, Stedtfeld RD, et al. In-feed antibiotic effects on the swine intestinal microbiome. *Proc Natl Acad Sci U S A.* 2012;109(5):1691–6.

39. Saari A, Virta LJ, Sankilampi U, Dunkel L, Saxen H. Antibiotic exposure in infancy and risk of being overweight in the first 24 months of life. *Pediatrics.* 2015;135(4):617–26.

40. Azad MB, Bridgman SL, Becker AB, Kozyrskyj AL. Infant antibiotic exposure and the development of childhood overweight and central adiposity. *Int J Obes (Lond).* 2014;38(10):1290–8.

22 Adipose Tissue Development

Michael E. Symonds, Shalini Ojha, and Helen Budge

CONTENTS

INTRODUCTION

Adipose tissue is composed of at least three different types of depot (i.e., brown, beige, and white), which can differ with the stage of development and anatomical location in individuals and between species [1]. In addition, the distribution and composition of adipose tissue changes throughout the life span of individuals (Figure 22.1). Generally, the most abundant fat is white adipose tissue, which comprises ~95% of fat mass in children and adults, with obesity being accompanied with an increased number and size of white adipocytes [2]. It not only serves as an energy reserve in the form of lipid but also can act as an important endocrine organ with a number of roles, of which the best documented is appetite regulation via the release of leptin [3]. Brown adipose tissue (BAT) is only ever present in comparatively small quantities and, even in the newborn, when it is most abundant, it comprises just up to ~4% of total body weight [4]. However, as a consequence of its unique location(s), protein composition (including a substantial mitochondrial component), and high rate of blood supply, it is capable of using/dissipating exceptional amounts of energy and releasing heat when maximally stimulated [5]. This capacity is rarely, if ever, reached again in later life [6].

BROWN ADIPOSE TISSUE AND ITS UNIQUE ROLE AT BIRTH

The role of adipose tissue in the fetus and newborn is very different compared with childhood, adolescence, and adulthood with the largest transitions in its appearance and function occurring during late gestation and around the time of birth [7]. In large mammals, including humans, birth is characterized by the rapid initiation of nonshivering thermogenesis [1] that is recruited through the activation of the BAT-specific uncoupling protein (UCP)1, a protein present on the inner mitochondrial membrane [8]. Once activated, UCP1 allows the free flow of protons across the inner mitochondrial membrane that results in the rapid release of heat without the need to convert adenosine diphosphate (ADP) to adenosine triphosphate (ATP) [5]. This process is dependent on the amount of UCP1, together with its capacity for unmasking guanosine diphosphate (GDP) binding sites [8]. As a consequence of the relatively high mass of BAT in the newborn and the maximal appearance of UCP1 at this age [9], BAT attains a near-maximal capacity to generate heat up to a rate of 300 W/kg compared with 1 W/kg in all other tissues [10]. BAT then gradually disappears after birth although UCP1 containing adipocytes is retained within a number of depots into adulthood [11,12]. The main depot in children and adults is believed to be within the supraclavicular region. This region

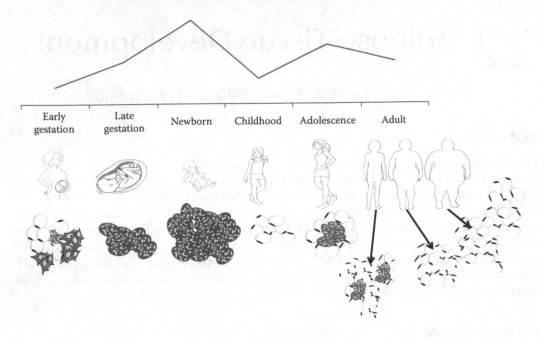

FIGURE 22.1 Summary of relative changes in the abundance of brown adipose tissue–specific mitochondrial uncoupling protein 1 during development, together with the changes in the appearance of brown fat.

is characterized as being hotter than most other regions of the body [13]. It does, however, also contain discrete depots that have much lower UCP1 abundance than classical BAT and is, therefore, considered to be beige fat [14]. In adults, it is clear that there is considerable variability in the characteristics of adipose tissue, both between depots and individuals, which can be observed in both preadipocytes [15] and adipocytes [16]. These differences may represent genetic determinants of adipocyte function, as recently suggested for single nucleotide polymorphism (SNP) related to fat mass and obesity-associated (FTO) obesity variant circuitry [17]. The extent to which these highly variable characteristics relate to early adipose tissue development or function remains completely unknown, which is perhaps surprising given the unprecedented rise in childhood obesity.

ADIPOSE TISSUE LINEAGE AND ITS POTENTIAL RELATIONSHIP WITH SKELETAL MUSCLE PRECURSORS

Our understanding of adipose tissue biology has been transformed over the past few years and one especially exciting discovery has been the suggestion that BAT may share a common lineage with skeletal muscle rather than white adipose tissue [18]. This new concept resulted from a series of lineage-tracing studies that can only be conducted in mice [19], so their translational relevance to larger mammals remains unknown. The first publication to suggest a new origin for BAT demonstrated that cells expressing engrailed 1 (*En1*; a homeobox transcription factor gene expressed in the central dermomyotome) not only gave rise to epaxial muscle, but also to interscapular BAT [20]. Furthermore, the fate of *En1*-expressing cells transformed from BAT alone at an early stage of embryo development, to BAT, dermis, and muscle as the embryo developed. Complementary studies then showed that newborn mice lacking both myogenic factor 5 (*Myf5*), which has a unique role in muscle development (and arises after the translocation of epithelial cells along the edge of the somite to the subjacent myotome), and another myoblast precursor factor, *MyoD*, which similarly plays a unique role in muscle development from migratory cells [21], not only have reduced muscle mass but also excessive amounts of white adipose tissue [22]. These studies ultimately led to the discovery of transcriptional regulator *Prdm16* (PRD1-BF1-RIZ1 homologous domain-containing 16), which was considered to be specific to a BAT rather than a myogenic (or skeletal muscle) lineage. Importantly, both arise from a myoblast progenitor and are distinct from the white adipogenic pathway [23].

The full extent to which BAT has a distinct lineage is now being questioned as depending on the depot. White adipocytes can have more diverse origins and be a mix of both Myf5– and Myf+ cells [24,25]. Indeed, comparable studies conducted using Pax3 tracing demonstrated a clear overlap between the origins of both brown and white adipocytes [26]. Additional populations of adipocytes have now been identified, that is, beige or brite, that are characterized as containing small groups of UCP1-expressing cells surrounded by large amounts of white adipocytes [27,28]. The thermogenic relevance of these cells remains to be established as the abundance of UCP1 is ~10% of classical BAT [29]. To date, a majority of studies investigating beige fat have been largely confined to adult rodents in which "almost everything" examined to date, browns white adipose tissue [30]. Furthermore, a diverse range of other markers for beige adipocytes have been suggested, but their applicability across species is now being questioned [31], together with the optimal conditions in which these classifications are defined [32]. White adipose tissue in humans now appears to have the capacity to undergo browning, as recently shown in children that were severely burnt [33]. This process took at least 1 month to develop but importantly was associated with an increase in energy expenditure. This raises the possibility that UCP1 can be reactivated in the postneonatal period.

FETAL ADIPOSE TISSUE DEVELOPMENT

The ontogeny of fetal BAT has been best described in sheep which, like humans, are born with a mature hypothalamic–pituitary–adrenal axis after a long gestation and with the majority of adipose tissue deposition having occurred during the final third of gestation [34]. With respect to adipose tissue distribution, the main difference between the human fetus and all other species is that fat is present around all internal organs and significant amounts of subcutaneous fat are also deposited up to term [35]. The best-studied fat depot in the fetus is the perirenal-abdominal, which constitutes at least 60% of fat in newborn sheep. It shows two distinct phases during fetal development, an early proliferative phase that commences around midgestation, followed by a second preparatory stage (i.e., for the transition at birth) [36]. This is characterized by a gradual rise in the abundance of adipocytes that show both brown and white characteristics [36]. The abundance of UCP1, therefore, gradually increases together with the main component of adipose tissue, that is, lipid [37]. The extent of the growth of perirenal adipose tissue is related to skeletal muscle development but whether other depots, such as those in the pericardial, sternal, and clavicular regions, demonstrate similar growth patterns remain to be established. The latter depots are of particular interest as in sheep they retain UCP1 into young adulthood [38] and possibly into old age.

Adipose tissue, which first appears in the sheep fetus, has a dense cellular structure but does not express UCP1 or related genes that characterize BAT [36]. Rapid cellular multiplication then occurs in conjunction with maximal gene expression of KI-67. In parallel with this process, genes normally abundant in developing cells are highly expressed, including HOXA1, HOXC9, and BMP4 and 7, that also regulate adipogenesis [39]. The growth of adipose tissue then continues up to term (~147 days gestation) when a majority of established BAT markers reach maximal abundance and the depot also contains a significant amount of white adipocytes [36]. Despite the relatively small fraction of fat (i.e., on a g/kg body-weight basis) present in most mammalian species at birth, both the amount and composition are highly sensitive to modulations in the maternal metabolic environment [38].

ADAPTATION OF ADIPOSE TISSUE AT BIRTH AND RECRUITMENT OF NONSHIVERING THERMOGENESIS

The primary role of BAT is to enable an effective thermoregulatory response following the cold exposure experienced in the transition from the uterine to extrauterine environments. Maturation of the hypothalamic–pituitary–adrenal axis largely determines the onset of nonshivering thermogenesis [7]. A compromised BAT function, as illustrated by studies in newborn sheep, results in pronounced hypothermia, as seen with preterm delivery [40] and/or cesarean-section birth [9]. Both these conditions prevent the normal rapid increase in BAT activity and body temperature rapidly falls after birth. This is because the onset of nonshivering thermogenesis is compromised due to a markedly slower rate of the appearance of several endocrine stimulatory factors that occurs after vaginal birth at term [9]. These effects are similar to those seen in humans [38]. An injection of triiodothyronine, norepinephrine, or both, into cesarean section–delivered sheep stimulates BAT function; responses are enhanced by delivery into a cool, rather than warm, ambient temperature [41]. The extent to which this further compromises adipose tissue development is not known but is of particular interest given the increased risk these offspring exhibit with respect to being overweight or obese [42,43]. Defective BAT development in early life could potentially contribute to excess adiposity. However, as with a majority of the factors that can modulate BAT function in early life, the longer-term consequences of cesarean-section birth for adipose tissue distribution have yet to be examined longitudinally.

Previously, it has been erroneously considered that factors released from the placenta actively inhibit the onset of nonshivering thermogenesis in fetal adipose tissue [44]. This was based on measuring changes in circulating concentrations of nonesterified fatty acids (NEFA), as a marker of lipolysis, rather than direct and/or functional measurements of UCP1 [45]. Both prostaglandins and adenosine were considered to inhibit BAT function, but these have now unequivocally been shown to be stimulators of BAT function [46,47]. The fetus is of course maintained within a metabolically constrained environment, which is characterized by basal concentrations of oxygen, glucose, and NEFA [1], and its temperature is ~1°C higher than that of the mother [48]. All these factors would constrain any activation of UCP1. In a normal pregnancy, the fetus has no need to thermoregulate, although when chronically stimulated, the thermogenic potential of BAT can be enhanced [49]. Furthermore, the increase in fetal plasma cortisol and catecholamine concentrations brought about by prolonged hypoxia also enhances the abundance of UCP1, but it still remains well below that present after birth [50].

MATERNAL DIETARY EFFECTS ON FETAL ADIPOSE TISSUE DEVELOPMENT

Maternal diet can have a profound effect on fetal adipose tissue growth and development as illustrated in sheep studies, of which the timing of any maternal intervention is critical in determining the newborn outcome [51]. To date, these have primarily focused on the perirenal-abdominal depot [38], although other depots, such as the pericardial, can be as responsive [52]. The main effects are seen on UCP1; reduced maternal food consumption in late gestation reduces UCP1 in fetal fat [52], although this does not always persist after birth [53]. In contrast, enhanced maternal food intake, such as allowing the mother to eat to appetite, increases both the amount of adipose tissue [54] and UCP1 in late gestation [55,56]. The extent to which these types of adaptations are specific to brown, as opposed to white and/or beige, adipocytes remains unclear because of the diffuse nature of their distribution within different depots [36,56]. It has been suggested that epigenetics provides a primary link between changes in the early nutritional environment and later outcomes [57], but the identification of a clear pathway remains elusive especially with regard to excess adiposity [58].

EPIGENETIC MECHANISMS IMPLICATED IN ADIPOSE TISSUE DEVELOPMENT

One reason why a more precise role for epigenetic regulation of adipose tissue development is currently unavailable is the very limited amount of measurements made at this stage of life. Most longitudinal studies in humans have simply focused on changes in gene methylation in blood as an indirect measure of epigenetic adaptation without a distinct adverse phenotype (e.g., [59]). One epigenetic mechanism recruited during preadipocyte differentiation involves acetylation and deacetylation [60], reversible processes controlled by competing enzymatic activities, namely, histone acetyltransferase (HAT) and histone deacetylase (HDAC) [61]. These, respectively, promote or inhibit adipocyte development [60]. There are at least 18 HDACs, subdivided into four classes [62]. When genes encoding individual HDACs are deleted, the offspring are often not viable, with the exceptions of HDAC5, 6, and 9. These types of studies have yet to show a direct role for HDAC on adipose tissue development, although it is known that HDACs are involved in development elsewhere. For example, HDAC2 is involved in heart growth and HDAC4 in bone development [62]. Class I HDACs appear to be more important in regulating adipose tissue metabolism. Inhibition of class I HDAC activity in obese mice has distinct metabolic benefits that are not seen using a class II inhibitor [63]. These differential outcomes appear to be mediated through increased BAT [63], although a complementary inhibition of adipogenesis may also occur [61]. The precise mechanisms involved have yet to be elucidated but short-chain fatty acids are inhibitors of class I HDACs and acetylation regulates the β-oxidation of NEFA [64]. Given the pronounced changes in their concentration around birth [1], they may be important epigenetic regulators of adipose tissue development.

CONCLUSION

We are now in a new and vibrant period of adipose tissue biology for which a greater understanding of the complex process in which it grows and develops could hold the key to preventing the annual rise in people who are overweight and obese. Clearly this problem starts early in life, perhaps before birth, and as such needs to be tackled at these early stages of development.

REFERENCES

1. Symonds ME, Pope M, Budge H. The ontogeny of brown adipose tissue. *Annu Rev Nutr.* 2015;35:295–320.
2. Spalding KL, Arner E, Westermark PO, Bernard S, Buchholz BA, Bergmann O, et al. Dynamics of fat cell turnover in humans. *Nature.* 2008;453(7196):783–7.
3. Ahima RS, Flier JS. Leptin. *Annu Rev Physiol.* 2000;62:413–37.
4. Mellor DJ, Cockburn F. A comparison of energy metabolism in the new-born infant, piglet and lamb. *Q J Exp Physiol.* 1986;71:361–79.
5. Cannon B, Nedergaard J. Brown adipose tissue: Function and physiological significance. *Phys Rev.* 2004;84(1):277–359.
6. Symonds ME, Andrews DC, Johnson PJ. The control of thermoregulation in the developing lamb during slow wave sleep. *J Dev Physiol.* 1989;11:289–98.
7. Symonds ME. Brown adipose tissue growth and development. *Scientifica.* 2013;2013:14.
8. Cannon B, Connoley E, Obregon M-J, Nedergaard J. Perinatal activation of brown adipose tissue. In Kunzel W, Jesen A, eds. *The Endocrine Control of the Fetus.* Berlin: Springer Verlag, pp. 306–20, 1988.
9. Clarke L, Heasman L, Firth K, Symonds ME. Influence of route of delivery and ambient temperature on thermoregulation in newborn lambs. *Am J Physiol Regul Integr Comp Physiol.* 1997;272(6 Pt 2):R1931–9.
10. Power G. Biology of temperature: The mammalian fetus. *J Dev Physiol.* 1989;12:295–304.
11. Cypess AM, Lehman S, Williams G, Tal I, Rodman D, Goldfine AB, et al. Identification and importance of brown adipose tissue in adult humans. *N Engl J Med.* 2009;360(15):1509–17.
12. Au-Yong IT, Thorn N, Ganatra R, Perkins AC, Symonds ME. Brown adipose tissue and seasonal variation in humans. *Diabetes.* 2009;58(11):2583–7.
13. Symonds ME, Henderson K, Elvidge L, Bosman C, Sharkey D, Perkins AC, et al. Thermal imaging to assess age-related changes of skin temperature within the supraclavicular region co-locating with brown adipose tissue in healthy children. *J Pediatr.* 2012;161(5):892–8.
14. Cypess AM, White AP, Vernochet C, Schulz TJ, Xue R, Sass CA, et al. Anatomical localization, gene expression profiling and functional characterization of adult human neck brown fat. *Nat Med.* 2013;19(5):635–9.
15. Xue R, Lynes MD, Dreyfuss JM, Shamsi F, Schulz TJ, Zhang H, et al. Clonal analyses and gene profiling identify genetic biomarkers of the thermogenic potential of human brown and white preadipocytes. *Nat Med.* 2015;21(7):760–8.

16. Shinoda K, Luijten IH, Hasegawa Y, Hong H, Sonne SB, Kim M, et al. Genetic and functional characterization of clonally derived adult human brown adipocytes. *Nat Med.* 2015;21(4):389–94.

17. Claussnitzer M, Dankel SN, Kim KH, Quon G, Meuleman W, Haugen C, et al. FTO obesity variant circuitry and adipocyte browning in humans. *N Engl J Med.* 2015;373(10):895–907.

18. Sanchez-Gurmaches J, Guertin DA. Adipocyte lineages: Tracing back the origins of fat. *Biochim Biophys Acta.* 2014;1842(3):340–51.

19. Schulz TJ, Tseng YH. Brown adipose tissue: Development, metabolism and beyond. *Biochem J.* 2013;453(2):167–78.

20. Atit R, Sgaier SK, Mohamed OA, Taketo MM, Dufort D, Joyner AL, et al. Beta-catenin activation is necessary and sufficient to specify the dorsal dermal fate in the mouse. *Dev Biol.* 2006;296(1):164–76.

21. Rudnicki MA, Schnegelsberg PN, Stead RH, Braun T, Arnold HH, Jaenisch R. MyoD or Myf-5 is required for the formation of skeletal muscle. *Cell.* 1993;75(7):1351–9.

22. Kablar B, Krastel K, Tajbakhsh S, Rudnicki MA. Myf5 and MyoD activation define independent myogenic compartments during embryonic development. *Dev Biol.* 2003;258(2):307–18.

23. Seale P, Bjork B, Yang W, Kajimura S, Chin S, Kuang S, et al. PRDM16 controls a brown fat/skeletal muscle switch. *Nature.* 2008;454(7207):961–7.

24. Shan T, Liang X, Bi P, Zhang P, Liu W, Kuang S. Distinct populations of adipogenic and myogenic Myf5-lineage progenitors in white adipose tissues. *J Lipid Res.* 2013;54(8):2214–24.

25. Sanchez-Gurmaches J, Hung CM, Sparks CA, Tang Y, Li H, Guertin DA. PTEN loss in the Myf5 lineage redistributes body fat and reveals subsets of white adipocytes that arise from Myf5 precursors. *Cell Metab.* 2012;16(3):348–62.

26. Sanchez-Gurmaches J, Guertin DA. Adipocytes arise from multiple lineages that are heterogeneously and dynamically distributed. *Nat Comm.* 2014;5:4099.

27. Petrovic N, Walden TB, Shabalina IG, Timmons JA, Cannon B, Nedergaard J. Chronic peroxisome proliferator-activated receptor gamma activation of epididymally derived white adipocyte cultures reveals a population of thermogenically competent, UCP1-containing adipocytes molecularly distinct from classic brown adipocytes. *J Biol Chem.* 2010;285(10):7153–64.

28. Harms M, Seale P. Brown and beige fat: Development, function and therapeutic potential. *Nat Med.* 2013;19(10):1252–63.

29. Nedergaard J, Cannon B. UCP1 mRNA does not produce heat. *Biochim Biophys Acta.* 2013;1831(5):943–9.

30. Nedergaard J, Cannon B. The browning of white adipose tissue: Some burning issues. *Cell Metab.* 2014;20(3):396–407.

31. Scheele C, Larsen TJ, Nielsen S. Novel nuances of human brown fat. *Adipocyte.* 2014;3(1):54–7.

32. de Jong JM, Larsson O, Cannon B, Nedergaard J. A stringent validation of mouse adipose tissue identity markers. *Am J Physiol Endocrinol Metab.* 2015;308(12):E1085–105.

33. Sidossis LS, Porter C, Saraf MK, Borsheim E, Radhakrishnan RS, Chao T, et al. Browning of subcutaneous white adipose tissue in humans after severe adrenergic stress. *Cell Metab.* 2015;22(2):219–27.

34. Symonds ME, Mostyn A, Pearce S, Budge H, Stephenson T. Endocrine and nutritional regulation of fetal adipose tissue development. *J Endocrinol.* 2003;179(3):293–9.

35. Widdowson EM. Chemical composition of newly born animals. *Nature.* 1950;116:626–8.

36. Pope M, Budge H, Symonds ME. The developmental transition of ovine adipose tissue through early life. *Acta Physiol (Oxf).* 2014;210(1):20–30.

37. Clarke L, Bryant MJ, Lomax MA, Symonds ME. Maternal manipulation of brown adipose tissue and liver development in the ovine fetus during late gestation. *Br J Nutr.* 1997;77(6):871–83.

38. Symonds ME, Pope M, Sharkey D, Budge H. Adipose tissue and fetal programming. *Diabetologia.* 2012;55(6):1597–606.

39. Zhang H, Schulz TJ, Espinoza DO, Huang TL, Emanuelli B, Kristiansen K, et al. Cross talk between insulin and bone morphogenetic protein signaling systems in brown adipogenesis. *Mol Cell Biol.* 2010;30(17):4224–33.

40. Clarke L, Bird JA, Lomax MA, Symonds ME. Effect of ß₃-adrenergic agonist (Zeneca D7114) on thermoregulation in near-term lambs delivered by cesarean section. *Pediatr Res.* 1996;40:330–6.

41. Symonds ME, Bird JA, Sullivan C, Wilson V, Clarke L, Stephenson T. Effect of delivery temperature on endocrine stimulation of thermoregulation in lambs born by cesarean section. *J Appl Physiol.* 2000;88(1):47–53.

42. Li HT, Zhou YB, Liu JM. The impact of cesarean section on offspring overweight and obesity: A systematic review and meta-analysis. *Int J Obes (Lond).* 2013;37(7):893–9.

43. Barros FC, Matijasevich A, Hallal PC, Horta BL, Barros AJ, Menezes AB, et al. Cesarean section and risk of obesity in childhood, adolescence, and early adulthood: Evidence from 3 Brazilian birth cohorts. *Am J Clin Nutr.* 2012;95(2):465–70.

44. Gunn TR, Gluckman PD. Perinatal thermogenesis. *Early Hum Dev.* 1995;42(3):169–83.

45. Symonds ME, Bird JA, Clarke L, Gate JJ, Lomax MA. Nutrition, temperature and homeostasis during perinatal development. *Exp Physiol.* 1995;80:907–40.

46. Gnad T, Scheibler S, von Kugelgen I, Scheele C, Kilic A, Glode A, et al. Adenosine activates brown adipose tissue and recruits beige adipocytes via A receptors. *Nature.* 2014;516(7531):395–9.

47. Vegiopoulos A, Muller-Decker K, Strzoda D, Schmitt I, Chichelnitskiy E, Ostertag A, et al. Cyclooxygenase-2 controls energy homeostasis in mice by *de novo* recruitment of brown adipocytes. *Science.* 2010;328(5982):1158–61.

48. Abrams R, Caton D, Curet LB, Crenshaw C, Mann L, Barron DH. Fetal brain-maternal aorta temperature differences in sheep. *Am J Physiol.* 1969;217(6):1619–22.

49. Bassett JM, Symonds ME. ß$_2$-Agonist ritodrine, unlike natural catecholamines, activates thermogenesis prematurely in utero in fetal sheep. *Am J Physiol Regul Integr Comp Physiol.* 1998;275:R112–9.

50. Gnanalingham MG, Giussani DA, Sivathondan P, Forhead AJ, Stephenson T, Symonds ME, et al. Chronic umbilical cord compression results in accelerated maturation of lung and brown adipose tissue in the sheep fetus during late gestation. *Am J Physiol Endocrinol Metab.* 2005;289(3):E456–65.

51. Symonds ME, Sebert SP, Budge H. Nutritional regulation of fetal growth and implications for productive life in ruminants. *Animal.* 2010;4(7):1057–83.

52. Ojha S, Robinson L, Yazdani M, Symonds ME, Budge H. Brown adipose tissue genes in pericardial adipose tissue of newborn sheep are downregulated by maternal nutrient restriction in late gestation. *Pediatr Res.* 2013;74(3):246–51.

53. Pearce S, Budge H, Mostyn A, Symonds ME, Stephenson T. Differential effects of maternal cold exposure and nutrient restriction on prolactin receptor and uncoupling protein 1 abundance in adipose tissue during development in young sheep. *Adipocytes.* 2005;1:57–64.

54. Bispham J, Gopalakrishnan GS, Dandrea J, Wilson V, Budge H, Keisler DH, et al. Maternal endocrine adaptation throughout pregnancy to nutritional manipulation: Consequences for maternal plasma leptin and cortisol and the programming of fetal adipose tissue development. *Endocrinology.* 2003;144(8):3575–85.

55. Budge H, Bispham J, Dandrea J, Evans E, Heasman L, Ingleton PM, et al. Effect of maternal nutrition on brown adipose tissue and its prolactin receptor status in the fetal lamb. *Pediatr Res.* 2000;47(6):781–6.

56. Ojha S, Symonds ME, Budge H. Suboptimal maternal nutrition during early-to-mid gestation in the sheep enhances pericardial adiposity in the near-term fetus. *Reprod Fertil Dev.* 2014;27(8):1205–12.

57. Sebert S, Sharkey D, Budge H, Symonds ME. The early programming of metabolic health: Is epigenetic setting the missing link? *Am J Clin Nutr.* 2011;94(6 Suppl):1953S–8S.

58. Symonds ME, Budge H, Frazier-Wood AC. Epigenetics and obesity: A relationship waiting to be explained. *Hum Hered.* 2013;75(2–4):90–7.

59. Godfrey KM, Sheppard A, Gluckman PD, Lillycrop KA, Burdge GC, McLean C, et al. Epigenetic gene promoter methylation at birth is associated with child's later adiposity. *Diabetes.* 2011;60(5):1528–34.

60. Zhou Y, Peng J, Jiang S. Role of histone acetyltransferases and histone deacetylases in adipocyte differentiation and adipogenesis. *Eur J Cell Biol.* 2014;93(4):170–7.

61. Catalioto RM, Maggi CA, Giuliani S. Chemically distinct HDAC inhibitors prevent adipose conversion of subcutaneous human white preadipocytes at an early stage of the differentiation program. *Exp Cell Res.* 2009;315(19):3267–80.

62. Haberland M, Montgomery RL, Olson EN. The many roles of histone deacetylases in development and physiology: Implications for disease and therapy. *Nat Rev Genet.* 2009;10(1):32–42.

63. Galmozzi A, Mitro N, Ferrari A, Gers E, Gilardi F, Godio C, et al. Inhibition of class I histone deacetylases unveils a mitochondrial signature and enhances oxidative metabolism in skeletal muscle and adipose tissue. *Diabetes.* 2013;62(3):732–42.

64. Ye J. Improving insulin sensitivity with HDAC inhibitor. *Diabetes.* 2013;62(3):685–7.

Section IV

---

*Behavioral and Metabolic
Consequences of Childhood Obesity*

23 Self-Esteem and Health-Related Quality of Life in Childhood Obesity

Andrew J. Hill

CONTENTS

INTRODUCTION

Body weight affects people's perception of themselves and others. While attitudes to obesity are shaped by age, gender, and cultural background, the prevailing climate in the developed world is antifat [1]. These negative attitudes lead to assumptions about the character and psychological state of people with obesity. However, the relationship between obesity and psychological well-being is neither linear nor uniform. Some children and adolescents with obesity have serious psychological problems. Others have mild problems, and some very few at all [2]. The purpose of this chapter is to summarize evidence on the core psychological well-being of an increasing section of children and youth. What does it mean to grow up and live as a young person seen and described as fat?

SELF-ESTEEM

Self-esteem is a long established psychological construct with a huge attendant literature. Self-esteem refers to how people perceive and value themselves. In a more elaborated form it is, "the extent to which a person believes himself to be capable, significant, successful and worthy" [3]. As Emler notes in his hugely influential review [4], the public discourse about self-esteem has moved on. In current usage, self-esteem is about psychological health and identity. It is a resource and an asset. High self-esteem is something we should have by right, as it is good for the individual and for society.

Opinion differs as to how to determine this (favorable) valuation of self. These differing perspectives offer an elaborated view of the relationship between obesity and self-esteem, and help to organize the published literature. Distinction will be made, here, between self-esteem as a generalized self-appraisal, a competence in externally (and internally) valued domains, and a metric of social acceptance (or likely rejection).

GLOBAL SELF-ESTEEM

The idea that self-esteem can be assessed as an evaluative attitude to the self has been attributed to Rosenberg [5], and his scale has become the gold standard in self-esteem research [4]. The Rosenberg self-esteem scale concerns very general evaluations of oneself. The 10-item scale yields a single score, a sum of positive statements. The popularity of the scale is, in part, due to its simplicity and brevity.

Unsurprisingly, this scale is prominent in evidence reviews of the relationship between obesity and global self-esteem. In a meta-analysis of research looking at global self-esteem in all age groups, Miller and Downey [6] found an effect size of -0.36 (95% CI -0.33 to -0.40), a robust but small- to moderate-sized relationship. Important influences on the strength of this relationship were age and gender. The correlation between overweight and self-esteem increased up to early adulthood, from -0.12 to -0.22 to -0.28 in children, adolescents, and young college-age adults, respectively. In addition, the relationship was significantly stronger in females (-0.23) than males (-0.09). More recently, a systematic review of studies comparing youth with obesity and healthy-weight controls found lower self-esteem scores in those with obesity in 17 of the 21 included studies [7]. The four exceptions had a feature in common. They all reported in nonwhite ethnic groups; either samples from Asia or minority ethnic groups in the United States. The review authors urged caution, however, noting that there are other studies of youth and adults from the same countries and ethnicity/income groups that do show lower self-esteem in individuals with obesity [8].

PERCEIVED SELF-COMPETENCE

The global perspective of self-esteem is in fact predated by an elaborated conceptualization. The representation of self-esteem as the ratio of a person's successes to his or her pretensions has been attributed to William James [4]. From this viewpoint, self-esteem is a personal evaluation of competence in areas that are important to a person. So there are two parts to this formulation of self-esteem: the multiple domains in which the self is evaluated and a likelihood that they are not all equal in perceived importance. Indeed, it is the discrepancy between competence and importance that defines overall self-worth. Only when a person feels low competence in an area of high importance is his or her self-worth jeopardized.

There are only a handful of commonly used multidimensional measures of self-esteem for children and adolescents [9]. Susan Harter has done most to develop the Jamesian conceptualization and assessment of perceived self-competence [10]. She argues that for children the necessary domains of competence are set by parents (scholastic competence, behavioral conduct) and peers (physical appearance, social, and athletic competence). These domains expand in number and range through adolescence into adulthood, incorporating attributes such as job competence, romantic appeal, and a sense of humor.

We conducted a systematic review of multicompetence assessments in young people with defined obesity. There were 17 studies, of which 9 were cross-sectional and 7 were weight management interventions [11]. Most had used Harter's questionnaires. All of the studies that assessed physical appearance and athletic/physical competence found lower scores in youth with obesity. Obesity also impacted on perceived social acceptance, with lower scores reported in half of those measuring this domain. In contrast, few differences were observed in scholastic competence or behavioral conduct. Global self-worth was lower in children with obesity compared with those of healthy weight in six of the nine cross-sectional studies, a finding comparable with that of the global self-esteem literature discussed in the last section. There were insufficient studies to detect any effects of age or sex. Likewise, comparisons based on race or ethnicity were infrequent in this literature. But the observation that in younger (9–12 years old) minority children from low-income families, all, regardless of their weight status, had lower global self-worth than a reference white population [12] is a reminder of the inherent complexities in this area.

Domain Importance

Thus far, this literature says much more about successes than pretensions in children with obesity. The competencies included in Harter's self-perception profiles may indeed be those most important to today's youth. Harter, herself, has written about how perceived physical appearance is the number one predictor of self-esteem [13]. This is true from age 5 through to adulthood. It raises the issue of how to help children value competencies other than appearance. But given that one way of managing poor competence is to diminish the importance of that feature, it is surprising that perceived importance has not been more thoroughly investigated. An assessment of domain importance is included in the manuals for Harter's scales but rarely used in research. Our own unpublished work suggests that for a community sample of 12-year-olds, at least, healthy-weight children and those with obesity do not differ in how important they rate appearance and athletic competencies. However, and in accord with the evidence presented earlier in this section, they do perceive themselves very differently on these features.

Low Self-Esteem

The response format of the Harter measures permits one further and rarely reported feature of self-esteem; the assessment of self-defined low self-esteem. One of the criticisms of the self-esteem literature generally is that too much attention is given to mean values on scales that are statistically different but of questionable functional difference. Requiring respondents to identify with either a high or low self-esteem characterization (as in Harter's questionnaires) addresses this issue.

In a state-wide survey of 9–13-year-olds from New South Wales, Australia, we found that the perception of physical appearance was particularly affected, with 63% of girls and 33% of boys with obesity identifying with the depiction of an unattractive child [14]. In contrast, the proportion of low scorers on the global measure of self-worth was smaller. Although the relative risk of low global self-worth in girls with obesity was 4.1 times more than normal-weight peers, only 20% of the group scored in this range. Danielsen et al. [15], using the same approach to define low self-esteem, also found higher proportions of overweight/obese Norwegian 10–13-year-olds to have low physical appearance and athletic competence perception. For this population sample, the difference from healthy weight children extended to low social acceptance and scholastic competence, although the proportions were smaller than observed in the Australian children.

Complementing this, in the Australian sample, girls with obesity were more than five times less likely to have high global self-worth, something achieved by around 70% of their peers. So, while it would be unwise to assume low self-esteem in every person with obesity, the consequences of not holding oneself in high self-regard should also be recognized. In practical terms, this may flag problems with confidence and self-efficacy, issues key to behavior change and its maintenance.

THE LOOKING-GLASS SELF

The "looking-glass self" framing of self-esteem is attributed to Charles Cooley, and again it is a long-standing and highly influential theory. Its basis is that our assessments of our own worth are based on the judgments we imagine *others* make of us [4]. Moreover, our predictions about these judgments depend upon the qualities we see in these other people. So, what shapes self-esteem are not our accomplishments objectively and directly appraised, but the anticipated judgments of these accomplishments by other people. Hence, self-esteem is what we expect will be reflected by this social mirror, and the intensity of reflection depends on whom we choose as our social referents.

Mark Leary has taken this social view in a particular direction, one very relevant to obesity. Sociometer theory proposes that the self-esteem system evolved primarily as a monitor of social acceptance, the motivation being not to maintain self-esteem, *per se*, but to avoid social devaluation and rejection [16]. He argues that people are particularly sensitive to changes in relational evaluation or the degree to which others regard their relationship with the individual as valuable, important, or close. Accordingly, self-esteem is lowered by failure, criticism, or rejection and raised by success, praise, and events associated with relational appreciation. Even the possibility of rejection can lower self-esteem. Two areas of research are particularly relevant to youth with obesity—interpersonal relations and victimization.

Interpersonal Relations

Sociometric procedures using peer-nominated friendships have shown little impact of being obese in community samples of primary school–aged children. Some 20 years ago, for example, young children with obesity were just as likely to be chosen as their lean peers as people to socialize with both inside and outside of school [17]. The situation is likely to be different now, as has been observed for teenagers. Data from the US National Longitudinal Study of Adolescent Health (Add Health) showed overweight adolescents were overrepresented in categories of no or few peer friendship nominations and underrepresented in the most popular categories [18]. Most importantly, they received fewer reciprocal nominations: that is, nominations by peers they themselves had nominated. Further analysis of this cohort indicated that overweight adolescents whose friendship attempts with nonoverweight peers were not reciprocated would turn to other overweight peers [19]. In another, smaller sample of US teenagers, friendship choices showed overweight youth were twice as likely to have overweight friends as their nonoverweight peers [20].

The relative failure to be named a friend by people you nominate suggests that the friendship ties of adolescents with obesity are less plentiful, potentially weaker, and more directed to others with obesity. In terms of self-esteem, the peer referent for self-evaluation chosen by teenagers with obesity determines their social standing: valued and held in esteem by others of similar weight but likely rejected and so of low self-esteem in the eyes of those of healthy weight (see Chapter 16 for further consideration of social networks).

Victimization

Peer difficulties and rejection have been observed in very young children. By age 5, parents of children with obesity are more likely to report peer relationship problems in their girls and boys than parents of healthy-weight children [21]. Five-year-olds themselves reject story characters drawn as fat as people they would choose to be friends with [22]. Rejection may be a very small step from perceived victimization.

The research evidence is unequivocal regarding the association between obesity and victimization. A meta-analysis of 16 studies and 28 effect sizes showed a significant relationship between being obese and being victimized (OR = 1.51 [1.32–1.71]; [23]). Most of these studies were of children aged 11 and upward. In an interesting development, observations of primary school teachers in the Netherlands and the children themselves revealed that children with obesity were more likely to be victimized by their peers and also more likely to bully others [24]. Indeed, there was a small group of children referred to as "bully-victims" who were both recipients and perpetrators of victimization. Children with obesity were twice as likely to be in this category as healthy-weight peers.

Restricting this to weight-related victimization, we have reported that some 42% of 9–12-year-olds with obesity identify themselves as fat victimized compared with 7% of their healthy-weight peers [25,26]. Being fat victimized was strongly associated with being victimized generally. In terms of self-esteem, those who were fat victimized scored lower in social acceptance, athletic competence, school competence, physical appearance, and global self-worth, compared with children

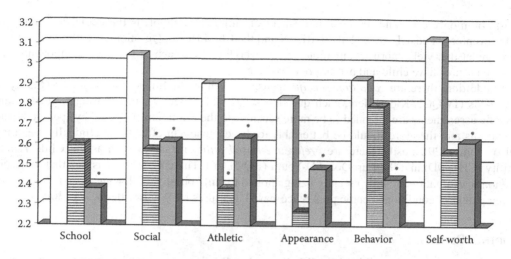

FIGURE 23.1 Perceived self-competence in eight hundred and thirty-two 9–12-year-olds who were not involved in fat victimization (open columns), were fat victimized (horizontally shaded columns), and who were both fat-victimized and fat bullies (gray columns); columns with an * indicate perceived self-competence that is significantly different from those not involved, $p < .05$. (From Hill, A.J., and Murphy, J.A., *International Journal of Obesity*, 24(Suppl. 1), 161, 2000; Hill, A.J., and Waterston, C.L., *International Journal of Obesity*, 26(Suppl. 1), 20, 2002.)

not involved in victimization (Figure 23.1). Children who bullied others for being fat had high self-competence on every domain other than behavioral conduct and global self-worth. The small group of bully-victims scored low on every measure of competence and global self-worth. Two additional points are noteworthy. First, while being fat teased was more common in children with obesity, at least half of obese children did not report these experiences. We know very little about what protects these children or what makes the other half vulnerable. Second, victimization did not impact the perceived importance of any of these domains. Once more, it would appear that these children were not managing their low self-esteem by modifying the importance of domains in which they judged themselves less competent.

QUALITY OF LIFE

Quality of life is a much younger and broader concept than self-esteem. Indeed, assessments of quality of life often include scales related to contentment with self. Health-related quality of life (HRQoL) is what is assessed in the context of obesity and, while variously defined, it describes the functional effect of a health condition on a person. HRQoL includes subjective assessments of present physical, psychological, and social state. The value of its measurement is the quantification of the impact of a health condition (and its treatment) on a person's life in a standard and reproducible way. For health economists, HRQoL provides the basis for calculating quality-adjusted life years (QALYs) that, in turn, permit the assessment of cost-effectiveness of health interventions. For researchers and clinicians, HRQoL measures provide broad-brush characterization of subjective health impact that can be compared across health conditions, assess the burden of preventable health conditions, and guide interventions to improve people's well-being [27].

MEASURES OF HRQoL

With HRQoL so central to evaluations of treatment outcomes and effectiveness it should be of little surprise that there is a variety of instruments to use with children [28]. There has been a surge in the number of studies on child obesity and its treatment that have included HRQoL. The most commonly used and reported assessment of children's HRQoL is the Pediatric Quality of Life Inventory (PedsQL). Like KIDSCREEN and the Child Health Questionnaire, this is a *generic* assessment that yields norm-comparable scores overall and for each of the main components. All these measures have child and parent-proxy versions.

In addition, there are *condition-specific* measures such as the Impact of Weight on Quality of Life-Kids (IWQOL-Kids). Here, each question starts with, "Because of my weight." Condition-specific assessments are intended to be more sensitive to the limitations imposed by specific health conditions and therefore should be better able to detect treatment effects and clinically meaning-ful outcomes [29]. Lastly, there are *preference-based utility* measures such as the Child Health Utility (CHU-9D) and the EuroQoL-5D-Youth (EQ-5D-Y). These generic measures that underpin economic evaluation are only recently being applied to child obesity. Following close behind is the development of condition-specific preference-based measures for youth with obesity [30].

EVIDENCE REVIEWS

The surge of interest in children's well-being and well-being as an obesity treatment outcome is reflected in updated evidence syntheses. Tsiros et al. [29] identified 28 studies, 15 of which had used the PedsQL. Pooling these data showed strong inverse linear relationships between body mass index (BMI) and physical and social functioning. The relationship was more moderate with emotional functioning and marginal for school functioning. Parent-proxy completions scored lower (i.e., lower HRQoL) than children's own ratings of their quality of life, although there was evidence of parents being more extreme in both low and high HRQoL. In an updated meta-analysis, children and adolescents with obesity scored lower on total, physical, and psychosocial PedsQL summary scores, with parent-proxy values again being lower than children's [31].

Our systematic review considered only children defined as obese [11]. The great majority of studies found lower scores on physical and social functioning and on physical/general health. Six of the nine cross-sectional studies that collected data on school or work functioning reported lower scores in youth with obesity. The difference from the scholastic competence outcomes observed by Tsiros et al. in the context of self-esteem could be related to scale content. For example, two of the five scale items in PedsQL ask about absence from school, while all questions in Harter's assessment are directed at perceived school achievement or performance.

The most recent published review at the time of writing this chapter included 34 studies and noted the use of 10 different HRQoL measures [32]. Despite this variety, there was good congruence observed. For example, only two studies failed to report a significant difference in overall scores between healthy-weight youth and those with obesity. One of these was in preschoolers but again there are other studies in this age group that do show a parentally assessed difference [33]. Clear differences were observed on each of the subdimensions of social, physical, emotional, and school functioning, with confirmation of an impact on school functioning (13 of 18 studies). As may be expected, scores in nearly all HRQoL dimensions were lower in clinical than community samples and worsened with the degree of obesity.

No information was presented on possible race/ethnicity differences. However, recent research parallels that on self-esteem in terms of apparently contradictory outcomes. For example, analysis of a multiethnic US cohort of 10–11-year-olds showed lower psychosocial PedsQL scores in children with obesity, regardless of whether they were white, black, or Hispanic [34]. In contrast, PedsQL scores of a large sample of Fijian 12–18-year-olds showed no meaningful association between obesity and HRQoL scores, although there was some variation by age [35].

CONSEQUENCES OF WEIGHT MANAGEMENT

In a review of the literature on structured weight management programs for children and adolescents that included a measure of self-esteem, 18 of 21 studies were observed to report some end of intervention improvement in self-esteem [36]. This improvement appeared to be related to the following intervention components: consistent parental involvement, group-based interventions, and actual weight loss.

The importance of the degree of weight loss is emphasized in reviews of studies that have included an assessment of HRQoL. Multidisciplinary interventions, that is those that included some sort of behavioral therapy, dietary advice, and/or physical activity, and the input of multiple health-care professionals showed no overall significant differences in HRQoL in short- or long-term follow-up [37]. Importantly, the change in both HRQoL and body weight was modest. The trend to improved HRQoL was paralleled by small reductions in BMI, mostly between −0.06 and −0.15 BMI standard deviation score (SDS) at around 6 months. Bariatric surgery, however, yields appreciable weight loss. In the 23 studies included in a meta-analysis by Black et al. [38], BMI decreased by 13.5 kg/m² at 12 months. The six studies that assessed HRQoL all showed significant improvements from baseline to postsurgery follow-up.

Returning to the self-esteem literature, we have previously noted the inconsistencies in associations between weight loss and self-esteem improvements in the intervention literature [11]. When interventions result in weight loss, most studies also observe improvements in global self-esteem and the competencies most affected, that is, physical appearance, athletic competence, and social acceptance [39]. It is surprising therefore that the degree of weight loss was correlated with self-esteem improvement in only one of the five studies that reported these associations. More recently, in an intensive, residential weight loss program for youth with obesity, attendees lost 5.5 kg (−0.25 BMI SDS) in just over 4 weeks [40]. Weight loss was positively associated with improvements in athletic competence and physical appearance but not global self-worth. The sample size was large ($n = 303$) but the correlation coefficients small (0.13 and 0.19). Overall, this is suggestive that psychological benefit may be as dependent on some feature of the environment or supportive network as it is on weight reduction. In the context of group interventions such as residential camps, these may include the daily company of others who have obesity in common, improvements in competence or self-efficacy in newly prioritized areas (such as exercising regularly), the establishment of new friendships, or fewer experiences of weight-related victimization. And these are experienced before adolescents notice levels of weight loss that have either clinical or personal significance.

CONCLUSIONS AND IMPLICATIONS

The relationship between obesity and impaired well-being in youth is present but modest in strength. Consider the key constituents. Psychological features such as low self-esteem are likely minor contributors to the development and maintenance of obesity, albeit with the potential to interact with other risk factors. And overweight is undoubtedly only one of several influences, although an important one, on an individual's sense of self-value. Additionally, both obesity and self-esteem are resistant to change. Longitudinally, any association will be bidirectional, in the same manner to that proposed for the relationship between obesity and depression [41]. This bidirectionality is more apparent in adults than in youth [42]. However, evidence that bidirectionality between obesity and impaired HRQoL emerges as children get older suggests that middle childhood is a key period for children in economically developed countries [43]. Changing peer relationships in the teenage years and priorities for physical attractiveness underpin this.

Mood disorders and eating disorders are other markers of impaired well-being, alongside low self-esteem and HRQoL. They are undoubtedly all interrelated. Furthermore, given that obesity persists, then the negativity associated with being fat is likely to accumulate. Unsurprisingly, therefore, those who remain obese from early childhood into adolescence have the highest levels of depressive symptoms [44] and binge eating [45]. This is a reminder that the priority for preventing obesity should never distract from addressing the needs of those already obese.

In terms of improving self-esteem and HRQoL, then, weight loss is undoubtedly important. But as reflected here, the child's environment and supportive network is equally important. As we have previously observed, many people with obesity, adults and children, have high self-esteem, do not suffer major depression, are in well-paid employment, and have good social relationships. This implies individual resistance or resilience. Resilience offers a different perspective to the more traditional risk-factor approach, focusing on strengths rather than deficits [46]. And it is concordant with assets-based approaches to health improvement that are extremely popular currently in public health. Assets exist within individuals (self-efficacy, drive), close community (family and friends, intergenerational), or are organizational or institutional (housing, representation/advocacy). Identifying and developing assets, many of which are external to the individual, is challenging, especially in an environment rife with antifat attitudes. But this is consistent with the view that targeting, personalization, and relationships are fundamental to improving the way that young people value themselves [4].

REFERENCES

1. Puhl RM, Heuer CA (2009). The stigma of obesity: A review and update. *Obesity (Silver Spring)*, 17, 941–964.
2. Walker L, Hill AJ (2009). Obesity: The role of child mental health services. *Child & Adolescent Mental Health*, 14, 114–120.
3. Coopersmith S (1967). *The Antecedents of Self-Esteem*. WH Freeman, San Francisco, CA.
4. Emler N (2001). *Self-Esteem: The Costs and Causes of Low Self-Worth*. Joseph Rowntree Foundation, New York.
5. Rosenberg M (1965). *Society and the Adolescent Self-Image*. Princeton University Press, Princeton, NJ.
6. Miller CT, Downey KT (1999). A meta-analysis of heavyweight and self-esteem. *Personality & Social Psychology Review*, 3, 68–84.
7. Sikorski C, Luppa M, Muck T, Riedel-Heller SG (2015). Weight stigma "gets under the skin": Evidence for an adapted mediation framework—A systematic review. *Obesity (Silver Spring)*, 23, 266–276.
8. Witherspoon D, Latta L, Wang Y, Black MM (2013). Do depression, self-esteem, body esteem, and eating attitudes vary by BMI among African American adolescents? *Journal of Pediatric Psychology*, 38, 112–120.
9. Butler RJ, Gasson SL (2005). Self esteem/self concept scales for children and adolescents: A review. *Child and Adolescent Mental Health*, 10, 190–201.
10. Harter S (1993). Causes and consequences of low self-esteem in children and adolescents. In RF Baumeister (ed.), *Self-Esteem: The Puzzle of Low Self-Regard*, pp. 87–116. Plenum, New York.
11. Griffiths LJ, Parsons TJ, Hill AJ (2010). Self-esteem and quality of life in obese children and adolescents: A systematic review. *International Journal of Pediatric Obesity*, 5, 282–304.
12. Wong WW, Mikhail C, Ortiz CL et al. (2014). Body weight has no impact on self-esteem of minority children living in inner city, low-income neighborhoods: A cross-sectional study. *BMC Pediatrics*, 14, 19.
13. Harter S (2000). Is self-esteem only skin deep? The inextricable link between physical appearance and self-esteem. *Reclaiming Children and Youth*, 9, 133–138.
14. Franklin J, Denyer G, Steinbeck KS, Caterson ID, Hill AJ (2006). Obesity and risk of low self-esteem: A state-wide survey of Australian children. *Pediatrics*, 118, 2481–2487.
15. Danielsen YS, Stormark KM, Nordhus IH et al. (2012). Factors associated with low self-esteem in children with overweight. *Obesity Facts*, 5, 722–733.
16. Leary M (1999). Making sense of self-esteem, *Current Directions in Psychological Science*, 8, 32–35.
17. Phillips RG, Hill AJ (1998). Fat, plain, but not friendless: Self-esteem and peer acceptance of obese preadolescent girls. *International Journal of Obesity*, 22, 287–293.
18. Strauss RS, Pollack HA (2003). Social marginalization of overweight children. *Archives of Pediatrics & Adolescent Medicine*, 157, 746–752.
19. Schaefer DR, Simpkins SD (2014). Using social network analysis to clarify the role of obesity in selection of adolescent friends. *American Journal of Public Health*, 107, 1223–1229.
20. Valente TW, Fujimoto K, Chou CP, Spruijt-Metz D (2009). Adolescent affiliations and adiposity: A social network analysis of friendships and obesity. *Journal of Adolescent Health*, 45, 202–204.
21. Griffiths LJ, Dezateux C, Hill AJ (2011). Is obesity associated with emotional and behavioural problems in children? Findings from the Millennium Cohort Study. *International Journal of Pediatric Obesity*, 6, e423–e432.
22. Harrison S, Rowlinson M, Hill AJ (2016). No fat friend of mine: Young children's responses to overweight and disability. *Body Image*, DOI: 10.1016/j.bodyim.2016.05.002.

23. van Geel M, Vedder P, Tanilon J (2014). Are overweight and obese youths more often bullied by their peers? A meta-analysis on the relation between weight status and bullying. *International Journal of Obesity*, 38, 1263–1267.

24. Jansen PW, Verlinden M, Dormisse-van Berkel A et al. (2014). Teacher and peer reports of overweight and bullying among young primary school children. *Pediatrics*, 134, 473–480.

25. Hill AJ, Murphy JA (2000). The psycho-social consequences of fat-teasing in young adolescent children. *International Journal of Obesity*, 24 (Suppl. 1), 161.

26. Hill AJ, Waterston CL (2002). Fat-teasing in pre-adolescent children: The bullied and the bullies. *International Journal of Obesity*, 26 (Suppl. 1), 20.

27. Centers for Disease Control and Prevention (2015). HRQOL concepts. http://www.cdc.gov/hrqol/concept.htm. Accessed November 18, 2015.

28. Solans M, Pane S, Estrada MD et al. (2008). Health-related quality of life measurement in children and adolescents: A systematic review of generic and disease-specific instruments. *Value in Health*, 11, 742–764.

29. Tsiros MD, Olds T, Buckley JD et al. (2009). Health-related quality of life in obese children and adolescents. *International Journal of Obesity*, 33, 387–400.

30. Oluboyede Y, Hulme C, Hill AJ (2016). Development and refinement of the WAItE: A new obesity specific quality of life measure for adolescents. *Quality of Life Research*, in review.

31. Ul-Haq Z, Mackay DF, Fenwick E, Pell JP (2013). Meta-analysis of the association between body mass index and health-related quality of life among children and adolescents, assessed using the Pediatric Quality of Life Index. *Journal of Pediatrics*, 162, 280–286.

32. Buttitta M, Iliescu C, Rousseau A, Guerrien A (2014). Quality of life in overweight and obese children and adolescents: A literature review. *Quality of Life Research*, 23, 1117–1139.

33. Kuhl ES, Rausch JR, Varni JW, Stark LJ (2012). Impaired health-related quality of life in preschoolers with obesity. *Journal of Pediatric Psychology*, 37, 1148–1156.

34. Wallander JL, Kerbawy S, Toomey S et al. (2013). Is obesity associated with reduced health-related quality of life in Latino, black and white children in the community? *International Journal of Obesity*, 37, 920–925.

35. Petersen S, Moodie M, Mavoa H et al. (2014). Relationship between overweight and health-related quality of life in secondary school children in Fiji: Results from a cross-sectional population-based study. *International Journal of Obesity*, 38, 539–546.

36. Lowry KW, Sallinen BJ, Janicke DM (2007). The effects of weight management programs on self-esteem in pediatric overweight populations. *Journal of Pediatric Psychology*, 32, 1179–1195.

37. Ligthart KAM, Paulis WD, Djasmo D, Koes BW, van Middelkoop M (2014). Effect of multidisciplinary interventions on quality of life in obese children: A systematic review and meta-analysis. *Quality of Life Research*, 24, 1635–1643.

38. Black JA, White B, Viner RM, Simmons RK (2013). Bariatric surgery for obese children and adolescents: A systematic review and meta-analysis. *Obesity Reviews*, 14, 634–644.

39. Danielsen YS, Nordhus IH, Juliusson PB, Maehle M, Pallesen S (2013). Effect of a family-based cognitive behavioural intervention on body mass index, self-esteem and symptoms of depression in children with obesity (aged 7–13): A randomised waiting list controlled study. *Obesity Research & Clinical Practice*, 7, e116–e128.

40. McGregor S, McKenna J, Gately P, Hill AJ (2016). Self-esteem outcomes over a summer camp for obese youth. *Pediatric Obesity*, DOI: 10.1111/ijpo.12093.

41. Napolitano MA, Foster GD (2008). Depression and obesity: Implications for assessment, treatment, and research. *Clinical Psychology: Science & Practice*, 15, 21–27.

42. Cameron AJ, Magliano DJ, Dunstan DW et al. (2012). A bi-directional relationship between obesity and health-related quality of life: Evidence from the longitudinal AusDiab study. *International Journal of Obesity*, 36, 295–303.

43. Jansen PW, Mensah FK, Clifford S, Nicholson JM, Wake M (2013). Bidirectional associations between overweight and health-related quality of life from 4–11 years: Longitudinal study of Australian children. *International Journal of Obesity*, 37, 1307–1313.

44. Martin-Storey A, Crosnoe R (2015). Trajectories of overweight and their association with adolescent depressive symptoms. *Health Psychology*, 34, 1004–1012.

45. Sonneville KR, Calzo JP, Horton NJ et al. (2012). Body satisfaction, weight gain and binge eating among overweight adolescents girls. *International Journal of Obesity*, 36, 944–949.

46. Russell-Mayhew S, McVey G, Bardick A, Ireland A (2012). Mental health, wellness, and childhood overweight/obesity. *Journal of Obesity*, 2012, DOI: 10.1155/2012/281801.

24 Childhood Obesity
Implications for Neurocognitive Functioning

Ashley A. Martin, Sara L. Hargrave, and Terry L. Davidson

CONTENTS

INTRODUCTION

It is well established that overweight and obese children and adolescents are at increased risk of many physical disorders (such as type 2 diabetes, hypertension, metabolic syndrome, and fatty liver) that were once largely confined to adults [1,2]. These are not short-term problems. Rather, it appears that the comorbidities of childhood obesity often extend into adulthood, where they can decrease both the length and the quality of life [3]. Unfortunately, data are accumulating that suggest such challenges to physical health are not the only, and are arguably not even the most serious, consequences of childhood obesity. This chapter summarizes findings that indicate that obesity, and the behaviors that produce it, may also have long-term adverse consequences for the cognitive and brain health of children.

The studies that we will review rely largely on standard measures related to body weight (e.g., percentile ranking in children, body mass index [BMI] in adolescents and adults) and adiposity as indices of obesity. We will also consider the effects of consuming diets high in saturated fat and sugar (aka Western diets) on cognitive function and brain health. The Western diet is of interest because it is known to promote obesity and cognitive dysfunction [4] and because its use is widespread in Western and Westernized societies where the incidence of obesity is high [5]. Further, the possibility that obesity and excess intake may be the result of impaired cognitive functioning is considered. We acknowledge that glucoregulatory disorders, inflammation, reduced cardiovascular fitness, and insulin resistance are prominent among the factors that have been linked to cognitive dysfunction and to abnormalities in brain substrates for cognition (for reviews see [4,6,7]). However, all of these problems are comorbid with obesity and with intake of the Western diet. Sorting out which disorders may be causes and which may be the effects of obesity and cognitive dysfunction is a long-standing challenge that remains outside the scope of this chapter.

CHILDHOOD OBESITY AND COGNITION

EXECUTIVE FUNCTION AND INHIBITORY CONTROL

Overweight and obese children exhibit deficits in a variety of cognitive capacities related to attention, inhibitory control/impulsivity, and memory. These types of deficits are often labeled as impairments in *executive function* (for a recent review, see [8]). Executive function includes a variety of diverse processes that are involved with cognitive and behavioral control. Tasks that require working memory, mental flexibility, task switching/multitasking, decision making, or delayed gratification are all thought to rely on executive functions [9].

Executive functions are also described as playing an inhibitory role in behavior and cognition. In this context, behavioral inhibition involves the ability to suppress prepotent responses that are incompatible with the performance of planned and situationally relevant goal-directed actions [10]. This type of inhibition also has a cognitive aspect in that it serves to suppress the ability of extraneous stimuli to attract our attention [11], or to retrieve unwanted or situationally inappropriate memories [12] that could underlie the impulsive evocation of behavior. Inhibitory control is a component of cognitive development that emerges in infancy and increases throughout childhood and adolescence [10]. Thus, there is a concern that events that impact the brain detrimentally early in life could produce impairments in behavioral and cognitive control that are exhibited throughout the lifespan.

EFFECTS OF OBESITY ON CHILDHOOD COGNITIVE FUNCTION

Overweight and obese children exhibit a number of cognitive-inhibitory problems that are associated with deficits in executive functioning. For example, a recent study conducted in 983 adolescents found that greater visceral adiposity was associated with lower performance on six measures of executive function [13]. Two of the most common measures of executive function are tasks that require mental flexibility and control over memory interference. Compared with children of lower body weight, children with higher body weights exhibit a higher number of perseverative errors on these tasks, which reflects a failure to adjust and update one's behavior in response to changing rules or task requirements [14]. This inflexible behavioral pattern appears to be at least partly due to impaired attentional processing [15]. Because attentional difficulty in early childhood has been found to predict impaired executive functioning later in childhood [16], this finding suggests that attentional difficulties may be an early warning sign of obesity-related inhibitory impairment.

Childhood obesity is also often associated with deficits related to impulsivity and a lack of inhibitory control. For example, in *delay discounting* tasks that measure participants' ability to delay a behavioral response in order to earn an incentive, obese children and adolescents appear to be less able to "wait" for the reward [17,18]. However, these deficits in behavioral control have also been observed in *no-go* or *stop signal* tasks that require participants to inhibit a prepotent behavioral response in the absence of any programed reward [19].

REDUCED INHIBITORY CONTROL AS A CAUSE AND A CONSEQUENCE OF CHILDHOOD OBESITY

Deficits in cognitive-inhibitory processes may compromise one's ability to resist thinking about food reward, thereby increasing one's risk of food cue reactivity, disinhibition, and ultimately weight gain (for a detailed discussion of this idea, see [20]). Thus, there is a concern that childhood obesity may promote cognitive impairments that could increase or exacerbate one's risk of obesity in adulthood. Consistent with this possibility, studies have shown that children who exhibit poor impulse control are also more responsive to food reward, being particularly poor at inhibiting responses to food versus nonfood incentives [21]. Others have found that children with a higher BMI show altered brain activation in response to food stimuli in brain areas typically associated with executive/inhibitory control (for a review, see [22]).

While these findings suggest that impulsivity is related to increased food cue reactivity, studies assessing actual food intake have yielded only equivocal evidence that impulsivity causally contributes to overeating in children. A recent cross-sectional study failed to find any significant relationships between children's impulsivity and snack intake or BMI [23]. Another study investigating eating in the absence of hunger found no relationship between executive function and intake in preschool children, but did find that lower cognitive performance, in general, was related to greater intake [24]. This is consistent with other studies showing that children with higher cognitive ability have a lower risk of becoming overweight and obese in the future [25].

Prospective studies have linked childhood inhibitory control to the development of weight gain over time. One study found that children with poorer inhibitory control had significantly higher body weights 6 and 12 months later, with the greatest weight gain occurring in the most impulsive children [26]. Indeed, a recent longitudinal study found that poor impulse control at age 4 was associated with a higher BMI 30 years later [27]. Poor inhibitory control has also been associated with resistance to weight loss for children participating in a weight intervention. Nederkoorn et al. [28] found that while obese children generally exhibited poorer inhibitory control than lean children, this was exacerbated even further in a subsample of obese children who exhibited binge-eating behavior (see also [29]). Together, these results suggest deficits in inhibitory processing may underlie aberrant eating behavior in children, and could be part of the etiology of their obesity.

INCONSISTENCIES AND CONTROVERSIES

Although deficits in executive-inhibitory functions have been frequently documented in overweight and obese children, the literature does not always tell a consistent story in regard to the specific underlying processes that are affected. For instance, tasks of working memory are thought to depend on the same kinds of inhibitory processes that are involved in other tasks of interference control (e.g., both require the suppression of no-longer-relevant information from memory), but obese children are not always impaired in both kinds of task (e.g., [14]). Thus, while executive function is indeed impaired in obese children, not all measures of executive function are equally sensitive to these impairments. Similarly, obese children exhibit abnormal neural activation in brain regions associated with inhibition/executive function (e.g., the prefrontal cortex [PFC]), but the direction of abnormality is inconsistent; some authors report hyperactivation of these areas [30], while others report hypoactivation [31].

Some of these discrepancies are probably due to the diverse nature of executive function that encompasses a number of potentially overlapping cognitive processes that may rely, in whole or in part, on different brain substrates. For example, while the PFC is often described as the brain site for executive function, recent reports indicate that diet and obesity are associated with impaired memory inhibitory functions that are thought to depend on the functional integrity of medial temporal lobe structures, most notably the hippocampus [32]. Moreover, reciprocal connections linking areas in the frontal cortex with the hippocampus complicate attempts to specify the neural basis for impairments in memory and executive functions [33]. Natural variations among obese children in metabolic disorder symptomology may also contribute to discrepancies in the literature, with certain biomarkers predicting neurological impairment (see [34]).

If cognitive deficits are either a cause or a consequence of childhood obesity, one might also expect that there would be a negative relationship between childhood body weight and measures of academic performance. While the data from some studies provide support for this relationship (e.g., [35]), other studies have questioned it [36]. One complication is that while academic performance relies on cognitive processes, it is also influenced by myriad factors both environmental (e.g., stress, school quality, parental support) and personal (e.g., physical health, intelligence, motivation). Thus, the relationship between underlying cognitive capacities and obesity could be obscured to the extent that such factors either enhance or interfere with a child's capacity to perform well in school. It also appears that physical fitness may be directly related to academic achievement. Therefore, normal-weight children in the population sample may reduce the correlation between body weight and scholastic performance to the extent that some of those children are not physically fit [37].

Obesity has also been linked to impairments in cognitive processes that are outside the normal rubric of executive function or inhibitory control. For example, recent findings indicate that in children 7–9 years old, both body adiposity [38] and self-reported saturated fat intake [39] were negatively correlated with relational memory (i.e., the ability to encode and remember relations [e.g., spatial, temporal, associative] between events). Because relational memory is also thought to rely on brain substrates that are anatomically distinct from those that appear to underlie executive function, these results suggest that obesity and diets associated with obesity may have an even broader impact on childhood cognitive and neural functioning than recognized previously.

CHILDHOOD OBESITY AND THE BRAIN

BRAIN DEVELOPMENT AND OBESITY

As indicated previously, research on the PFC has focused primarily on its role in executive function, whereas the hippocampus has largely been seen as a substrate for certain types of memory (e.g., episodic, contextual, relational, spatial). However, more recent work has identified both memory and inhibitory control functions that involve PFC and hippocampal integration [32,40]. It should not be surprising, then, that the PFC and the hippocampus have both been implicated in the cognitive/inhibitory control of food intake, and both show functional deficits in obese subjects [4,41,42].

During childhood, the brain undergoes pronounced neural proliferation, pruning, myelination, and synaptic organization [43,44]. In humans, the PFC is among the last regions to mature [45]. Interestingly, PFC development appears to be regulated at least in part by the hippocampus. Ventral hippocampal lesions during the neonatal period can induce myriad neural complications in the PFC of both rodents and primates [46,47]. These lesions are also associated with disruptions in ingestive behaviors, including increased meal duration and cumulative intake of a single food, and a distinct lack of sensory-specific satiety in the form of a rebound increase in novel food intake [48].

Perinatal lesions are rare and therefore unlikely to account for widespread increases in childhood obesity. However, there is evidence that brain pathologies may arise in response to normal events that are encountered at many stages of development. For example, prenatal stress exposure reduces hippocampal neurogenesis (which is thought to be required for adaptive memory functioning) throughout the lifespan, compromises hippocampal-dependent spatial learning [49], and increases susceptibility to diet-induced obesity [50].

DIET, OBESITY, AND BRAIN PATHOLOGY

Obesity and the Western diet have been associated with signs of structural and functional brain abnormalities that are found across the lifespan in both human and nonhuman animals. Neuroimaging studies have reported that high body adiposity in humans is accompanied by gray matter atrophy, although there is disagreement on the specific brain areas that are most affected (see [51] for a review). In adolescents, higher adiposity is predictive of reduced gray-matter volume in the PFC, which is associated with impaired cognitive function. For example, Maayan et al. [29] reported that obese adolescents scored significantly higher on measures of disinhibited eating, lower on tests of executive function, and exhibited reduced orbitofrontal cortex (a subregion of the PFC) volume compared with normal-weight controls. Another study found gray-matter volume to be reduced in the left hippocampus [52] of obese 6- to 8-year-old children.

Adult rats maintained on the Western diet develop hippocampal-dependent cognitive deficits and exhibit a cluster of symptoms consistent with neurodegenerative syndromes, including reductions in hippocampal brain-derived neurotrophic factor (BDNF; a protein involved with the growth, maturation, differentiation, and maintenance of neurons), perturbations in synaptic plasticity, nutrient transporter deficiencies, neuroinflammation, blood–brain barrier (BBB) breakdown, and impairments in hippocampal-dependent learning and memory processes [4,42,53].

Other evidence suggests that the pathology produced by the Western diet emerges early in development. Juvenile rats fed the Western diet for 2 months showed impairments in spatial reference memory in the Morris water maze and an elevated hippocampal inflammatory response [54]. In another study, 9-week-old mice were fed the Western diet until they were 24 weeks old, then returned to standard chow, which normalized their body weights [55]. At week 85, or 61 weeks following cessation of the Western diet, mice showed significant impairments in Morris water maze acquisition latency and performance, and reduced contextual fear conditioning. At week 90, these effects of the Western diet were accompanied by increased signs of inflammation and significant reductions in hippocampal gene expression for BDNF.

There are concerns that juvenile-onset diet- or obesity-induced brain pathologies may persist throughout the lifespan and lead to the development of more serious brain disease and cognitive dementias much later in life. A recent report from the Alzheimer's Association identified obesity at midlife and its associated metabolic factors as the primary modifiable risk of developing dementia [56]. Thus, preventing childhood obesity may be critical for preventing not only adult obesity but also more serious late-life cognitive disorders.

WESTERN DIET AND THE BLOOD–BRAIN BARRIER

Normal brain function depends on the stability of the neuronal microenvironment. The BBB regulates the chemical milieu of the brain, eliminating "noise" and prohibiting the entry of potentially neurotoxic humoral substances. Composed of neurovascular endothelial cells linked by tight-junction proteins, supported by astrocytes and pericytes, and reinforced by an enzymatic barrier, the BBB precludes most molecules from entering the brain interstitial fluid [57].

The integrity of the hippocampal BBB is compromised for obese rats maintained on the Western diet or similar high-energy diets [6]. We have repeatedly observed increases in hippocampal BBB permeability to sodium fluorescein (a small molecule dye that cannot cross an intact BBB) following exposure to the Western diet [58–60]. Furthermore, reductions in the expression of tight-junction proteins in both the BBB and the choroid plexus (which comprises a brain–cerebrospinal fluid barrier) have been reported for rats maintained on the Western diet [60]. In most instances, changes in BBB permeability were observed after 90 days of maintenance on the Western diet, though one study using somewhat older rats detected increases in permeability after just 28 days of diet exposure [59].

In two studies [58,59], significantly increased hippocampal BBB permeability was observed only in rats that gained the most weight and body fat (diet-induced obese rats) on the Western diet compared with rats fed standard low-fat chow. Rats that were more resistant to the obesity-promoting effects of the Western diet (diet-resistant rats) failed to show increased BBB leakage relative to chow-fed controls. Interestingly, these studies also found that diet-induced obese, but not diet-resistant, rats showed impaired performance on behavioral tasks that depend on the functional integrity of the hippocampus, whereas neither group performed worse than chow-fed controls on hippocampal-*independent* learning and memory problems. The results of these studies provide evidence that the Western diet compromises the hippocampal BBB and selectively impairs hippocampal-dependent cognitive functioning.

Even subtle damage to the BBB may set the stage for neurodegeneration by permitting the influx of harmful substances into the brain interstitial fluid. Accordingly, individuals who consume the Western diet may be more vulnerable to the harmful effects of environmental contaminants (e.g., air pollution, pesticides, bisphenol A, lead) and therefore at increased risk of developing hippocampal and other brain pathologies that lead to cognitive impairment. Although definitive data does not yet exist, it is plausible that the BBB in children and adolescents is also vulnerable to the adverse effects of the Western diet and/or obesity. The extent to which impaired PFC and hippocampal function is based on a weakening of the BBB that occurs as a consequence of childhood obesity and exposure to the Western diet is an important open research question.

POTENTIAL VICIOUS CYCLE OF OBESITY AND COGNITIVE DECLINE

Based on findings such as those described previously, we have proposed that consuming the Western diet may initiate a *vicious cycle* in which cognitive processes that are involved in the inhibition of intake are impaired as a result of pathologies that develop in brain areas that serve as substrates for those processes [61]. Our current environment is rich with high–energy palatable foods and beverages, and cues that entice us to eat and drink are abundant. A reduced capacity to resist such environmental enticements would lead to increased intake, resulting in weight gain and further deterioration of brain substrates underlying the cognitive inhibition of eating and drinking, thereby resulting in progressively more intake, weight gain, and neurodegeneration (see Figure 24.1).

How might this vicious cycle begin? Reminiscent of ideas expressed previously in Schachter's 1968 externality theory [62], it seems reasonable that the capacity of environmental cues to evoke eating is countered by physiological "satiety signals" arising from one's internal milieu. One way that satiety signals promote inhibitory function is by informing animals that their energy needs have been met and that either the continuation or the initiation of intake will have nonrewarding and even aversive postingestive consequences. Recent research in our laboratory by Sample et al. [63] suggests that intake of the Western diet reduces the ability of rats to use their interoceptive satiety cues to control their appetitive behavior, while leaving control by external food-related cues relatively intact. In that study, rats maintained on standard chow were first trained to use different levels of food deprivation (internal cues corresponding to hunger and satiety) as discriminative signals for the delivery of sucrose pellets. After asymptotic discrimination performance was achieved, half of the rats were shifted to the Western diet and half remained on chow. When discrimination performance was tested 42 days later, results showed that maintenance on the Western diet weakened the rats' ability to use their interoceptive "hunger" cues to solve the discrimination, whereas chow-fed rats were unimpaired. However, when external cues (tones, lights) were introduced along with the interoceptive cues and trained as discriminative stimuli, both diet groups showed comparable and

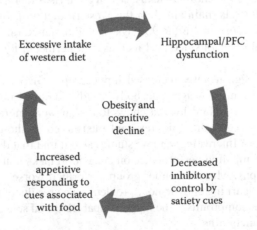

FIGURE 24.1 The "vicious cycle" model of obesity and cognitive decline. (Adapted from Davidson, T.L., et al., *Neurobiol Learn Mem.*, 108, 172–84, 2014; Kanoski, S.E., and Davidson, T.L., *Physiol Behav.*, 103[1], 59–68, 2011.)

significant discriminative responding. In a final test, when the external stimuli were removed, rats fed the Western diet were once again unable to solve the discrimination. This outcome indicated that the Western diet did not have strong global or nonspecific effects (e.g., sensory, motivational) on performance or learning, but selectively impacted rats' ability to utilize internal state cues to guide their food-oriented behavior.

These results indicate that intake of the Western diet reduces rats' ability to use interoceptive cues but spares their ability to use environmental cues for control of behavior. A similar degradation of sensitivity to interoceptive cues was reported for obese human adolescents. Mata et al. [64] found that for overweight but not normal-weight adolescents, activation of the insula, a brain area thought to be important for the detection of interoceptive stimulation, was positively correlated with external eating and negatively correlated with sensitivity to interoceptive cues (in this case heart rate monitoring). This finding suggests that excess weight may be related to neurocognitive adaptations that interfere more with the utilization of interceptive stimuli than with external cues. Considered together, the results reported by Sample et al. and Mata et al. are consistent with the hypothesis that interference with the utilization of internal satiety cues represents an early loss of inhibitory control in a vicious cycle of obesity and cognitive decline.

CONCLUSIONS

In children and adolescents, obesity and the Western diet are associated with cognitive impairments in inhibitory and executive-like processes. These deficits can increase a child's susceptibility to memory deficits, distractions, and impulsivity, thereby interfering with normal cognitive development. Moreover, these inhibitory deficits can promote excess intake by making children more responsive to food and food cues. In addition, considerable evidence from humans and rodents link obesity and the intake of a Western diet to abnormalities (e.g., inflammation, atrophy, BBB disruption) in brain areas that are known to be important substrates for these cognitive processes (e.g., PFC, hippocampus). Beginning in childhood, a vicious cycle of diet-induced deterioration of brain function and inhibitory control could set the stage not only for adult obesity but also for serious cognitive decline much later in life.

REFERENCES

1. Estrada E, Eneli I, Hampl S, Mietus-Snyder M, Mirza N, Rhodes E, et al. Children's Hospital Association consensus statements for comorbidities of childhood obesity. *Child Obes.* 2014;10(4):304–17.
2. Pulgaron ER. Childhood obesity: A review of increased risk for physical and psychological comorbidities. *Clin Ther.* 2013;35(1):A18–32.
3. Barton M. Childhood obesity: A life-long health risk. *Acta Pharmacol Sin.* 2012;33(2):189–93.
4. Kanoski SE, Davidson TL. Western diet consumption and cognitive impairment: Links to hippocampal dysfunction and obesity. *Physiol Behav.* 2011;103(1):59–68.
5. Popkin BM. The world is fat. *Sci Am.* 2007;297(3):88–95.
6. Freeman LR, Haley-Zitlin V, Rosenberger DS, Granholm AC. Damaging effects of a high-fat diet to the brain and cognition: A review of proposed mechanisms. *Nutr Neurosci.* 2014;17(6):241–51.
7. Stranahan AM. Models and mechanisms for hippocampal dysfunction in obesity and diabetes. *Neuroscience.* 2015;309:125–39.
8. Reinert KR, Po'e FK, Barkin SL. The relationship between executive function and obesity in children and adolescents: A systematic literature review. *J Obes.* 2013;2013:820956.
9. Diamond A. Executive functions. *Annu Rev Psychol.* 2013;64:135–68.
10. Luna B. Developmental changes in cognitive control through adolescence. *Adv Child Dev Behav.* 2009;37:233–78.
11. Houghton G, Tipper SP. Inhibitory mechanisms of neural and cognitive control: Applications to selective attention and sequential action. *Brain Cogn.* 1996;30(1):20–43.
12. Storm BC, Levy BJ. A progress report on the inhibitory account of retrieval-induced forgetting. *Mem Cognit.* 2012;40(6):827–43.

13. Schwartz DH, Leonard G, Perron M, Richer L, Syme C, Veillette S, et al. Visceral fat is associated with lower executive functioning in adolescents. *Int J Obes (Lond)*. 2013;37(10):1336–43.

14. Verdejo-Garcia A, Perez-Exposito M, Schmidt-Rio-Valle J, Fernandez-Serrano MJ, Cruz F, Perez-Garcia M, et al. Selective alterations within executive functions in adolescents with excess weight. *Obesity (Silver Spring)*. 2010;18(8):1572–8.

15. Cserjesi R, Molnar D, Luminet O, Lenard L. Is there any relationship between obesity and mental flexibility in children? *Appetite*. 2007;49(3):675–8.

16. Friedman NP, Haberstick BC, Willcutt EG, Miyake A, Young SE, Corley RP, et al. Greater attention problems during childhood predict poorer executive functioning in late adolescence. *Psychol Sci*. 2007;18(10):893–900.

17. Epstein LH, Dearing KK, Temple JL, Cavanaugh MD. Food reinforcement and impulsivity in overweight children and their parents. *Eat Behav*. 2008;9(3):319–27.

18. Johnson WG, Parry W, Drabman RS. The performance of obese and normal size children on a delay of gratification task. *Addict Behav*. 1978;3(3–4):205–8.

19. Wirt T, Hundsdorfer V, Schreiber A, Kesztyus D, Steinacker JM. Associations between inhibitory control and body weight in German primary school children. *Eat Behav*. 2014;15(1):9–12.

20. Martin AA, Davidson TL. Human cognitive function and the obesogenic environment. *Physiol Behav*. 2014;136:185–93.

21. Folkvord F, Anschutz DJ, Nederkoorn C, Westerik H, Buijzen M. Impulsivity, "advergames," and food intake. *Pediatrics*. 2014;133(6):1007–12.

22. Bruce AS, Martin LE, Savage CR. Neural correlates of pediatric obesity. *Prev Med*. 2011;52(Suppl. 1):S29–35.

23. Scholten EW, Schrijvers CT, Nederkoorn C, Kremers SP, Rodenburg G. Relationship between impulsivity, snack consumption and children's weight. *PLoS One*. 2014;9(2):e88851.

24. Pieper JR, Laugero KD. Preschool children with lower executive function may be more vulnerable to emotional-based eating in the absence of hunger. *Appetite*. 2013;62:103–9.

25. Guxens M, Mendez MA, Julvez J, Plana E, Forns J, Basagana X, et al. Cognitive function and overweight in preschool children. *Am J Epidemiol*. 2009;170(4):438–46.

26. Nederkoorn C, Jansen E, Mulkens S, Jansen A. Impulsivity predicts treatment outcome in obese children. *Behav Res Ther*. 2007;45(5):1071–5.

27. Schlam TR, Wilson NL, Shoda Y, Mischel W, Ayduk O. Preschoolers' delay of gratification predicts their body mass 30 years later. *J Pediatr*. 2013;162(1):90–3.

28. Nederkoorn C, Braet C, Van Eijs Y, Tanghe A, Jansen A. Why obese children cannot resist food: The role of impulsivity. *Eat Behav*. 2006;7(4):315–22.

29. Maayan L, Hoogendoorn C, Sweat V, Convit A. Disinhibited eating in obese adolescents is associated with orbitofrontal volume reductions and executive dysfunction. *Obesity (Silver Spring)*. 2011;19(7):1382–7.

30. Davids S, Lauffer H, Thoms K, Jagdhuhn M, Hirschfeld H, Domin M, et al. Increased dorsolateral prefrontal cortex activation in obese children during observation of food stimuli. *Int J Obes (Lond)*. 2010;34(1):94–104.

31. Bruce AS, Lepping RJ, Bruce JM, Cherry JB, Martin LE, Davis AM, et al. Brain responses to food logos in obese and healthy weight children. *J Pediatr*. 2013;162(4):759–64.e2.

32. Wimber M, Rutschmann RM, Greenlee MW, Bauml KH. Retrieval from episodic memory: Neural mechanisms of interference resolution. *J Cogn Neurosci*. 2009;21(3):538–49.

33. Chudasama Y, Doobay VM, Liu Y. Hippocampal-prefrontal cortical circuit mediates inhibitory response control in the rat. *J Neurosci*. 2012;32(32):10915–24.

34. Miller AL, Lee HJ, Lumeng JC. Obesity-associated biomarkers and executive function in children. *Pediatr Res*. 2015;77(1–2):143–7.

35. Torrijos-Nino C, Martinez-Vizcaino V, Pardo-Guijarro MJ, Garcia-Prieto JC, Arias-Palencia NM, Sanchez-Lopez M. Physical fitness, obesity, and academic achievement in schoolchildren. *J Pediatr*. 2014;165(1):104–9.

36. Baxter SD, Guinn CH, Tebbs JM, Royer JA. There is no relationship between academic achievement and body mass index among fourth-grade, predominantly African-American children. *J Acad Nutr Diet*. 2013;113(4):551–7.

37. Burkhalter TM, Hillman CH. A narrative review of physical activity, nutrition, and obesity to cognition and scholastic performance across the human lifespan. *Adv Nutr*. 2011;2(2):201S–6S.

38. Khan NA, Baym CL, Monti JM, Raine LB, Drollette ES, Scudder MR, et al. Central adiposity is negatively associated with hippocampal-dependent relational memory among overweight and obese children. *J Pediatr*. 2015;166(2):302–8.e1.

39. Baym CL, Khan NA, Monti JM, Raine LB, Drollette ES, Moore RD, et al. Dietary lipids are differentially associated with hippocampal-dependent relational memory in prepubescent children. *Am J Clin Nutr.* 2014;99(5):1026–32.
40. Preston AR, Eichenbaum H. Interplay of hippocampus and prefrontal cortex in memory. *Curr Biol.* 2013;23(17):R764–73.
41. Batterink L, Yokum S, Stice E. Body mass correlates inversely with inhibitory control in response to food among adolescent girls: An fMRI study. *Neuroimage.* 2010;52(4):1696–703.
42. Hargrave SL, Davidson TL, Lee TJ, Kinzig KP. Brain and behavioral perturbations in rats following Western diet access. *Appetite.* 2015;93:35–43.
43. Bourgeois JP, Goldman-Rakic PS, Rakic P. Synaptogenesis in the prefrontal cortex of rhesus monkeys. *Cereb Cortex.* 1994;4(1):78–96.
44. Huttenlocher PR. Synaptic density in human frontal cortex: Developmental changes and effects of aging. *Brain Res.* 1979;163(2):195–205.
45. Casey BJ, Giedd JN, Thomas KM. Structural and functional brain development and its relation to cognitive development. *Biol Psychol.* 2000;54(1–3):241–57.
46. Lipska BK, Khaing ZZ, Weickert CS, Weinberger DR. BDNF mRNA expression in rat hippocampus and prefrontal cortex: Effects of neonatal ventral hippocampal damage and antipsychotic drugs. *Eur J Neurosci.* 2001;14(1):135–44.
47. O'Donnell P, Lewis BL, Weinberger DR, Lipska BK. Neonatal hippocampal damage alters electrophysiological properties of prefrontal cortical neurons in adult rats. *Cereb Cortex.* 2002;12(9):975–82.
48. Macedo CE, Angst MJ, Gobaille S, Schleef C, Guignard B, Guiberteau T, et al. Prefrontal dopamine release and sensory-specific satiety altered in rats with neonatal ventral hippocampal lesions. *Behav Brain Res.* 2012;231(1):97–104.
49. Lemaire V, Koehl M, Le Moal M, Abrous DN. Prenatal stress produces learning deficits associated with an inhibition of neurogenesis in the hippocampus. *Proc Natl Acad Sci USA.* 2000;97(20):11032–7.
50. Li J, Olsen J, Vestergaard M, Obel C, Baker JL, Sorensen TI. Prenatal stress exposure related to maternal bereavement and risk of childhood overweight. *PLoS One.* 2010;5(7):e11896.
51. Willette AA, Kapogiannis D. Does the brain shrink as the waist expands? *Ageing Res Rev.* 2015;20:86–97.
52. Bauer CC, Moreno B, Gonzalez-Santos L, Concha L, Barquera S, Barrios FA. Child overweight and obesity are associated with reduced executive cognitive performance and brain alterations: A magnetic resonance imaging study in Mexican children. *Pediatr Obes.* 2015;10(3):196–204.
53. Freeman LR, Granholm AC. Vascular changes in rat hippocampus following a high saturated fat and cholesterol diet. *J Cereb Blood Flow Metab.* 2012;32(4):643–53.
54. Boitard C, Cavaroc A, Sauvant J, Aubert A, Castanon N, Laye S, et al. Impairment of hippocampal-dependent memory induced by juvenile high-fat diet intake is associated with enhanced hippocampal inflammation in rats. *Brain Behav Immun.* 2014;40:9–17.
55. Dong W, Wang R, Ma LN, Xu BL, Zhang JS, Zhao ZW, et al. Influence of age-related learning and memory capacity of mice: Different effects of a high and low caloric diet. *Aging Clin Exp Res.* 2015;28:303–11.
56. Baumgart M, Snyder HM, Carrillo MC, Fazio S, Kim H, Johns H. Summary of the evidence on modifiable risk factors for cognitive decline and dementia: A population-based perspective. *Alzheimers Dement.* 2015;11(6):718–26.
57. Abbott NJ, Friedman A. Overview and introduction: The blood–brain barrier in health and disease. *Epilepsia.* 2012;53(Suppl. 6):1–6.
58. Davidson TL, Hargrave SL, Swithers SE, Sample CH, Fu X, Kinzig KP, et al. Inter-relationships among diet, obesity and hippocampal-dependent cognitive function. *Neuroscience.* 2013;253:110–22.
59. Davidson TL, Monnot A, Neal AU, Martin AA, Horton JJ, Zheng W. The effects of a high-energy diet on hippocampal-dependent discrimination performance and blood–brain barrier integrity differ for diet-induced obese and diet-resistant rats. *Physiol Behav.* 2012;107:26–33.
60. Kanoski SE, Zhang Y, Zheng W, Davidson TL. The effects of a high-energy diet on hippocampal function and blood–brain barrier integrity in the rat. *J Alzheimers Dis.* 2010;21:207–19.
61. Davidson TL, Sample CH, Swithers SE. An application of Pavlovian principles to the problems of obesity and cognitive decline. *Neurobiol Learn Mem.* 2014;108:172–84.
62. Schachter S. Obesity and eating: Internal and external cues differentially affect the eating behavior of obese and normal subjects. *Science.* 1968;161(3843):751–6.
63. Sample CH, Martin AA, Jones S, Hargrave SL, Davidson TL. Western-style diet impairs stimulus control by food deprivation state cues: Implications for obesogenic environments. *Appetite.* 2015;93:13–23.
64. Mata F, Verdejo-Roman J, Soriano-Mas C, Verdejo-Garcia A. Insula tuning towards external eating versus interoceptive input in adolescents with overweight and obesity. *Appetite.* 2015;93:24–30.

25 Insulin Resistance and Type 2 Diabetes in Pediatric Populations

Nicola Santoro and Sonia Caprio

CONTENTS

INTRODUCTION

The prevalence of childhood obesity has progressively increased in the last four decades [1]. In 2010, it was estimated that 43 million children were overweight worldwide, and this number is expected to increase up to 60 million by 2020 [1]. This increase in pediatric obesity is accompanied by an increased prevalence of type 2 diabetes (T2D) in adolescents [2]. T2D usually occurs after 10 years of age, after the onset of puberty, with an incidence estimated between 7.0 and 49.4 per 100,000 person-years in subjects between 10 and 19 years of age in the United States [2]. Recent data indicate that in the United States in 2010 about 20,000 subjects below the age of 20 showed T2D and that this number may increase up to ~84,000 by 2050 [3]. In this chapter, we will discuss the current knowledge and the future perspectives concerning the pathophysiology and therapy of pediatric T2D.

DEFINITION OF TYPE 2 DIABETES AND PREDIABETES

According to American Diabetes Association (ADA) criteria, T2D is defined as fasting plasma glucose levels higher than 125 mg/dL or plasma glucose levels higher than 200 mg/dL 2 hours after an oral glucose tolerance test (OGTT), while impaired glucose tolerance (IGT) is defined as when plasma glucose levels are higher than 140 mg/dL after an OGTT [4] (Table 25.1). Along with IGT, another prediabetic state has been defined: impaired fasting glucose (IFG). IFG is defined as serum fasting glucose levels between 100 and 125 mg/dL [4] (Table 25.1). Epidemiological studies indicate that IFG and IGT are two distinct categories of glucose tolerance that overlap only to a very limited extent in children [5]. Recently, the ADA has published recommendations to use hemoglobin A1c (HbA1c) to diagnose diabetes [4]. In particular, it has suggested a cutoff point of 6.5% to diagnose T2D. This cutoff point was chosen on the basis of cross-sectional and longitudinal studies

TABLE 25.1

Criteria for Diagnosis of Prediabetes and Diabetes

Criteria for Diagnosis of Increased Risk for Diabetes (Prediabetes)	Criteria for Diagnosis of Diabetes
HbA1c 5.7%–6.4%	HbA1c ≥6.5%
Fasting plasma glucose ≥100 mg/dL: IFG	Fasting plasma glucose ≥126 mg/dL
2-hour plasma glucose ≥140 mg/dL: IGT	2-hour plasma glucose ≥200 mg/dL
	Random plasma glucose ≥200 mg/dL in patients with symptoms

Source:　Criteria for the diagnosis of type 2 diabetes and prediabetes according to the American Diabetes Association. Imperatore G et al., *Diabetes Care*, 2012;35(12):2515–20.

Note:　IFG, impaired fasting glucose; IGT, impaired glucose tolerance.

conducted in adults showing that it identifies about one-third of cases of undiagnosed diabetes and that subjects with HbA1c higher than that cutoff show higher prevalence of microvascular complications in the long term [6]. Subjects with HbA1c between 5.7% and 6.4% are identified as being "at increased risk of diabetes" [4]. It has to be noted that the measure of 2-hour glucose and the measure of HbA1c are not mutually exclusive as diagnostic tools of diabetes; in fact, there is little agreement between them [7]. Thus, for a correct diagnosis and to avoid missing some patients it would be useful to measure them both.

LINK BETWEEN OBESITY AND T2D: ECTOPIC FAT ACCUMULATION

Obesity-related ectopic fat accumulation in key insulin-sensitive organs such as skeletal muscles and the liver causes alterations of the insulin-signaling pathway, leading to increased insulin resistance, characterized by defects in the nonoxidative pathway of glucose metabolism, higher intramyocellular lipid content, and higher visceral and hepatic fat content [8]. Fat accumulation in the liver is an important trigger of insulin resistance and its severity is associated with the presence of prediabetes in adolescents [9]. Recent studies in obese children and adolescents have elucidated the effect of hepatic steatosis on insulin sensitivity and metabolic syndrome. In a multiethnic group of 118 obese adolescents, Cali et al. observed that, independent of obesity, the severity of fatty liver was associated with the presence of prediabetes (IGT and IFG/IGT) [9] (Figure 25.1). Paralleling the severity of hepatic steatosis, there was a significant decrease in insulin sensitivity and impairment in beta cell function, as indicated by the fall in the disposition index [9]. Moreover, the authors observed that, paralleling the severity of fatty liver, there was a significant increase in the prevalence of the metabolic syndrome, suggesting that hepatic steatosis may be a predictive factor of metabolic syndrome in children [9] (Figure 25.1). Importantly, in obese adolescents the negative effect of fatty liver on insulin sensitivity is independent of the degree of visceral fat and intramyocellular lipid content [10]. A longitudinal study has shown that baseline hepatic fat content correlates with 2-hour glucose, insulin sensitivity, and insulin secretion at 2 years follow-up [11]. These data indicate that intrahepatic fat accumulation is more deleterious than ectopic fat accumulation elsewhere in the body [12].

PUBERTY AND ETHNICITY AS MAJOR RISK FACTORS FOR T2D IN CHILDREN

T2D usually manifests during puberty together with a peak of transient insulin resistance, probably as a consequence of the rise in growth hormone [13,14]. Previous data suggest that insulin resistance during puberty is restricted to peripheral glucose metabolism and that selective insulin resistance leading to compensatory hyperinsulinemia may serve to amplify insulin's effect on amino acid metabolism, thereby facilitating protein anabolism during this period of rapid growth [15]. Gender

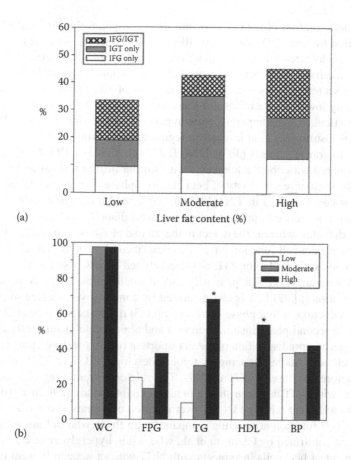

FIGURE 25.1 (a) Prevalence of prediabetes in obese adolescents according to the degree of liver fat content (%) measured by fast magnetic resonance imaging (MRI). The prevalence rates of impaired glucose regulation (IFG, IGT, IFG/IGT) tended to rise across tertiles (p for trend = .07). (b) Prevalence rate of each component of the metabolic syndrome (Ford's criteria) according to the degree of liver fat content (%) measured by fast MRI. There were no differences in waist circumference (WC), fasting plasma glucose (FPG), or blood pressure (BP) across categories. The prevalence rates for triglycerides (TG) and large high-density lipoprotein (L-HDL) levels showed significant differences between low liver fat content and the remaining groups (p = .000). p values were adjusted for age, gender, and race/ethnicity. White box = low liver fat content; light gray = moderate liver fat content; dark gray = high liver fat content. (Reproduced with permission of John Wiley and Sons: license no. 3646730552564, released 06/12/2015. From Cali, A.M., et al., *Hepatology*, 49, 1896–903, 2009.)

and ethnicity represent additional risk factors. In fact, African American, Hispanic, Asian/Pacific Islander, and American Indian adolescents have a much higher incidence and prevalence of T2D than non-Hispanic whites, and this is independent of any ethnic difference in overall adiposity or fat distribution [2]. Within each ethnic group, girls show a higher risk than boys, which could be because adolescent girls experience a more severe degree of insulin resistance than boys [2].

BETA CELL IMPAIRMENT AS A KEY DETERMINANT OF TYPE 2 DIABETES DEVELOPMENT

The relationship between insulin demand and secretion is a key factor regulating the maintenance of NGT. In fact, the beta cell response to insulin resistance results in hyperinsulinemia, which is needed to maintain normal glucose levels. In the long term, however, beta cell function tends to deteriorate and insulin secretion may not be sufficient to maintain glucose levels within the normal range [16]. The deterioration of beta cells occurs faster in youth than in adults; in fact, while in adults the transition toward T2D takes about 10 years with an ~7%-per-year reduction in beta cell function, in obese adolescents beta cells deteriorate at a rate of ~20%–30% per year [17], with a mean transition time from prediabetes to overt diabetes of about 2.5 years [18].

When insulin secretion is estimated in the context of the "resistant milieu," IGT subjects show a significantly lower degree of insulin secretion than a group with normal glucose tolerance (NGT) [19]. In particular, using hyperglycemic hyperinsulinemic clamp studies, Weiss et al. investigated the role of insulin secretion in glucose regulation in a group of 62 obese adolescents with different glucose tolerance statuses (30 with NGT, 22 with IGT, and 10 with T2D) [19]. This study showed that, compared with obese adolescents with similar insulin resistance, those with IGT have a progressive loss of glucose sensitivity of beta cell first-phase secretion and that beta cell second-phase secretion is compromised in T2D [19]. This observation recognizes that the decline of the first phase of insulin secretion is present before the overt diabetes and that it may be considered a fingerprint of prediabetes, whereas the defect in the second phase is required for the development of T2D. Differences in beta cell function have been described in various prediabetic conditions seen in obese adolescents, such as IFG or IGT, or the combined IFG/IGT states. Cali et al. documented that in obese adolescents (1) IFG is primarily linked to alterations in glucose sensitivity of first-phase insulin secretion [5], (2) IGT is characterized by a more severe degree of peripheral insulin resistance and a reduction in first-phase secretion, and (3) the co-occurrence of IFG and IGT is the result of a defect in second-phase insulin secretion and of profound insulin resistance [5].

The idea that genetic predisposition plays an important role in the development of pediatric T2D is supported by clinical studies showing that youth developing IGT or T2D show a lower insulin secretion even before the onset of IGT or T2D. The role of a *preexisting* beta cell dysfunction in obese adolescents with NGT has been shown in a longitudinal study [20]. In a group of obese NGT adolescents who underwent repeated OGTT over a period of 3 years, those who progressed to IGT had a lower beta cell function at baseline compared with those who did not progress. These data have recently been confirmed by Giannini et al., who, using hyperglycemic clamp studies, showed an early impairment of beta cells in subjects with NGT who subsequently went on to develop IGT or T2D [16].

COMPLICATIONS OF PEDIATRIC TYPE 2 DIABETES

Microalbuminuria and hypertension have been reported in cross-sectional studies in youth with T2D [21,22]. Hypertension is present in 11.6% of youth with T2D, but this number increases to 33.8% about 3.9 years after the diagnosis [23], with males showing a much higher risk than females of developing hypertension [23].

The prevalence of retinopathy in youth with T2D has been estimated at around 13.7% [24], similar to adult data from the Diabetes Prevention Program (12.6% after 3 years of T2D) [25]. A higher prevalence of retinopathy has been observed in subjects with older age, a longer duration of diabetes, and poorer glycemic control [24].

Microalbuminuria is usually seen in about 6% of youth with T2D, but this increases by about three times approximately 3.9 years after the diagnosis [23]. Moreover, an elevation of HbA1c level is strongly correlated with microalbuminuria, with every 1% increase in HbA1c level increasing the risk of microalbuminuria by 17% [23].

Along with microvascular complications, macrovascular issues are already present in youth with T2D. In fact, pediatric T2D is associated with an abnormal vascular stiffness, as measured by aortic pulse wave velocity [26]. In the SEARCH for Diabetes in Youth study, 43% of youth with poorly controlled T2D had a low-density lipoprotein cholesterol level higher than 130 mg/dL, and 40% had a triglyceride level greater than 200 mg/dL [27]. These data clearly indicate that complications of T2D are already present in the pediatric population and that their degree of severity might progress much faster than in adults.

GENETIC STUDIES IN PEDIATRIC PREDIABETES AND TYPE 2 DIABETES

So far, several genome-wide association studies (GWAS) have helped to highlight the genetic bases of T2D, and several single-nucleotide polymorphisms (SNPs) have been discovered to be associated with T2D [36]. The majority of them are intronic or nearby a gene and only a few of them are missense mutations (such as rs1801282 in PPAR-gamma, characterized by a C-to-G substitution encoding a proline-to-alanine substitution at codon 12) [37]. The majority of gene variants associated with T2D are in genes expressed in beta cells. Because of the lack of very large pediatric cohorts, the majority of GWAS have been conducted in adults and information on the genetics of T2D in youth is limited to few studies. Recently, Dabelea et al. genotyped the rs12255372 and rs7903146 variants in/or near the *TCF7L2* gene in a multiethnic cohort of 1239 youths (240 cases and 999 controls) enrolled in the SEARCH study, and observed that in African Americans the rs7903146 variant was associated with an almost twofold increase in odds of showing T2D [28]. Barker et al. genotyped 16 SNPs, previously found to be associated with diabetes by GWAS, in 6000 children and adolescents and determined whether they were also associated with fasting glucose levels [29]. The authors observed that nine loci were associated with fasting glucose levels; in particular, they confirmed five previously discovered SNPs and discovered four more loci associated with fasting glucose.

More recently, it has been shown that common variants in or near genes modulating insulin secretion are associated with a higher risk of developing prediabetes and T2D in youth [30]. In particular, Giannini et al. have shown that the co-occurrence of risk alleles in or near genes expressed in beta cells is associated with a defect of insulin secretion, resulting, in conditions of extreme insulin resistance, in the development of prediabetes and T2D [30]. Similarly, Zheng et al. have observed that genetic variants in the *MTNR1B* gene, which is involved in modulating fasting glucose levels, are associated with the development of IFG and IGT [31]. These observations support the theory that a predisposed genetic background is associated with the onset of prediabetes and T2D at a lower age.

Despite the strength of these associations, the portion of heritability explained by the identified loci has been estimated to be around 10%. Although the sample size of GWAS continues to increase, revealing new associations, each newly associated variant has an incrementally smaller effect size and contributes only marginally to the cumulative variation of the phenotype. GWAS may be reaching the limits of their ability to reveal genetic variations underlying complex traits, and additional genetic variations, such as rare variants with large individual effects, may contribute to the heritability of complex traits such as T2D. Therefore, very recently, it has been proposed that rare variants may explain the *missing heritability* of T2D.

THERAPEUTIC STRATEGIES FOR YOUTH WITH TYPE 2 DIABETES

In the pediatric population, only two drugs are approved for the therapy of T2D—insulin and metformin—and the best approach to this disease in the pediatric population remains unclear. Recently, the pediatric trial Treatment Options for Type 2 Diabetes in Adolescents and Youth (TODAY) was completed [32]. The TODAY study was a 15-center clinical trial, sponsored by the National Institute of Diabetes and Digestive and Kidney Diseases, that examined the efficacy of three approaches to the treatment of T2D in youth: metformin alone, metformin plus rosiglitazone, and metformin plus an intensive lifestyle intervention called the TODAY Lifestyle Program [32]. The authors studied 699 subjects between 10 and 17 years of age; the patients were randomized to each arm and followed up for about 3.86 years. Although the rate of failure in each arm was quite high (51.7% metformin alone, 38.6% metformin plus rosiglitazone, 46.6% metformin plus lifestyle), treatment with metformin and rosiglitazone was more effective in maintaining glycemic control than the treatment with metformin alone ($p = .006$), and although it seemed to be better also than the metformin and lifestyle treatment, this difference was not statistically significant ($p = .16$) [32]. Interestingly, performing subgroup analyses, the authors observed that metformin alone was less effective in non-Hispanic blacks than in non-Hispanic whites or Hispanics [32].

In general, what is really striking from the TODAY study is the high rate of failure in each arm. As it has been observed [33], this study was dealing with a highly complex population: adolescents with T2D who grew up in a very sedentary environment [32]. The data seem to suggest that any intervention in this population may be extremely challenging, thus more effort should be put into the prevention of obesity and T2D.

More recently, another multicenter effort to assess the best strategy to treat subjects with T2D has started. The Restoring Insulin Secretion (RISE) study, which involves an adult and a pediatric population, is testing interventions designed to preserve or improve beta cell function in prediabetes or early T2D [34]. Although the design has been published, the study is still ongoing and will answer a very important question: can we restore beta cell responsivity in obese kids by using insulin in the early stages of T2D or even in the prediabetic stage?

Although progress has been made over decades toward a better understanding of the pathophysiology of T2D in youth, additional research addressing how certain gene variants modulate pathogenetic mechanisms may advance the current state of knowledge and provide new insights for the prevention and the treatment of T2D in youth. There is an urgent need for novel prevention and intervention strategies to curb youth-onset T2D.

CONCLUSIONS

This overview shows that T2D can be particularly aggressive in youth. Moreover, this is the first generation in which this phenomenon is so diffuse; therefore, longitudinal data showing the long-term natural history of early onset T2D are not available yet. That is why it is important to bear in mind that childhood obesity represents a major problem for public health to be fought not only from a medical point of view but mainly from a political perspective [35,36].

REFERENCES

1. de Onis M, Blossner M, Borghi E. Global prevalence and trends of overweight and obesity among preschool children. *The American Journal of Clinical Nutrition*. 2010;92(5):1257–64.
2. Dabelea D, Mayer-Davis EJ, Saydah S, Imperatore G, Linder B, Divers J, et al. Prevalence of type 1 and type 2 diabetes among children and adolescents from 2001 to 2009. *JAMA: The Journal of the American Medical Association*. 2014;311(17):1778–86.
3. Imperatore G, Boyle JP, Thompson TJ, Case D, Dabelea D, Hamman RF, et al. Projections of type 1 and type 2 diabetes burden in the U.S. population aged <20 years through 2050: Dynamic modeling of incidence, mortality, and population growth. *Diabetes Care*. 2012;35(12):2515–20.
4. American Diabetes Association. Diagnosis and classification of diabetes mellitus. *Diabetes Care*. 2010;33(Suppl. 1):S62–9.
5. Cali AM, Bonadonna RC, Trombetta M, Weiss R, Caprio S. Metabolic abnormalities underlying the different prediabetic phenotypes in obese adolescents. *The Journal of Clinical Endocrinology and Metabolism*. 2008;93(5):1767–73.
6. Selvin E, Steffes MW, Zhu H, Matsushita K, Wagenknecht L, Pankow J, et al. Glycated hemoglobin, diabetes, and cardiovascular risk in nondiabetic adults. *The New England Journal of Medicine*. 2010;362(9):800–11.
7. Nowicka P, Santoro N, Liu H, Lartaud D, Shaw MM, Goldberg R, et al. Utility of hemoglobin A1c for diagnosing prediabetes and diabetes in obese children and adolescents. *Diabetes Care*. 2011;34(6):1306–11.
8. Petersen KF, Dufour S, Savage DB, Bilz S, Solomon G, Yonemitsu S, et al. The role of skeletal muscle insulin resistance in the pathogenesis of the metabolic syndrome. *Proceedings of the National Academy of Sciences of the United States of America*. 2007;104(31):12587–94.
9. Cali AM, De Oliveira AM, Kim H, Chen S, Reyes-Mugica M, Escalera S, et al. Glucose dysregulation and hepatic steatosis in obese adolescents: Is there a link? *Hepatology*. 2009;49(6):1896–903.
10. D'Adamo E, Cali AM, Weiss R, Santoro N, Pierpont B, Northrup V, et al. Central role of fatty liver in the pathogenesis of insulin resistance in obese adolescents. *Diabetes Care*. 2010;33(8):1817–22.
11. Kim G, Giannini C, Pierpont B, Feldstein AE, Santoro N, Kursawe R, et al. Longitudinal effects of MRI-measured hepatic steatosis on biomarkers of glucose homeostasis and hepatic apoptosis in obese youth. *Diabetes Care*. 2013;36(1):130–6.

12. Fabbrini E, Magkos F, Mohammed BS, Pietka T, Abumrad NA, Patterson BW, et al. Intrahepatic fat, not visceral fat, is linked with metabolic complications of obesity. *Proceedings of the National Academy of Sciences of the United States of America.* 2009;106(36):15430–5.

13. Amiel SA, Sherwin RS, Simonson DC, Lauritano AA, Tamborlane WV. Impaired insulin action in puberty: A contributing factor to poor glycemic control in adolescents with diabetes. *The New England Journal of Medicine.* 1986;315(4):215–9.

14. Caprio S, Boulware S, Diamond M, Sherwin RS, Carpenter TO, Rubin K, et al. Insulin resistance: An early metabolic defect of Turner's syndrome. *The Journal of Clinical Endocrinology and Metabolism.* 1991;72(4):832–6.

15. Amiel SA, Caprio S, Sherwin RS, Plewe G, Haymond MW, Tamborlane WV. Insulin resistance of puberty: A defect restricted to peripheral glucose metabolism. *The Journal of Clinical Endocrinology and Metabolism.* 1991;72(2):277–82.

16. Giannini C, Weiss R, Cali A, Bonadonna R, Santoro N, Pierpont B, et al. Evidence for early defects in insulin sensitivity and secretion before the onset of glucose dysregulation in obese youths: A longitudinal study. *Diabetes.* 2012;61(3):606–14.

17. Narasimhan S, Weinstock RS. Youth-onset type 2 diabetes mellitus: Lessons learned from the TODAY study. *Mayo Clinic Proceedings.* 2014;89(6):806–16.

18. Weiss R, Taksali SE, Tamborlane WV, Burgert TS, Savoye M, Caprio S. Predictors of changes in glucose tolerance status in obese youth. *Diabetes Care.* 2005;28(4):902–9.

19. Weiss R, Caprio S, Trombetta M, Taksali SE, Tamborlane WV, Bonadonna R. Beta-cell function across the spectrum of glucose tolerance in obese youth. *Diabetes.* 2005;54(6):1735–43.

20. Cali AM, Man CD, Cobelli C, Dziura J, Seyal A, Shaw M, et al. Primary defects in beta-cell function further exacerbated by worsening of insulin resistance mark the development of impaired glucose tolerance in obese adolescents. *Diabetes Care.* 2009;32(3):456–61.

21. Ettinger LM, Freeman K, DiMartino-Nardi JR, Flynn JT. Microalbuminuria and abnormal ambulatory blood pressure in adolescents with type 2 diabetes mellitus. *The Journal of Pediatrics.* 2005;147(1):67–73.

22. Maahs DM, Snively BM, Bell RA, Dolan L, Hirsch I, Imperatore G, et al. Higher prevalence of elevated albumin excretion in youth with type 2 than type 1 diabetes: The SEARCH for Diabetes in Youth study. *Diabetes Care.* 2007;30(10):2593–8.

23. Treatment Options for Type 2 Diabetes in Adolescents and Youth. Rapid rise in hypertension and nephropathy in youth with type 2 diabetes: The TODAY clinical trial. *Diabetes Care.* 2013;36(6):1735–41.

24. Treatment Options for Type 2 Diabetes in Adolescents and Youth. Retinopathy in youth with type 2 diabetes participating in the TODAY clinical trial. *Diabetes Care.* 2013;36(6):1772–4.

25. Diabetes Prevention Program Research Group. The prevalence of retinopathy in impaired glucose tolerance and recent-onset diabetes in the Diabetes Prevention Program. *Diabetic Medicine: A Journal of the British Diabetic Association.* 2007;24(2):137–44.

26. Davis PH, Dawson JD, Riley WA, Lauer RM. Carotid intimal-medial thickness is related to cardiovascular risk factors measured from childhood through middle age: The Muscatine Study. *Circulation.* 2001;104(23):2815–9.

27. Petitti DB, Imperatore G, Palla SL, Daniels SR, Dolan LM, Kershnar AK, et al. Serum lipids and glucose control: The SEARCH for Diabetes in Youth study. *Archives of Pediatrics & Adolescent Medicine.* 2007;161(2):159–65.

28. Dabelea D, Dolan LM, D'Agostino R, Jr, Hernandez AM, McAteer JB, Hamman RF, et al. Association testing of TCF7L2 polymorphisms with type 2 diabetes in multi-ethnic youth. *Diabetologia.* 2011;54(3):535–9.

29. Barker A, Sharp SJ, Timpson NJ, Bouatia-Naji N, Warrington NM, Kanoni S, et al. Association of genetic Loci with glucose levels in childhood and adolescence: A meta-analysis of over 6,000 children. *Diabetes.* 2011;60(6):1805–12.

30. Giannini C, Dalla Man C, Groop L, Cobelli C, Zhao H, Shaw MM, et al. Co-occurrence of risk alleles in or near genes modulating insulin secretion predisposes obese youth to prediabetes. *Diabetes Care.* 2014;37(2):475–82.

31. Zheng C, Dalla Man C, Cobelli C, Groop L, Zhao H, Bale AE, et al. A common variant in the MTNR1b gene is associated with increased risk of impaired fasting glucose (IFG) in youth with obesity. *Obesity (Silver Spring).* 2015;23(5):1022–9.

32. Zeitler P, Hirst K, Pyle L, Linder B, Copeland K, Arslanian S, et al. A clinical trial to maintain glycemic control in youth with type 2 diabetes. *The New England Journal of Medicine.* 2012;366(24):2247–56.

33. Allen DB. TODAY: A stark glimpse of tomorrow. *The New England Journal of Medicine.* 2012;366(24):2315–6.

34. RISE Consortium. Restoring Insulin Secretion (RISE): Design of studies of beta-cell preservation in prediabetes and early type 2 diabetes across the life span. *Diabetes Care.* 2014;37(3):780–8.

35. Van Name M, Santoro N. Type 2 diabetes mellitus in pediatrics: A new challenge. *World Journal of Pediatrics: WJP.* 2013;9(4):293–9.

36. Franks PW, Pearson E, Florez JC. Gene-environment and gene-treatment interactions in type 2 diabetes: Progress, pitfalls, and prospects. *Diabetes Care.* 2013;36(5):1413–21.

37. Santoro N. Childhood obesity and type 2 diabetes: The frightening epidemic. *World Journal of Pediatrics: WJP.* 2013;9(2):101–2.

26 Childhood Obesity and Cardiovascular Risk

P. Babu Balagopal

CONTENTS

INTRODUCTION

Obesity prevalence in children and adolescents has dramatically increased in the past 30 years [1]. Despite the more vigorous efforts over the last decade to prevent and control obesity, it remains at a disturbingly high state in children and adolescents. The relationship between early body mass index (BMI) and adult cardiovascular disease (CVD) risk is very complex. However, the severity of obesity, its presence for a longer period, and its tracking into adulthood are of concern because adult obesity directly portends and escalates metabolic and cardiovascular consequences. Despite the recent notion of a stabilization of obesity trends in children and adolescents [1], the issue continues to be troubling because of the concerns it raises about accelerated development of type 2 diabetes mellitus (T2DM) and CVD [2–7]. Obese children are, to a large extent, more likely than normal-weight children to become obese adults [8]. What is particularly worrisome is the fast-increasing prevalence of *severe obesity* in children, with an enhanced potential for the development of cardiometabolic diseases at an early age [9]. The central premise of this chapter is to briefly discuss the effect of child obesity on the development of CVD and the role of potential mediators of the relationship between childhood obesity and CVD risk (Figure 26.1). In doing so, the role of dysfunctional adipose tissue and obesity-driven biomarkers (Figure 26.2) that increase CVD risk will also be discussed.

TRACKING OF OBESITY FROM CHILDHOOD TO ADULTHOOD

An imminent risk of clinical events such as coronary heart disease (CHD) death is extremely low among youth. This notion, however, is gradually being modified because of the potential impact of obesity on early derangements in the metabolic framework of children and adolescents. Longitudinal

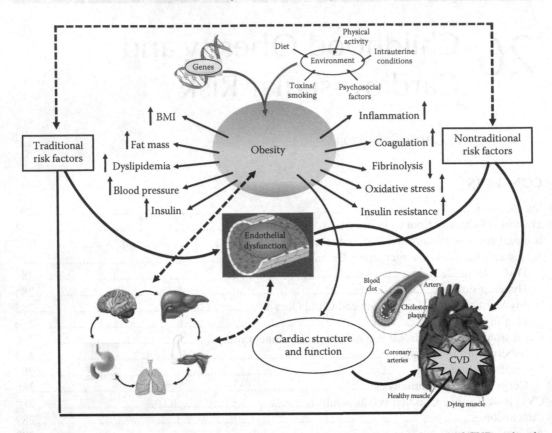

FIGURE 26.1   Overall conceptual framework of obesity-related biomarkers/risk factors of CVD and pathways that lead to CVD.

studies have frequently demonstrated the persistence of childhood obesity into adulthood, with increased risk of adverse consequences in terms of chronic diseases in adulthood, T2DM and CVD being the most ominous [10]. Studies including the Bogalusa Heart Study and the Coronary Artery Risk Development in Young Adults (CARDIA) study have consistently shown the adverse effects of progressive weight gain. Excess weight, once gained, is difficult to manage and tracks into adulthood. Yet, the independent contribution of early obesity to CVD risk remains inconclusive and not explicitly established. The majority of metabolic and cardiovascular complications related to obesity, however, appear to be already present at an early age in the clinical course of obesity. These include unfavorable levels of blood pressure, insulin, high-density lipoprotein cholesterol (HDL-C), low-density lipoprotein (LDL) cholesterol, and triglyceride levels [3,11,12]. More recent studies have reported alterations in various nontraditional risk factors or biomarkers of CVD [7,13]. Cardiac structure and function, including left ventricular hypertrophy (LVH) and excess left ventricular mass relative to cardiac workload, has also been reported to be adversely affected by excess fat mass in children and adolescents [11,14,15].

The risk of obesity-related comorbidities is amplified owing to various factors. The severity of obesity in childhood and its duration and persistence over many years are crucial factors that are involved in the progression of obesity to overt CVD [16]. More than two decades of obesity duration doubled the mortality risk, as reported in a recent analysis of the Framingham data [17]. An inverse association between birth weight and the development of various disorders such as CHD, hypertension, T2DM, and CVD has been suggested [5]. Although the relationship between birth weight and later obesity is less clear, it appears that a "u-shaped" curve exists [11]. While high birth weight appears to predict obesity in children and adults, low birth weight has been linked to lower lean

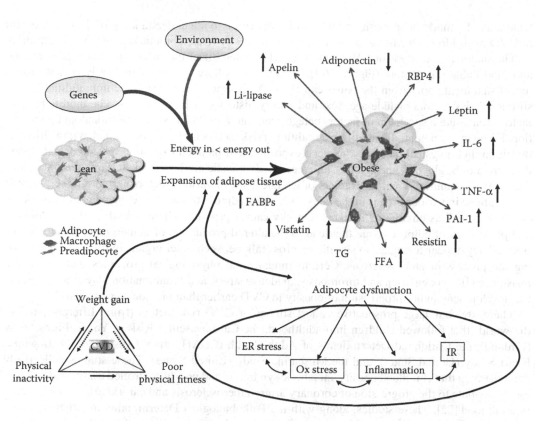

FIGURE 26.2 Expansion of the adipose tissue and consequent adipocyte dysfunction in an obesogenic environment.

body mass (mainly muscle) and increased abdominal obesity and higher body fat percentage later in life [18], leading to significant health problems and adult morbidity and mortality.

Obesity is an extraordinarily complex phenotype and its silent progression to various chronic diseases is intricate. A cascade of events contribute, mostly in concert; obesity-related comorbidities can be considered the accumulated result of a range of both genetic and environmental factors (Figure 26.1). Fortunately, overt CVD is rare in children and/or young people, but many of the underlying traits and exposures that lead to CVD and related comorbidities in later life are acquired in childhood. In fact, the complex framework and the track toward CVD appear to start from the preconception period and pass through fetal development, postnatal life, childhood, adulthood, and old age [7,18]. High adolescent BMI significantly increased adult diabetes and coronary artery disease risks in Israeli military recruits who were followed from late adolescence to adulthood [19]. Some studies, however, have shown that BMI in early childhood (<9 years) is less predictive of future risk compared with BMI in the adolescent period [20]. Notwithstanding the debate on the threshold age at which obesity makes a larger contribution to future CVD risk, it is obvious that the exposures at various stages of life result in small and large insults/injuries to the system. The cumulative effects of various exposures over time lead to chronic diseases, including T2DM and CVD.

BIOMARKERS/RISK FACTORS AND SURROGATE END POINTS IN CVD

Because CVD is silently progressive and the atherosclerotic process takes decades to manifest into overt disease, the final disease end points are not easily detectable in children. Clinical and biological risk factors associated with CVD have been identified in children using surrogate anatomic and physiological markers and have been tracked into adulthood [21]. In this context, reliable risk factors and biomarkers of obesity-related CVD are central to the understanding of the development of CVD in children. One focus of this chapter is on obesity-related biomarkers of CVD in children.

The major risk factors for CVD can be roughly categorized into nonmodifiable/constitutional and modifiable risk factors (Figure 26.1). These aspects have been systematically reviewed in a recent statement paper from the American Heart Association [7]. In brief, the nonmodifiable/constitutional risk factors include age, sex, and family history of atherosclerosis. The modifiable risk factors constitute a spectrum of factors categorized into two broad types: traditional and nontraditional. The major potentially modifiable traditional risk factors for CVD include behavioral/lifestyle (nutrition/diet, physical inactivity, tobacco exposure, and prenatal exposure), physiological (blood pressure, lipids, glucose, and insulin), and medical diagnostic markers (diabetes and chronic kidney disease). The nontraditional risk factors of CVD consist of various factors and biomarkers related to alterations in various organs in the body, especially adipose tissue. These include both functional markers as well as circulating markers. Obesity causes profound changes both in the vasculature and physiology of adipose tissue that lead to the altered production of numerous molecules in the tissue. They appear to engage in significant cross talk between other organs in the body, accelerating the process of atherosclerosis. Certain fundamental physiological processes such as insulin resistance (IR), coagulation and thrombosis, oxidative stress, and inflammation play crucial roles in the development and/or progression of obesity to CVD earlier than previously considered.

There are four large prospective cohort studies of CVD risk factors (from different parts of the world) that followed children into adulthood: the Cardiovascular Risk in Young Finns Study (Finland), the Childhood Determinants of Adult Health (CDAH) study (Australia), the Bogalusa Heart Study (United States), and the Muscatine Study (United States). These studies collectively demonstrated that childhood obesity, metabolic syndrome, and poorly controlled traditional risk factors contribute to the progression of coronary artery atherosclerosis and carotid artery calcification in adulthood [22]. These studies, along with the Pathobiological Determinants of Atherosclerosis in Youth (PDAY) studies, provide support for earlier observations that atherosclerosis begins in childhood and progresses mutely through adolescence and young adulthood into middle age; a high relative risk at young age likely will be transformed into high absolute risk of advanced coronary artery lesions later in life [23].

SURROGATE MEASURES OF TARGET ORGAN DAMAGE

Since overt CVD events remain extremely rare in children and adolescents, surrogate CVD markers are used as alternative indicators of CVD events. Biomarkers of CVD are useful at multiple points as indicators of disease traits, disease state, rate of progression, or surrogate end points for monitoring treatment outcomes [11]. These surrogate biomarkers used for CVD include anatomical measures (carotid intima-media thickness [cIMT] and coronary artery calcification [CAC]), noninvasive assessment of vascular function and physiological measures (vascular structure, arterial stiffness, endothelial function, and blood pressure), and circulating biomarkers (lipids and markers of inflammation, oxidative stress, and IR). Recently, the American Heart Association published recommendations/statements regarding these surrogate markers and their use in the pediatric population [7,24].

DISLIPIDEMIA

Over the past several decades, data have accumulated linking adverse levels and patterns of lipids and lipoproteins to the initiation and progression of the atherosclerotic process in children and adolescents [2]. Atherogenic dyslipidemia is characterized by an assemblage of abnormalities that include elevated triglycerides (TG), apolipoprotein B (apoB), small LDL (sLDL) particles, and a reduced level of HDL-C [11]. No direct data from longitudinal population-based studies are available that link the absolute levels of lipids and lipoproteins in childhood to overt CVD in adulthood. However, various reports, including the Third National Health and Nutritional Examination Survey

(NHANES III), the Bogalusa Heart Study, and the Lipid Research Clinics Population Studies, have shown that, compared with children and adolescents with normal body weight, their obese counterparts have a more unfavorable profile of the preceding factors. Magnussen et al. analyzed data from the Bogalusa Heart, Young Finns, and CDAH studies and concluded that adolescent dyslipidemia combined with obesity was most strongly associated with adult cIMT [25]. The pathophysiology still remains unclear, but lifestyle, rather than genetic influences, predominate the atherogenic-type dyslipidemia phenotype [11,26]. Childhood non-HDL-C level and change in BMI over time predicted adult dyslipidemia, but was not independent of adult obesity, as shown from the Bogalusa Heart Study data [10]. Combined data from the Young Finns, Bogalusa Heart, and CDAH studies suggested that childhood BMI was the best predictor of adult HDL-C levels [25,27].

HYPERTENSION

Hypertension is one the major cardiovascular complications associated with obesity. Contrary to the typical notion that essential or primary hypertension affects only adults, increased rates of hypertension are evident at early age in the clinical course of obesity [28]. In 2004, the NHANES data demonstrated the first hint of a shift in the epidemiology of childhood hypertension and showed that overall blood pressure levels in US children and adolescents have increased [29,30]. In autopsy studies, elevated childhood BP has been associated with atherosclerotic lesions [31]. The Bogalusa Heart Study has also demonstrated that children with elevated blood pressure are several times more likely to develop essential hypertension as a young adult [28]. The risk of hypertension in children appears to increase across the spectrum of BMI values rather than having a specific threshold effect [28]. In adults, persistent hypertension has a significant impact on health, including coronary artery disease, stroke, and kidney diseases. However, the natural history of primary hypertension in children is not available, but insights have been gleaned from data on pediatric secondary hypertension and health consequences that include aortic coarctation and chronic kidney disease [30]. Hypertension in cross-sectional studies of obese youth with T2DM has been shown to coexist with LVH as early as adolescence [11,30]. Therefore, obesity-related hypertension in the pediatric population cannot be ignored, and additional data are needed to assess the independent relationship between obesity in childhood and hypertension in adulthood.

MYOCARDIAL TISSUE REMODELING AND CHILD OBESITY

Intermediate end points between conventional risk assessment and overt disease events include left atrial enlargement, LVH, coronary calcium, increased carotid wall thickness, and abnormal endothelial function. These intermediate risk assessment points are not only related to conventional risk factors, but are also independent predictors themselves. LVH, or increased thickness of the heart's main pumping chamber, is an essential manifestation of hypertensive damage to the organ and has been recognized as an independent contributor to increased cardiovascular morbidity and mortality. Daniels et al. showed a high prevalence of severe LVH and abnormal geometry in children and adolescents with essential hypertension [14]. This finding has been corroborated in various subsequent studies [32,33]. Gidding et al. reported coronary artery calcium and increased carotid wall thickness in adolescents with heterozygous familial hypercholesterolemia [34]. A recent study showed an association with the degree of adiposity and concentric left ventricular remodeling in midlife, whereas the cumulative effects of a longer duration of overall obesity during young adulthood contribute to eccentric remodeling, predominantly by increasing left ventricular mass [35]. Epidemiological and clinical studies have indicated that LVH in children worsened with the dual burden of obesity and elevated blood pressure than with blood pressure elevation alone. Recent data from the Bogalusa Heart Study have indicated that the process of LVH and subclinical changes in cardiac structure are influenced by excess adiposity and hypertension, both cumulatively and independently from early life [33]. These data support the presence of end organ injury in youth

(Figure 26.1). Therefore, good cardiovascular health cannot be assumed in obese children and adolescents. While there are no longitudinal data on weight trends in children with congenital heart disease, recent studies indicate a relationship between congenital heart disease and overweight/obesity [36].

INSULIN RESISTANCE

Although IR can be broadly characterized as an impaired biological response to insulin, it is the product of various processes. These processes are mediated at the level of cellular mitochondria that produce endoplasmic reticulum (ER) stress, oxidative stress, and adipocyte dysfunction that leads to alterations in the release of numerous adipokines. Systemic manifestation of these processes is evident mainly in fat, muscle, and liver. The direct relationship between IR and fatness is well known and it is considered the most ominous abnormality related to obesity [3,6,37]. In adults, IR is well recognized as a cardinal feature in the development of T2DM. In children and adolescents, IR is related to obesity and various metabolic and cardiovascular complications [3,6,7,13]. Obesity in children frequently persists into adulthood with increased risk of the development of IR, which is the consequence of various interrelated processes. IR is considered not only to be the key link between adiposity and T2DM, but it accelerates the progression of obesity to CVD and worsens its outcomes [11]. Despite these strong relationships, the assessment of IR in children is challenging and still lacks clarity. The hyperinsulinemic euglycemic clamp and the frequently sampled intravenous glucose tolerance test (FSIVGTT) with modeling are generally accepted as valid and reliable for the measurement of insulin sensitivity [3,38]. However, these methods pose various technical challenges for frequent use in children, such as the fact that they are time consuming, they are relatively invasive in nature, and a research setting is required to perform the studies. Despite their limitations, less invasive, surrogate estimates of IR, such as insulinemia and homeostatic model assessment (HOMA)-IR have been used in numerous studies in children. Although studies have demonstrated childhood obesity correlates with IR, assessed using various estimates of IR, obesity is not synonymous with IR [11]; studies have demonstrated that despite an equal degree of adiposity, the extent of IR is significantly higher in obese youth with impaired glucose tolerance (IGT) compared with those with normal glucose tolerance (NGT) [39]. Similarly, obese youth with T2DM are significantly more insulin resistant that those without diabetes, matched for age, sex, and BMI [40]. Further, IR in obese youth varies by ethnicity and studies have also shown the direct effects of IR on CVD outcomes, independent of BMI [3]. The association between IR and traditional risk factors such as hyperglycemia, dyslipidemia, and hypertension is well established. Recent studies have suggested strong associations between IR and various nontraditional risk factors, such as those related to inflammation, thrombosis, and oxidative stress [7,13]. Further, it appears that there is an interaction between traditional and nontraditional risk factors, and both can worsen IR, consequently leading to a vicious cycle that promotes the development of atherothrombotic disease.

EXPANSION OF ADIPOSE TISSUE AND ADIPOCYTE DYSFUNCTION

Insights into adipose tissue biology and metabolism in humans have rapidly evolved during the last several years. The stature of adipose tissue has been transformed from an inert organ for energy homeostasis to a biologic reservoir for nutrient storage that expands in response to overnutrition and releases lipids, various hormones, and an array of cytokines, commonly referred to as adipokines. Excess adiposity/expansion of the adipose tissue, especially its storage in specific depots of body fat, appears to be central to shifts in the metabolic and pathophysiological pathways, leading to increased risk of cardiometabolic diseases. A simplistic portrayal of this excess fat can be linked to an imbalance between energy intake and energy expenditure. Children are growing and they need to have a positive energy balance for tissue growth. How the excess energy will be partitioned and stored is crucial. It appears that, in an obesogenic environment, the surplus energy is stored as fat cells, leading to an increase either in number (hyperplasia) or size/volume (hypertrophy), or often in both [8,41]. When the hyperplasia and hypertrophy are inadequate for the absorption of the excess circulating nutrients, the capacity of the adipocyte to store glucose and TG is also compromised, leading to dysfunctional adipose tissue (Figure 26.2). The dysfunction of the adipose tissue channels into a variety of stresses and inflammatory processes within the tissue, causing alterations in the production and regulation of numerous molecules. Some of these molecules are shown in Figure 26.2. Unfortunately, obesity-related alterations in these molecules arise quite early in life, with a profound impact on overall health, leading to cardiometabolic disease. The Bogalusa Heart Study provided the earliest evidence of the contribution of adipose tissue to increased risk of T2DM and CVD in children and adolescents [21].

The expansion of adipose tissue has profound effects not only within the adipose tissue, but on the function of most other organ systems in the body as well. The cross talk between organs is orchestrated by diverse metabolites and secretomes produced in the adipose tissue, leading to various physiological abnormalities such as ER stress and oxidative stress, and alterations in inflammatory signals, prothrombotic factors, and IR (Figure 26.2). For example, inflammatory molecules such as IL-6 stimulate the production of various acute-phase proteins such as fibrinogen, CRP, and RBP4 in the liver. Further, it appears that a vicious connection exists between weight gain, poor physical fitness, and physical inactivity; each separately or in concert reinforces the path toward CVD [7,41].

SUBCLINICAL INFLAMMATION

Multiple lines of evidence indicate that the presence of an obesity-related inflammatory state not only plays a crucial role in the evolution of CVD, but is central to all stages of atherosclerosis, including plaque development, disruption, and thrombosis [42]. In recent years, the pivotal role of inflammation in obesity-related CVD has become more widely appreciated in children [7]. The dysfunction of the adipose tissue results in the altered secretion of an array of molecules that are crucial in the regulation of many metabolic, hormonal, and inflammatory signals in humans (Figure 26.2). Although numerous biomarkers related to inflammation have been proposed and their predictive roles are being vigorously investigated [7,43], C-reactive protein (CRP) is probably the most studied biomarker for inflammation in children [44–47]. Studies in children have also reported a coordinated elevation in CRP, IL-6, and fibrinogen in the setting of obesity and IR [7,46]. Increases in the levels of CRP and oxidized LDL as a function of the degree of obesity has also been reported [9]. Despite the consistent finding of a raised inflammatory state in obese children [7], the relationship between childhood CRP levels and vascular function (cIMT) in adults remains uncertain [47,48]. Since a state of sustained exposure to subclinical inflammation results in cardiovascular end organ injury [42], the presence of an inflammatory state in obese children is perturbing. Although not universal, it appears that lifestyle interventions early in the clinical course of obesity reduce the elevated levels of these inflammatory factors (recently reviewed in [7,9,43]).

OXIDATIVE STRESS

Different pathways and mechanisms are involved in the complex link between obesity and CVD (Figure 26.1). Oxidative stress may be involved in the pathogenesis of CVD and atherosclerosis via the oxidation of LDL particles and their uptake by macrophages, as well as the production of reactive oxygen species (ROS) that cause localized damage to cells [49–52]. Oxidative stress involves an imbalance in the net concentration of ROS relative to the body's capacity to offset their damaging effects. ER and the mitochondria play crucial roles in the production of ROS. In obesity, adipocyte dysfunction due to nutrient excess triggers the mitochondria to produce adenosine triphosphate (ATP) at a more rapid rate via the uncoupling of oxidative phosphorylation, leading to the increased production and accumulation of ROS. This could result from unfolded-protein response

(UPR)-regulated oxidative folding machinery in the ER, superoxide anion produced mainly in mitochondria, nitric oxide produced during arginine metabolism, α-ketoglutarate dehydrogenase in the tricarboxylic acid (TCA) cycle, complexes I and III of the mitochondrial respiratory chain, and several other factors [50]. With the increase in ROS production, the overall antioxidant defense mechanism is compromised, thus magnifying oxidative stress in the system, leading to mitochondrial DNA damage and IR. The direct measurement of *in vivo* oxidative stress is problematic. Although several markers have been suggested, whole-body oxidative stress is best reflected by systemic levels of lipid peroxidation, for example, F2-isoprostanes. Little is known about oxidative stress in the pediatric age range, but most available studies have shown concurrent elevations in inflammatory and oxidative status, paralleled by marked alterations in IR [7,43,49–51].

COAGULATION AND FIBRINOLYSIS

Coagulation and fibrinolysis are two key components of thrombosis. The balance between these two dynamic processes is essential to maintain the fluidity of blood, and it determines the propensity for clot formation and removal [53]. The process of coagulation and the formation of a clot involve the thrombin-induced formation of insoluble fibrin strands from soluble fibrinogen. Plasminogen activator inhibitor 1 (PAI-1) is a marker of fibrinolysis, which is the basic defense mechanism of organisms for removing the clot and controlling the deposition of fibrin in the vascular system [54]. Hyperfibrinogenemia and hypofibrinolysis (enhanced levels of PAI-1) reflect a prothrombotic state en route to cardiovascular events. The manifestation of such a thrombotic state related to obesity has been reported in children and adolescents [7,55,56]. Although obesity-related derangements in coagulation and fibrinolysis systems have been consistently reported in animal and adult studies [57], the data in children are somewhat limited and mixed [7]. A recent advance in the field has been the proposed role of gamma prime (γ') fibrinogen (an isoform of fibrinogen), which forms clots that are more resistant to fibrinolysis [58]. Elevated levels of γ' fibrinogen have been recently reported in obese children compared with their lean counterparts [59]. Although the data on the effect of lifestyle-based interventions in obese children are consistent on the coagulation system [46,55], they are mixed with respect to its effect on the fibrinolysis system [7,55,56,59]. There is a clear gap in our understanding of the role of a hypercoagulable and hypofibrinolytic state early in the clinical course of obesity and its impact on future thrombotic events.

CVD RISK FACTORS: CHILDREN VERSUS ADULTS

While the risk factors and biomarkers are evident at early age in obese children, it is less clear whether the mechanistic regulation of these risk factors is similar in adults and children. This is important because such an understanding will help in the development of more directed therapies to prevent and/or reverse the progression of obesity into overt disease conditions. Unfortunately, studies exploring the underlying mechanisms in children are sparse. Although direct comparisons of studies in children and adults and/or the elderly are not viable, there are some glimpses of data showing potential differences in the regulation of risk factors of CVD in children and adults/the elderly [7]. For example, while hyperfibrinogenemia in children and its reduction by physical activity are mainly regulated by changes in fibrinogen fractional synthesis rates [56], elevated levels of fibrinogen in the elderly appear to be due to its deceased breakdown [60]. Elevated levels of retinol binding protein 4 (RBP4) are related to obesity-related IR in children [61] and adults [62]. An unexpected, perhaps counterintuitive, direct relationship between RBP4 and inflammation was also observed in obese children, unlike that found in disease-related inflammation [61]. These suggest that the potential regulation of biomarkers or risk factors of CVD in obese children may be different from that reported in adults and/or disease conditions other than obesity. Indeed, as far as obesity and certain CVD risk factors are concerned, children are not little adults. Thus, therapies developed in adults for reducing obesity-related CVD risk cannot be directly translated to children. Recent studies suggest that medications approved for long-term obesity treatment, when used as an adjunct to lifestyle intervention, lead to greater mean weight loss and an increased likelihood of achieving clinically meaningful, longer-term weight loss [63]. Further studies are warranted on such adjunct therapeutic approaches that are useful in CVD risk reduction in obese children.

CONCLUSION

Childhood obesity tracks into adulthood and adult obesity directly impacts metabolic and cardio-vascular consequences. The relationship between early obesity and adult CVD risk is complex, but many obese children and adolescents already manifest various metabolic complications, and these children are at high risk of developing cardiometabolic diseases with increased morbidity. As is obvious from the available literature, a complex interplay among biological and physiologic factors promotes the initiation and progression of obesity into metabolic and vascular diseases. Understanding the underlying mechanisms of the pathogenesis of the obese phenotype with early derangements in insulin sensitivity, oxidative stress, and subclinical inflammation is of critical importance. There is a gradation in understanding the long-term CVD risk in children, and bio-markers of CVD are important when considering the magnitude of risk and the effectiveness of interventions at different stages of the lifespan. The long-term consequences of childhood obesity are avoidable, with the available data supporting this positive message, and there remains an oppor-tunity for intervention across the lifespan. However, better understanding of the pathophysiology and underlying mechanisms regulating the different pathways of progression from obesity to CVD is required for the development of more directed therapies in children.

ACKNOWLEDGMENTS

I wish to acknowledge Dr. James Sylvester for the helpful comments on the manuscript draft.

REFERENCES

1. Ogden CL, Carroll MD, Kit BK, Flegal KM 2014 Prevalence of childhood and adult obesity in the United States, 2011–2012. *JAMA* 311:806–814.
2. Daniels SR, Arnett DK, Eckel RH, Gidding SS, Hayman LL, Kumanyika S, Robinson TN, Scott BJ, St. Jeor S, Williams CL 2005 Overweight in children and adolescents: Pathophysiology, consequences, prevention, and treatment. *Circulation* 111:1999–2012.
3. Cruz ML, Shaibi GQ, Weigensberg MJ, Spruijt-Metz D, Ball GDC, Goran MI 2005 Pediatric obesity and insulin resistance: Chronic disease risk and implications for treatment and prevention beyond body weight modification. *Annu Rev Nutr* 25:435–468.
4. Poirier P, Giles TD, Bray GA, Hong Y, Stern JS, Pi-Sunyer FX, Eckel RH 2006 Obesity and cardiovas-cular disease: Pathophysiology, evaluation, and effect of weight loss: An update of the 1997 American Heart Association Scientific Statement on Obesity and Heart Disease from the Obesity Committee of the Council on Nutrition, Physical Activity, and Metabolism. *Circulation* 113:898–918.
5. Juonala M, Magnussen CG, Berenson GS, Venn A, Burns TL, Sabin MA, Srinivasan SR, et al. 2011 Childhood adiposity, adult adiposity, and cardiovascular risk factors. *N Engl J Med* 365:1876–1885.
6. Weiss R, Dziura J, Burgert TS, Tamborlane WV, Taksali SE, Yeckel CW, Allen K, et al. 2004 Obesity and the metabolic syndrome in children and adolescents. *N Engl J Med* 350:2362–2374.
7. Balagopal P, de Ferranti SD, Cook S, Daniels SR, Gidding SS, Hayman LL, McCrindle BW, Mietus-Snyder ML, Steinberger J, on behalf of the American Heart Association Committee on Atherosclerosis HaOiYotCoCDitYCoNPAaMaCoEaP 2011 Nontraditional risk factors and biomarkers for cardiovas-cular disease: Mechanistic, research, and clinical considerations for youth: A scientific statement from the American Heart Association. *Circulation* 123:2749–2769.
8. Bray GA 2003 Risks of obesity. *Prim Care* 30:281–299, v–vi.
9. Kelly AS, Barlow SE, Rao G, Inge TH, Hayman LL, Steinberger J, Urbina EM, Ewing LJ, Daniels SR 2013 Severe obesity in children and adolescents: Identification, associated health risks, and treatment approaches: A scientific statement from the American Heart Association. *Circulation* 128:1689–1712.

10. Freedman DS, Khan LK, Dietz WH, Srinivasan SR, Berenson GS 2001 Relationship of childhood obesity to coronary heart disease risk factors in adulthood: The Bogalusa Heart Study. *Pediatrics* 108:712–718.

11. Nadeau KJ, Maahs DM, Daniels SR, Eckel RH 2011 Childhood obesity and cardiovascular disease: Links and prevention strategies. *Nat Rev Cardiol* 8:513–525.

12. Gidding SS, McMahan CA, McGill HC, Colangelo LA, Schreiner PJ, Williams OD, Liu K 2006 Prediction of coronary artery calcium in young adults using the Pathobiological Determinants of Atherosclerosis in Youth (PDAY) risk score: The CARDIA study. *Arch Intern Med* 166:2341–2347.

13. Steinberger J, Daniels SR, Eckel RH, Hayman L, Lustig RH, McCrindle B, Mietus-Snyder ML 2009 Progress and challenges in metabolic syndrome in children and adolescents: A scientific statement from the American Heart Association Atherosclerosis, Hypertension, and Obesity in the Young Committee of the Council on Cardiovascular Disease in the Young; Council on Cardiovascular Nursing; and Council on Nutrition, Physical Activity, and Metabolism. *Circulation* 119:628–647.

14. Daniels SR, Loggie JM, Khoury P, Kimball TR 1998 Left ventricular geometry and severe left ventricular hypertrophy in children and adolescents with essential hypertension. *Circulation* 97:1907–1911.

15. Gidding SS, Liu K, Colangelo LA, Cook NL, Goff DC, Glasser SP, Gardin JM, Lima JA 2013 Longitudinal determinants of left ventricular mass and geometry: The Coronary Artery Risk Development in Young Adults (CARDIA) Study. *Circ Cardiovasc Imaging* 6:769–775.

16. Must A, Jacques PF, Dallal GE, Bajema CJ, Dietz WH 1992 Long-term morbidity and mortality of overweight adolescents: A follow-up of the Harvard Growth Study of 1922 to 1935. *N Engl J Med* 327:1350–1355.

17. Abdullah A, Amin FA, Stoelwinder J, Tanamas SK, Wolfe R, Barendregt J, Peeters A 2014 Estimating the risk of cardiovascular disease using an obese-years metric. *BMJ Open* 4:e005629.

18. Yliharsila H, Kajantie E, Osmond C, Forsen T, Barker DJ, Eriksson JG 2007 Birth size, adult body composition and muscle strength in later life. *Int J Obes (Lond)* 31:1392–1399.

19. Tirosh A, Shai I, Afek A, Dubnov-Raz G, Ayalon N, Gordon B, Derazne E, Tzur D, Shamis A, Vinker S, Rudich A 2011 Adolescent BMI trajectory and risk of diabetes versus coronary disease. *N Engl J Med* 364:1315–1325.

20. Lawlor DA, Leon DA 2005 Association of body mass index and obesity measured in early childhood with risk of coronary heart disease and stroke in middle age: Findings from the Aberdeen children of the 1950s prospective cohort study. *Circulation* 111:1891–1896.

21. Berenson GS, Srnivasan SR 2005 Cardiovascular risk factors in youth with implications for aging: The Bogalusa Heart Study. *Neurobiol Aging* 26:303–307.

22. Juonala M, Magnussen CG, Venn A, Dwyer T, Burns TL, Davis PH, Chen W, et al. 2010 Influence of age on associations between childhood risk factors and carotid intima-media thickness in adulthood/clinical perspective. *Circulation* 122:2514–2520.

23. McGill HC, Jr, McMahan CA, Gidding SS 2008 Preventing heart disease in the 21st century: Implications of the Pathobiological Determinants of Atherosclerosis in Youth (PDAY) study. *Circulation* 117:1216–1227.

24. Urbina EM, Williams RV, Alpert BS, Collins RT, Daniels SR, Hayman L, Jacobson M, et al., on behalf of the American Heart Association Atherosclerosis HaOiYCotCoCDitY 2009 Noninvasive assessment of subclinical atherosclerosis in children and adolescents: Recommendations for standard assessment for clinical research; A scientific statement from the American Heart Association. *Hypertension* 54:919–950.

25. Magnussen CG, Venn A, Thomson R, Juonala M, Srinivasan SR, Viikari JSA, Berenson GS, Dwyer T, Raitakari OT 2009 The association of pediatric low- and high-density lipoprotein cholesterol dyslipidemia classifications and change in dyslipidemia status with carotid intima-media thickness in adulthood: Evidence from the Cardiovascular Risk in Young Finns Study, the Bogalusa Heart Study, and the CDAH (Childhood Determinants of Adult Health) study. *J Am Coll Cardiol* 53:860–869.

26. Juonala M, Viikari JS, Ronnemaa T, Marniemi J, Jula A, Loo BM, Raitakari OT 2008 Associations of dyslipidemias from childhood to adulthood with carotid intima-media thickness, elasticity, and brachial flow-mediated dilatation in adulthood: The Cardiovascular Risk in Young Finns Study. *Arterioscler Thromb Vasc Biol* 28:1012–1017.

27. Magnussen CG, Raitakari OT, Thomson R, Juonala M, Patel DA, Viikari JS, Marniemi J, Srinivasan SR, Berenson GS, Dwyer T, Venn A 2008 Utility of currently recommended pediatric dyslipidemia classifications in predicting dyslipidemia in adulthood: Evidence from the Childhood Determinants of Adult Health (CDAH) study, Cardiovascular Risk in Young Finns Study, and Bogalusa Heart Study. *Circulation* 117:32–42.

28. Sorof J, Daniels S 2002 Obesity hypertension in children: A problem of epidemic proportions. *Hypertension* 40:441–447.

29. Muntner P, He J, Cutler JA, Wildman RP, Whelton PK 2004 Trends in blood pressure among children and adolescents. *JAMA* 291:2107–2113.

30. Flynn JT 2009 Hypertension in the young: Epidemiology, sequelae and therapy. *Nephrol Dial Transplant* 24:370–375.

31. Berenson GS, Srinivasan SR, Bao W, Newman WP, Tracy RE, Wattigney WA 1998 Association between multiple cardiovascular risk factors and atherosclerosis in children and young adults: The Bogalusa Heart Study. *N Engl J Med* 338:1650–1656.

32. Hanevold C, Waller J, Daniels S, Portman R, Sorof J 2004 The effects of obesity, gender, and ethnic group on left ventricular hypertrophy and geometry in hypertensive children: A collaborative study of the International Pediatric Hypertension Association. *Pediatrics* 113:328–333.

33. Lai CC, Sun D, Cen R, Wang J, Li S, Fernandez-Alonso C, Chen W, Srinivasan SR, Berenson GS 2014 Impact of long-term burden of excessive adiposity and elevated blood pressure from childhood on adulthood left ventricular remodeling patterns: The Bogalusa Heart Study. *J Am Coll Cardiol* 64:1580–1587.

34. Gidding SS, Bookstein LC, Chomka EV 1998 Usefulness of electron beam tomography in adolescents and young adults with heterozygous familial hypercholesterolemia. *Circulation* 98:2580–2583.

35. Reis JP, Allen N, Gibbs BB, Gidding SS, Lee JM, Lewis CE, Lima J, et al. 2014 Association of the degree of adiposity and duration of obesity with measures of cardiac structure and function: The CARDIA study. *Obesity (Silver Spring)* 22:2434–2440.

36. Pemberton VL, McCrindle BW, Barkin S, Daniels SR, Barlow SE, Binns HJ, Cohen MS, et al. 2010 Report of the National Heart, Lung, and Blood Institute's Working Group on obesity and other cardiovascular risk factors in congenital heart disease. *Circulation* 121:1153–1159.

37. Berenson GS 2005 Obesity: A critical issue in preventive cardiology; The Bogalusa Heart Study. *Prev Cardiol* 8:234–241.

38. Levy-Marchal C, Arslanian S, Cutfield W, Sinaiko A, Druet C, Marcovecchio ML, Chiarelli F 2010 Insulin resistance in children: Consensus, perspective, and future directions. *J Clin Endocrinol Metab* 95:5189–5198.

39. Weiss R, Dufour S, Taksali SE, Tamborlane WV, Petersen K, Bonadonna RC, Boselli L, et al. 2003 Prediabetes in obese youth: A syndrome of impaired glucose tolerance, severe insulin resistance, and altered myocellular and abdominal fat partitioning. *Lancet* 362:951–957.

40. Nadeau KJ, Zeitler PS, Bauer TA, Brown MS, Dorosz JL, Draznin B, Reusch JE, Regensteiner JG 2009 Insulin resistance in adolescents with type 2 diabetes is associated with impaired exercise capacity. *J Clin Endocrinol Metab* 94:3687–3695.

41. Gutin B 2011 The role of nutrient partitioning and stem cell differentiation in pediatric obesity: A new theory. *Int J Pediatr Obes* 6(Suppl. 1):7–12.

42. Libby P, Ridker PM, Hansson GK 2009 Inflammation in atherosclerosis: From pathophysiology to practice. *J Am Coll Cardiol* 54:2129–2138.

43. Canas JA, Sweeten S, Balagopal PB 2013 Biomarkers for cardiovascular risk in children. *Curr Opin Cardiol* 28:103–114.

44. Ford ES, Giles WH, Myers GL, Rifai N, Ridker PM, Mannino DM 2003 C-reactive protein concentration distribution among US children and young adults: Findings from the National Health and Nutrition Examination Survey, 1999–2000. *Clin Chem* 49:1353–1357.

45. Visser M, Bouter LM, McQuillan GM, Wener MH, Harris JB 2001 Low-grade systemic inflammation in overweight children. *Pediatrics* 107:E13.

46. Balagopal P, George D, Patton N, Yarandi H, Roberts WL, Bayne E, Gidding S 2005 Lifestyle-only intervention attenuates the inflammatory state associated with obesity: A randomized controlled study in adolescents. *J Pediatr* 146:342–348.

47. Juonala M, Viikari JSA, Ronnemaa T, Taittonen L, Marniemi J, Raitakari OT 2006 Childhood C-reactive protein in predicting CRP and carotid intima-media thickness in adulthood: The Cardiovascular Risk in Young Finns Study. *Arterioscler Thromb Vasc Biol* 26:1883–1888.

48. Jarvisalo MJ, Harmoinen A, Hakanen M, Paakkunainen U, Viikari J, Hartiala J, Lehtimaki T, Simell O, Raitakari OT 2002 Elevated serum C-reactive protein levels and early arterial changes in healthy children. *Arterioscler Thromb Vasc Biol* 22:1323–1328.

49. Wildman RP, McGinn AP, Lin J, Wang D, Muntner P, Cohen HW, Reynolds K, Fonseca V, Sowers MR 2011 Cardiovascular disease risk of abdominal obesity vs. metabolic abnormalities. *Obesity (Silver Spring)* 19:853–860.

50. Montero D, Walther G, Perez-Martin A, Roche E, Vinet A 2012 Endothelial dysfunction, inflammation, and oxidative stress in obese children and adolescents: Markers and effect of lifestyle intervention. *Obes Rev* 13:441–455.

51. Gross M, Steffes M, Jacobs DR, Jr, Yu X, Lewis L, Lewis CE, Loria CM 2005 Plasma F2-isoprostanes and coronary artery calcification: The CARDIA Study. *Clin Chem* 51:125–131.

52. Warolin J, Coenen KR, Kantor JL, Whitaker LE, Wang L, Acra SA, Roberts LJ, Buchowski MS 2014 The relationship of oxidative stress, adiposity and metabolic risk factors in healthy black and white American youth. *Pediatr Obes* 9:43–52.

53. Fibrinogen Studies Collaboration 2007 Associations of plasma fibrinogen levels with established cardiovascular disease risk factors, inflammatory markers, and other characteristics: Individual participant meta-analysis of 154,211 adults in 31 prospective studies. *Am J Epidemiol* 166:867–879.

54. Vaughan DE 2005 PAI-1 and atherothrombosis. *J Thromb Haemost* 3:1879–1883.

55. Ferguson MA, Gutin B, Owens S, Barbeau P, Tracy RP, Litaker M 1999 Effects of physical training and its cessation on the hemostatic system of obese children. *Am J Clin Nutr* 69:1130–1134.

56. Balagopal P, George D, Sweeten S, Mann KJ, Yarandi H, Mauras N, Vaughan DE 2008 Response of fractional synthesis rate (FSR) of fibrinogen, D-dimer and fibrinolytic balance to physical activity-based intervention in obese children. *J Thromb Haemost* 6:1296–1303.

57. Giannini C, Mohn A, Chiarelli F, Kelnar CJH 2011 Macrovascular angiopathy in children and adolescents with type 1 diabetes. *Diabetes Metab Res Rev* 27:436–460.

58. Farrell DH 2004 Pathophysiologic roles of the fibrinogen gamma chain. *Curr Opin Hematol* 11:151–155.

59. Lovely RS, Hossain J, Ramsey JP, Komakula V, George D, Farrell DH, Balagopal PB 2013 Obesity-related increase of γ' fibrinogen concentration in children and its reduction by physical activity-based lifestyle intervention: A randomized controlled study. *J Pediatr* 163:333–338.

60. Fu AZ, Nair KS 1998 Age effect on fibrinogen and albumin synthesis in humans. *Am J Physiol* 275:E1023–E1030.

61. Balagopal P, Graham TE, Kahn BB, Altomare A, Funanage V, George D 2007 Reduction of elevated serum retinol binding protein in obese children by lifestyle intervention: Association with subclinical inflammation. *J Clin Endocrinol Metab* 92:1971–1974.

62. Graham TE, Yang Q, Bluher M, Hammarstedt A, Ciaraldi TP, Henry RR, Wason CJ, Oberbach A, Jansson PA, Smith U, Kahn BB 2006 Retinol-binding protein 4 and insulin resistance in lean, obese, and diabetic subjects. *N Engl J Med* 354:2552–2563.

63. Yanovski SZ, Yanovski JA 2014 Long-term drug treatment for obesity: A systematic and clinical review. *JAMA* 311:74–86.

27 Pediatric Nonalcoholic Fatty Liver Disease
Recent Advances in Diagnostics and Emerging Therapeutics

Elizabeth L. Yu, Kimberly P. Newton, Jonathan A. Africa, and Jeffrey B. Schwimmer

CONTENTS

INTRODUCTION

Nonalcoholic fatty liver disease (NAFLD) is the most common cause of liver disease in children and adolescents.[1] NAFLD encompasses a spectrum of diseases, from isolated steatosis to steatohepatitis and fibrosis. Histological examination is required for definitive diagnosis of NAFLD. Though NAFLD is often suspected in obese children with elevated liver enzymes, it is important to recognize that obesity and NAFLD are not necessarily concomitant. In fact, NAFLD is present in only a minority of children with obesity. However, obese children with NAFLD are at a higher risk of morbidity and mortality. NAFLD also occurs in nonobese children, with average estimates of ~5% prevalence of NAFLD in normal-weight children.[2–4] The pathophysiology of NAFLD, though still incompletely understood, is multifactorial. This chapter highlights pediatric NAFLD (epidemiology, diagnostic approaches, pathophysiology, the impact of NAFLD, and emerging treatments) and more closely examines the relationship between obesity and NAFLD in children.

DIAGNOSIS OF NAFLD

Histology

Clinical Histopathologic Diagnosis

NAFLD is defined as 5% or greater macrovesicular steatosis in hepatocytes after exclusion of other causes of steatosis.[5] Hepatic histology is key in the diagnosis of NAFLD. Liver histology can also determine the presence of other findings in addition to steatosis, which may lean toward diagnoses other than NAFLD.[5]

Components of Nonalcoholic Steatohepatitis

The diagnosis of nonalcoholic steatohepatitis (NASH) is determined by a constellation of different components of a biopsy, not one single finding, in contrast to diseases such as cancer. In NASH, steatosis is present along with a multitude of other findings that are indicative of hepatic inflammation and cell injury. *Hepatocyte ballooning* is a manifestation of liver injury and refers to the swelling of hepatocytes. *Inflammation* refers to the presence of inflammatory cells, including polymorphonuclear leukocytes, lymphocytes, mononuclear cells, eosinophils, and microgranulomas.[6] These hepatic changes can be either around the central vein or around the portal triad, which includes the portal vein, hepatic artery, and bile duct. *Fibrosis* is collagen deposition in the areas around the sinusoids (*perisinusoidal*) or around the cells (*pericellular*). *Advanced fibrosis* is characterized by bridging fibrosis and, at its worst, cirrhosis.

Scoring Systems

Pathologists have tried to tie the findings of NASH into semiquantitative scoring systems to correlate clinical findings with histology. However, none of these are used in clinical practice as of yet. The Brunt system attempts to categorize patients with NASH as mild, moderate, or severe based on histological findings and a corresponding numerical score.[6] However, this system does not account for pediatric pathology as it was derived from adult data. The NAFLD Activity Score (NAS), developed by the NASH Clinical Research Network, is a modified version of the Brunt system and is based on three factors: steatosis grade (minimum of >5% for NAFLD) (0–3), lobular inflammation (0–3), and hepatocellular ballooning (0–2).[6] This scoring system is exclusively used in the research setting to evaluate change, not to grade severity; higher scores are not always indicative of NASH, nor is a lower score benign.[7]

Fatty Liver Disease in Children versus Adults

Pediatric NAFLD has many subphenotypes that are still beginning to be understood and which differ from adults. Hence, what is known about NAFLD in adults cannot be extrapolated to children. Histologically, there are differences in the location of fat and fibrosis along with differences in where inflammation is noted. At this point, it is unclear if the differences are part of a continuum of disease, with pediatric histology transitioning to adult histology, or if the differences are actually representative of two or more different disease processes.

Other Diseases with Steatosis

It is important to note that not all liver steatosis is NAFLD. Other etiologies that can have hepatic steatosis include: Wilson's disease, hepatitis C, drugs/toxins, metabolic disorders, hepatic ischemia, and disorders of lipid metabolism. Hourigan et al. reviewed liver biopsies of 155 children with steatosis and only 37% were diagnosed with NAFLD, with other diagnoses including metabolic disease (9%), oncologic (8.4%), and viral hepatitis (6.5%).[8] Some children who have NAFLD may have concurrent liver disease, with the most common being autoimmune hepatitis.[9]

Overall, liver histology is an integral part of the diagnosis of NAFLD and NASH. Hepatic histology provides information on a microscopic level that has yet to be derived from noninvasive measures. Furthermore, hepatic histology helps better define whether a patient has NAFLD or more progressive NASH and fibrosis.

IMAGING

To date, no imaging modality has been shown to be uniformly useful to diagnose NAFLD. This includes ultrasound. Ultrasound was found to have a positive predictive value of 47%–62%,[10,11] and did not have a consistent correlation with findings on hepatic biopsy. In a recent systematic review[12] evaluating the imaging of liver fat in pediatric patients, evidence did not support the use of ultrasound for the diagnosis or grading of fatty liver in a pediatric population.

An advanced MRI measure of steatosis called *proton density fat fraction* (PDFF) is an emerging imaging modality that has demonstrated accurate correlation with the histologic degree of steatosis. In a recent study evaluating the correlation and diagnostic accuracy of PDFF measured by MRI compared with the grade of histologic steatosis in 174 children, liver PDFF was significantly correlated with steatosis grade ($p < .01$) and had an overall accuracy of 56% in predicting histologic steatosis grade.[13] Though MRI is not yet sufficient to replace histologic examination for diagnosis in children, further studies are underway at this time.

EPIDEMIOLOGY

In the Study of Child and Adolescent Liver Epidemiology (SCALE), a 2006 study based on autopsies over a 10-year period (1993–2003) of 742 children aged 2–19 after sudden death, the overall prevalence of NAFLD was demonstrated to be 9.6% when adjusted for age, race, gender, and ethnicity.[1] The prevalence of NAFLD increased to 20%–33% in obese or overweight children (Table 27.1).[1] On one extreme of the spectrum, a recent study evaluating the prevalence of NAFLD among severely obese adolescents (mean body mass index [BMI] 52 kg/m^2) undergoing bariatric surgery demonstrated a 59% prevalence of NAFLD.[2] Of note, patients included in this study were older adolescents who were on the maximum end of the spectrum of obesity compared with other typical study populations.

The prevalence of pediatric NASH in the general population was demonstrated to be 23% (SCALE), whereas the prevalence of NASH in adolescents undergoing bariatric surgery was similar, at 24%.[2,14] In a separate study for the NASH Clinical Research Network (NASH CRN), 36% of children with NAFLD were found to have NASH.[15]

Pediatric obesity is an emerging epidemic with ever-rising rates. As demonstrated by the National Health and Nutrition Examination Survey (NHANES), childhood obesity rates rose from 5.0% in 1960 to 15.4% in 2001 and 16.9% in 2009–2010.[16] Though the prevalence of NAFLD is higher in children with obesity, an important distinction is that NAFLD and obesity are not interchangeable. NAFLD can also occur in normal-weight children. In SCALE, the prevalence of NAFLD in normal-weight children was 5%. In a 2012 Turkish autopsy study in 340 children aged 2–20 years with normal weight, the prevalence of NAFLD was also 5%.[17] In a clinical study of children with NAFLD, the prevalence of normal weight ranged from 1% to 8%.[3,4] The prevalence of overweight body habitus in children with NAFLD is 5%–21%, and the prevalence of obesity among pediatric patients with NAFLD is 72%–92% (Table 27.1).

Sex, age, race, and ethnicity are other factors affecting the prevalence of NAFLD. Male sex, older age, Hispanic ethnicity, and Asian race are factors significantly associated with a higher risk of fatty liver.[1] As demonstrated in multiple studies, boys have a higher prevalence of NAFLD (11.1% in SCALE) than girls (7.9% in SCALE). NAFLD prevalence also increases with increasing age. In SCALE, the prevalence of NAFLD in children aged 2–4 was 1%, 3% in children aged 5–9, 11% in children aged 10–14, and increased to 17% of children aged 15–19.[1] The prevalence of NAFLD is highest in Hispanic (12%) and Asian (11%) children and lowest in African American children (1.5%). The prevalence of NAFLD in Caucasian children is 9%.[1]

TABLE 27.1
Weight Distribution in Pediatric NAFLD

Author	Publication Year	Sample Size	Population	Location	Underweight (BMI <5%)	Normal Weight (BMI >5% and <85%)	Overweight (BMI 85% and <95%)	Obese (BMI 95%)	Mean BMI of NAFLD Cohort
NAFLD Cohorts									
Schwimmer et al.[3]	2005	100	Children with NAFLD	San Diego	1%	1%	6%	92%	30.7
Nobili et al.[4]	2006	85	Children with NAFLD	Rome		8%	51%	41%	26.3
Manco et al.[50]	2008	120	Children with NAFLD	Rome		7%			
Mager et al.[69]	2008	53	Suspected NAFLD (U/S)	Toronto		8%	21%	72%	29.7
A-Kader et al.[70]	2008	106	Children with NAFLD	Arizona	0%	2%	10%	88%	32.8
Carter-Kent et al.[46]	2009	130	Children with NAFLD	Cleveland, Mayo, Cincinnati, Chicago, Toronto		13%	6%	82%	31
NAFLD Prevalence Study									
Schwimmer et al.[1]	2006	742 (97 [13%] with NAFLD)	General population autopsy study	San Diego	0%	20%	20%	60%	30.2 (NAFLD) 33.6 (NASH)
Yuksel et al.[17]	2012	330	General population autopsy study	Turkey		5%		11%	23
NAFLD Cohorts Not Subdivided into Weight Categories									
Schwimmer et al.[45]	2008	150	Children with NAFLD	San Diego					33.8
Ko et al.[71]	2009	80	Children with NAFLD	Seoul					27.6
Fitzpatrick et al.[72]	2010	45	Children with NAFLD	London					25.3
Takahashi et al.[73]	2011	34	Children with NAFLD	Japan					26.7
Schwimmer et al.[9]	2013	193	Children with NAFLD	San Diego					31.5
Schwimmer et al.[51]	2014	494	Children with NAFLD	NASH CRN					32.7
Alkhouri et al.[74]	2014	302	Children with NAFLD	Rome					25.5 (NAFLD) 26.3 (NASH)

PATHOPHYSIOLOGY

Multiple factors interplay in the pathophysiology of NAFLD: genetics, inflammatory cytokines, insulin resistance, microbiome, and perinatal and environmental factors.

GENETICS

Genetics also play a key role in the pathophysiology of NAFLD. Prior studies have demonstrated differences in the prevalence of NAFLD between racial and ethnic groups. Although the latest NHANES data from 2011–2012 demonstrate that girls of black race or Hispanic ethnicity have the highest rates of obesity (both at 20.4%),[18] pediatric NAFLD rates are the lowest in African Americans, at 1.5% compared with 11.8% in Hispanics.[1] The importance of genetics in NAFLD risk has been demonstrated by studies of heritability. In a 2009 study by Schwimmer et al., obese children with and without NAFLD and their family members (parents, siblings, second- and third-degree relatives) underwent MRI to assess PDFF. Fatty liver was found in parents (78%) and siblings (59%) of obese children with NAFLD, compared with 37% of parents and 17% of siblings in obese children without NAFLD. Adjusting for age, sex, race, and BMI, heritability of liver fat fraction was .386 or 38.6%.[19]

The discovery in 2008 of rs738409, a common variant allele in the patatin-like phospholipase 3 (PNPLA3) gene that increases susceptibility to NAFLD, has led to multiple genetic studies.[20] PNPLA3 was the first polymorphism, independent of BMI or insulin resistance, to be highly correlated with the onset and progression of NAFLD. This SNP is highly associated with hepatic fat content, as measured by magnetic resonance spectroscopy (MRS), and is independent of BMI, diabetes, or alcohol use. The highest frequency of this allele is present in Hispanics (0.49), followed by European Americans (0.23) and African Americans (0.17). In a study of 153 obese Hispanic children and adolescents, HFF, as measured by MRI, was positively related to total sugar and carbohydrate intake in patients with the *GG* PNPLA3 genotype.[21] Furthermore, in a study composed of 475 obese children and adolescents, higher levels of alanine aminotransferase (ALT) were seen for each mutant allele of the PNPLA3 locus present.[22] In an Italian study, the PNPLA34 variant allele was associated with steatosis severity, the presence of fibrosis, lobular inflammation, and hepatocellular ballooning in 149 pediatric NAFLD patients.[23] In a contrasting study in 223 children with NAFLD from the NASH CRN, no association between PNPLA3 loci and histologic severity of NAFLD was found.[24] Thus, further studies are needed regarding the genetics of NAFLD.

INSULIN RESISTANCE

Systemic insulin resistance is hypothesized to play a key role in the pathogenesis of pediatric NAFLD via increased free fatty-acid circulation and increased *de novo* lipogenesis.[25] Insulin resistance affects hepatocyte lipid accumulation and the resultant oxidative stress, which in turn incites an inflammatory response.[26]

INFLUENCE OF MATERNAL FACTORS AND BREAST-FEEDING ON NAFLD

Recently, it has been proposed that NAFLD may have *in utero* origins.[27] Patel et al.[28] demonstrated that fetal hepatic steatosis was significantly higher in infants born to mothers with gestational diabetes mellitus (GDM) (79%) compared with women without GDM (17%). Brumbaugh et al. demonstrated that infants born to obese mothers with GDM had 68% greater liver hepatic fat fraction (HFF) compared with those born to normal-weight mothers.[29]

After birth, neonatal feeding practices, especially overfeeding, may have long-term consequences on *de novo* lipogenesis.[30] Breast-feeding, on the other hand, may be protective in the prevention of hepatic steatosis. Nobili et al. demonstrated that in children with NAFLD, steatosis distribution, inflammation, ballooning of hepatocytes, and fibrosis were all more severe in children who were *not* breast-fed compared with their breast-fed counterparts.[31] Thus, the origins of NAFLD are affected by maternal factors; GDM, maternal obesity, and neonatal feeding habits may all play a role in the development of NAFLD.

SCREENING FOR NAFLD

The prevailing recommendations regarding the prevention, assessment, and treatment of child and adolescent overweight and obesity were published in 2007 by an expert committee.[32] These guidelines recommend screening for NAFLD by evaluating serum ALT and aspartate aminotransferase (AST) levels. The expert committee suggests biannual screening starting at age 10 years in obese children and overweight children with additional risk factors. The guidelines further suggest referral to a pediatric hepatologist if AST or ALT levels are twice the upper limit of normal.

The ideal age at which initial screening takes place is debated. In a recent study, Beacher et al. demonstrated that ALT elevation was found in 25% of children aged 2–5 years referred to a tertiary care clinic, and concluded that, instead of starting to screen for NAFLD via AST/ALT at age 10 years and above, as currently recommended in obese children, screening severely obese children (BMI ≥99%) should begin at age 2.[33] ALT elevation can be common even at very young ages. Whether this is due to NAFLD is unknown.

As screening is based on laboratory results, it is important to define what is normal. The Screening ALT for Elevation in Today's Youth (SAFETY) study demonstrated that conventional ALT cutoff values of normal used in children's hospitals varies widely and is too high for reliable detection of chronic liver disease. The median upper limit of normal ALT used by children's hospitals in the United States was found to be 53 U/L, with a range of 30–90 U/L.[34] In a large, nationally representative sample, the 95th percentiles for ALT levels for healthy-weight, metabolically normal children without liver disease were 25.8 U/L in boys and 22.1 U/L in girls. According to these data, the median normal ALT used in many laboratories today would actually fall into the category of twice the upper limit of normal for biologically based ALT. Thus, interpretation of aminotransferases with biologically based values in mind will assist in detecting patients who may have liver disease with higher sensitivity and specificity (sensitivity of 72% in boys and 82% in girls, and specificity of 79% in boys and 85% in girls). Sensitivity in the detection of NAFLD was lower using current children's hospitals ALT levels (32%–48%).

In order to evaluate the prevailing guidelines, a study prospectively evaluated 347 children ≥10 years of age who were overweight or obese and who were screened for NAFLD via aminotransferases by their primary care provider and referred to pediatric gastroenterology for suspected NAFLD. In this cohort of patients referred to tertiary care, only 55% had NAFLD and the remainder were almost equally divided between not having any liver disease or having liver disease attributed to another reason besides NAFLD. Thus, we cannot conclude that elevated transaminases in obese children are automatically indicative of NAFLD.[9]

IMPACT OF NONALCOHOLIC FATTY LIVER DISEASE

Advanced fibrosis is demonstrated in 5%–15% of children with NAFLD at the time of diagnosis.[15,23] In a recent study in overweight and obese children referred from primary care to pediatric gastroenterology for suspected NAFLD, 33 out of 193 patients (17%) had advanced fibrosis on initial diagnostic liver biopsy.[9] Advanced fibrosis and cirrhosis increase the risk of hepatocellular carcinoma (HCC) and the need for liver transplant. NASH-associated cirrhosis is now the second-most common cause of liver transplantation in adults[35] and is anticipated to overtake the hepatitis C virus (HCV) and alcohol-induced cirrhosis as the leading cause of hepatic transplantation within the next decade.[36] The risk of HCC can be present even in childhood, based on a recent report of a 7-year-old child developing HCC in association with NAFLD.[37] It is anticipated that NAFLD-associated HCC will increase as the prevalence of obesity and NAFLD continue to rise.

Although mortality data in pediatric NAFLD are limited, a 2009 natural history study following pediatric NAFLD (mean follow-up time of 6.4 years) found children with NAFLD to be at higher risk of mortality in comparison with the general population.[38] The standardized mortality ratio in NAFLD patients was 13.6%, with significantly shorter observed survival free of liver transplantation in the NAFLD cohort, compared with the expected survival of the general US population with similar age and sex.

Children with NAFLD are at greater risk of cardiopulmonary, endocrinologic, and psychologic comorbidities compared with children with obesity alone and children without NAFLD (Table 27.2).

Obstructive sleep apnea (OSA) is a condition whereby recurrent partial or complete upper airway obstruction occurs during sleep, leading to hypoxic events, oxidative stress, and ischemic and reperfusional tissue injury. Obesity is a risk factor for OSA. Symptoms of OSA manifest as snoring, daytime sleepiness, and poor school performance.[39,40] Two recent studies[41,42] have demonstrated an OSA prevalence of 60% in mainly obese children with NAFLD, which is much higher than the prevalence of OSA in the general population of 1.2%–5.7%.[43] Moreover, in children with NAFLD, the presence of OSA may impact disease severity. For instance, in a study with 65 NAFLD patients, Nobili et al. demonstrated that the presence of NASH (compared with NAFLD) and fibrosis was associated with more severe OSA.[42] Hypoxemia, defined as oxygen saturation <90%, was correlated with increased activation of intrahepatic inflammatory cells and increased circulating markers of hepatocyte fibrosis and fibrogenesis. Similarly, Sundaram et al. demonstrated that NAFLD in association with OSA had more severe hepatic fibrosis.[41] Thus, OSA is an important comorbidity in NAFLD and screening questions should include the presence of snoring and/or daytime sleepiness.

NAFLD is associated with type 2 diabetes; however, the prevalence of type 2 diabetes among children with NAFLD is not yet certain. In a case series of pediatric NAFLD, the frequency of type 2 diabetes has ranged from 2% to 14%.[4,15,44–49] Larger studies to allow a more stable estimate are still needed. Insulin resistance is a major common factor between NAFLD and type 2 diabetes, as it plays a role in the pathogenesis of both.

Dyslipidemia is also commonly associated with NAFLD. In a study of 120 children with NAFLD from Italy,[50] over 60% had elevated serum triglycerides and 45% had low high-density lipoprotein (HDL). Furthermore, fibrosis was associated with higher total serum cholesterol and triglycerides. The dyslipidemia that occurs in children with NAFLD in conjunction with obesity appears to be more severe than in children with obesity alone. This was shown in a study by Schwimmer et al. that compared 150 children with NAFLD with 150 overweight and obese children without NAFLD. Children with NAFLD had significantly higher total cholesterol, low-density lipoprotein (LDL), and triglycerides.[45]

Hypertension is another comorbidity in patients with NAFLD, independent of BMI and obesity. In a study comparing 150 children with overweight or obese body habitus without NAFLD with 150 children with NAFLD, children with NAFLD had higher rates of elevated systolic blood pressure (SBP) than similarly overweight children.[45] In a 2014 study from the NASH CRN evaluating 382 children with NAFLD, higher rates of high blood pressure were demonstrated both cross-sectionally and longitudinally in NAFLD patients compared with patients with obesity alone. In this study, 36% of the patients had elevated blood pressure at baseline, and 21% had persistent high blood pressure over the 48-week follow-up period. Furthermore, children with high blood pressure were more likely to have more severe steatosis (mild 19.8%, moderate 35%, severe 45.2%) than children without high blood pressure (mild 34.2%, moderate 30.7%, severe 35.1%).[51]

In addition to physical impacts, NAFLD also has a substantial psychological burden. A study from the NASH CRN demonstrated impaired quality of life (QOL) in children with NAFLD compared with healthy children.[48] More than one-third of children with NAFLD were found to have impaired QOL. Not surprisingly, children with NAFLD had worse total physical and psychosocial health scores compared with healthy children. Difficulty sleeping, sadness, and fatigue constituted

TABLE 27.2
Co-Morbidities in Pediatric NAFLD

Diabetes

Author	Publication Year	Location	Sample Size	Age	Children with NASH (%)	NAFLD Criteria	Children with Diabetes (%)
Schwimmer et al.[44]	2003	San Diego	43	2–17 years	Nonstated	Biopsy	14%
Nobili et al.[4]	2006	Italy	84	3–18 years	26%, 5% advanced fibrosis	Biopsy	2%
Carter-Kent et al.[46]	2009	5 centers in US/Canada	130	3–18 years	82% NASH, 20% advanced fibrosis	Biopsy	7%
Patton et al.[47]	2010	NASH CRN	254	6–17 years	35% NASH, 14% advanced fibrosis	Biopsy	3%
Kistler et al.[48]	2010	NASH CRN	239	5–17 years	39% NASH, 14% advanced fibrosis	Biopsy	4%

Dyslipidemia

Study	Publication Year	Location	Sample Size	Age	Population	NAFLD Criteria	Results
Cali et al.[75]	2007	New Haven	49	Mean 15 years	BMI >95%	Fast MRI	If HFF >5.5%, higher TG and very low density lipoprotein (VLDL), lower HDL
Manco et al.[50]	2008	Italy	120	3–18 years	NAFLD	Biopsy	63% with high TG, 45% with low HDL, fibrosis assoc. with higher TC and TG
Schwimmer et al.[45]	2008	San Diego	300	5–17 years	NAFLD vs. BMI >85%	Biopsy	Higher TC, LDL, TG in NAFLD patients
Pacifico et al.[76]	2014	Italy	136	Mean 12 years	Lean, obese, obese + NAFLD	Biopsy	NAFLD/obese group with higher TG, lower HDL

Cardiovascular Disease

Study	Publication Year	Location	Sample Size	Age	Population	NAFLD Criteria	Results
Schwimmer et al.[45]	2008	San Diego	300	5–17 years	NAFLD vs. BMI >85%	Biopsy	Higher SBP, TC, LDL, TG in NAFLD patients
Manco et al.[77]	2010	Italy	80	9–16 years	Obese vs. obese + NAFLD	Biopsy	No relation to liver disease; carotid intima-media thickness (CIMT) elevated in obese and obese plus NAFLD
Singh et al.[78]	2013	St Louis	44	Mean 15 years	Lean, obese, obese + NAFLD	MRS	NAFLD/obese group with higher SBP, DBP, and LV strain compared with obese/no NAFLD
Pacifico et al.[76]	2014	Italy	136	Mean 12 years	Lean, obese, obese + NAFLD	Biopsy	NAFLD/obese group with higher SBP, TB, lower HDL, more LV dysfunction, higher LV mass
Schwimmer et al.[51]	20.4	NASH CRN	382	2–17 years	NAFLD	Biopsy	Prevalence of HTN = 36% at baseline, persistent HTN = 21%, patients with HTN more likely to have steatosis

almost half of the variances in QOL scores. In another study comparing children with NAFLD with obese children, children with NAFLD were found to have higher levels of depression and lower self-esteem compared with their obese control counterparts.[52] Furthermore, this study demonstrated that postdiagnosis standard-care counseling on lifestyle and dietary changes had no impact on QOL or other psychosocial measures longitudinally.

APPROACH TO CARE

Weight loss, through lifestyle modifications in the form of increased activity and healthier dietary choices, is the most commonly recommended first-line treatment of NAFLD. Other emerging treatment modalities that require additional study are pharmacologic therapies, with targets ranging from the intestinal microbiome to insulin resistance, and bariatric surgery.

Weight loss improves insulin sensitivity, decreases reactive oxygen species and delivery of free fatty acids to the liver, and thus should counteract predominant mechanisms involved in the pathogenesis of NAFLD. It is hypothesized that a 3%–5% reduction in total body weight decreases hepatic steatosis, but a 10% or more reduction in total body weight may be required to prevent progression and result in improvement in steatohepatitis.[53] In a recent study of 293 adults with NAFLD, the highest rates of NASH resolution and fibrosis regression occurred in patients with a loss of 10% or more of their total body weight.[54] Of the patients who lost 10% or more of their total body weight, 90% had complete resolution of NASH, compared with 58% NASH resolution in patients who lost 5%–10% of their total body weight. In a recent pediatric study, for those children who were adherent to a 2-year lifestyle intervention, there was improvement in weight, aminotransferases, and liver histology.[55] An earlier study also demonstrated that an uncontrolled, 12-month lifestyle modification program (a balanced, low-calorie diet tailored to individual preferences and moderate physical activity of 30–45 minutes a day, three times a week) was associated with significant decreases in BMI (average BMI decreasing from 25.9 to 23.8) and ALT (average ALT decreasing from 62 to 33 IU/L).[4] Notably, there is a lack of randomized controlled trials with evidence to show that lifestyle interventions are effective for the treatment of NAFLD in children. Thus, there is a need for large randomized controlled trials that investigate specific dietary interventions and exercise regimens in children with carefully staged NAFLD, in order to have specific evidence-based recommendations for the treatment of NAFLD.

Bariatric surgery is increasingly performed on adolescents for weight reduction.[56] The impact of bariatric surgery on children with NAFLD, however, is not entirely clear. Moreover, it is not known whether bariatric surgery improves histologically severe NASH. A recent study evaluating pre- and postsurgery NAFLD scores among adolescents with preexisting NAFLD undergoing laparoscopic adjustable gastric banding demonstrated significant improvements in NAFLD scores, which decreased by an average of 0.68 ($p < .01$) 2 years postoperatively.[57] In 2015, the hepatology committee of the European Society for Paediatric Gastroenterology, Hepatology and Nutrition (ESPGHAN) published a position paper regarding bariatric intervention in severely obese children and adolescents.[56] A BMI >97% with major comorbidities (including NASH with significant fibrosis) was recommended as a criteria for bariatric surgery. Though multiple studies have demonstrated improvement in liver histology in adults following bariatric surgery, outcome data in adolescents are currently lacking.

Though pharmacologic therapy is not uniformly recommended in pediatric NAFLD, avid interest and evaluation of multiple medications as potential therapeutic targets is underway. Metformin, an insulin-sensitizing agent, was proposed as a therapeutic target for NAFLD, as insulin resistance is believed to play a major role in the pathogenesis of NAFLD. Additionally, metformin has previously been demonstrated to reduce body weight, improve insulin resistance, and have chemoprotective benefits in decreasing HCC.[58] Initial pilot studies were promising.[59,60] After 24 weeks of therapy, 40% of subjects with NAFLD had normalization of ALT. Additionally, 90% of subjects had a significant reduction in hepatic signal fat fraction via MRS signal fat fraction imaging.[59] In a separate study in 30 children with NAFLD, 24 months of therapy with metformin as well as lifestyle interventions was compared with lifestyle interventions alone. Metformin was not more effective than lifestyle intervention in improving transaminase levels and hepatic steatosis.[60] Treatment of NAFLD in Children (TONIC), a large, multicenter, double-blind, placebo-controlled trial by the NASH CRN, evaluated the efficacy of metformin and vitamin E over 96 weeks of therapy in patients with NAFLD. Metformin was associated with significant improvement in hepatocellular ballooning compared with placebo, but did not improve ALT, steatosis, inflammation, or fibrosis.[61]

The TONIC trial also evaluated the efficacy of vitamin E, an antioxidant, as a potential therapeutic, given oxidative stress is believed to be a contributor to the pathogenesis of NAFLD. After 96 weeks of vitamin E treatment, pediatric patients with NAFLD did not have any significant decrease in ALT compared with placebo.[61] Similar to metformin, vitamin E was associated with significant improvement in hepatocellular ballooning but not steatosis, inflammation, or fibrosis.

Cysteamine, another antioxidant, is also a potential therapy for NAFLD as it readily enters into hepatocytes and can replete glutathione, which may be therapeutic as glutathione depletion contributes to hepatocellular injury and fibrosis.[62] In a small pilot study, 11 children with NAFLD received cysteamine therapy for 24 weeks. Significant reductions were demonstrated in serum transaminases (ALT decreased from 120.2 IU/L at baseline to 55 IU/L at week 24), serum adiponectin, and CK-18 levels. Currently, the NASH CRN is in the process of completing a multicenter, placebo-controlled clinical trial in children aged 8–17 with NAFLD to evaluate whether 52 weeks of cysteamine treatment will result in an improvement in the severity of liver disease.

Dietary docosahexaenoic acid (DHA), a major dietary long-chain polyunsaturated fatty acid, lowers serum triglycerides and has both insulin-sensitizing and anti-inflammatory properties. Thus, dietary DHA supplementation is of interest as a possible therapeutic target for NAFLD. In a clinical trial by Nobili et al.,[63] children aged 6–16 years with NAFLD received DHA 250 mg/day, DHA 500 mg/day, or placebo ($n = 20$/group). No effect was noted on BMI or ALT after DHA treatment. In a continuation study of 20 children with NAFLD, treatment with DHA for 18 months was associated with the modulation of hepatic progenitor cells and prolonged hepatocyte survival.[64]

Recent studies have suggested a role for microbiome gut dysbiosis in the development of NAFLD in children.[65] In animal models, the composition of gut microbiota can influence intrahepatic fat accumulation via mechanisms such as increased monosaccharide absorption from the intestinal lumen and the production of hepatotoxic products.[66] Though multiple studies in humans have been performed, outcomes in regard to whether modification of the gut microbiome can impact obesity and NAFLD are currently mixed. In a recent randomized clinical trial, the effects of VSL#3 in obese children with NAFLD were evaluated.[67] A total of 44 children were enrolled, with 22 receiving VSL#3 and 22 receiving a placebo for 4 months. There was an 8% decrease in BMI noted with probiotic treatment, with no change in the placebo group. There was no improvement in ALT or insulin sensitivity in either group.

A separate study of 21 obese children with persistently elevated hepatic transaminases and increased echogenicity on ultrasound evaluated the effect of *Lactobacillus rhamnosus*.[68] After 8 weeks of therapy with *L. rhamnosus*, ALT was noted to decrease significantly (70 to 40 U/L on average) in the treatment group. In the control group, ALT was unchanged. These preliminary studies provide a rationale for further studies of the impact of dysbiosis and the microbiome on NAFLD in children.

SUMMARY

NAFLD is a frequent cause of chronic liver disease in children. Although the prevalence of NAFLD and NASH is higher in obese children, NAFLD occurs in both obese and nonobese children. Multiple factors play a role in the pathophysiology of NAFLD, including maternal and neonatal factors, insulin resistance, and genetics. Multiple studies are currently underway to gain additional insight into the complex relationships between these multiple factors and NAFLD.

NAFLD can be associated with many negative health consequences, from increased risk of cirrhosis and HCC to multiple extrahepatic comorbidities such as OSA, diabetes, dyslipidemia, and hypertension. Effective treatment modalities for NAFLD are more important than ever. Lifestyle modifications, such as improved diet and increased physical activity, are the recommended first line of treatment. Multiple pharmacologic and surgical options are being evaluated. Pediatric NAFLD is likely to play an increasingly important role in the care and management of obese children.

REFERENCES

1. Schwimmer J, Deutsch R, Kahen T, Lavine J, Stanley C, Behling C. Prevalence of fatty liver in children and adolescents. *Pediatrics.* 2006;118(4):1388–1393.
2. Xanthakos S, Jenkins T, Kleiner D, Boyce T, Mourya R, Karns R, et al. High prevalence of non-alcoholic fatty liver disease in adolescents undergoing bariatric surgery. *Gastroenterology.* 2015;149(3):623–634.e8.
3. Schwimmer J, Behling C, Newbury R, Deutsch R, Nievergelt C, Schork N, et al. Histopathology of pediatric nonalcoholic fatty liver disease. *Hepatology.* 2005;42:641–649.
4. Nobili V, Marcellini M, Devito R, Ciampalini P, Piemonte F, Comparcola D, et al. NAFLD in children: A prospective clinical-pathological study and effect of lifestyle advice. *Hepatology.* 2006;44:458–465.
5. Brunt E, Ramrakhiani S, Cordes B, Neuschwander-Tetri B, Janney C, Bacon B, et al. Concurrence of histologic features of steatohepatitis with other forms of chronic liver disease. *Modern Pathology.* 2003;16(1):49–56.
6. Brunt E, Janney C, Bisceglie A, Neuschwander-Tetri B, Bacon B. Nonalcoholic steatohepatitis: A proposal for grading and staging the histological lesions. *The American Journal of Gastroenterology.* 1999;94(9):2467–2474.
7. Brunt E, Kleiner D, Wilson L, Belt P, Neuschwander-Tetri B. Nonalcoholic fatty liver disease (NAFLD) activity score and the histopathologic diagnosis in NAFLD: Distinct clinicopathologic meanings. *Hepatology.* 2011;53(3):810–820.
8. Hourigan S, Torbenson M, Tibesar E, Scheimann A. The full spectrum of hepatic steatosis in children. *Clinical Pediatrics.* 2015;54(7):635–642.
9. Schwimmer J, Newton K, Awai H, Choi L, Garcia M, Ellis L, et al. Paediatric gastroenterology evaluation of overweight and obese children referred from primary care for suspected non-alcoholic fatty liver disease. *Alimentary Pharmacology & Therapeutics.* 2013;38(10):1267–1277.
10. El-Koofy N, El-Karaksy H, El-Akel W, Helmy H, Anwar G, El-Sayed R, et al. Ultrasonography as a non-invasive tool for detection of nonalcoholic fatty liver disease in overweight/obese Egyptian children. *European Journal of Radiology.* 2012;81(11):3120–3123.
11. Shannon A, Alkhouri N, Carter-Kent C, Monti L, Devito R, Lopez R, et al. Ultrasonographic quantitative estimation of hepatic steatosis in children with NAFLD. *Journal of Pediatric Gastroenterology and Nutrition.* 2011;53(2):190–195.
12. Awai H, Newton K, Sirlin C, Behling C, Schwimmer J. Evidence and recommendations for imaging liver fat in children, based on systematic review. *Clinical Gastroenterology and Hepatology.* 2014;12(5):765–773.
13. Schwimmer J, Middleton M, Behling C, Newton K, Awai H, Paiz M, et al. Magnetic resonance imaging and liver histology as biomarkers of hepatic steatosis in children with nonalcoholic fatty liver disease. *Hepatology.* 2015;61(6):1887–1895.
14. Xanthakos S, Daniels S, Inge T. Bariatric surgery in adolescents: An update. *Adolescent Medicine Clinics.* 2006;17(3):589–612.
15. Patton H, Lavine J, Van Natta M, Schwimmer J, Kleiner D, Molleston J. Clinical correlates of histopathology in pediatric nonalcoholic steatohepatitis. *Gastroenterology.* 2008;135(6):1961–1971.e2.
16. Ogden C, Carroll M, Kit B, Flegal K. Prevalence of childhood and adult obesity in the United States, 2011–2012. *Journal of the American Medical Association.* 2014;311(8):806.
17. Yuksel F, Turkkan D, Yuksel I, Kara S, Celik N, Samdanci E. Fatty liver disease in an autopsy series of children and adolescents. *Hippokratia.* 2012;16(1):61–65.
18. Skinner A, Skelton J. Prevalence and trends in obesity and severe obesity among children in the United States, 1999–2012. *JAMA Pediatrics.* 2014;168(6):561.
19. Schwimmer JB, Celadon MA, Lavine JE, Salem R, Campbell N, Schork NJ, et al. Heritability of nonalcoholic fatty liver disease. *Gastroenterology.* 2009;136(5):1585–1592.

20. Romeo S, Kozlitina J, Xing C, Pertsemlidis A, Cox D, Pennacchio LA, et al. Genetic variation in PNPLA3 confers susceptibility to nonalcoholic fatty liver disease. *Nature Genetics.* 2008;40:1461–1465.

21. Davis JN, Le KA, Walker RW, Vikman S, Spruijt-Metz D, et al. Increased hepatic fat in overweight Hispanic youth influenced by interaction between genetic variation in *PNPLA3* and high diet carbohydrate and sugar consumption. *American Journal of Clinical Nutrition.* 2010;92:1522–1527.

22. Romeo S, Sentinelli F, Cambuli VM, Incani M, Congiu T, Matta V, et al. The 148M allele of the PNPLA3 gene is associated with indices of liver damage early in life. *Journal of Hepatology.* 2010;53:335–338.

23. Valenti L, Alisi A, Galmozzi E, Bartuli A, Del Menico B, Alterio A, et al. I148M patatin-like phosphpolipase domain-containing 3 gene variant and severity of pediatric nonalcoholic fatty liver disease. *Hepatology.* 2010;52(4):1274–1280.

24. Speliotes EK, Butler JL, Palmer CD, Voight BF, GIANT Consortium, MIGen consortium, et al. PNPLA3 variants specifically confer increased risk for histologic nonalcoholic fatty liver disease but not metabolic disease. *Hepatology.* 2010;52(3):904–912.

25. Heptulla R, Stewart A, Enocksson S, Rife F, Ma T, Sherwin R, et al. *In situ* evidence that peripheral insulin resistance in adolescents with poorly controlled type 1 diabetes is associated with impaired suppression of lipolysis: A microdialysis study. *Pediatric Research.* 2003;53(5):830–835.

26. Ferolla SM, Armiliato GN, Couto CA, Ferrari TC. Probiotics as a complementary therapeutic approach in nonalcoholic fatty liver disease. *World Journal of Hepatology.* 2015;7(3):559–565.

27. Brumbaugh D, Friedman J. Developmental origins of nonalcoholic fatty liver disease. *Pediatric Research.* 2013;75(1–2):140–147.

28. Patel K, White F, Deutsch G. Hepatic steatosis is prevalent in stillborns delivered to women with diabetes mellitus. *Journal of Pediatric Gastroenterology and Nutrition.* 2015;60(2):152–158.

29. Brumbaugh D, Tearse P, Cree-Green M, Fenton L, Brown M, Scherzinger A, et al. Intrahepatic fat is increased in the neonatal offspring of obese women with gestational diabetes. *The Journal of Pediatrics.* 2013;162(5):930–936.e1.

30. Ugalde-Nicalo P, Schwimmer JB. On the origin of pediatric nonalcoholic fatty liver disease. *Journal of Pediatric Gastroenterology and Nutrition.* 2015;60(2):147–148.

31. Nobili V, Bedogni G, Alisi A, Pietrobattista A, Alterio A, Tiribelli C, et al. A protective effect of breastfeeding on the progression of non-alcoholic fatty liver disease. *Archives of Disease in Childhood.* 2009;94(10):801–805.

32. Barlow SE, Expert Committee. Expert committee recommendations regarding the prevention, assessment, and treatment of child and adolescent overweight and obesity: Summary report. *Pediatrics.* 2007;120(Suppl. 4):S164–S192.

33. Beacher D, Ariza A, Fishbein M, Binns H. Screening for elevated risk of liver disease in preschool children (aged 2–5 years) being seen for obesity management. *SAGE Open Medicine.* 2014;2.

34. Schwimmer JB, Dunn W, Norman GJ, Pardee PE, Middleton MS, Kerkar N, et al. SAFETY Study: Alanine aminotransferase cutoff values are set too high for reliable detection of pediatric chronic liver disease. *Gastroenterology.* 2010;138:1357–1364.

35. Kim WR, Lake JR, Smith JM, Skeans MA, Schladt DP, Edwards EB, Harper AM, Wainright JL, Snyder JJ, Israni AK, Kasiske BL. OPTN/SRTR 2013 Annual Data Report: Liver. *American Journal of Transplantation* 2015;15(Suppl. 2):1–28.

36. Zezos P. Liver transplantation and non-alcoholic fatty liver disease. *World Journal of Gastroenterology.* 2014;20(42):15532.

37. Nobili V, Alisi A, Grimaldi C, Liccardo D, Francalanci P, Monti L, et al. Non-alcoholic fatty liver disease and hepatocellular carcinoma in a 7-year-old obese boy: Coincidence or comorbidity? *Pediatric Obesity.* 2014;9(5):e99–e102.

38. Feldstein AE, Charatcharoenwitthaya P, Treeprasertsuk S, Benson JT, Enders FB, Augulo P. The natural history of non-alcoholic fatty liver disease in children: A follow-up study for up to 20 years. *Gut.* 2009;58:1538–1544.

39. Mathurin P, Durand F, Ganne N, Mollo JL, Lebrec D, Degott C, et al. Ischemic hepatitis due to obstructive sleep apnea. *Gastroenterology.* 1995;109:1682–1684.

40. Henrion J, Colin L, Schapira M, Heller FR. Hypoxic hepatitis caused by severe hypoxemia from obstructive sleep apnea. *Journal of Clinical Gastroenterology.* 1997;24:245–249.

41. Sundaram SS, Sokol RJ, Capocelli KE, Pan Z, Sullivan JS, Robbins K, et al. Obstructive sleep apnea and hypoxemia are associated with advanced liver histology in pediatric nonalcoholic fatty liver disease. *Journal of Pediatrics.* 2014;164(4):699–706.

42. Nobili V, Cutrera R, Liccardo D, Pavone M, Devito R, Giorgio V, et al. OSAS affects liver histology and inflammatory cell activation in paediatric NAFLD, regardless of obesity/insulin resistance. *American Journal of Respiratory Critical Care Medicine*. 2014;189(1):66–76.

43. Marcus C, Brooks L, Ward S, Draper K, Gozal D, Halbower A, et al. Diagnosis and management of childhood obstructive sleep apnea syndrome. *Pediatrics*. 2012;130(3):e714–e755.

44. Schwimmer JB, Deutsch R, Rauch JB, Behling C, Newbury R, Lavine JE. Obesity, insulin resistance, and other clinicopathological correlates of pediatric nonalcoholic fatty liver disease. *Journal of Pediatrics*. 2003;143(4):500–505.

45. Schwimmer JB, Pardee PE, Lavine JE, Blumkin AK, Cook S. Cardiovascular risk factors and the metabolic syndrome in pediatric nonalcoholic fatty liver disease. *Circulation*. 2008;118(3):277–283.

46. Carter-Kent C, Yerian LM, Brunt EM, Angulo P, Kohli R, Ling SC, et al. Nonalcoholic steatohepatitis in children: A multicenter clinicopathological study. *Hepatology*. 2009;50(4):1113–1120.

47. Patton HM, Yates K, Unalp-Arida A, Behling CA, Huang TT, Rosenthal P, et al. Association between metabolic syndrome and liver histology among children with nonalcoholic fatty liver disease. *American Journal of Gastroenterology*. 2010;105(9):2093–2102.

48. Kistler K, Molleston J, Unalp A, Abrams S, Behling C, Schwimmer J. Symptoms and quality of life in obese children and adolescents with non-alcoholic fatty liver disease. *Alimentary Pharmacology & Therapeutics*. 2010;31(3):396–406.

49. Nobili V, Alkhouri N, Bartuli A, Manco M, Lopez R, Alisi A, et al. Severity of liver injury and atherogenic lipid profile in children with nonalcoholic fatty liver disease. *Pediatric Research*. 2010;67(6):665–670.

50. Manco M, Marcellini M, DeVito R, Comparcola D, Sartorelli M, Nobili V. Metabolic syndrome and liver histology in paediatric non-alcoholic steatohepatitis. *International Journal of Obesity*. 2008;32:381–387.

51. Schwimmer J, Zepeda A, Newton K, Xanthakos S, Behling C, Hallinan E, et al. Longitudinal assessment of high blood pressure in children with nonalcoholic fatty liver disease. *PLoS ONE*. 2014;9(11):e112569.

52. Kerkar N, D'Urso C, Nostrand K, Kochin I, Gault A, Suchy F, et al. Psychosocial outcomes for children with nonalcoholic fatty liver disease over time and compared with obese controls. *Journal of Pediatric Gastroenterology and Nutrition*. 2013;56:77–82.

53. Perito ER, Rodriguez LA, Lustig RH. Dietary treatment of nonalcoholic steatohepatitis. *Current Opinion Gastroenterology*. 2013;29(2):170–176.

54. Vilar-Gomez E, Martinez-Perez Y, Calzadilla-Bertrot L, Torees-Gonzalez A, Gra-Oramas B, Gonzalez-Fabian L, et al. Weight loss via Lifestyle modification significantly reduces features of nonalcoholic steatohepatitis. *Gastroenterology*. 2015;149(2): 367–378.

55. Nobili V, Manco M, Devito R, DiCiommo V, Comparcola D, Sartorelli MR, et al. Lifestyle intervention and antioxidant therapy in children with nonalcoholic fatty liver disease: A randomized, controlled trial. *Hepatology*. 2008;48:119–128.

56. Nobili V, Vajro P, Dezsofi A, Fischler B, Hadzic N, Jahnel J, et al. Indications and limitations of bariatric intervention in severely obese children and adolescents with and without nonalcoholic steatohepatitis: ESPGHAN Hepatology Committee Position Statement. *Journal of Pediatric Gastroenterology and Nutrition*. 2015;60:550–561.

57. Loy J, Youn H, Schwack B, Kurian M, Ren Fielding C, Fielding G. Improvement in nonalcoholic fatty liver disease and metabolic syndrome in adolescents undergoing bariatric surgery. *Surgery for Obesity and Related Diseases*. 2015;11(2):442–449.

58. Doycheva I, Loomba R. Effect of metformin on ballooning degeneration in nonalcoholic steatlhepatitis (NASH): When to use metformin in nonalcoholic fatty liver disease (NAFLD). *Advanced Therapeutics*. 2014;31:30–43.

59. Schwimmer JB, Middleton MS, Deutsch R, Lavine JE. A phase 2 clinical trial of metformin as a treatment for non-diabetic paediatric non-alcoholic steatohepatitis. *Alimentary Pharmacologics and Therapeutics*. 2005;21:871–879.

60. Nobili V, Manco M, Ciampalini P, Alisi A, Devito R, Bugianesi E, et al. Metformin use in children with nonalcoholic fatty liver disease: An open-label, 24-month, observational pilot study. *Clinical Therapeutics*. 2008;30(6):1168–1176.

61. Lavine JE, Scwimmer JB, Van Natta ML, Molleston NP, Murphy KF, Abrams RP, et al. NASH CRN. Effect of vitamin E or metformin for treatment of nonalcoholic fatty liver disease in children and adolescents: The TONIC randomized controlled trial. *Journal of the American Medical Association*. 2011;305(16):1659–1668.

62. Dohil R, Schmeltzer S, Cabera BL, Wang T, Durelle J, Duke KB, et al. Enteric-coated cysteamine for the treatment of paediatric non-alcoholic fatty liver disease. *Alimentary Pharmacologics and Therapeutics*. 2011;33:1036–1044.

63. Nobili V, Alisi A, Della Corte C, Risé P, Galli C, Agostoni C, et al. Docosahexaenoic acid for the treatment of fatty liver: Randomised controlled trial in children. *Nutrition, Metabolism and Cardiovascular Diseases.* 2013;23(11):1066–1070.

64. Nobili V, Carpino G, Alisi A, De Vito R, Franchitto A, Alpini G, et al. Role of docosahexaenoic acid treatment in improving liver histology in pediatric nonalcoholic fatty liver disease. *PLoS ONE.* 2014;9(2):e88005.

65. Zhu L, Baker SS, Gill C, Liu W, Alkhouri R, Baker RD, et al. Characterization of gut microbiomes in noalcoholic steatohepatitis (NASH) patients: A connection between endogenous alcohol and NASH. *Hepatology.* 2013;57(2):601–609.

66. Backhed F, Ding H, Wang T, Hooper LV, Koh GY, Nagy A, et al. The gut microbiota as an environmental factor that regulates fat storage. *Proceedings of the National Academy of Science USA* 2004;101(44):15718–15723.

67. Alisi A, Bedogni G, Baviera G, Giogio V, Porro E, Paris C, et al. Randomised clinical trial: The beneficial effects of VSL#3 in obese children with non-alcocholic steatohepatitis. *Alimentary Pharmacologics and Therapeutics.* 2014;39(11):1276–1285.

68. Vajro P, Mandato C, Licenziati M, Franzese A, Vitale D, Lenta S, et al. Effects of *Lactobacillus rhamnosus* strain GG in pediatric obesity-related liver disease. *Journal of Pediatric Gastroenterology and Nutrition.* 2011;52(6):740–743.

69. Mager D, Ling S, Roberts EA. Anthropometric and metabolic characteristics in children with clinically diagnosed nonalcoholic fatty liver disease. *Paediatric and Child Health.* 2008;13(2):111–117.

70. A-Kader HH, Henderson J, Vanhoesen K, Ghishan F, Bhattacharyya A. Nonalcoholic fatty liver disease in children: A single center experience. *Clinical Gastroenterology and Hepatology.* 2008;6:799–802.

71. Ko J, Yoon J, Yang H, Myung J, Kim H, Kang G, et al. Clinical and histological features of nonalcoholic fatty liver disease in children. *Digestive Diseases and Sciences.* 2009;54(10):2225–2230.

72. Fitzpatrick E, Mitry RR, Quaglia A, Hussain MJ, deBruyne R, Dhawan A. Serum levels of CK18 M30 and leptin are useful predictors of steatohepatitis and fibrosis in pediatric NAFLD. *Journal of Pediatric Gastroenterology and Nutrition.* 2010;51:500–506.

73. Takahashi Y, Inui A, Fujisawa T, Takikawa H, Fukusato T. Histopathological characteristics of non-alcoholic fatty liver disease in children: Comparison with adult cases. *Hepatology Research.* 2011;41:1066–1074.

74. Alkhouri N, Eng K, Lopez R, Nobili V. Non-high-density lipoprotein cholesterol (non-HDL-C) levels in children with nonalcoholic fatty liver disease (NAFLD). *SpringerPlus.* 2014;3(1):407.

75. Cali AM, Zern TL, Taksali SE, de Oliveira AM, Dufour S, Otvos JD, et al. Intrahepatic fat accumulation and alterations in lipoprotein composition in obese adolescents: A perfect proatherogenic state. *Diabetes Care.* 2007;30(12):3093–3098.

76. Pacifico L, Bonci E, Andreoli G, Romaggioli S, Di Miscio R, Lombardo C, et al. Association of serum triglyceride-to-HDL cholesterol ratio with carotid artery intima-media thickness, insulin resistance and nonalcoholic fatty liver disease in children and adolescents. *Nutrition, Metabolism and Cardiovascular Diseases.* 2014;24(7):737–743.

77. Manco M, Bedogni G, Monti L, Morino G, Natali G, Nobili V. Intima-media thickness and liver histology in obese children and adolescents with non-alcoholic fatty liver disease. *Atherosclerosis.* 2010;209(2):463–468.

78. Singh GK, Vitola BE, Holland MR, Sekarski T, Patterson BW, Magkos F, et al. Atlerations in ventricular structure and function in obese adolescents with nonalcoholic fatty liver disease. *Journal of Pediatrics.* 2013;162(6):1160–1168.

28 Sleep Outcomes and Childhood Obesity

Kristie R. Ross and Susan Redline

CONTENTS

INTRODUCTION

As the prevalence of childhood obesity has increased, so has our understanding of the relationship between adiposity and sleep disorders in children and adolescents. Obesity is associated with sleep-disordered breathing (SDB), daytime sleepiness, short sleep duration, and hypersomnolence disorders. These associations are complex, with evidence of bidirectional relationships between obesity and sleep disorders that are modified by age and other comorbidities. The focus of this chapter is to review the sleep-related consequences of childhood obesity, with a focus on SDB.

EPIDEMIOLOGY OF SDB

Sleep-disordered breathing (SDB) is a term that is used broadly to describe abnormal breathing and/or gas exchange during sleep. SDB includes a spectrum of severity from primary snoring to upper-airway resistance syndrome (UARS) to obstructive sleep apnea syndrome (OSAS). Untreated SDB is associated with behavioral and neurocognitive effects across its spectrum, and metabolic and cardiovascular effects in its more severe form. Methodologic challenges in describing the epidemiology of SDB are reviewed in detail elsewhere [1].

Primary snoring refers to the presence of snoring—a cardinal symptom of turbulent nasopharyngeal airflow—occurring without gas exchange abnormalities or significant sleep fragmentation. The prevalence of snoring, as reported by caregivers, is highly variable depending on the definition used, but a meta-analysis of studies that included over 95,000 children worldwide found the prevalence to be 7.45% (95% CI 5.75–9.61) [1].

In OSAS and UARS, there is recurrent intermittent partial or complete collapse of the upper airway during sleep, which results in arousals (UARS and OSAS) or impaired gas exchange (OSAS). The severity, frequency, and consequences of the airway collapse separate OSAS from UARS. While the American Academy of Pediatrics clinical practice guideline recommends that polysomnography (PSG) be performed to diagnose OSAS in children [2], the definition of OSAS using

PSG-measured variables is not consistent across studies. In addition, for practical reasons (including cost and the limited availability of pediatric sleep laboratories), many children are diagnosed with and referred for treatment of OSAS without undergoing PSG. Most studies suggest an OSAS prevalence of 4%–11% using questionnaires and 1%–4% using PSG in otherwise healthy children [1].

ROLE OF OBESITY IN CHILDHOOD SDB

Obesity has long been recognized as an important risk factor for SDB in adults [3]. More than 50% of the attributable risk of SDB in individuals less than 50 years of age has been attributed to obesity [4], and the growing obesity epidemic has been identified as a contributor to a 14%–55% relative increase in SDB prevalence over the last 10 years [5]. In children, while there are case reports of hypoventilation during sleep associated with morbid obesity going back 50 years, early reports of pediatric OSAS did not describe obesity as a common feature [6,7]. Instead, the children in these series had high rates of adenotonsillar hypertrophy (66%–72%) and failure to thrive (27%). As the prevalence of childhood obesity rose, researchers began reporting an association between obesity and SDB. In 1989, Mallory et al. reported a series of 41 children and adolescents with greater than 150% ideal body weight, of whom 37% had an abnormal PSG, most indicating mild-to-moderate SDB [8]. Silvestri and others studied 32 obese children, and found high rates of symptoms of SDB as well as polysomnographic evidence of OSAS (59%) [9]. In this series, children with an ideal body weight of 200% or more and adenotonsillar hypertrophy were at particularly high risk of OSAS [9].

The first large study to suggest an association between obesity and SDB in children was the Cleveland Family Study, in which 399 children aged 2–18 years were studied with in-home PSG [10]. SDB was characterized using a relatively high apnea–hypopnea index (AHI) of 10 or higher. Obesity (body mass index [BMI] >28) was associated with 4.69 (95% CI 1.59–14.15) increased odds of moderate-to-severe SDB after adjusting for race. In a case control study conducted in Asia published in 2003, 46 obese otherwise healthy children (>120% ideal body weight) and 44 age- and sex-matched controls were studied using fiber-optic upper-airway examinations and PSG [11]. Sleep architecture was similar in both normal-weight and obese children. However, SDB was much more common in the obese children. Consistent with other studies of snoring in healthy children, 15.9% of the normal-weight children in this series had habitual snoring and 2.3% had evidence for OSAS (obstructive apnea index ≥1). Obese children had a higher prevalence of snoring and OSAS, at 34.8% and 26.1%, respectively. Adenoidal enlargement and a narrow velopharyngeal space were also more common in the obese participants. Verhulst and colleagues subsequently published a series of studies further establishing a relationship between obesity and SDB in children and adolescents, including evidence that, as in adults, SDB is associated with several inflammatory and metabolic abnormalities [12,13]. This relationship, confirmed by others, is explored further in another section of this chapter. In a large population-based cohort study in the United Kingdom of children aged 6 months to 6 years, those with early evidence of SDB had higher standardized BMI scores than nonsnorers or children with later onset of snoring [14].

Obesity and SDB likely share many risk factors, including race, socioeconomic status, genetic markers, prematurity, and chronic respiratory conditions [15–17]. Many of these processes share proinflammatory and oxidative signaling pathways, potentially resulting in additive or synergistic effects, or the modification of risk or outcomes. Thus, discerning the causal relationships between obesity and SDB can be challenging. The Cleveland Children's Sleep and Health Study was a population-based cohort of 907 children with stratified sampling to achieve a study population composed of approximately 50% children who had been born preterm and with overrepresentation of minority children [18]. Investigators used questionnaires and in-home overnight cardiorespiratory studies to estimate the prevalence of SDB and to understand how risk factors including race, sex, prematurity, and obesity affected the risk of SDB. SDB was measured longitudinally over three examinations: when children were aged 8–11 years, 13–16 years, and 16–19 years. Obesity was not associated with SDB at ages 8–11 years. In contrast, among adolescents aged 16–19 years,

BMI z-score was associated with a significant 2.7-fold increased odds of SDB (per unit change in z-score) [19]. Similar to the latter finding, a study of 234 Caucasian children aged 2–18 years studied with overnight PSG found a relationship between OSAS and obesity only in adolescents 12 years of age and older who had a 3.5-fold increased risk of OSAS with each standard deviation increase in BMI z-score [20]. In another study that included Caucasian and Hispanic children, obesity was more common in children with SDB that persisted during a 5-year study period from mid-childhood to very early adolescence [21]. The evidence for relatively stronger associations between obesity and SDB in older children and adolescents compared with younger children may be based on several factors, including differences in the magnitude and distribution of adiposity and underlying differences in anatomic susceptibility as airway structures develop and lymphoid hyperplasia changes.

The importance of distinguishing between *classic* pediatric OSAS and *obesity-related* OSAS was proposed in 2007, with the suggestion that this distinction may help understand the long-term impact of the disorder and suggest treatment strategies [17]. Further delineation of subgroups defined by anatomic risk factors, neuromuscular activation of the airway, central components of ventilatory control, and arousal thresholds, may help with strategies for "personalizing" treatment strategies. Additionally, elucidating how these risk factors relate to obesity may be important, given that obesity may influence allergic/lymphatic tissues and airway inflammation (see Figure 28.1). While rigorously designed clinical trials to test the hypothesis that treatment responses vary based on phenotype have not been done, there are data supporting this concept. In particular, there is some evidence that daytime sleepiness may be greater in children with SDB who are obese, compared with their nonobese peers. Furthermore, the level of objectively measured sleepiness was significantly correlated with the level of BMI ($r = .44$, $p = .001$) [22]. Excessive daytime sleepiness has been linked to inflammation, and the authors postulate that the inflammatory dysregulation that occurs in both obesity and SDB interact to result in augmented sleepiness. Similarly, it has been suggested that obese children with SDB may also have poorer cognitive outcomes than nonobese children with SDB. In a study that compared nonobese children with OSAS, obese children with OSAS, and age- and sex-matched healthy control children, those with both obesity and OSAS had lower scores on the Weschler Intelligence Scale for Children compared with nonobese children with OSAS. Both groups were lower than healthy controls [23].

The presence of obesity may impact not only the presentation but also the severity of OSAS. In the Childhood Adenotonsillectomy Trial (CHAT)—a randomized, controlled trial of children aged 5–9 years in which early adenotonsillectomy was compared with watchful waiting in the treatment

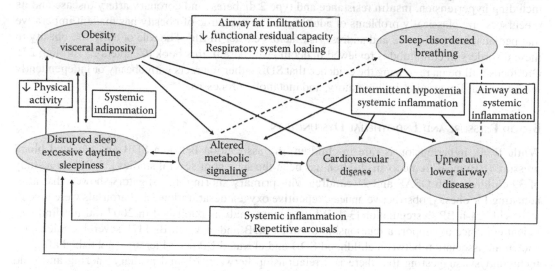

FIGURE 28.1   Theoretical scheme showing complex and bidirectional relationships between sleep-disordered breathing, obesity, and comorbidities. Dotted lines represent relationships that are less well established.

of mild-to-moderate OSAS—obesity, along with race and the score of a validated SDB screening questionnaire, were the only significant predictors of OSAS severity in children. In this study population, children with a BMI z-score of 2 or higher had a 1.22 (95% CI 1.02–1.45) increased likelihood of more severe OSAS (defined by an oxygen desaturation index >10) [24].

Characterizing the distribution of fat may be important in understanding SDB risk and outcomes. In adults, measures of central adiposity are more closely related to OSAS than BMI. There is early evidence that there are similar patterns in children. In the CHAT study, an elevated waist circumference, but not BMI, was associated with the persistence of SDB in the watchful waiting group [25]. A pilot study of 20 otherwise healthy obese adolescents showed that the AHI was not correlated with BMI but was strongly correlated with visceral fat volume measured by computed tomography (CT) of the abdomen ($r = .73$, $p < .001$) [26].

The presence of asthma and allergic upper-airway disease may also provide insight into SDB and obesity phenotypes, and shed light on genetic susceptibility and proinflammatory and oxidative signaling derangements that occur in the airway and systemically [27]. In the Cleveland Family Study, multiple upper- and lower-airway symptoms were independently associated with moderate SDB after adjusting for obesity and race [10]. Analysis of the relationship between obesity, wheezing, and SDB in participants in the Cleveland Children's Sleep and Health Study showed that while SDB and obesity were each independently associated with asthma and wheezing, the relationship between obesity and lower-airway symptoms was partly mediated by SDB [28]. Similarly, in a longitudinal cohort study in which SDB was strongly associated with severe asthma, BMI z-score modified the relationship between SDB and asthma severity [29]. Others have shown that markers of airway inflammation (exhaled nitric oxide) and airway obstruction (pulmonary function testing) are more consistently abnormal in children with both SDB and obesity than in either process alone [30,31].

METABOLIC AND CARDIOVASCULAR CONSEQUENCES OF SDB

Untreated SDB is associated with neurocognitive and behavioral problems, endothelial dysfunction and hypertension, systemic inflammation, cardiac dysfunction, and metabolic abnormalities, prompting recommendations that all children be screened during routine well-child care [32]. However, a major challenge is the lack of data that identify which threshold levels of SDB confer increased risk of these chronic health conditions. This is particularly relevant given that SDB may remit or change in severity during development [19]. Cardiovascular and metabolic diseases, including hypertension, insulin resistance and type 2 diabetes, and coronary artery disease and its precursors, are classically problems of adulthood. The epidemic of obesity has made it imperative that pediatricians recognize and address risk factors earlier in life. The role of early-life obesity in these disorders in childhood is reviewed in detail elsewhere in this book (Chapters 25 through 27). Our focus will be on reviewing the evidence that SDB either interacts with obesity or independently influences cardiovascular, inflammatory, and metabolic processes.

BLOOD PRESSURE AND ENDOTHELIAL DYSFUNCTION

While frank hypertension is rare in children, the association between SDB and elevated blood pressure (BP) measurements in children has been the subject of several studies [33–36]. In a study of 39 children with OSAS and 21 children with primary snoring, investigators showed that after adjusting for obesity, obstructive apneas, repetitive oxygen desaturations, and arousals were associated with 24-h BP dysregulation [34]. While a meta-analysis published in 2007 did not find sufficient evidence to support a relationship between SDB and elevated BP [37], several studies have shown an association between childhood SDB and elevated BP, with literature published after the meta-analysis suggesting that there is a relationship between BP and primary snoring and mild OSAS [35,36,38]. In a study of 105 children with SDB (ranging in severity from primary snoring to moderate-to-severe OSAS) and 35 nonsnoring controls, BP during waking and during overnight monitoring was 10–15 mm higher across the SDB groups compared with healthy controls [35]. In another study in which children in Hong Kong were followed prospectively for 4 years after initial diagnosis of OSAS, the baseline AHI was associated with BP during wake and sleep after 4 years [36]. Treatment rates of OSAS were low in this community-based sample of predominantly mild OSAS, and the findings were independent of obesity.

Endothelial dysfunction may occur prior to the onset of hypertension, is a marker of cardiovascular risk, is associated with OSAS in adults, can be measured noninvasively, and can provide information on preclinical risk of cardiovascular outcomes. In a case control study of 108 obese and nonobese prepubertal children without hypertension or other chronic cardiovascular or metabolic diseases (54 with OSAS and 54 without OSAS, matched based on age, sex, and race), endothelial function was measured using a modified hyperemic test [39]. OSAS and obesity were both associated with endothelial dysfunction, in a severity-dependent manner. Children with both OSAS and obesity had substantially higher rates of endothelial dysfunction (62.5%) than those with only OSAS (AHI >5, 20%) or obesity (38.7%) alone. In a study of 59 children with habitual snoring, this group also found that, similar to adults with OSAS, endothelial function deteriorates during the night in an OSAS severity-dependent manner [40]. Others have shown that endothelial dysfunction is more prevalent and that markers of oxidative stress are higher in children with primary snoring and OSAS, compared with healthy controls [41]. Furthermore, both improved following adenotonsillectomy.

Metabolic syndrome, characterized by visceral adiposity and a cluster of abnormalities in glucose and lipid regulation, is a risk factor for future cardiovascular morbidity in both adults and children. OSAS is associated with insulin resistance and metabolic syndrome in adults [42]. In the Cleveland Children's Sleep and Health Study there was a close association between SDB and metabolic syndrome. After adjusting for age, race, sex, and prematurity, adolescent children with SDB (AHI ≥5) had a 6.49 (95% CI 2.52–16.7) increased odds of having metabolic syndrome [33]. The intermittent hypoxemia seen in OSAS may be the strongest driver of this relationship [12]. Gozal et al. demonstrated an improvement in lipid homeostasis and inflammatory profiles in children with OSAS following adenotonsillectomy [43]. These findings were seen only in obese children, and an improvement in glycemic control was seen primarily in obese children in whom adenotonsillectomy resulted in the resolution of OSAS. Visceral adiposity is more closely correlated with insulin resistance and OSAS in adults than total body fat. Further research is needed to tease apart the influences of visceral adiposity and SDB on metabolism in children.

NONALCOHOLIC FATTY LIVER DISEASE

As reviewed in the previous chapter, nonalcoholic fatty liver disease (NAFLD) is an obesity-associated condition characterized by a spectrum of histological changes ranging from steatosis to nonalcoholic steatohepatitis (NASH) that can progress to cirrhosis and end stage liver disease. In adults with NAFLD, the presence of OSAS predicts more advanced disease (fibrosis) independently of obesity and metabolic syndrome [44]. The first study to report an association in children was published in 2008, in which 518 children evaluated for SDB underwent liver enzyme measurement [45]. Of the 376 nonobese children enrolled, <1% had elevated liver enzymes. In contrast, among the 142 overweight or obese children, 32% had elevated liver enzymes, and 91% of those children had OSAS, compared with 72% in the obese children without elevated liver enzymes. Verhulst and colleagues also reported an association between SDB and fatty liver disease (elevated transaminases and/or abnormal abdominal ultrasound) in a clinical sample of overweight children and adolescents [46]. More recent work has shown relationships between biopsy-proven NAFLD and OSAS in children [47,48]. In a series of 25 children (mean age 12.8 ± 1.9 years) with NAFLD who underwent PSG, while there was no relationship between OSAS/hypoxemia and the presence of NASH on biopsy, there was an association between OSAS/hypoxemia and more advanced liver fibrosis stages. Consistent with the hypothesis that oxidative stress due to intermittent hypoxemia may drive the progression of NAFLD, there was a correlation between oxygen nadir and the

NAFLD fibrosis stage [47]. Among 65 children with biopsy-proven NAFLD, the presence and severity of OSAS was associated with 4.8-fold increased odds of NASH on biopsy as well as nearly 6-fold increased odds of significant fibrosis, independent of measures of adiposity and metabolic abnormalities [48].

IMPACT OF OBESITY ON TREATMENT FOR CHILDHOOD SDB

Adenotonsillectomy is a first-line treatment for children with OSAS and adenotonsillar hypertrophy, irrespective of the presence of obesity. Obesity has long been recognized as a condition that may confer elevated risk of perioperative complications and as a risk factor for the failure for OSAS to resolve completely after surgery.

PERIOPERATIVE COMPLICATIONS

In 1994, obesity was identified as a potential risk factor for perioperative respiratory complications following adenotonsillectomy based on a small series that included one morbidly obese child [49]. Subsequent larger studies have been mixed, with some confirming evidence of increased perioperative risk in obese children compared with their normal-weight peers, and others failing to find a difference. In a retrospective review of 2170 children undergoing PSG at a single center, overweight and obese children were more likely than normal-weight children to have oxygen desaturation below 90% during surgery (40.4% vs. 30.9%, $p = .004$) as well as experience upper-airway obstruction intraoperatively (5.9% vs. 0.2%, $p = .001$) and during recovery (3.7% vs. 0.3%, $p = .001$). BMI independently predicted the need for admission ($p < .001$) [50].

OBESITY AND RESPONSE TO ADENOTONSILLECTOMY

In 2004, Mitchell and Kelly published an uncontrolled series of 30 obese children with OSAS aged 3–17 years. Adenotonsillectomy resulted in an improvement in the respiratory disturbance index from 30.0 to 11.6 ($p <.001$), with corresponding improvements in quality of life, but 53% of participants had evidence of persistent OSAS on postoperative PSG [51]. In another uncontrolled series of 18 obese children with OSAS and 22 nonobese children with OSAS, 5% of the nonobese children had an AHI of more than 3 six weeks after adenotonsillectomy, compared with 35 of obese children ($p = .03$). More striking was the finding that after 1 year following adenotonsillectomy, 79% of obese children had either persistence or recurrence of SDB, compared with 27% of nonobese children ($p = .004$). African American children and those with a more rapid gain in BMI during the follow-up period were at particularly high risk of persistence or recurrence [52]. Others have shown that quality of life measures show less improvement in obese children following surgery compared with nonobese children [53]. A meta-analysis published in 2009 that included four studies with 110 children showed a significant reduction in AHI in obese children following adenotonsillectomy (by 18.3 events per hour, 95% CI 11.2–25.5), but 51% of children had persistent evidence for OSAS on PSG (AHI $\geq$5). One study showed that waist circumference was negatively correlated with response to adenotonsillectomy, independent of BMI, OSAS severity, neck circumference, and demographic factors [54], suggesting the potential importance of central obesity in influencing OSAS treatment outcomes. These data, however, are from uncontrolled studies and have potential for selection and information bias.

The CHAT study is the first randomized, controlled study to evaluate early adenotonsillectomy compared with watchful waiting in children with OSAS [55]. Children with significant comorbidities, very severe OSAS (AHI >30, significant hypoxemia), very severe obesity (BMI z-score >3), and who used medications for attention deficit hyperactivity disorder were excluded. PSG, neuropsychological testing, behavior rating scores, and health outcomes were measured as outcomes. Investigators were blinded to the study group assignment. Compared with surgical treatment, watchful waiting did not improve the primary outcome of neuropsychological testing but did improve the secondary outcomes of PSG findings, parent behavior ratings, and quality of life. The AHI improved in both the early adenotonsillectomy and watchful waiting groups during the study, but significantly more so in the surgical group. In both the surgery and control arms, obesity was associated with a lower likelihood that OSAS improved [56]. Of the nonobese children, 54% had normalization of the AHI in the watchful waiting group and 85% had normalization in the early adenotonsillectomy group. Obese children were significantly less likely to have normalization of PSG findings in either group, with 29% normalizing in the watchful waiting group and 67% in the early adenotonsillectomy group. However, the relative benefit of surgery versus watchful waiting was similar in both arms, suggesting that surgery is a reasonable option for obese children with OSAS, but follow-up evaluation is important.

Uncontrolled studies have suggested that adenotonsillectomy is associated with accelerated weight gain in children with failure to thrive where it would be considered beneficial, but also in normal-weight and obese children. Better understanding of the role of postoperative weight gain across children with different weight levels could influence the risk/benefit assessment of surgery, as well as assist with strategies for long-term postoperative monitoring. The CHAT study design allowed investigators to determine if early adenotonsillectomy was associated with weight gain compared with watchful waiting across a spectrum of baseline BMIs [57]. After adjustment for baseline weight and other relevant covariates, early surgery was associated with larger increases in multiple measures of weight compared with watchful waiting during the 7-month follow-up period, including BMI z-score. BMI z-score change was associated with early adenotonsillectomy, being overweight or obese at baseline, and baseline AHI. It was not associated with AHI at follow-up. While BMI z-score increased in normal-weight children during the study, there was no difference in the proportion who became overweight or obese at follow-up (15% in early adenotonsillectomy group vs. 17% in watchful waiting, $p = .72$). However, among children who were overweight at baseline, 52% became obese in the early adenotonsillectomy group vs. 21% in the watchful waiting group ($p < .05$). Longer follow-up periods would be needed to determine if these weight changes persist or worsen, but these findings suggest that preoperative counseling about the risk of weight gain and need for follow-up should be incorporated into practice.

Weight loss in obese adults is associated with an improvement and in some cases the resolution of OSAS [58]. There are limited data that weight loss is an effective treatment for OSAS in adolescents [59]. However, given the elevated perioperative risks and the longer-term risk of accelerated weight gain, referral to medically supervised weight management programs in obese children with mild-to-moderate OSAS may be a reasonable approach. Close follow-up with repeated testing to monitor for worsening of OSAS would be important components of this approach. Referral to a pediatric sleep medicine specialist for evaluation and treatment with positive airway pressure should be strongly considered in children with moderate to severe residual OSAS following surgical treatment or in those who are not surgical candidates.

SUMMARY

Screening for SDB is recommended for all children [32], with a need for particular vigilance in the growing population of overweight and obese children. The presence of additional risk factors, including asthma, prematurity, and neighborhood-level factors, may further increase the risk. When obesity and SDB coexist, the presenting symptoms and complications may be more severe due to either additive or synergistic interactions of proinflammatory and oxidative signaling pathways. Further work is needed to establish the relevance of the patterns of adiposity to SDB and its consequences in children. Risk related to treatment and response to treatment may differ in obese children, and further work is needed to understand the best long-term strategies to treat OSAS in obese children.

REFERENCES

1. Lumeng JC, Chervin RD. Epidemiology of pediatric obstructive sleep apnea. *Proceedings of the American Thoracic Society.* 2008;5(2):242–52.
2. Marcus CL, Brooks LJ, Draper KA, Gozal D, Halbower AC, Jones J, et al. Diagnosis and management of childhood obstructive sleep apnea syndrome. *Pediatrics.* 2012;130(3):e714–55.
3. Wolk R, Shamsuzzaman AS, Somers VK. Obesity, sleep apnea, and hypertension. *Hypertension.* 2003;42(6):1067–74.
4. Young T, Peppard PE, Taheri S. Excess weight and sleep-disordered breathing. *Journal of Applied Physiology.* 2005;99(4):1592–9.
5. Peppard PE, Young T, Barnet JH, Palta M, Hagen EW, Hla KM. Increased prevalence of sleep-disordered breathing in adults. *American Journal of Epidemiology.* 2013;177(9):1006–14.
6. Brouillette RT, Fernbach SK, Hunt CE. Obstructive sleep apnea in infants and children. *The Journal of Pediatrics.* 1982;100(1):31–40.
7. Frank Y, Kravath RE, Pollak CP, Weitzman ED. Obstructive sleep apnea and its therapy: Clinical and polysomnographic manifestations. *Pediatrics.* 1983;71(5):737–42.
8. Mallory GB, Jr, Fiser DH, Jackson R. Sleep-associated breathing disorders in morbidly obese children and adolescents. *The Journal of Pediatrics.* 1989;115(6):892–7.
9. Silvestri JM, Weese-Mayer DE, Bass MT, Kenny AS, Hauptman SA, Pearsall SM. Polysomnography in obese children with a history of sleep-associated breathing disorders. *Pediatric Pulmonology.* 1993;16(2):124–9.
10. Redline S, Tishler PV, Schluchter M, Aylor J, Clark K, Graham G. Risk factors for sleep-disordered breathing in children: Associations with obesity, race, and respiratory problems. *American Journal of Respiratory and Critical Care Medicine.* 1999;159(5 Pt 1):1527–32.
11. Wing YK, Hui SH, Pak WM, Ho CK, Cheung A, Li AM, et al. A controlled study of sleep related disordered breathing in obese children. *Archives of Disease in Childhood.* 2003;88(12):1043–7.
12. Verhulst SL, Schrauwen N, Haentjens D, Rooman RP, Van Gaal L, De Backer WA, et al. Sleep-disordered breathing and the metabolic syndrome in overweight and obese children and adolescents. *The Journal of Pediatrics.* 2007;150(6):608–12.
13. Verhulst SL, Rooman R, Van Gaal L, De Backer W, Desager K. Is sleep-disordered breathing an additional risk factor for the metabolic syndrome in obese children and adolescents? *International Journal of Obesity.* 2009;33(1):8–13.
14. Freeman K, Bonuck K. Snoring, mouth-breathing, and apnea trajectories in a population-based cohort followed from infancy to 81 months: A cluster analysis. *International Journal of Pediatric Otorhinolaryngology.* 2012;76(1):122–30.
15. Kohler MJ, van den Heuvel CJ. Is there a clear link between overweight/obesity and sleep disordered breathing in children? *Sleep Medicine Reviews.* 2008;12(5):347–61.
16. Patel SR, Larkin EK, Redline S. Shared genetic basis for obstructive sleep apnea and adiposity measures. *International Journal of Obesity.* 2008;32(5):795–800.
17. Dayyat E, Kheirandish-Gozal L, Gozal D. Childhood obstructive sleep apnea: One or two distinct disease entities? *Sleep Medicine Clinics.* 2007;2(3):433–44.
18. Rosen CL, Larkin EK, Kirchner HL, Emancipator JL, Bivins SF, Surovec SA, et al. Prevalence and risk factors for sleep-disordered breathing in 8- to 11-year-old children: Association with race and prematurity. *The Journal of Pediatrics.* 2003;142(4):383–9.
19. Spilsbury JC, Storfer-Isser A, Rosen CL, Redline S. Remission and incidence of obstructive sleep apnea from middle childhood to late adolescence. *Sleep.* 2015;38(1):23–9.
20. Kohler MJ, Thormaehlen S, Kennedy JD, Pamula Y, van den Heuvel CJ, Lushington K, et al. Differences in the association between obesity and obstructive sleep apnea among children and adolescents. *Journal of Clinical Sleep Medicine.* 2009;5(6):506–11.
21. Goodwin JL, Vasquez MM, Silva GE, Quan SF. Incidence and remission of sleep-disordered breathing and related symptoms in 6- to 17-year old children: The Tucson Children's Assessment of Sleep Apnea Study. *The Journal of Pediatrics.* 2010;157(1):57–61.
22. Gozal D, Kheirandish-Gozal L. Obesity and excessive daytime sleepiness in prepubertal children with obstructive sleep apnea. *Pediatrics.* 2009;123(1):13–8.
23. Vitelli O, Tabarrini A, Miano S, Rabasco J, Pietropaoli N, Forlani M, et al. Impact of obesity on cognitive outcome in children with sleep-disordered breathing. *Sleep Medicine.* 2015;16(5):625–30.
24. Mitchell RB, Garetz S, Moore RH, Rosen CL, Marcus CL, Katz ES, et al. The use of clinical parameters to predict obstructive sleep apnea syndrome severity in children: The Childhood Adenotonsillectomy (CHAT) study randomized clinical trial. *JAMA Otolaryngology: Head & Neck Surgery.* 2015;141(2):130–6.

25. Chervin RD, Ellenberg SS, Hou X, Marcus CL, Garetz SL, Katz ES, et al. Prognosis for spontaneous resolution of obstructive sleep apnea in children. *Chest.* 2015;148(5):1204–13.
26. Hannon TS, Lee S, Chakravorty S, Lin Y, Arslanian SA. Sleep-disordered breathing in obese adolescents is associated with visceral adiposity and markers of insulin resistance. *International Journal of Pediatric Obesity.* 2011;6(2):157–60.
27. Mehra R, Redline S. Sleep apnea: A proinflammatory disorder that coaggregates with obesity. *The Journal of Allergy and Clinical Immunology.* 2008;121(5):1096–102.
28. Sulit LG, Storfer-Isser A, Rosen CL, Kirchner HL, Redline S. Associations of obesity, sleep-disordered breathing, and wheezing in children. *American Journal of Respiratory and Critical Care Medicine.* 2005;171(6):659–64.
29. Ross KR, Storfer-Isser A, Hart MA, Kibler AM, Rueschman M, Rosen CL, et al. Sleep-disordered breathing is associated with asthma severity in children. *The Journal of Pediatrics.* 2012;160(5):736–42.
30. Verhulst SL, Aerts L, Jacobs S, Schrauwen N, Haentjens D, Claes R, et al. Sleep-disordered breathing, obesity, and airway inflammation in children and adolescents. *Chest.* 2008;134(6):1169–75.
31. Van Eyck A, Van Hoorenbeeck K, De Winter BY, Van Gaal L, De Backer W, Verhulst SL. Sleep-disordered breathing and pulmonary function in obese children and adolescents. *Sleep Medicine.* 2014;15(8):929–33.
32. Marcus CL, Brooks LJ, Draper KA, Gozal D, Halbower AC, Jones J, et al. Diagnosis and management of childhood obstructive sleep apnea syndrome. *Pediatrics.* 2012;130(3):576–84.
33. Redline S, Storfer-Isser A, Rosen CL, Johnson NL, Kirchner HL, Emancipator J, et al. Association between metabolic syndrome and sleep-disordered breathing in adolescents. *American Journal of Respiratory and Critical Care Medicine.* 2007;176(4):401–8.
34. Amin RS, Carroll JL, Jeffries JL, Grone C, Bean JA, Chini B, et al. Twenty-four-hour ambulatory blood pressure in children with sleep-disordered breathing. *American Journal of Respiratory and Critical Care Medicine.* 2004;169(8):950–6.
35. Horne RS, Yang JS, Walter LM, Richardson HL, O'Driscoll DM, Foster AM, et al. Elevated blood pressure during sleep and wake in children with sleep-disordered breathing. *Pediatrics.* 2011;128(1):e85–92.
36. Li AM, Au CT, Ng C, Lam HS, Ho CK, Wing YK. A 4-year prospective follow-up study of childhood OSA and its association with BP. *Chest.* 2014;145(6):1255–63.
37. Zintzaras E, Kaditis AG. Sleep-disordered breathing and blood pressure in children: A meta-analysis. *Archives of Pediatrics & Adolescent Medicine.* 2007;161(2):172–8.
38. Li AM, Au CT, Ho C, Fok TF, Wing YK. Blood pressure is elevated in children with primary snoring. *The Journal of Pediatrics.* 2009;155(3):362–8.e1.
39. Bhattacharjee R, Kim J, Alotaibi WH, Kheirandish-Gozal L, Capdevila OS, Gozal D. Endothelial dysfunction in children without hypertension: Potential contributions of obesity and obstructive sleep apnea. *Chest.* 2012;141(3):682–91.
40. Kheirandish-Gozal L, Etzioni T, Bhattacharjee R, Tan HL, Samiei A, Molero Ramirez H, et al. Obstructive sleep apnea in children is associated with severity-dependent deterioration in overnight endothelial function. *Sleep Medicine.* 2013;14(6):526–31.
41. Loffredo L, Zicari AM, Occasi F, Perri L, Carnevale R, Angelico F, et al. Endothelial dysfunction and oxidative stress in children with sleep disordered breathing: Role of NADPH oxidase. *Atherosclerosis.* 2015;240(1):222–7.
42. Punjabi NM, Shahar E, Redline S, Gottlieb DJ, Givelber R, Resnick HE. Sleep-disordered breathing, glucose intolerance, and insulin resistance: The Sleep Heart Health Study. *American Journal of Epidemiology.* 2004;160(6):521–30.
43. Gozal D, Capdevila OS, Kheirandish-Gozal L. Metabolic alterations and systemic inflammation in obstructive sleep apnea among nonobese and obese prepubertal children. *American Journal of Respiratory and Critical Care Medicine.* 2008;177(10):1142–9.
44. Agrawal S, Duseja A, Aggarwal A, Das A, Mehta M, Dhiman RK, et al. Obstructive sleep apnea is an important predictor of hepatic fibrosis in patients with nonalcoholic fatty liver disease in a tertiary care center. *Hepatology International.* 2015;9(2):283–91.
45. Kheirandish-Gozal L, Sans Capdevila O, Kheirandish E, Gozal D. Elevated serum aminotransferase levels in children at risk for obstructive sleep apnea. *Chest.* 2008;133(1):92–9.
46. Verhulst SL, Jacobs S, Aerts L, Schrauwen N, Haentjens D, Rooman RP, et al. Sleep-disordered breathing: A new risk factor of suspected fatty liver disease in overweight children and adolescents? *Sleep & Breathing (Schlaf & Atmung).* 2009;13(2):207–10.
47. Sundaram SS, Sokol RJ, Capocelli KE, Pan Z, Sullivan JS, Robbins K, et al. Obstructive sleep apnea and hypoxemia are associated with advanced liver histology in pediatric nonalcoholic fatty liver disease. *The Journal of Pediatrics.* 2014;164(4):699–706.e1.

48. Nobili V, Cutrera R, Liccardo D, Pavone M, Devito R, Giorgio V, et al. Obstructive sleep apnea syndrome affects liver histology and inflammatory cell activation in pediatric nonalcoholic fatty liver disease, regardless of obesity/insulin resistance. *American Journal of Respiratory and Critical Care Medicine*. 2014;189(1):66–76.

49. Rosen GM, Muckle RP, Mahowald MW, Goding GS, Ullevig C. Postoperative respiratory compromise in children with obstructive sleep apnea syndrome: Can it be anticipated? *Pediatrics*. 1994;93(5):784–8.

50. Nafiu OO, Green GE, Walton S, Morris M, Reddy S, Tremper KK. Obesity and risk of peri-operative complications in children presenting for adenotonsillectomy. *International Journal of Pediatric Otorhinolaryngology*. 2009;73(1):89–95.

51. Mitchell RB, Kelly J. Adenotonsillectomy for obstructive sleep apnea in obese children. *Otolaryngology Head Neck Surgery*. 2004;131(1):104–8.

52. Amin R, Anthony L, Somers V, Fenchel M, McConnell K, Jefferies J, et al. Growth velocity predicts recurrence of sleep-disordered breathing 1 year after adenotonsillectomy. *American Journal of Respiratory and Critical Care Medicine*. 2008;177(6):654–9.

53. Mitchell RB, Boss EF. Pediatric obstructive sleep apnea in obese and normal-weight children: Impact of adenotonsillectomy on quality-of-life and behavior. *Developmental Neuropsychology*. 2009;34(5):650–61.

54. Nino G, Gutierrez MJ, Ravindra A, Nino CL, Rodriguez-Martinez CE. Abdominal adiposity correlates with adenotonsillectomy outcome in obese adolescents with severe obstructive sleep apnea. *Pulmonary Medicine*. 2012;2012:351037.

55. Marcus CL, Beck SE, Traylor J, Cornaglia MA, Meltzer LJ, DiFeo N, et al. Randomized, double-blind clinical trial of two different modes of positive airway pressure therapy on adherence and efficacy in children. *Journal of Clinical Sleep Medicine*. 2012;8(1):37–42.

56. Marcus CL, Moore RH, Rosen CL, Giordani B, Garetz SL, Taylor HG, et al. A randomized trial of adenotonsillectomy for childhood sleep apnea. *The New England Journal of Medicine*. 2013;368(25):2366–76.

57. Katz ES, Moore RH, Rosen CL, Mitchell RB, Amin R, Arens R, et al. Growth after adenotonsillectomy for obstructive sleep apnea: An RCT. *Pediatrics*. 2014;134(2):282–9.

58. Peppard PE, Young T, Palta M, Dempsey J, Skatrud J. Longitudinal study of moderate weight change and sleep-disordered breathing. *JAMA*. 2000;284(23):3015–21.

59. Verhulst SL, Franckx H, Van Gaal L, De Backer W, Desager K. The effect of weight loss on sleep-disordered breathing in obese teenagers. *Obesity*. 2009;17(6):1178–83.

Section V

---

*Treatment and Prevention
of Childhood Obesity*

29 Family-Based Behavioral Treatment for Childhood Obesity

Dorothy J. Van Buren, Katherine N. Balantekin,
Sara D. McMullin, and Denise E. Wilfley

CONTENTS

INTRODUCTION

Childhood is an opportune time to address the serious disease of obesity. Since children are still growing, slowing their rate of weight gain or encouraging modest weight losses can help children normalize their weight [1]. However, it is this very fact that children are still growing that has often resulted in obesity in childhood not being treated seriously. The assumption has been that a child who is overweight or obese will "grow out of it," but this is not the case. Without effective intervention, an estimated 82% of children who are obese, defined as having a body mass index (BMI) at or above the 95th percentile for sex and age [2], will track obesity into adulthood [3]. As reviewed in other chapters in this book, obesity at any age is associated with major physical (e.g., type 2 diabetes, cardiovascular disease) and psychological health burdens (e.g., depression) [4,5] that are costly to the individual as well as to society. For example, current health-care costs related to obesity are estimated to be $315.8 billion annually or 27.5% of health-care spending in the United States [6]. By successfully addressing obesity in childhood, not only do we help children lead healthier, happier lives but we may also be engaging in a form of indicated or targeted prevention of obesity and its costly comorbidities in adulthood [7]. Fortunately, effective treatments for childhood obesity have been developed, and in this chapter we will (1) provide a brief review of the literature in support of treatment of childhood obesity, (2) describe the components of family-based behavioral treatments for childhood obesity, (3) summarize the factors found to impact or predict the effectiveness of these treatments, and (4) explore future directions in the management of childhood obesity.

CURRENT TREATMENT RECOMMENDATIONS FOR CHILDHOOD OBESITY

The US Preventive Services Task Force (USPSTF) recommends that clinicians start tracking BMI percentiles at 2 years of age, that they screen children aged 6 years and older for obesity, and offer them or refer them to a comprehensive, behavioral intervention to promote improvement in weight status [3]. These recommendations are based on the results of a rigorous scientific review that demonstrated the efficacy of interventions of moderate (26–75 contact hours) to high (>75 contact hours) intensity that include dietary, physical activity, and behavioral counseling components [8]. Other organizations and professional groups have issued similar recommendations or treatment guidelines (i.e., the National Institute on Care and Excellence [NICE]; the Expert Committee on Childhood Obesity) [9–11].

Underpinning these recommendations and guidelines is a significant body of research pointing to the superiority of intensive, multicomponent lifestyle interventions in inducing weight loss in children and in reducing medical and psychological comorbidities associated with obesity compared with no-treatment controls, education only, or single-component conditions. The amount or duration of treatment contact has also been found to be a consistent predictor of long-term weight outcomes in children [12,13]. Furthermore, the inclusion of parents or caregivers in the treatment of childhood obesity improves weight loss outcomes in comparison with interventions that only target the child. In fact, interventions with a family-based component result in a 6% greater mean reduction in percentage overweight compared with those without [14]. A representative sample of these reviews and meta-analyses and their main findings are summarized in Table 29.1.

When obesity is addressed at an early age, weight loss outcomes are more robust and enduring [15–17]. These findings highlight the importance of catching obesity early in childhood and responding with a treatment of sufficient scope and intensity to help prevent children from tracking obesity into adolescence. Unfortunately, treatment for older children and adolescents with extreme obesity and severe medical comorbidities is somewhat more complicated. For this population, the use of pharmacotherapy (Chapter 30) and/or weight loss surgery (Chapter 31) in combination with evidence-based behavioral weight loss treatment may be considered [10]. However, there are few studies evaluating the long-term outcomes and safety of pharmacological and surgical treatments for pediatric obesity. Also, adherence to lifestyle behavior changes is still necessary following weight loss surgery and to potentiate the success of pharmacotherapy [18]. Therefore, even youth who meet the criteria for these more invasive interventions will benefit from participation in multicomponent, behavioral weight control interventions.

FAMILY-BASED BEHAVIORAL WEIGHT LOSS

Family-based behavioral weight loss treatment (FBT) is a multicomponent behavioral weight control intervention developed and refined by Leonard Epstein, Denise Wilfley, and colleagues [19,20]. FBT targets both parents and children and is considered a first-line treatment for this population [1]. Not only does FBT have a positive impact on weight, but improvements in other health parameters such as reductions in blood pressure and cholesterol levels and psychological well-being are associated with FBT [21,22]. Although the majority of the research base for FBT rests on work done with children of elementary to middle school age [19], it has also been successfully adapted for use with preschoolers [23] and adolescents [24].

To improve a child's weight status, FBT targets the modification of energy balance behaviors (i.e., decreasing caloric intake and increasing caloric expenditure) through the use of behavioral treatment techniques and the active involvement of a parent or caregiver. In FBT, the parent or caregiver, who is often also overweight or obese, is encouraged to change his or her own energy balance behaviors as well as support the child in these endeavors. Furthermore, the parent or caregiver is charged with the task of engineering the home environment so that it is conducive to

TABLE 29.1

Relevant Reviews and Meta-analyses of Childhood Weight Loss Studies

Authors	Type of Review and Number of Studies	Target Population	Conclusions
Altman et al., 2015	Systematic review of 53 studies	Children (2–18 years) with overweight and obesity	This review found that multicomponent treatments that include a parent component are the most efficacious.
Epstein et al., 2007	Targeted systematic review of 8 studies	Children (5–12 years) with overweight and obesity	This review demonstrates a consistent pattern of weight loss results across efficacy studies across time, an important step in preparing interventions for translation to wider-spread clinical care.
Hayes et al., 2015	Systematic review of 22 studies	Children and adolescents (2–18 years) with overweight and obesity	This review found that behavioral interventions that include individual family sessions achieve a greater magnitude of weight loss than those with only group sessions.
Ho et al., 2013	Systematic review of 38 randomized control trials	Children and adolescents (≤18 years) with overweight and obesity	This review concluded that weight loss was greater when the duration of treatment was longer than 6 months.
Janicke et al., 2014	Meta-analysis of 20 randomized control trials	Children and adolescents (≤19 years) with overweight and obesity	This meta-analysis found that dose (duration, number of sessions, time in treatment) was positively related to effect size, and individual and in-person comprehensive family interventions were associated with larger effect sizes.
Whitlock et al., 2010	Targeted systematic review of 16 studies	Children (5–18 years) with overweight and obesity	This review confirmed that comprehensive moderate-to-high intensity behavioral interventions can be effective at producing significant weight loss in children.
Wilfley et al., 2007	Meta-analysis of 14 randomized control trials	Children (≤19 years) with overweight	This meta-analysis concluded that lifestyle interventions produce significant changes in weight status in the short term, with evidence suggesting results persist in the long term.
Young et al., 2007	Meta-analysis of 16 studies	Children (5–12 years) with overweight and obesity	This meta-analysis found that interventions with a family component achieve a greater magnitude of weight loss than those using an alternative treatment approach.

healthy energy balance behaviors for the entire family. This focus on making changes throughout the household is an important tenet of FBT. Although significant weight change can occur within the first few months of FBT, weight losses are better maintained over the long term by extending treatment contact to allow for the focus on both the continued practice of behavioral change skills and the development of family and social networks in support of weight loss maintenance behaviors [25]. The components of FBT are described in the following sections and in Table 29.2.

TABLE 29.2

Family-Based Behavioral Treatment Components

Goal	Strategies
Dietary Modification	
Decrease caloric intake	• Define appropriate calorie range.
	• Increase intake of Green foods (i.e., highly nutritious, low-calorie-dense foods).
	• Decrease intake of Red foods (i.e., high-fat, high-sugar foods).
Energy Expenditure Modification	
Increase energy expenditure	• Increase physical activity (goal: 60 min/day, 5 days/week).
	• Decrease sedentary activity (goal: <2 h/day outside of school time).
Behavior Modification	
Goal setting	• Dietary goals (e.g., <15 Red foods/week, calorie range 1200–1500).
	• Physical activity goals (e.g., >60 min activity/day, reduce sedentary activity by 50%).
	• Weight goals (e.g., weight loss of 0.5 lb/week).
Self-monitoring	• Record daily food intake (e.g., calorie intake, number of Red foods, fruit and vegetable intake).
	• Record activity (e.g., time spent in moderate-to-vigorous activity and sedentary activity).
	• Record weight (e.g., weekly weighing).
Reward systems	• Rewards based on goal achievement.
	• Rewards based on weight achievement.
Stimulus control	• Restructure home environment (e.g., increase availability of Green foods) to increase chance of success.
Parental Involvement	
Shape home environment	• Make the healthy choice the easy choice in home (limit Red foods, etc.).
	• Parent models healthy eating and physical activity lifestyle.
Model healthy eating and activity parenting skills	• Develop skills to support healthy lifestyle for family (e.g., problem solve solutions).
Limit setting	• Parents set limits to help create structure around eating, activity, and sleep behaviors.
Goals	• Diet, physical activity, and weight goals are set for both parents and children.
Socioenvironmental Contexts	
Peer level	• Parents help children establish healthy peer networks.
	• Techniques to help deal with weight-based teasing and improve body image and self-esteem.
Community level	• Families are encouraged to become advocates for increased access to healthy foods in their schools and communities.
	• Problem solve ways to work with built environment.

Dietary Modification

There are three primary goals in FBT regarding dietary modification: (1) decrease caloric intake, (2) improve nutritional quality, and (3) shift food preferences. To facilitate a decrease in caloric intake while improving nutritional quality, FBT uses a family-friendly method of categorizing foods according to traffic light colors [26]. In this way, families learn to gradually adopt healthier eating habits through decreasing portion sizes, decreasing their intake of high–energy dense, low–nutrient dense foods (Red foods), increasing their intake of lower-calorie, more nutritious foods (Green foods), and by regularly consuming three meals a day. In FBT, families are discouraged from "swapping" high-calorie, non-nutritious foods (e.g., soft drinks, cookies) with calorie-free or low-fat substitutes to help shift taste preferences away from "junk" foods to more nutritious food choices. Additionally, families are encouraged to eat more meals at home, since this change in eating pattern has been found to be positively associated not only with improvements in the nutritional quality of foods eaten but also with improvements in weight status [27].

ENERGY EXPENDITURE MODIFICATION

FBT's primary goals related to shifting energy expenditure are to increase moderate-to-vigorous physical activity and to decrease engagement in sedentary pursuits (e.g., non-school- or work-related screen time). Again, the colors of the traffic light are useful in helping families differentiate among activities to increase (Green: moderate-to-vigorous physical activity) and those to decrease (Red: sedentary pursuits). In addition to being encouraged to increase time spent in moderate-to-vigorous physical activities, families are also encouraged to increase lifestyle activities such as using stairs instead of elevators, or walking or riding a bike to school rather than taking a car. Since sedentary activities are often accompanied by eating, decreasing sedentary time helps decrease caloric intake while also creating opportunities for greater energy expenditure [28]. Increasing physical activity not only facilitates weight change in the short term, regular physical activity is predictive of percentage overweight in treated children 10 years after their participation in FBT [29].

BEHAVIOR MODIFICATION

FBT is first and foremost a behavioral intervention employing such techniques as self-monitoring, goal setting, shaping, modeling, reward systems, and stimulus control to effect changes in energy balance behaviors. Self-monitoring is a mainstay of behavioral change efforts [30]. In addition to its utility in helping individuals develop awareness of behavioral patterns and choices, it aids in establishing baseline rates of target behaviors to facilitate goal setting and the implementation of reward systems. The value of self-monitoring is highlighted by research that has demonstrated greater decreases in child percentage overweight with increased frequency of self-monitoring [31], and research with adults suggests that the number of behavioral change techniques an individual reports using is associated with weight loss success [32]. FBT has an advantage in that it employs a variety of behavioral change techniques, and current advances in the basic cognitive and behavioral sciences are informing the development of additional behavioral change tools for use in FBT. For example, techniques have been developed to improve episodic future-thinking skills in children and their parents to improve impulse control, and implementation intention procedures may be used to improve prospective thinking or memory, which in turn may strengthen goal-setting skills [33].

PARENTAL INVOLVEMENT

While parental participation during multicomponent childhood obesity treatments has been shown to be positively related to child weight loss outcomes [34], in FBT, participating parents and caregivers are also taught to systematically use behavioral principles and positive parenting approaches to help shape and support their child's weight change efforts [1]. For example, through the use of stimulus control and positive parenting techniques, such as allowing children latitude in making choices among a variety of healthy foods, parents are able to support their children in reducing energy intake without using restrictive feeding practices, which in turn results in better weight loss outcomes [35]. Parents are also encouraged to use limit setting to help create structure and routines around eating, activity, and sleep behaviors. Since parents or caregivers participating in FBT are often overweight or obese themselves, they are also encouraged to actively work toward changing their own weight status in addition to supporting their child's efforts. Parental weight loss is positively associated with child weight loss, perhaps through changes made to the shared environment as well as through parental use and modeling of healthy weight-regulating behaviors [36,37]. In fact, children who are overweight or obese may be particularly sensitive to adult influence in terms of the transmission of healthy behaviors [38], underscoring the importance of active parental or caregiver involvement in FBT.

SOCIOENVIRONMENTAL CONTEXTS

A child's weight-related dietary and physical activity behaviors are developed and maintained in the context of the family home as well as the broader community within which children and their families live, work, study, and play [39]. When new weight control behaviors are acquired during the course of FBT, these new behaviors do not replace the old behaviors associated with weight gain but rather coexist with them [40]. Unfortunately, new behaviors are not very generalizable outside of the setting in which they were learned; however, old learning or old behaviors are easily activated across the different contexts of our obesogenic world. As a result of this contextual influence on the acquisition and practice of energy balance behaviors, FBT takes a socioenvironmental or multilevel approach to behavioral change in order to improve maintenance of weight loss over time [41]. To address these challenges to the maintenance of newly learned weight-regulating behaviors, FBT teaches families to be aware of the impact these various contexts have on them and to identify and plan for the different constraints or barriers to maintaining a healthy energy balance across these different levels of influence. In addition, they learn how to identify and capitalize on facilitators or supports for healthy living, not only within the family but also within peer networks and the community.

Peer Level

Peer interactions are naturally reinforcing to children and good peer relationships have a positive influence on overall quality of life. When peers are supportive of healthy energy balance behaviors, weight loss maintenance efforts are enhanced [42]. Conversely, a lack of peer support for physical activity and healthy eating are likely to contribute to weight gain [25]. Therefore, in FBT, families are encouraged to establish healthy peer networks and to disentangle socializing from unhealthy activities such as eating high–energy dense, low–nutrient dense foods and sedentary pursuits such as playing video games. Unfortunately, weight-related teasing and bullying from peers can be a source of great distress, and children with severe social problems have been less successful in weight loss maintenance [20]. In an effort to improve children's confidence in their ability to relate positively to peers, FBT includes training in prosocial techniques for dealing with teasing and cognitive-behavioral techniques to improve body image and self-esteem.

Community Level

The community or *built environment* offers many opportunities as well as challenges to families participating in FBT as they attempt to maintain healthy energy balance behaviors. For example, Epstein and colleagues [43] found that families with greater access to parks and open spaces were more likely to maintain their weight losses up to 2 years, compared with families with less access to parks and open spaces but with greater access to grocery and convenience stores. Families are often unaware of the ways in which their communities impact their behavioral choices. In FBT, families engage in a number of activities to help increase their familiarity with what their built environment has to offer and in what ways it might interfere with the establishment of healthy habits over the long term. Problem solving, goal setting, and stimulus control are techniques that families can use in FBT to better work around or with their built environments. In addition, families are encouraged to become advocates for increased access to healthy foods and activity choices in their schools, their work places, and other community settings. In FBT, families are encouraged to build a culture of health in their homes, in their relationships, and in their communities to provide support for the difficult challenge of healthy weight maintenance in our obesogenic world.

TREATMENT DURATION, MODALITY, AND SETTING

Reviews of the literature on childhood obesity interventions (e.g., [12]) support the importance of treatment duration (26–75 h of contact) to achieving successful weight loss maintenance, especially when multiple levels of influence are addressed and there are strong behavioral and family components to the intervention, such as are found in FBT [25,29]. Given its efficacy and congruence with current USPSTF and Expert Committee guidelines for the treatment of pediatric obesity, there is a desire to make FBT more broadly available to children and their families.

One way to *scale up* treatment and make family-based weight loss interventions more available would be to deliver treatment in a group format. However, a recent review of group-based childhood weight loss programs found that group-only treatment formats may not achieve clinically significant weight changes [44]. Decreases in BMI z-scores of greater than 0.25 have been linked to changes in cardiometabolic outcomes in children, and thus are considered to have clinical significance. In this review, the median decrease in BMI z-score for group-only interventions was 0.15. Outcomes improved when an individual family component was included in the treatment along with group sessions (mixed format). These mixed-format programs had median BMI z-score changes of 0.2, closer to clinically significant outcomes than the group-only treatments. It is possible that in group-only interventions without an individualized behavioral component, families do not have sufficient support from the interventionist to make the necessary changes in their energy balance behaviors to realize clinically significant weight losses.

Another way to improve the availability of FBT while preserving its potency would be to conduct FBT with individual families within primary care settings. Colocation is a model of coordinated health care that places a behavioral health-care provider within the same location as the primary care physician. Preliminary research suggests that FBT interventionists can be successfully colocated within pediatric primary care practices and weight losses can be achieved in both the parent and the child [45]. However, an abbreviated form of FBT in terms of both treatment content and intensity was used in this study. Although further research is needed to test the efficacy of full-dose FBT in the primary care setting, the colocation of a behavioral health interventionist within primary care would allow pediatricians to more easily utilize the algorithm created by the American Academy of Pediatrics Institute for Healthy Childhood Weight for the assessment and management of childhood obesity in children 2 years of age and older using the 2007 Expert Committee recommendations [46].

This algorithm includes three important pretreatment components for the pediatrician: assessment of healthy eating and active living behaviors, prevention counseling on healthy eating and active behaviors, and the accurate determination of weight classification. After completion of the pretreatment components, patients move through a stepped-care approach of four stages, starting at the least intensive stage and advancing through the stages as necessary, based on the response to treatment, age, BMI, health, risks, and motivation. In Stage 1, "Prevention Plus," the primary care provider helps the family create positive behavioral change regardless of change in BMI, with an aim for weight maintenance or a decrease in BMI velocity. After 3–6 months without weight status improvement, children advance to Stage 2, "Structured Weight Management." This builds on Stage 1 by including more intensive support and structure to help achieve healthy behavioral change. After 3–6 months without weight status improvement, children advance to Stage 3, "Comprehensive Multidisciplinary Intervention," which involves more structured behavioral modification, including food and physical activity monitoring and goal setting. Given the constraints on primary care physicians' time and training, Stage 3 will typically involve referral to a weight management clinic with a multidisciplinary team. After 3–6 months without weight status improvement, children advance to Stage 4, "Tertiary Care Intervention." Stage 4 is designed for children with a BMI of ≥95% with significant comorbidities and children with a BMI of ≥99% who do not show improvement in Stage 3. Stage 4 consists of intensive diet and physical activity counseling, with the use of medication and surgery when appropriate. With a colocated behavioral health interventionist, families advancing to Stage 3 and beyond can continue their behavioral weight loss treatment in the familiar setting of the pediatrician's office, which they may prefer over being referred to an outside facility [47]. Colocation also allows for easier coordination of care, which is important given obesity's potential for medical comorbidities. It should be noted that the "wait and see" components as outlined in Stages 1 and 2 (i.e., after 3–6 months without weight status improvement children advance to the next stage or intensity of treatment) could result in an additional 12 months of weight gain for a given child. Weight gain is more difficult to address than to prevent [7] and valuable intervention time could be lost by taking this "wait and see" approach [48].

CONCLUSIONS AND FUTURE DIRECTIONS

Childhood obesity poses a significant public health concern and, left untreated, tracks into adulthood, with all its associated comorbidities placing a tremendous burden on our health-care system and causing significant emotional distress to those affected by obesity. Evidence supports early intervention for obesity during childhood, as robust and sustainable changes can be made at this time. Family-based behavioral treatment for childhood obesity, a multicomponent treatment that intervenes across several contexts, has demonstrated effectiveness in reducing weight and improving physiological and psychosocial outcomes in children and their parents. Given its reach beyond the target child, FBT may be a very cost-effective way to treat obesity across multiple generations. Since siblings of overweight/obese children are at greater risk of overweight/obesity themselves [49], the potential for FBT's impact to generalize to other family members' health is an important area for future research.

Although FBT is a very effective treatment for childhood obesity, transdisciplinary research is needed to facilitate our understanding of individual, modifiable factors that can affect treatment response and to contribute to the development of even more potent, personalized, and efficient forms of FBT. For example, we know that a child's weight loss by the eighth week of FBT predicts long-term treatment success [48]. Given this knowledge, advances in educational and systems sciences [50,51] could be brought to bear to assist in the development of mastery learning models [52] or adaptive treatment algorithms [53] that would allow the intensity or direction of FBT to adjust to the needs of individual families, thus conserving resources and improving treatment outcomes. Also, appetitive traits such as high food reinforcement, binge or loss-of-control eating, and impulsivity are associated with weight gain and may inhibit treatment response [1]. Learning theory and behavioral economics can inform the development and assessment of cognitive and behavioral interventions to address these traits within FBT to improve weight loss maintenance in this subset of families [50,54].

FBT is an effective behavioral health treatment that is uniquely well suited for implementation within primary care settings using colocated behavioral health providers. As insurers and medical service delivery systems shift toward a health-care market that incentivizes prevention and the effective management of complex, multilevel diseases such as obesity, interventions such as FBT will be in demand to meet this need. In anticipation of this shift in the health-care system, and to make effective care more broadly available to children who are overweight or obese and their families, it will be necessary to determine how best to scale up FBT for broader implementation without losing its potency. Feasible and effective approaches to training interventionists to deliver FBT on a large scale with a high degree of fidelity, such as web-based learning systems and patient simulation methods, will need to be developed and tested to ensure high-quality delivery of FBT to more children and their families.

REFERENCES

1. Wilfley DE, Kass AE, Kolko RP. Counseling and behavior change in pediatric obesity. *Pediatric Clinics of North America*. 2011;58(6):1403–24.
2. Kuczmarski RJ, Ogden CL, Grummer-Strawn LM, Flegal KM, Guo SS, Wei R, et al. CDC growth charts: United States. *Advance Data*. 2000;(314):1–27.

3. Juonala M, Magnussen CG, Berenson GS, Venn A, Burns TL, Sabin MA, et al. Childhood adiposity, adult adiposity, and cardiovascular risk factors. *The New England Journal of Medicine.* 2011;365(20):1876–85.

4. Daniels S. Complications of obesity in children and adolescents. *International Journal of Obesity.* 2009;33:S60–5.

5. Sanders RH, Han A, Baker JS, Cobley S. Childhood obesity and its physical and psychological comorbidities: A systematic review of Australian children and adolescents. *European Journal of Pediatrics.* 2015;174(6):715–46.

6. Cawley J, Meyerhoefer C, Biener A, Hammer M, Wintfeld N. Savings in medical expenditures associated with reductions in body mass index among US adults with obesity, by diabetes status. *PharmacoEconomics.* 2014;33(7):707–22.

7. Goldschmidt AB, Wilfley DE, Paluch RA, Roemmich JN, Epstein LH. Indicated prevention of adult obesity: How much weight change is necessary for normalization of weight status in children? *Journal of the American Medical Association Pediatrics.* 2013;167(1):21–6.

8. Whitlock EP, O'Connor EA, Williams SB, Beil TL, Lutz KW. Effectiveness of weight management interventions in children: A targeted systematic review for the USPSTF. *Pediatrics.* 2010;125(2):e396–418.

9. United States Preventative Services Task Force. Screening for obesity in children and adolescents: US Preventive Services Task Force recommendation statement. *Pediatrics.* 2010;125(2):361–7.

10. Barlow SE and Expert Committee. Expert committee recommendations regarding the prevention, assessment, and treatment of child and adolescent overweight and obesity: Summary report. *Pediatrics.* 2007;120(Suppl. 4):S164–92.

11. NICE. Weight management: Lifestyle services for overweight or obese children and young people. NICE guidelines [PH47]. October 2013. Available from: http://www.nice.org.uk/guidance/PH47.

12. Janicke DM, Steele RG, Gayes LA, Lim CS, Clifford LM, Schneider EM, et al. Systematic review and meta-analysis of comprehensive behavioral family lifestyle interventions addressing pediatric obesity. *Journal of Pediatric Psychology.* 2014;39(8):809–25.

13. Ho M, Garnett SP, Baur LA, Burrows T, Stewart L, Neve M, Collins C. Impact of dietary and exercise interventions on weight change and metabolic outcomes in obese children and adolescents: A systematic review and meta-analysis of randomized trials. *JAMA Pediatrics.* 2013;167(8):759–68.

14. Young KM, Northern JJ, Lister KM, Drummond JA, O'Brien WH. A meta-analysis of family-behavioral weight-loss treatments for children. *Clinical Psychology Review.* 2007;27(2):240–9.

15. Danielsson P, Svensson V, Kowalski J, Nyberg G, Ekblom Ö, Marcus C. Importance of age for 3-year continuous behavioral obesity treatment success and dropout rate. *Obesity Facts.* 2012;5(1):34–44.

16. Reinehr T, Kleber M, Lass N, Toschke AM. Body mass index patterns over 5 y in obese children motivated to participate in a 1-y lifestyle intervention: Age as a predictor of long-term success. *The American Journal of Clinical Nutrition.* 2010;91(5):1165–71.

17. McGovern L, Johnson JN, Paulo R, Hettinger A, Singhal V, Kamath C, et al. Treatment of pediatric obesity: A systematic review and meta-analysis of randomized trials. *The Journal of Clinical Endocrinology & Metabolism.* 2008;93(12):4600–5.

18. Berkowitz RI, Wadden TA, Tershakovec AM, Cronquist JL. Behavior therapy and sibutramine for the treatment of adolescent obesity: A randomized controlled trial. *Journal of the American Medical Association.* 2003;289(14):1805–12.

19. Epstein LH, Paluch RA, Roemmich JN, Beecher MD. Family-based obesity treatment, then and now: Twenty-five years of pediatric obesity treatment. *Health Psychology.* 2007;26(4):381.

20. Wilfley DE, Tibbs TL, Van Buren D, Reach KP, Walker MS, Epstein LH. Lifestyle interventions in the treatment of childhood overweight: A meta-analytic review of randomized controlled trials. *Health Psychology.* 2007;26(5):521.

21. Gunnarsdottir T, Einarsson SM, Njardvik U, Olafsdottir AS, Gunnarsdottir AB, Helgason T, et al. Family-based behavioral treatment for obese children: Results and two year follow up. *Laeknabladid.* 2014;100(3):139–45.

22. Gunnarsdottir T, Njardvik U, Olafsdottir AS, Craighead L, Bjarnason R. Childhood obesity and co-morbid problems: Effects of Epstein's family-based behavioural treatment in an Icelandic sample. *Journal of Evaluation in Clinical Practice.* 2012;18(2):465–72.

23. Quattrin T, Roemmich JN, Paluch R, Yu J, Epstein LH, Ecker MA. Efficacy of family-based weight control program for preschool children in primary care. *Pediatrics.* 2012;130(4):660–6.

24. Jelalian E, Lloyd-Richardson EE, Mehlenbeck RS, Hart CN, Flynn-O'Brien K, Kaplan J, et al. Behavioral weight control treatment with supervised exercise or peer-enhanced adventure for overweight adolescents. *Pediatrics.* 2010;157(6):923–8.e1.

25. Wilfley DE, Stein RI, Saelens BE, Mockus DS, Matt GE, Hayden-Wade HA, et al. Efficacy of maintenance treatment approaches for childhood overweight: A randomized controlled trial. *Journal of the American Medical Association.* 2007;298(14):1661–73.

26. Epstein LH, Squires S. *The Stoplight Diet for Children.* Boston, MA: Little, Brown, 1988.

27. Altman M, Holland JC, Lundeen D, Kolko RP, Stein RI, Saelens BE, et al. Reduction in food away from home is associated with improved child relative weight and body composition outcomes and this relation is mediated by changes in diet quality. *Journal of the Academy of Nutrition and Dietetics.* 2015;115(9):1400–7.

28. Epstein LH, Paluch RA, Gordy CC, Dorn J. Decreasing sedentary behaviors in treating pediatric obesity. *Archives of Pediatrics & Adolescent Medicine.* 2000;154(3):220–6.

29. Epstein LH, Valoski A, Wing RR, McCurley J. Ten-year outcomes of behavioral family-based treatment for childhood obesity. *Health Psychology.* 1994;13(5):373–83.

30. Burke LE, Wang J, Sevick MA. Self-monitoring in weight loss: A systematic review of the literature. *Journal of the American Dietetic Association.* 2011;111(1):92–102.

31. Mockus DS, Macera CA, Wingard DL, Peddecord M, Thomas RG, Wilfley DE. Dietary self-monitoring and its impact on weight loss in overweight children. *International Journal of Pediatric Obesity.* 2011;6(3–4):197–205.

32. Hankonen N, Sutton S, Prevost AT, Simmons RK, Griffin SJ, Kinmonth AL, et al. Which behavior change techniques are associated with changes in physical activity, diet and body mass index in people with recently diagnosed diabetes? *Annals of Behavioral Medicine.* 2014;49(1):7–17.

33. Daniel TO, Stanton CM, Epstein LH. The future is now: Comparing the effect of episodic future thinking on impulsivity in lean and obese individuals. *Appetite.* 2013;71:120–5.

34. Wrotniak BH, Epstein LH, Paluch RA, Roemmich JN. Parent weight change as a predictor of child weight change in family-based behavioral obesity treatment. *Archives of Pediatrics & Adolescent Medicine.* 2004;158(4):342–7.

35. Holland JC, Kolko RP, Stein RI, Welch RR, Perri MG, Schechtman KB, et al. Modifications in parent feeding practices and child diet during family-based behavioral treatment improve child zBMI. *Obesity.* 2014;22(5):E119–26.

36. Best JR, Goldschmidt AB, Mockus-Valenzuela DS, Stein RI, Epstein LH, Wilfley DE. Shared weight and dietary changes in parent–child dyads following family-based obesity treatment. *Health Psychology.* 2016;35(1):92–5.

37. Theim KR, Sinton MM, Stein RI, Saelens BE, Thekkedam SC, Welch RR, et al. Preadolescents' and parents' dietary coping efficacy during behavioral family-based weight control treatment. *Journal of Youth and Adolescence.* 2012;41(1):86–97.

38. Frerichs LM, Araz OM, Huang TTK. Modeling social transmission dynamics of unhealthy behaviors for evaluating prevention and treatment interventions on childhood obesity. *PloS One.* 2013;8(12):e82887.

39. Davison KK, Birch LL. Childhood overweight: A contextual model and recommendations for future research. *Obesity Reviews.* 2001;2(3):159–71.

40. Bouton ME. Context, ambiguity, and unlearning: Sources of relapse after behavioral extinction. *Biological Psychiatry.* 2002;52(10):976–86.

41. Wilfley DE, Buren DJ, Theim KR, Stein RI, Saelens BE, Ezzet F, et al. The use of biosimulation in the design of a novel multilevel weight loss maintenance program for overweight children. *Obesity.* 2010;18(S1):S91–8.

42. Salvy S-J, Bowker JW, Roemmich JN, Romero N, Kieffer E, Paluch R, et al. Peer influence on children's physical activity: An experience sampling study. *Journal of Pediatric Psychology.* 2007;33(1):39–49.

43. Epstein LH, Raja S, Daniel TO, Paluch RA, Wilfley DE, Saelens BE, et al. The built environment moderates effects of family-based childhood obesity treatment over 2 years. *Annals of Behavioral Medicine.* 2012;44(2):248–58.

44. Hayes JF, Altman M, Coppock JH, Wilfley DE, Goldschmidt AB. Recent updates on the efficacy of group-based treatments for pediatric obesity. *Current Cardiovascular Risk Reports.* 2015;9(4):1–10.

45. Quattrin T, Roemmich JN, Paluch R, Yu J, Epstein LH, Ecker MA. Treatment outcomes of overweight children and parents in the medical home. *Pediatrics.* 2014;134(2):290–7.

46. Institute for Healthy Childhood Weight. Algorithm for the assessment and management of childhood obesity in patients 2 years and older. Available from: https://ihcw.aap.org/Documents/Assessment%20 and%20Management%20of%20Childhood%20Obesity%20Algorithm_v1015.pdf.

47. Melnyk BM, Grossman DC, Chou R, Mabry-Hernandez I, Nicholson W, DeWitt TG, et al. USPSTF perspective on evidence-based preventive recommendations for children. *Pediatrics.* 2012;130(2):e399–407.

48. Goldschmidt AB, Stein RI, Saelens BE, Theim KR, Epstein LH, Wilfley DE. Importance of early weight change in a pediatric weight management trial. *Pediatrics*. 2011;128(1):e33–9.
49. Pachucki MC, Lovenheim MF, Harding M. Within-family obesity associations: Evaluation of parent, child, and sibling relationships. *American Journal of Preventive Medicine*. 2014;47(4):382–91.
50. Epstein LH, Wrotniak BH. Future directions for pediatric obesity treatment. *Obesity*. 2010;18(S1):S8–12.
51. Savage JS, Downs DS, Dong Y, Rivera DE. Control systems engineering for optimizing a prenatal weight gain intervention to regulate infant birth weight. *American Journal of Public Health*. 2014;104(7):1247–54.
52. Epstein LH, McKenzie SJ, Valoski A, Klein KR, Wing RR. Effects of mastery criteria and contingent reinforcement for family-based child weight control. *Addictive Behaviors*. 1994;19(2):135–45.
53. Lavori PW, Dawson R. Adaptive treatment strategies in chronic disease. *Annual Review of Medicine*. 2008;59:443.
54. Best JR, Theim KR, Gredysa DM, Stein RI, Welch RR, Saelens BE, et al. Behavioral economic predictors of overweight children's weight loss. *Journal of Consulting and Clinical Psychology*. 2012;80(6):1086–96.

30 Advances in Pharmacological Treatment of Pediatric Obesity

Ovidiu A. Galescu and Jack A. Yanovski

CONTENTS

This work was supported by the Intramural Research Programs of NICHD (ZIAHD00641 to JAY). JAY is a commissioned officer in the US Public Health Service. The opinions and assertions expressed herein are those of the authors and are not to be construed as reflecting the views of the US Public Health Service.

Disclosures: JAY has received grant support from Zafgen, Inc. (beloranib) and Roche (orlistat) for clinical studies of pediatric obesity.

INTRODUCTION

Because comprehensive lifestyle interventions may have insufficient impact on body weight and medical comorbid conditions among severely obese children and adolescents [1–4], there is abiding interest in adjuvant therapies, including pharmacotherapy, for pediatric obesity. This chapter reviews medications that are either approved by the US Food and Drug Administration (FDA) for use in pediatric patients aged <16 years, are not FDA approved but have undergone pediatric trials, or, because they are approved by the FDA to be used in adults for obesity management [5,6], are considered by the FDA to be approved for use in adolescents aged ≥16 years. Some medications in late-stage clinical trials for obesity treatment are also discussed. Pharmacotherapy for the treatment of childhood obesity is generally prescribed only after 3–6 months of lifestyle modification has not been sufficiently successful at reducing weight. Nevertheless, pharmacotherapy is always considered an adjunct, to be administered together with intensive lifestyle modification [7]. Limited data suggest that, as in adults [8], pharmacotherapy without a concurrent behavioral modification program for adolescent obesity is less successful [9]. Finally, although there are few pediatric data on this issue, it is recommended that, as in adults [5], clinicians can maximize the likelihood of long-term positive outcomes by discontinuing obesity pharmacotherapy in those without sufficient early weight loss (4%–5% of initial body weight after 12–16 weeks' therapy). In this chapter, both FDA-approved and candidate medications have been organized according to their major mechanism of action; when insufficient pediatric data are available, adult studies are discussed. Common side effects, contraindications, and necessary monitoring for each agent are described in Table 30.1.

DRUGS DECREASING ENERGY INTAKE

CENTRALLY ACTING ANOREXIANT AGENTS

Norepinephrine, serotonin, and dopamine are neurotransmitters implicated in reward and appetite control pathways. The classical anorexiants act within the central nervous system to modulate these neurotransmitters and their receptors. There are currently no long-term pediatric safety or efficacy data for any of these drugs. However, the FDA has approved several drugs that exert anorexiant effects by stimulating adrenergic tone [10,11] for short-term use in adults. Phentermine, diethylpropion, and the other amphetamine-related drugs (Table 30.1) have been studied only in small pediatric trials [12–17] lasting no more than 12 weeks. The adverse effect profiles of both of these drugs are related to their amphetamine-like structure. All three drugs are Drug Enforcement Administration (DEA) Schedule IV controlled substances with a relatively low potential for abuse [18,19]. Because of their adverse effect profile [20] and the absence of trials showing long-term weight loss efficacy, none of the amphetamine-like agents are recommended or approved for obesity management in children. Other compounds such as *fenfluramine* and its stereoisomer *dexfenfluramine* affect appetite through their serotonergic effects [21–26]. These drugs increase serotonin release and inhibit its reuptake [11,27]. Although some large trials found fenfluramine was significantly more effective than placebo in adolescents in decreasing body mass index (BMI) [24], both agents increased the risk of valvular heart disease and have been removed from use [28]. *Lorcaserin* is a selective serotonergic $5HT_{2C}$ receptor agonist that decreases food intake [29]. Adults treated with lorcaserin lose an additional 3.2% of initial body weight versus placebo [30–32]. The FDA approved lorcaserin to treat adults with BMI ≥ 30 kg/m^2 or BMI ≥ 27 kg/m^2 accompanied with at least one comorbid condition, with the specification that patients who have not lost $\geq 5\%$ of their baseline body weight by 12 weeks should discontinue therapy [33]. There are limited data suggesting that combining lorcaserin with phentermine may improve short-term weight loss in adults [34]. There are no published pediatric data using lorcaserin, although trials are underway [35]. Given its limited efficacy in adults, lorcaserin is unlikely to be highly effective as a monotherapy in pediatric samples.

AGENTS WITH PRIMARILY DOPAMINERGIC EFFECTS

Methylphenidate and *dextroamphetamine* are amphetamines that inhibit dopamine reuptake, thus increasing the dopaminergic tone [36,37]. Most medications in this class are DEA Schedule II controlled substances and are considered to have a high potential for abuse [20]. The anorexic effect of these drugs has been observed in many adult [38,39] and pediatric [40,41] samples. Apart from their abuse potential, these drugs also have a significant side-effect profile including agitation, insomnia, tachycardia, hypertension, and hyperhidrosis [42–44]. This and the absence of trials showing long-term weight loss efficacy make this class not recommended for obesity management. *Lisdexamfetamine dimesylate* inhibits the reuptake of dopamine (and, to a lesser extent, norepinephrine) and deceases food intake [45]. In a 12-week trial of adults with binge-eating disorder, lisdexamfetamine produced a weight loss of 4.3 kg (vs. −0.1 kg in the placebo group) [46]. Lisdexamfetamine is FDA approved for the treatment of attention deficit hyperactivity disorder (ADHD) in patients aged 6 and older and for binge-eating disorder in adults. However, it is not approved for the management of obesity.

TABLE 30.1

Medications for Obesity

Drug	Status	Common Side Effects	Monitoring and Contraindications
Centrally Acting Anorexiant Agents			
Phentermine, diethylpropion, and mazindol	FDA-approved only for short-term use in adults.	Insomnia, elevation in heart rate, dry mouth, taste alterations, dizziness, tremors, headache, diarrhea, constipation, vomiting, gastro-intestinal distress, anxiety, restlessness	Monitor HR, BP. Contraindicated in uncontrolled hypertension, hyperthyroidism, glaucoma, agitated states, history of drug abuse, MAOIs. Caution prescribing to patients with even mild hypertension.
Fenfluramine, dexfenfluramine	Not FDA-approved for weight loss; voluntarily removed from the US market.	Drowsiness, dry mouth, headache, abdominal pain, insomnia, increased activity, irritability	Associated with an increased incidence of primary pulmonary hypertension. Associated with valvular heart disease.
Lisdexamfetamine dimesylate	Not FDA-approved for weight loss; approved for binge-eating disorder in adults and for attention deficit hyperactivity disorder in patients aged 6 years and older.	Dry mouth, sleeplessness (insomnia), increased heart rate, jittery feelings, constipation, anxiety	Contraindicated with MAOIs. Risk of sudden death in people who have heart problems or heart defects, and stroke and heart attack in adults. Monitor blood pressure and heart rate. Psychotic or manic symptoms such as hallucinations, delusional thinking, or mania may occur. May worsen peripheral vasculopathy, including Raynaud's phenomenon.
Sibutramine	Withdrawn in the United States (increased risk of serious cardiovascular events); still available in some countries such as Brazil.	Tachycardia, hypertension, palpitations, insomnia, anxiety, nervousness, depression, diaphoresis	Monitor HR, BP. Do not use with other drugs, MAO inhibitors.
Naltrexone ER + Bupropion ER	Approved for long-term use in adults.	Nausea, constipation, headache, vomiting, dizziness, insomnia, dry mouth, and diarrhea	Monitor HR, BP. Do not administer to patients with a history of seizure disorders or with anorexia or bulimia nervosa, to patients who are using opioids or abruptly discontinuing the use of alcohol, benzodiazepines, barbiturates, or antiseizure medications. There is potential increased risk of suicidality.
Lorcaserin	Approved for long-term use in adults.	Headache, dizziness, fatigue, nausea, dry mouth, cough, constipation; back pain, cough and hypoglycemia in patients with type 2 diabetes	Risk of serotonin syndrome or neuroleptic malignant syndrome-like reactions. Evaluate patients for signs or symptoms of valvular heart disease. Euphoria, hallucination, and dissociation have been seen with supratherapeutic doses. Interactions with triptans, MAOIs including linezolid, SSRIs, SNRIs, dextromethorphan, tricyclic antidepressants, bupropion, lithium, tramadol, tryptophan, and St John's wort.

(Continued)

TABLE 30.1 (CONTINUED)
Medications for Obesity

Drug	Status	Common Side Effects	Monitoring and Contraindications
Phentermine + Topiramate SR	Approved for long-term use in adults.	Paresthesia, dizziness, taste alterations, insomnia, constipation, dry mouth, elevation in heart rate, memory or cognitive changes	Contraindicated in glaucoma, hyperthyroidism, MAOIs. Concerns about teratogenicity (increased risk of oral clefts) mandate effective contraceptive use and pregnancy test monitoring in females. Metabolic acidosis, hypokalemia, and elevated creatinine have been reported, and periodic monitoring is advised. Abrupt withdrawal of topiramate may cause seizures
Liraglutide	Approved for long-term use in adults.	Nausea, diarrhea, constipation, vomiting, headache, decreased appetite, dyspepsia, fatigue, dizziness, abdominal pain, increased lipase	Monitor HR at regular intervals. Contraindicated in patients with a history of medullary thyroid carcinoma or in patients with multiple endocrine neoplasia syndrome type 2. Discontinue promptly if pancreatitis is suspected.

Drugs in Development or Used Off-Label That May Act Centrally as Anorexiant Medications

Drug	Status	Common Side Effects	Monitoring and Contraindications
Recombinant human leptin, metreleptin	Investigational for use in obesity; FDA approved for generalized lipodystrophy.	Hypoglycemia, headache, abdominal pain	Useful only in leptin deficiency. Antibodies with neutralizing activity have been identified in patients treated with metreleptin. T-cell lymphoma has been reported in patients with acquired generalized lipodystrophy. A risk evaluation and mitigation strategy is in place to prevent inappropriate prescription.
Exenatide	Not FDA-approved for obesity.	Nausea, vomiting, diarrhea, feeling jittery, dizziness, headache, dyspepsia	Acute pancreatitis, including fatal and nonfatal hemorrhagic or necrotizing pancreatitis has been reported. Observe patients carefully for signs and symptoms of pancreatitis; discontinue promptly if pancreatitis is suspected. Contraindicated in patients with severe renal impairment.
Beloranib	Investigational.	Sleep disturbance, headache, infusion site injury, nausea, diarrhea	Teratogenic in animal models. Induces dose-dependent azoospermia and other sperm abnormalities, leading to infertility in males.

Drugs Affecting Nutrient Trafficking

Drug	Status	Common Side Effects	Monitoring and Contraindications
Orlistat [132,134–139]	FDA-approved for treatment of obesity in adolescents ≥12 years old.	Oily spotting, flatus with discharge, fecal urgency, fatty/oily stool, increased defecation, fecal incontinence	Contraindicated in chronic malabsorption syndromes and cholestasis. Cholelithiasis and, rarely, severe liver injury, including hepatocellular necrosis and acute hepatic failure leading to death, have been reported. Decreases drug concentrations of cyclosporine and levothyroxine. Doses should be temporally separated from orlistat. Fat-soluble vitamin absorption is decreased by orlistat. Use with caution in those at risk of renal insufficiency. MVI supplementation is strongly recommended. A low-dose preparation is approved for over-the-counter sale.

TABLE 30.1 (CONTINUED)
Medications for Obesity

Drug	Status	Common Side Effects	Monitoring and Contraindications
Dapagliflozin	Not FDA-approved for obesity; approved for T2DM in adult population.	Vaginal yeast infections and yeast infections of the penis, stuffy or runny nose and sore throat, urinary tract infections, changes in urination, including urgent need to urinate more often, in larger amounts, or at night	Contraindicated in renal impairment, end-stage renal disease or dialysis, active or history of bladder cancer. Before initiating therapy, assess volume status and correct hypovolemia in the elderly, in patients with renal impairment or low systolic blood pressure, and in patients on diuretics. Monitor and treat for hypoglycemia, genital mycotic infections, increased LDL-C, bladder cancer.
Drugs Affecting Internal Milieu/Metabolic Control			
Metformin	Not FDA-approved for obesity; approved for ≥10 years of age for T2DM.	Nausea, flatulence, bloating, diarrhea; usually resolves	Do not use in renal failure or with IV contrast. MVI supplementation is strongly recommended. Potential risk of vitamin B12 deficiency when used long term.
Octreotide	Not FDA-approved for obesity.	Cholelithiasis (can be prevented by concurrent ursodiol), diarrhea, edema, abdominal cramps, nausea, bloating, reduction in T4 concentrations, decreased GH but normal IGF-I	Monitor fasting glucose, FT4, HbA1c. Useful only for hypothalamic obesity. Ursodiol coadministration is strongly recommended.
Recombinant human growth hormone	Not FDA-approved for obesity; FDA-approved in Prader–Willi syndrome to increase height velocity.	Edema, carpal tunnel syndrome, death in patients with preexisting obstructive sleep apnea	Growth hormone should be used only after screening to rule out obstructive sleep apnea in patients with Prader–Willi syndrome. Must closely monitor pulmonary function, glucose, HbA1c.

Note: Medications that are in late-phase clinical trials in adults, are FDA approved in adults or adolescents, or have been recently studied for their effects on body weight among children or adults. Please see the full prescribing information for all warnings, contraindications, adverse effects, and required monitoring.

GLUCAGON-LIKE PEPTIDE-1 ANALOGS (EXENATIDE, LIRAGLUTIDE)

These agents are administered by subcutaneous injection, are approved by the FDA for adjunctive treatment of type 2 diabetes mellitus in adults, and have been shown to produce dose-dependent weight loss in both diabetic and nondiabetic adults [47–55], likely through central anorectic effects mediated via glucagon-like peptide-1 (GLP-1) receptors [56]. Liraglutide 3 mg (but not exenatide) is FDA approved for obesity management in adults on the basis of trials finding weight losses of ~8.4 kg (vs. ~2.8 kg for placebo) after treatment for 1 year [55]. Recent trials of two once-weekly GLP-1 analogs, albiglutide and dulaglutide, have shown glycemic improvement in select adult diabetic populations with modest mean loss in body weight [57,58] when compared with sitagliptin and liraglutide, respectively. Several small cohort studies in adults have also investigated the effect of combined GLP-1 agonist and metformin therapy, with promising results in glucose metabolism and weight [59,60]. Exenatide has been studied in 26 adolescents with extreme obesity during a 3-month, randomized, double-blind, placebo-controlled, multicenter clinical trial followed by a 3-month open-label extension and produced weight loss of −2.9 kg versus a +0.32 kg weight gain in the placebo group, without regain during the open-label period [61,62]. One ongoing study examines the effects of exenatide on overweight adolescents with Prader–Willi syndrome [63]. At present, there are no pediatric liraglutide weight loss data available and insufficient long-term safety and efficacy data to recommend GLP-1 analogs for pediatric obesity.

AGENTS WITH ACTION AT MULTIPLE SITES/COMBINATION AGENTS

Sibutramine, a combined norepinephrine and serotonin reuptake inhibitor, has substantial data indicating it reduces appetite and promotes weight loss in obese adults [64] and adolescents [9,65–74]. The largest adolescent multicenter trial [66], which enrolled 498 adolescents with BMI at least 2 units more than the US 95th percentile based on age and sex, but less than 45 kg/m², found BMI decreased 2.9 kg/m² in the sibutramine (10–15 mg) group versus 0.3 kg/m² for placebo, after treatment for 1 year. Treatment with sibutramine also improved waist circumference, triglycerides, high-density lipoprotein cholesterol (HDL-C), insulin levels, and insulin sensitivity. However, cardiovascular adverse events (increased blood pressure [9,66,71] and heart rate [9,66,75–77]) were reported in sibutramine-treated patients, and the Sibutramine Cardiovascular Outcomes Trial (SCOUT) found that rates of nonfatal myocardial infarction and nonfatal stroke were significantly increased in adults treated with sibutramine [78]. Although withdrawn from the US market, sibutramine continues to be used and studied in other countries [74,79–81].

NALTREXONE PLUS BUPROPION

Naltrexone is an opioid receptor antagonist approved to treat alcohol and opioid dependence. Bupropion is an aminoketone antidepressant with a structure similar to the appetite suppressant diethylpropion [82] that enhances both noradrenergic and dopaminergic neurotransmission via reuptake inhibition [83]. Bupropion is approved by the FDA as monotherapy for smoking cessation. Combination therapy with naltrexone-SR 16–32 mg plus bupropion-SR 180–360 mg/d was approved for adults, based on studies finding a mean weight loss of ~6.8% of initial body weight (vs. ~2.2% for placebo) [6]. The proposed mechanism for the beneficial effects of this combination is that bupropion stimulates hypothalamic pro-opiomelanocortin-producing neurons to release alpha-MSH, while naltrexone interrupts the autoinhibitory feedback loop that the endorphin products of pro-opiomelanocortin can induce, leading to a long-term synergistic effect on energy balance [84]. There are some short-term open-label studies in pediatric samples finding that bupropion monotherapy decreases body weight in subjects who are not participating in lifestyle interventions [85,86], There are as yet no available pediatric data for combination naltrexone–bupropion therapy.

PHENTERMINE PLUS TOPIRAMATE

In adults, the combination of immediate-release phentermine (3.75–15 mg/d) plus the extended-release (ER) GABAergic [87] antiseizure medication topiramate (23–92 mg/d), produced, together with lifestyle intervention, weight loss of 10%–11% compared with 1%–2% for those who received placebo [88–91]. These results make phentermine plus ER topiramate the most effective obesity pharmacotherapy that is FDA approved for adults [5,6]. This combination also improved glycemia, lipids, blood pressure, sleep apnea, and quality-of-life measures in adults. Of note, there is a warning of potential increased risk of orofacial clefts in fetuses exposed to topiramate [92] and a required *risk evaluation and mitigation strategy* [93] requiring monthly pregnancy tests, which may limit its use in adolescent girls. There are currently no pediatric weight loss studies of this combination available; there appear to be two ongoing randomized placebo controlled trials examining topiramate monotherapy in children and adolescents [94,95]. The most common adverse events associated with topiramate include paresthesias, taste impairment, psychomotor disturbances, and impairment of cognitive function at dosages similar to those used to treat seizure disorders [96]. These adverse events limit the use of topiramate because of the higher doses needed for the medication to be effective as a stand-alone therapy for the treatment of obesity.

OTHER DRUGS IN DEVELOPMENT WITH POTENTIAL CENTRAL ANOREXIANT EFFECTS

The adipocyte-derived hormone *leptin* signals to brain regions that control energy intake, modifying the activity of hypothalamic appetite-regulating neurons [97]. In cases of congenital leptin deficiency, subcutaneous administration of leptin improves body composition, suppresses appetite, and normalizes the metabolic profiles [98–101] both short and long term. Leptin has also been used with some success to restore menses in leptin-insufficient women with hypothalamic amenorrhea [102] and to treat complete generalized lipodystrophy. In adult obesity trials, leptin has proved to be ineffective as monotherapy [103,104]. There is some evidence that leptin may reverse the muscular, neuroendocrine, and autonomic adaptations to the weight-reduced state in individuals who have achieved substantial weight loss [105–109]. However, in a small double-blind, placebo-controlled trial, when leptin was used in an attempt to promote further weight loss in the plateau phase following bariatric surgery, there were no significant effects of leptin treatment [110]. No trials have examined the effects of leptin in non-leptin-deficient obese children and teenagers attempting weight loss.

Tesofensine, like sibutramine, is a multiamine reuptake inhibitor. Due to its triple monoamine reuptake inhibitor properties, tesofensine blocks the presynaptic uptake of noradrenaline, dopamine, and serotonin, thus increasing satiety and energy expenditure [111–113]. In one 6-month phase II trial of 203 adults, this medication resulted in dose-related weight loss, with the highest dose producing over 10% weight loss (vs. 2% in placebo) [114]. However, as with sibutramine, there were increases in blood pressure and pulse. There are no pediatric studies to date.

Amylin is a 37-residue pancreatic β-cell hormone that is cosecreted with insulin from the pancreatic β-cells. Amylin plays a role in glycemic regulation by reducing food intake, slowing gastric emptying, and reducing postprandial glucagon secretion in humans. Amylin has its own receptors in the hind brain that are hetero-oligomers with calcitonin receptors [115]. Its anorexic effects seem to be modulated through amylin's interaction with other signals involved in the short-term control of food intake, including cholecystokinin, glucagon-like peptide 1, and peptide YY, by decreasing the expression of orexigenic neuropeptides in the lateral hypothalamus [116].

Pramlintide is a synthetic analog of amylin that has been approved for the treatment of both type 1 and type 2 diabetes and has been shown to result in small weight losses in obese and diabetic adults [117–120]. The main adverse effects of pramlintide are nausea and abdominal discomfort. There are a few pramlintide reports about adolescents with type 1 diabetes [121,122]; however, there appear to be no pediatric or adolescent weight loss studies.

Beloranib is a methionine aminopeptidase 2 (MetAP2) inhibitor and an analog of the natural compound fumagillin [123]. MetAP2 inhibition reduces fat biosynthesis and induces lipolysis and fat oxidation through unclear mechanisms [124]. It was originally developed as an angiogenesis inhibitor for the treatment of solid tumors [125] and it was observed to have weight-lowering effects at significantly lower doses than the ones used in cancer patients [126]. A phase II double-blind, randomized, placebo-controlled trial of three dose regimens of beloranib studying 147 obese adult patients (primarily women) showed weight loss of up to ~11 kg in the high-dose group versus −0.4 kg in the placebo group [127]. Beloranib was associated with a dose-dependent reduction in the sense of hunger in these trials, suggesting a central mechanism of action that has yet to be elucidated. Animals treated with beloranib also exhibit reduced food intake [128,129]. Beloranib has also been reported to decrease weight in adults with hypothalamic injury–associated obesity [130]. A phase III double-blind, placebo-controlled trial of beloranib in pediatric and adult patients with Prader–Willi syndrome is now complete; results should be available by mid-2016.

DRUGS AFFECTING NUTRIENT TRAFFICKING

Medications affecting digestion in the gut include the following:

- *Orlistat* is a gastric and pancreatic lipase inhibitor that reduces dietary fat absorption by approximately 30% [131,132]. Orlistat is the only FDA-approved agent for the management of obesity in adolescents 12–16 years of age. There are multiple short- and long-term trials using orlistat in adolescents [131,133–138]. One of the largest randomized, placebo-controlled trials showed an overall -0.55 kg/m^2 decrease in BMI with orlistat versus a $+0.31$ kg/m^2 increase with placebo after 52 weeks ($p < .001$) [137]. The side-effect profile is primarily related to gastrointestinal issues, with oily stools, abdominal pain, and fecal urgency most commonly reported. Orlistat appears to affect the absorption of fat-soluble vitamins E and D [139], and users should also take a multivitamin. Some studies have also reported small but significant increases in serum liver enzyme concentrations [140]. Although orlistat has undergone two label changes due to reports of liver injury, cholelithiasis, and pancreatitis, a cause-and-effect relationship of severe liver injury with orlistat use has not been established [141]. Orlistat is the only FDA-approved drug for treatment of obesity in children aged 12–17 years to date, despite limited data on long-term (beyond 1 year) efficacy and its limited overall benefits. Orlistat must be taken with each meal, thus reducing its feasibility for school-attending adolescents. Available community data suggest half of the pediatric patients prescribed orlistat discontinue it within 1 month, 75% stop by 3 months, and only 10% remain on orlistat after 6 months [142,143]. Given its limited efficacy and low long-term use, orlistat appears of little benefit in practice.
- *Cetilistat* is another gastrointestinal lipase inhibitor currently under investigation [144,145]. It has shown similar weight reduction effects when compared with orlistat over 12 weeks among obese adults with type 2 diabetes treated with metformin, but may have a milder side-effect profile [144]. Cetilistat is approved in Japan for use in adults [146].
- *Acarbose* is a pseudotetrasaccharide that acts as a competitive inhibitor of intestinal alpha-glucosidases and compromises the uptake of monosaccharides, leading to lower postprandial insulin and glucose [147]. It is approved for diabetes management and has been shown to produce small weight losses in some adult studies [148–150]. There are no published pediatric trials for acarbose as an antiobesity drug.

MEDICATIONS AFFECTING RENAL NUTRIENT REABSORPTION

These drugs include dapagliflozin, canagliflozin, and empagliflozin, which are selective inhibitors of the sodium-dependent glucose cotransporter 2 in the renal tubule. They cause dose-related glucosuria by suppressing renal glucose reabsorption [151] and are approved for treatment of type 2 diabetes. Dapagliflozin induces relatively small but significant reductions in body weight, ranging from 2 to 5 kg [152–155] (vs. 0.95–1.55 kg reductions for placebo) in patients with type 2 diabetes [151]. Side effects include urinary tract and genital infections, volume depletion leading to increases in hematocrit and blood urea nitrogen, and hypoglycemia in those with diabetes. These agents are not approved for weight reduction in adults or children.

DRUGS AFFECTING INTERNAL MILIEU/METABOLIC CONTROL

None of the following agents have proved sufficiently potent to become FDA approved as therapy for obesity. However, modulation of the *milieu intérieur* is conceptually an important approach to ameliorate obesity. These drugs include the following:

- *Metformin*, a biguanide that inhibits intestinal glucose absorption, reduces hepatic gluco-neogenesis, and increases peripheral insulin sensitivity [156,157]. It is one of the corner-stones of treatment of type 2 diabetes in adults and children over 10 years of age [158]; however, it is not approved for the treatment of obesity. In nondiabetic adults it has been associated with modest weight loss and a reduction of insulin resistance [156] as well as the prevention or delay of type 2 diabetes onset [159]. Its use as a weight loss agent in adolescents has been studied in relatively few long-term trials (6 months or more). The largest trial in adolescents (92 subjects) showed a BMI change of -0.9 kg/m^2 in the met-formin group versus $+2.2$ kg/m^2 in the placebo arm; however, metformin treatment did not produce a significant change in total fat mass, abdominal fat, or insulin [160]. A study of younger children aged 6–12 years with extreme obesity showed an average weight change over 6 months in the metformin group of $+1.47$ kg versus $+4.85$ kg in a placebo group in an intent-to-treat analysis [161]. The effect of metformin on BMI has also been studied in girls with polycystic ovary syndrome (PCOS) [162–168] and in adolescents receiving antipsy-chotic drugs [169,170], with similar efficacy. Metformin has a modest impact on weight; its metabolic effects in nondiabetic children and adolescents are also inconsistent between studies [160,161,171–173]. Metformin remains one of the most studied drugs in pediatric samples. Currently, there are insufficient data to recommend metformin for weight reduc-tion in children or adolescents.
- *Octreotide*, an octapeptide analog of somatostatin, is a potent inhibitor of growth hormone (GH), ghrelin, glucagon, cholecystokinin, and glucose-dependent insulin secretion [174]. Octreotide has been primarily studied for its weight loss properties in patients with hypo-thalamic obesity who are believed to have elevated insulin production in response to their brain injury–stimulated hepatic glucose production. In patients with Prader–Willi syn-drome (who have marked increases in circulating ghrelin concentrations [175]), octreotide suppresses ghrelin; however, after 16 weeks of monthly octreotide administration, there was no significant change in BMI compared with placebo [176]. A small cohort of patients with hypothalamic obesity following cranial insults appeared to benefit from 6 months of octreotide therapy, with weight loss when compared with 6 months of prestudy observa-tion [177], but a placebo-controlled trial suggested weight stabilization rather than weight loss in patients with hypothalamic obesity [178]. Among obese adults with insulin hyper-secretion, treatment with octreotide for 6 months resulted in only ~2% more weight loss than in controls [179]. Octreotide appears reasonable to consider only in those with hypo-thalamic obesity, for whom it may be modestly effective.
- *Growth hormone*, which has multiple metabolic functions, increases hormone-sensitive lipase, stimulates adipocyte lipolysis [180], stimulates protein synthesis, and increases fat-free mass (both muscle and bone mass). GH is currently FDA approved for the treat-ment of patients with Prader–Willi syndrome and has proved to be efficacious at increas-ing height velocity [181] while decreasing fat mass and increasing lean body mass in such patients [182–184]. In GH-deficient adults and children, GH therapy has consistently resulted in decreased fat mass [185–188]. Despite its efficacy in these subset populations, a review of clinical trials of GH administration in patients with obesity showed no better performance for GH than for a hypocaloric diet [189]. The use of GH as a weight loss agent has also been limited due to the concerns regarding tumor development [190], changes in glucose metabo-lism [191], increased cardiac diameter [192], and exacerbation of respiratory symptoms (spe-cifically sleep apnea) [193,194]. Thus, GH is not approved for use as obesity therapy.

CAFFEINE PLUS EPHEDRINE

Ephedrine enhances catecholaminergic tone, with resulting thermogenic effects. This is augmented by the coadministration of methylxanthines such as caffeine, which inhibit phosphodiesterases [195].

In adults, a herbal caffeine–ephedrine preparation produced significant weight loss when compared with placebo [196]. This effect has also been observed in hypothalamic obesity [197]. One small study that randomized 16 adolescents to caffeine plus ephedrine and 16 to placebo reported significant weight loss (2.9 vs. 0.5 kg/m^2 with placebo) in a 5-month trial [198]. The most frequent side effects were nausea, insomnia, tremors, dizziness, and palpitations [199]. Ephedrine, however, was removed from use when it was found to cause significant cardiovascular effects.

CONCLUSION

At present, the only medication approved in the United States for use among adolescents for the amelioration of obesity is orlistat, which, when combined with lifestyle modification, has a moderate efficacy of approximately 3% additional weight loss relative to placebo, and is generally not well tolerated among adolescents in practice. Thus, at present, pharmacotherapy cannot be recommended for pediatric or adolescent obesity. Given the limited efficacy of even intensive behavior modification programs, however, there is a clear need for effective and safe long-term adjunctive drug therapy for children with severe obesity. FDA-approved drugs for long-term weight loss therapy in adults include combinations of bupropion and naltrexone, phentermine and topiramate, and monotherapy with liraglutide and lorcaserin. The percentage of adult patients achieving clinically meaningful (at least 5%) weight loss ranges from 37% to 47% for lorcaserin, 48%–66% for Contrave, 67%–70% for Qsymia, and approximately 51% for liraglutide. These encouraging results make them good candidates to be studied in randomized, controlled trials in pediatric and adolescent samples. In 2015, however, the literature on drug treatment for pediatric obesity remains quite limited and rife with issues (short intervention periods, high attrition rates, inadequate description of methods, and data analyses that use biased approaches to dealing with missing data) [5]. It is to be hoped that carefully designed, adequately powered clinical trials of the medications recently approved for long-term adult use will be carried out among pediatric samples in the near future.

REFERENCES

1. Oude Luttikhuis H, Baur L, Jansen H, Shrewsbury VA, O'Malley C, Stolk RP, et al. Interventions for treating obesity in children. *Cochrane Database Syst Rev*. 2009;(1):CD001872.
2. Fowler-Brown A, Kahwati LC. Prevention and treatment of overweight in children and adolescents. *Am Fam Physician*. 2004;69(11):2591–8.
3. McGovern L, Johnson JN, Paulo R, Hettinger A, Singhal V, Kamath C, et al. Clinical review: Treatment of pediatric obesity; A systematic review and meta-analysis of randomized trials. *J Clin Endocrinol Metab*. 2008;93(12):4600–5.
4. Kalarchian MA, Levine MD, Arslanian SA, Ewing LJ, Houck PR, Cheng Y, et al. Family-based treatment of severe pediatric obesity: Randomized, controlled trial. *Pediatrics*. 2009;124(4):1060–8.
5. Yanovski SZ, Yanovski JA. Long-term drug treatment for obesity: A systematic and clinical review. *JAMA*. 2014;311(1):74–86.
6. Yanovski SZ, Yanovski JA. Naltrexone extended-release plus bupropion extended-release for treatment of obesity. *JAMA*. 2015;313(12):1213–4.
7. Peirson L, Fitzpatrick-Lewis D, Morrison K, Warren R, Usman Ali M, Raina P. Treatment of overweight and obesity in children and youth: A systematic review and meta-analysis. *CMAJ Open*. 2015;3(1):E35–46.
8. Wadden TA, Berkowitz RI, Womble LG, Sarwer DB, Phelan S, Cato RK, et al. Randomized trial of lifestyle modification and pharmacotherapy for obesity. *N Engl J Med*. 2005;353(20):2111–20.
9. Berkowitz RI, Wadden TA, Tershakovec AM, Cronquist JL. Behavior therapy and sibutramine for the treatment of adolescent obesity: A randomized controlled trial. *JAMA*. 2003;289(14):1805–12.
10. Alexander M, Rothman RB, Baumann MH, Endres CJ, Brasic JR, Wong DF. Noradrenergic and dopaminergic effects of (+)-amphetamine-like stimulants in the baboon *Papio anubis*. *Synapse (New York, NY)*. 2005;56(2):94–9.
11. Rothman RB, Baumann MH, Dersch CM, Romero DV, Rice KC, Carroll FI, et al. Amphetamine-type central nervous system stimulants release norepinephrine more potently than they release dopamine and serotonin. *Synapse*. 2001;39(1):32–41.

12. Lorber J. Obesity in childhood: A controlled trial of anorectic drugs. *Arch Dis Child*. 1966;41(217):309–12.

13. Spranger J. [Phentermine resinate in obesity: Clinical trial of Mirapront in adipose children]. *Munch Med Wochenschr*. 1965;107(38):1833–4.

14. Andelman MB, Jones C, Nathan S. Treatment of obesity in underprivileged adolescents: Comparison of diethylpropion hydrochloride with placebo in a double-blind study. *Clin Pediatr (Phila)*. 1967;6(6):327–30.

15. Stewart DA, Bailey JD, Patell H. Tenuate dospan as an appetite suppressant in the treatment of obese children. *Appl Ther*. 1970;12(5):34–6.

16. Golebiowska M, Chlebna-Sokol D, Kobierska I, Konopinska A, Malek M, Mastalska A, et al. [Clinical evaluation of Teronac (mazindol) in the treatment of obesity in children: Part II; Anorectic properties and side effects (author's trans.)]. *Przegl Lek*. 1981;38(3):355–8.

17. Golebiowska M, Chlebna-Sokol D, Mastalska A, Zwaigzne-Raczynska J. [The clinical evaluation of teronac (Mazindol) in the treatment of children with obesity: Part I; Effect of the drug on somatic patterns and exercise capacity (author's trans.)]. *Przegl Lek*. 1981;38(2):311–4.

18. Hendricks EJ, Srisurapanont M, Schmidt SL, Haggard M, Souter S, Mitchell CL, et al. Addiction potential of phentermine prescribed during long-term treatment of obesity. *Int J Obes*. 2014;38(2):292–8.

19. Caplan J. Habituation to diethylpropion (Tenuate). *Can Med Assoc J*. 1963;88:943–4.

20. Klein-Schwartz W. Abuse and toxicity of methylphenidate. *Curr Opin Pediatr*. 2002;14(2):219–23.

21. Malecka-Tendera E, Koehler B, Muchacka M, Wazowski R, Trzciakowska A. [Efficacy and safety of dexfenfluramine treatment in obese adolescents]. *Pediatr Pol*. 1996;71(5):431–6.

22. Bacon GE, Lowrey GH. A clinical trial of fenfluramine in obese children. *Curr Ther Res Clin Exp*. 1967;9(12):626–30.

23. Goldstein DJ, Rampey AH, Jr, Enas GG, Potvin JH, Fludzinski LA, Levine LR. Fluoxetine: A randomized clinical trial in the treatment of obesity. *Int J Obes Relat Metab Disord*. 1994;18(3):129–35.

24. Pedrinola F, Cavaliere H, Lima N, Medeiros-Neto G. Is DL-fenfluramine a potentially helpful drug therapy in overweight adolescent subjects? *Obes Res*. 1994;2(1):1–4.

25. Pedrinola F, Sztejnsznajd C, Lima N, Halpern A, Medeiros-Neto G. The addition of dexfenfluramine to fluoxetine in the treatment of obesity: A randomized clinical trial. *Obes Res*. 1996;4(6):549–54.

26. Rauh JL, Lipp R. Chlorphentermine as an anorexigenic agent in adolescent obesity: Report of its efficacy in a double-blind study of 30 teen-agers. *Clin Pediatr (Phila)*. 1968;7(3):138–40.

27. Rothman RB, Ayestas MA, Dersch CM, Baumann MH. Aminorex, fenfluramine, and chlorphentermine are serotonin transporter substrates: Implications for primary pulmonary hypertension. *Circulation*. 1999;100(8):869–75.

28. Centers for Disease Control and Prevention (CDC). Cardiac valvulopathy associated with exposure to fenfluramine or dexfenfluramine: U.S. Department of Health and Human Services interim public health recommendations, November 1997. *MMWR Morb Mortal Wkly Rep*. 1997;46(45):1061–6.

29. Martin CK, Redman LM, Zhang J, Sanchez M, Anderson CM, Smith SR, et al. Lorcaserin, a 5-HT(2C) receptor agonist, reduces body weight by decreasing energy intake without influencing energy expenditure. *J Clin Endocrinol Metab*. 2011;96(3):837–45.

30. Smith SR, Weissman NJ, Anderson CM, Sanchez M, Chuang E, Stubbe S, et al. Multicenter, placebo-controlled trial of lorcaserin for weight management. *N Engl J Med*. 2010;363(3):245–56.

31. Fidler MC, Sanchez M, Raether B, Weissman NJ, Smith SR, Shanahan WR, et al. A one-year randomized trial of lorcaserin for weight loss in obese and overweight adults: The BLOSSOM trial. *J Clin Endocrinol Metab*. 2011;96(10):3067–77.

32. O'Neil PM, Smith SR, Weissman NJ, Fidler MC, Sanchez M, Zhang J, et al. Randomized placebo-controlled clinical trial of lorcaserin for weight loss in type 2 diabetes mellitus: The BLOOM-DM study. *Obesity (Silver Spring)*. 2012;20(7):1426–36.

33. Eisai Inc. BELVIQ (lorcaserin hydrochloride) tablets, for oral use. 2012 (updated June 27, 2013). Available from: http://www.accessdata.fda.gov/drugsatfda_docs/label/2012/022529lbl.pdf.

34. ClinicalTrials.gov. A multicenter, double-blind, randomized, parallel-group, pilot study of 12-week duration to assess the short-term safety and tolerability of lorcaserin plus two doses of immediate-release phentermine-hcl compared with lorcaserin alone in overweight and obese adults. NCT01987427. November 12, 2013 (updated January 22, 2015). Available from: https://clinicaltrials.gov/ct2/show/NCT01987427.

35. ClinicalTrials.gov. Single dose study to determine the safety, tolerability, and pharmacokinetic properties of lorcaserin hydrochloride (BELVIQ) in obese adolescents from 12 to 17 years of age. NCT02022956. December 23, 2013 (updated March 28, 2014). Available from: https://clinicaltrials.gov/show/NCT02022956.

36. Schabram I, Henkel K, Mohammadkhani Shali S, Dietrich C, Schmaljohann J, Winz O, et al. Acute and sustained effects of methylphenidate on cognition and presynaptic dopamine metabolism: An [18F] FDOPA PET study. *J Neurosci.* 2014;34(44):14769–76.

37. Raiteri M, Bertollini A, Angelini F, Levi G. d-Amphetamine as a releaser or reuptake inhibitor of biogenic amines in synaptosomes. *Eur J Pharmacol.* 1975;34(1):189–95.

38. Davis C, Fattore L, Kaplan AS, Carter JC, Levitan RD, Kennedy JL. The suppression of appetite and food consumption by methylphenidate: The moderating effects of gender and weight status in healthy adults. *Int J Neuropsychopharmacol.* 2012;15(2):181–7.

39. Adler LA, Orman C, Starr HL, Silber S, Palumbo J, Cooper K, et al. Long-term safety of OROS methylphenidate in adults with attention-deficit/hyperactivity disorder: An open-label, dose-titration, 1-year study. *J Clin Psycho.* 2011;31(1):108–14.

40. Poulton A, Briody J, McCorquodale T, Melzer E, Herrmann M, Baur LA, et al. Weight loss on stimulant medication: How does it affect body composition and bone metabolism? A prospective longitudinal study. *Int J Pediatr Endocrinol.* 2012;2012(1):30.

41. Wigal T, Greenhill L, Chuang S, McGough J, Vitiello B, Skrobala A, et al. Safety and tolerability of methylphenidate in preschool children with ADHD. *J Am Acad Child Adolesc Psychiatry.* 2006;45(11):1294–303.

42. Fredriksen M, Dahl AA, Martinsen EW, Klungsoyr O, Haavik J, Peleikis DE. Effectiveness of one-year pharmacological treatment of adult attention-deficit/hyperactivity disorder (ADHD): An open-label prospective study of time in treatment, dose, side-effects and comorbidity. *Eur Neuropsychopharmacol.* 2014;24(12):1873–84.

43. Wigal SB, Greenhill LL, Nordbrock E, Connor DF, Kollins SH, Adjei A, et al. A randomized placebo-controlled double-blind study evaluating the time course of response to methylphenidate hydrochloride extended-release capsules in children with attention-deficit/hyperactivity disorder. *J Child Adolesc Psychopharmacol.* 2014;24(10):562–9.

44. Trenque T, Herlem E, Abou Taam M, Drame M. Methylphenidate off-label use and safety. *SpringerPlus.* 2014;3:286.

45. Heal DJ, Cheetham SC, Smith SL. The neuropharmacology of ADHD drugs *in vivo*: Insights on efficacy and safety. *Neuropharmacology.* 2009;57(7–8):608–18.

46. McElroy SL, Hudson JI, Mitchell JE, Wilfley D, Ferreira-Cornwell MC, Gao J, et al. Efficacy and safety of lisdexamfetamine for treatment of adults with moderate to severe binge-eating disorder: A randomized clinical trial. *JAMA Psychiatry.* 2015;72(3):235–46.

47. Astrup A, Rossner S, Van Gaal L, Rissanen A, Niskanen L, Al Hakim M, et al. Effects of liraglutide in the treatment of obesity: A randomised, double-blind, placebo-controlled study. *Lancet.* 2009;374(9701):1606–16.

48. Zinman B, Gerich J, Buse JB, Lewin A, Schwartz S, Raskin P, et al. Efficacy and safety of the human glucagon-like peptide-1 analog liraglutide in combination with metformin and thiazolidinedione in patients with type 2 diabetes (LEAD-4 Met+TZD). *Diabetes Care.* 2009;32(7):1224–30.

49. Russell-Jones D, Vaag A, Schmitz O, Sethi BK, Lalic N, Antic S, et al. Liraglutide vs. insulin glargine and placebo in combination with metformin and sulfonylurea therapy in type 2 diabetes mellitus (LEAD-5 met+SU): A randomised controlled trial. *Diabetologia.* 2009;52(10):2046–55.

50. Nauck MA, Ratner RE, Kapitza C, Berria R, Boldrin M, Balena R. Treatment with the human once-weekly glucagon-like peptide-1 analog taspoglutide in combination with metformin improves glycemic control and lowers body weight in patients with type 2 diabetes inadequately controlled with metformin alone: A double-blind placebo-controlled study. *Diabetes Care.* 2009;32(7):1237–43.

51. Nauck M, Frid A, Hermansen K, Shah NS, Tankova T, Mitha IH, et al. Efficacy and safety comparison of liraglutide, glimepiride, and placebo, all in combination with metformin, in type 2 diabetes: The LEAD (liraglutide effect and action in diabetes)-2 study. *Diabetes Care.* 2009;32(1):84–90.

52. Garber A, Henry R, Ratner R, Garcia-Hernandez PA, Rodriguez-Pattzi H, Olvera-Alvarez I, et al. Liraglutide versus glimepiride monotherapy for type 2 diabetes (LEAD-3 Mono): A randomised, 52-week, phase III, double-blind, parallel-treatment trial. *Lancet.* 2009;373(9662):473–81.

53. Taylor K, Gurney K, Han J, Pencek R, Walsh B, Trautmann M. Exenatide once weekly treatment maintained improvements in glycemic control and weight loss over 2 years. *BMC Endocr Disord.* 2011;11:9.

54. Rosenstock J, Klaff LJ, Schwartz S, Northrup J, Holcombe JH, Wilhelm K, et al. Effects of exenatide and lifestyle modification on body weight and glucose tolerance in obese subjects with and without prediabetes. *Diabetes Care.* 2010;33(6):1173–5.

55. Pi-Sunyer X, Astrup A, Fujioka K, Greenway F, Halpern A, Krempf M, et al. A randomized, controlled trial of 3.0 mg of liraglutide in weight management. *N Engl J Med.* 2015;373(1):11–22.

56. van Bloemendaal L, Ijzerman RG, Ten Kulve JS, Barkhof F, Konrad RJ, Drent ML, et al. GLP-1 receptor activation modulates appetite- and reward-related brain areas in humans. *Diabetes.* 2014;63(12):4186–96.

57. Leiter LA, Carr MC, Stewart M, Jones-Leone A, Scott R, Yang F, et al. Efficacy and safety of the once-weekly GLP-1 receptor agonist albiglutide versus sitagliptin in patients with type 2 diabetes and renal impairment: A randomized phase III study. *Diabetes Care.* 2014;37(10):2723–30.

58. Dungan KM, Povedano ST, Forst T, Gonzalez JG, Atisso C, Sealls W, et al. Once-weekly dulaglutide versus once-daily liraglutide in metformin-treated patients with type 2 diabetes (AWARD-6): A randomised, open-label, phase 3, non-inferiority trial. *Lancet.* 2014;384(9951):1349–57.

59. Rosenstock J, Hanefeld M, Shamanna P, Min KW, Boka G, Miossec P, et al. Beneficial effects of once-daily lixisenatide on overall and postprandial glycemic levels without significant excess of hypoglycemia in type 2 diabetes inadequately controlled on a sulfonylurea with or without metformin (GetGoal-S). *J Diabetes Complications.* 2014;28(3):386–92.

60. Jensterle Sever M, Kocjan T, Pfeifer M, Kravos NA, Janez A. Short-term combined treatment with liraglutide and metformin leads to significant weight loss in obese women with polycystic ovary syndrome and previous poor response to metformin. *Eur J Endocrinol.* 2014;170(3):451–9.

61. Kelly AS, Metzig AM, Rudser KD, Fitch AK, Fox CK, Nathan BM, et al. Exenatide as a weight-loss therapy in extreme pediatric obesity: A randomized, controlled pilot study. *Obesity (Silver Spring).* 2012;20(2):364–70.

62. Kelly AS, Rudser KD, Nathan BM, Fox CK, Metzig AM, Coombes BJ, et al. The effect of glucagon-like peptide-1 receptor agonist therapy on body mass index in adolescents with severe obesity: A randomized, placebo-controlled, clinical trial. *JAMA Pediatrics.* 2013;167(4):355–60.

63. ClinicalTrials.gov. Effects of exenatide on overweight adolescents with Prader–Willi syndrome. NCT01444898. September 27, 2011 (updated July 25, 2013). Available from: https://clinicaltrials.gov/ct2/show/NCT01444898?term=glp+1+agonist+weight+children&rank=2.

64. Ioannides-Demos LL, Piccenna L, McNeil JJ. Pharmacotherapies for obesity: Past, current, and future therapies. *J Obes.* 2011;2011:179674.

65. Godoy-Matos A, Carraro L, Vieira A, Oliveira J, Guedes EP, Mattos L, et al. Treatment of obese adolescents with sibutramine: A randomized, double-blind, controlled study. *J Clin Endocrinol Metab.* 2005;90(3):1460–5.

66. Berkowitz RI, Fujioka K, Daniels SR, Hoppin AG, Owen S, Perry AC, et al. Effects of sibutramine treatment in obese adolescents: A randomized trial. *Ann Intern Med.* 2006;145(2):81–90.

67. Garcia-Morales LM, Berber A, Macias-Lara CC, Lucio-Ortiz C, Del-Rio-Navarro BE, Dorantes-Alvarez LM. Use of sibutramine in obese Mexican adolescents: A 6-month, randomized, double-blind, placebo-controlled, parallel-group trial. *Clin Ther.* 2006;28(5):770–82.

68. Budd GM, Hayman LL, Crump E, Pollydore C, Hawley KD, Cronquist JL, et al. Weight loss in obese African American and Caucasian adolescents: Secondary analysis of a randomized clinical trial of behavioral therapy plus sibutramine. *J Cardiovasc Nurs.* 2007;22(4):288–96.

69. Daniels SR, Long B, Crow S, Styne D, Sothern M, Vargas-Rodriguez I, et al. Cardiovascular effects of sibutramine in the treatment of obese adolescents: Results of a randomized, double-blind, placebo-controlled study. *Pediatrics.* 2007;120(1):e147–57.

70. Danielsson P, Janson A, Norgren S, Marcus C. Impact sibutramine therapy in children with hypothalamic obesity or obesity with aggravating syndromes. *J Clin Endocrinol Metab.* 2007;92(11):4101–6.

71. Van Mil EG, Westerterp KR, Kester AD, Delemarre-van de Waal HA, Gerver WJ, Saris WH. The effect of sibutramine on energy expenditure and body composition in obese adolescents. *J Clin Endocrinol Metab.* 2007;92(4):1409–14.

72. Violante-Ortiz R, Del-Rio-Navarro BE, Lara-Esqueda A, Perez P, Fanghanel G, Madero A, et al. Use of sibutramine in obese Hispanic adolescents. *Adv Ther.* 2005;22(6):642–9.

73. Reisler G, Tauber T, Afriat R, Bortnik O, Goldman M. Sibutramine as an adjuvant therapy in adolescents suffering from morbid obesity. *Isr Med Assoc J.* 2006;8(1):30–2.

74. Franco RR, Cominato L, Damiani D. [The effect of sibutramine on weight loss in obese adolescents]. *Arq Bras Endocrinol Metabol.* 2014;58(3):243–50.

75. Pischon T, Sharma AM. Recent developments in the treatment of obesity-related hypertension. *Curr Opin Nephrol Hypertens.* 2002;11(5):497–502.

76. Torp-Pedersen C, Caterson I, Coutinho W, Finer N, Van Gaal L, Maggioni A, et al. Cardiovascular responses to weight management and sibutramine in high-risk subjects: An analysis from the SCOUT trial. *Eur Heart J.* 2007;28(23):2915–23.

77. Yanovski JA. Behavior therapy and sibutramine for the treatment of adolescent obesity. *J Pediatr.* 2003;143(5):686.

78. James WP, Caterson ID, Coutinho W, Finer N, Van Gaal LF, Maggioni AP, et al. Effect of sibutramine on cardiovascular outcomes in overweight and obese subjects. *N Engl J Med*. 2010;363(10):905–17.

79. Hayes JF, Bhaskaran K, Batterham R, Smeeth L, Douglas I. The effect of sibutramine prescribing in routine clinical practice on cardiovascular outcomes: A cohort study in the United Kingdom. *Int J Obes*. 2015;39(9):1359–64.

80. Al-Tahami BA, Ismail AA, Bee YT, Awang SA, Salha Wan Abdul Rani WR, Sanip Z, et al. The effects of anti-obesity intervention with orlistat and sibutramine on microvascular endothelial function. *Clin Hemorheol Microcirc*. 2015;59(4):323–34.

81. Pavlik V, Fajfrova J, Slovacek L, Drahokoupilova E. The role of sibutramine in weight reduction. *Bratisl Lek Listy*. 2013;114(3):155–7.

82. Billes SK, Cowley MA. Inhibition of dopamine and norepinephrine reuptake produces additive effects on energy balance in lean and obese mice. *Neuropsychopharmacology*. 2007;32(4):822–34.

83. Anderson JW, Greenway FL, Fujioka K, Gadde KM, McKenney J, O'Neil PM. Bupropion SR enhances weight loss: A 48-week double-blind, placebo-controlled trial. *Obes Res*. 2002;10(7):633–41.

84. Ornellas T, Chavez B. Naltrexone SR/Bupropion SR (Contrave): A new approach to weight loss in obese adults. *P T*. 2011;36(5):255–62.

85. Glod CA, Lynch A, Flynn E, Berkowitz C, Baldessarini RJ. Open trial of bupropion SR in adolescent major depression. *J Child Adolesc Psychiatr Nurs*. 2003;16(3):123–30.

86. Becker EA, Shafer A, Anderson R. Weight changes in teens on psychotropic medication combinations at Austin State Hospital. *Tex Med*. 2005;101(3):62–70.

87. Perucca E, Bialer M. The clinical pharmacokinetics of the newer antiepileptic drugs: Focus on topiramate, zonisamide and tiagabine. *Clin Pharmacokinet*. 1996;31(1):29–46.

88. Gadde KM, Allison DB, Ryan DH, Peterson CA, Troupin B, Schwiers ML, et al. Effects of low-dose, controlled-release, phentermine plus topiramate combination on weight and associated comorbidities in overweight and obese adults (CONQUER): A randomised, placebo-controlled, phase 3 trial. *Lancet*. 2011;377(9774):1341–52.

89. Allison DB, Gadde KM, Garvey WT, Peterson CA, Schwiers ML, Najarian T, et al. Controlled-release phentermine/topiramate in severely obese adults: A randomized controlled trial (EQUIP). *Obesity (Silver Spring)*. 2012;20(2):330–42.

90. Garvey WT, Ryan DH, Look M, Gadde KM, Allison DB, Peterson CA, et al. Two-year sustained weight loss and metabolic benefits with controlled-release phentermine/topiramate in obese and overweight adults (SEQUEL): A randomized, placebo-controlled, phase 3 extension study. *Am J Clin Nutr*. 2012;95(2):297–308.

91. Winslow DH, Bowden CH, DiDonato KP, McCullough PA. A randomized, double-blind, placebo-controlled study of an oral, extended-release formulation of phentermine/topiramate for the treatment of obstructive sleep apnea in obese adults. *Sleep*. 2012;35(11):1529–39.

92. Roberts MD. US Food and Drug Administration: Endocrinologic and Metabolic Drugs Advisory Committee Meeting, Clinical Briefing Document, February 22, 2012. VIVUS, Inc. New Drug Application 22580: VI-0521 QNEXA (phentermine/topiramate). 2012 (updated March 30, 2012). Available from: http://www.fda.gov/downloads/AdvisoryCommittees/CommitteesMeetingMaterials/Drugs/EndocrinologicandMetabolicDrugsAdvisoryCommittee/UCM292315.pdf.

93. VIVUS Inc. NDA 22580: QSYMIA (phentermine and topiramate extended-release) Capsules. Risk Evaluation and Mitigation Strategy (REMS). Reference ID: 3294731. 2013 (updated July 3, 2013). Available from: http://www.fda.gov/downloads/Drugs/DrugSafety/PostmarketDrugSafetyInformationfor PatientsandProviders/UCM312598.pdf.

94. ClinicalTrials.gov. Topiramate and severe obesity (TOBI). NCT02273804. October 22, 2014. Available from: https://clinicaltrials.gov/ct2/show/NCT02273804.

95. ClinicalTrials.gov. Topiramate in adolescents with severe obesity. NCT01859013. May 9, 2013 (updated February 24, 2016). Available from: https://clinicaltrials.gov/ct2/show/NCT01859013?term=topiramate +children&rank=15.

96. Nathan PJ, O'Neill BV, Napolitano A, Bullmore ET. Neuropsychiatric adverse effects of centrally acting antiobesity drugs. *CNS Neurosci Ther*. 2011;17(5):490–505.

97. Schwartz MW. Brain pathways controlling food intake and body weight. *Exp Biol Med (Maywood)*. 2001;226(11):978–81.

98. Farooqi IS, Jebb SA, Langmack G, Lawrence E, Cheetham CH, Prentice AM, et al. Effects of recombinant leptin therapy in a child with congenital leptin deficiency. *N Engl J Med*. 1999;341(12):879–84.

99. Farooqi IS, Matarese G, Lord GM, Keogh JM, Lawrence E, Agwu C, et al. Beneficial effects of leptin on obesity, T cell hyporesponsiveness, and neuroendocrine/metabolic dysfunction of human congenital leptin deficiency. *J Clin Invest*. 2002;110(8):1093–103.

100. Gibson WT, Farooqi IS, Moreau M, DePaoli AM, Lawrence E, O'Rahilly S, et al. Congenital leptin deficiency due to homozygosity for the Delta133G mutation: Report of another case and evaluation of response to four years of leptin therapy. *J Clin Endocrinol Metab.* 2004;89(10):4821–6.

101. Paz-Filho G, Wong ML, Licinio J. Ten years of leptin replacement therapy. *Obes Rev.* 2011;12(5):e315–23.

102. Chou SH, Chamberland JP, Liu X, Matarese G, Gao C, Stefanakis R, et al. Leptin is an effective treatment for hypothalamic amenorrhea. *Proc Natl Acad Sci USA.* 2011;108(16):6585–90.

103. Heymsfield SB, Greenberg AS, Fujioka K, Dixon RM, Kushner R, Hunt T, et al. Recombinant leptin for weight loss in obese and lean adults: A randomized, controlled, dose-escalation trial. *JAMA.* 1999;282(16):1568–75.

104. Moon HS, Matarese G, Brennan AM, Chamberland JP, Liu X, Fiorenza CG, et al. Efficacy of metreleptin in obese patients with type 2 diabetes: Cellular and molecular pathways underlying leptin tolerance. *Diabetes.* 2011;60(6):1647–56.

105. Rosenbaum M, Murphy EM, Heymsfield SB, Matthews DE, Leibel RL. Low dose leptin administration reverses effects of sustained weight-reduction on energy expenditure and circulating concentrations of thyroid hormones. *J Clin Endocrinol Metab.* 2002;87(5):2391–4.

106. Rosenbaum M, Goldsmith R, Bloomfield D, Magnano A, Weimer L, Heymsfield S, et al. Low-dose leptin reverses skeletal muscle, autonomic, and neuroendocrine adaptations to maintenance of reduced weight. *J Clin Invest.* 2005;115(12):3579–86.

107. Rosenbaum M, Sy M, Pavlovich K, Leibel RL, Hirsch J. Leptin reverses weight loss-induced changes in regional neural activity responses to visual food stimuli. *J Clin Invest.* 2008;118(7):2583–91.

108. Goldsmith R, Joanisse DR, Gallagher D, Pavlovich K, Shamoon E, Leibel RL, et al. Effects of experimental weight perturbation on skeletal muscle work efficiency, fuel utilization, and biochemistry in human subjects. *Am J Physiol Regul Integr Comp Physiol.* 2010;298(1):R79–88.

109. Baldwin KM, Joanisse DR, Haddad F, Goldsmith RL, Gallagher D, Pavlovich KH, et al. Effects of weight loss and leptin on skeletal muscle in human subjects. *Am J Physiol Regul Integr Comp Physiol.* 2011;301(5):R1259–66.

110. Korner J, Conroy R, Febres G, McMahon DJ, Conwell I, Karmally W, et al. Randomized double-blind placebo-controlled study of leptin administration after gastric bypass. *Obesity (Silver Spring).* 2013;21(5):951–6.

111. Gilbert JA, Gasteyger C, Raben A, Meier DH, Astrup A, Sjodin A. The effect of tesofensine on appetite sensations. *Obesity.* [Research Support, Non-US Govt]. 2012;20(3):553–61.

112. Sjodin A, Gasteyger C, Nielsen AL, Raben A, Mikkelsen JD, Jensen JK, et al. The effect of the triple monoamine reuptake inhibitor tesofensine on energy metabolism and appetite in overweight and moderately obese men. *Int J Obes.* 2010;34(11):1634–43.

113. Appel L, Bergstrom M, Buus Lassen J, Langstrom B. Tesofensine, a novel triple monoamine re-uptake inhibitor with anti-obesity effects: Dopamine transporter occupancy as measured by PET. *Eur Neuropsychopharmacol.* 2014;24(2):251–61.

114. Astrup A, Madsbad S, Breum L, Jensen TJ, Kroustrup JP, Larsen TM. Effect of tesofensine on body-weight loss, body composition, and quality of life in obese patients: A randomised, double-blind, placebo-controlled trial. *Lancet.* 2008;372(9653):1906–13.

115. Hay DL, Christopoulos G, Christopoulos A, Sexton PM. Amylin receptors: Molecular composition and pharmacology. *Biochem Soc Trans.* 2004;32(Pt 5):865–7.

116. Potes CS, Lutz TA. Brainstem mechanisms of amylin-induced anorexia. *Physiol Behav.* 2010;100(5):511–8.

117. Singh-Franco D, Perez A, Harrington C. The effect of pramlintide acetate on glycemic control and weight in patients with type 2 diabetes mellitus and in obese patients without diabetes: A systematic review and meta-analysis. *Diabetes Obes Metab.* 2011;13(2):169–80.

118. Maggs D, Shen L, Strobel S, Brown D, Kolterman O, Weyer C. Effect of pramlintide on A1C and body weight in insulin-treated African Americans and Hispanics with type 2 diabetes: A pooled post hoc analysis. *Metabolism.* 2003;52(12):1638–42.

119. Aronne L, Fujioka K, Aroda V, Chen K, Halseth A, Kesty NC, et al. Progressive reduction in body weight after treatment with the amylin analog pramlintide in obese subjects: A phase 2, randomized, placebo-controlled, dose-escalation study. *J Clin Endocrinol Metab.* 2007;92(8):2977–83.

120. Smith SR, Aronne LJ, Burns CM, Kesty NC, Halseth AE, Weyer C. Sustained weight loss following 12-month pramlintide treatment as an adjunct to lifestyle intervention in obesity. *Diabetes Care.* 2008;31(9):1816–23.

121. Chase HP, Lutz K, Pencek R, Zhang B, Porter L. Pramlintide lowered glucose excursions and was well-tolerated in adolescents with type 1 diabetes: Results from a randomized, single-blind, placebo-controlled, crossover study. *J Pediatr.* 2009;155(3):369–73.

122. Kishiyama CM, Burdick PL, Cobry EC, Gage VL, Messer LH, McFann K, et al. A pilot trial of pramlintide home usage in adolescents with type 1 diabetes. *Pediatrics.* 2009;124(5):1344–7.

123. Chun E, Han CK, Yoon JH, Sim TB, Kim YK, Lee KY. Novel inhibitors targeted to methionine aminopeptidase 2 (MetAP2) strongly inhibit the growth of cancers in xenografted nude model. *Int J Cancer.* 2005;114(1):124–30.

124. Rupnick MA, Panigrahy D, Zhang CY, Dallabrida SM, Lowell BB, Langer R, et al. Adipose tissue mass can be regulated through the vasculature. *Proc Natl Acad Sci USA.* 2002;99(16):10730–5.

125. Shin SJ, Ahn JB, Park KS, Lee YJ, Hong YS, Kim TW, et al. A Phase Ib pharmacokinetic study of the anti-angiogenic agent CKD-732 used in combination with capecitabine and oxaliplatin (XELOX) in metastatic colorectal cancer patients who progressed on irinotecan-based chemotherapy. *Invest New Drugs.* 2012;30(2):672–80.

126. Hughes TE, Kim DD, Marjason J, Proietto J, Whitehead JP, Vath JE. Ascending dose-controlled trial of beloranib, a novel obesity treatment for safety, tolerability, and weight loss in obese women. *Obesity (Silver Spring).* 2013;21(9):1782–8.

127. Kim DD, Krishnarajah J, Lillioja S, de Looze F, Marjason J, Proietto J, et al. Efficacy and safety of beloranib for weight loss in obese adults: A randomized controlled trial. *Diabetes Obes Metab.* 2015;17(6):566–72.

128. Kim YM, An JJ, Jin YJ, Rhee Y, Cha BS, Lee HC, et al. Assessment of the anti-obesity effects of the TNP-470 analog, CKD-732. *J Mol Endocrinol.* 2007;38(4):455–65.

129. Lijnen HR, Frederix L, Van Hoef B. Fumagillin reduces adipose tissue formation in murine models of nutritionally induced obesity. *Obesity (Silver Spring).* 2010;18(12):2241–6.

130. Zafgen. Zafgen announces positive results from phase 2 clinical trial of beloranib in hypothalamic injury associated obesity. Press release. January 7, 2015. Available from: http://ir.zafgen.com/releasedetail.cfm?releaseid=889999.

131. McDuffie JR, Calis KA, Uwaifo GI, Sebring NG, Fallon EM, Hubbard VS, et al. Three-month tolerability of orlistat in adolescents with obesity-related comorbid conditions. *Obes Res.* 2002;10(7):642–50.

132. FDA. Highlights of prescribing information. Reference ID: 3391274. October 2013. Available from: http://www.accessdata.fda.gov/drugsatfda_docs/label/2013/020766s033lbl.pdf.

133. Zhi J, Moore R, Kanitra L. The effect of short-term (21-day) orlistat treatment on the physiologic balance of six selected macrominerals and microminerals in obese adolescents. *J Am Coll Nutr.* 2003;22(5):357–62.

134. Norgren S, Danielsson P, Jurold R, Lotborn M, Marcus C. Orlistat treatment in obese prepubertal children: A pilot study. *Acta Paediatr.* 2003;92(6):666–70.

135. Ozkan B, Bereket A, Turan S, Keskin S. Addition of orlistat to conventional treatment in adolescents with severe obesity. *Eur J Pediatr.* 2004;163(12):738–41.

136. McDuffie JR, Calis KA, Uwaifo GI, Sebring NG, Fallon EM, Frazer TE, et al. Efficacy of orlistat as an adjunct to behavioral treatment in overweight African American and Caucasian adolescents with obesity-related co-morbid conditions. *J Pediatr Endocrinol Metab.* 2004;17(3):307–19.

137. Chanoine JP, Hampl S, Jensen C, Boldrin M, Hauptman J. Effect of orlistat on weight and body composition in obese adolescents: A randomized controlled trial. *JAMA.* 2005;293(23):2873–83.

138. Maahs D, de Serna DG, Kolotkin RL, Ralston S, Sandate J, Qualls C, et al. Randomized, double-blind, placebo-controlled trial of orlistat for weight loss in adolescents. *Endocr Pract.* 2006;12(1):18–28.

139. McDuffie JR, Calis KA, Booth SL, Uwaifo GI, Yanovski JA. Effects of orlistat on fat-soluble vitamins in obese adolescents. *Pharmacotherapy.* 2002;22(7):814–22.

140. Yanovski JA, McDuffie JR, Salaita CS, Tanofsky-Kraff M, Sebring NG, Young-Hyman D, et al. A randomized, placebo-controlled trial of the effects of orlistat on body weight and body composition in African American and Caucasian adolescents with obesity-related comorbid conditions. *Obesity.* 2008;16(Suppl. 1):S63.

141. Mathis LL. US Food and Drug Administration: Pediatric Advisory Committee Meeting, March 22, 2010. Orlistat Update. 2010 (updated March 22, 2010). Available from: http://www.fda.gov/downloads/AdvisoryCommittees/CommitteesMeetingMaterials/PediatricAdvisoryCommittee/UCM205380.pdf.

142. Viner RM, Hsia Y, Neubert A, Wong IC. Rise in antiobesity drug prescribing for children and adolescents in the UK: A population-based study. *Br J Clin Pharmacol.* 2009;68(6):844–51.

143. Sun AP, Kirby B, Black C, Helms PJ, Bennie M, McLay JS. Unplanned medication discontinuation as a potential pharmacovigilance signal: A nested young person cohort study. *BMC Pharmacol Toxicol.* 2014;15:11.

144. Kopelman P, Bryson A, Hickling R, Rissanen A, Rossner S, Toubro S, et al. Cetilistat (ATL-962), a novel lipase inhibitor: A 12-week randomized, placebo-controlled study of weight reduction in obese patients. *Int J Obes (Lond).* 2007;31(3):494–9.

145. Kopelman P, Groot Gde H, Rissanen A, Rossner S, Toubro S, Palmer R, et al. Weight loss, HbA 1c reduction, and tolerability of cetilistat in a randomized, placebo-controlled phase 2 trial in obese diabetics: Comparison with orlistat (Xenical). *Obesity.* 2010;18(1):108–15.

146. Gras J. Cetilistat for the treatment of obesity. *Drugs Today.* 2013;49(12):755–9.

147. Salvatore T, Giugliano D. Pharmacokinetic-pharmacodynamic relationships of Acarbose. *Clin Pharmacokinet.* 1996;30(2):94–106.

148. Wang JS, Lin SD, Lee WJ, Su SL, Lee IT, Tu ST, et al. Effects of acarbose versus glibenclamide on glycemic excursion and oxidative stress in type 2 diabetic patients inadequately controlled by metformin: A 24-week, randomized, open-label, parallel-group comparison. *Clin Ther.* [Research Support, Non-US Govt]. 2011;33(12):1932–42.

149. Wolever TM, Chiasson JL, Josse RG, Hunt JA, Palmason C, Rodger NW, et al. Small weight loss on long-term acarbose therapy with no change in dietary pattern or nutrient intake of individuals with non-insulin-dependent diabetes. *Int J Obes Relat Metab Disord.* 1997;21(9):756–63.

150. Tugrul S, Kutlu T, Pekin O, Baglam E, Kiyak H, Oral O. Clinical, endocrine, and metabolic effects of acarbose, a alpha-glucosidase inhibitor, in overweight and nonoverweight patients with polycystic ovarian syndrome. *Fertil Steril.* 2008;90(4):1144–8.

151. Komoroski B, Vachharajani N, Boulton D, Kornhauser D, Geraldes M, Li L, et al. Dapagliflozin, a novel SGLT2 inhibitor, induces dose-dependent glucosuria in healthy subjects. *Clin Pharmacol Ther.* 2009;85(5):520–6.

152. Zhang L, Feng Y, List J, Kasichayanula S, Pfister M. Dapagliflozin treatment in patients with different stages of type 2 diabetes mellitus: Effects on glycaemic control and body weight. *Diabetes Obes Metab.* 2010;12(6):510–6.

153. Strojek K, Yoon KH, Hruba V, Elze M, Langkilde AM, Parikh S. Effect of dapagliflozin in patients with type 2 diabetes who have inadequate glycaemic control with glimepiride: A randomized, 24-week, double-blind, placebo-controlled trial. *Diabetes Obes Metab.* 2011;13(10):928–38.

154. Nauck MA, Del Prato S, Meier JJ, Duran-Garcia S, Rohwedder K, Elze M, et al. Dapagliflozin versus glipizide as add-on therapy in patients with type 2 diabetes who have inadequate glycemic control with metformin: A randomized, 52-week, double-blind, active-controlled noninferiority trial. *Diabetes Care.* 2011;34(9):2015–22.

155. Bolinder J, Ljunggren O, Kullberg J, Johansson L, Wilding J, Langkilde AM, et al. Effects of dapagliflozin on body weight, total fat mass, and regional adipose tissue distribution in patients with type 2 diabetes mellitus with inadequate glycemic control on metformin. *J Clin Endocrinol Metab.* 2012;97(3):1020–31.

156. Mehnert H. Metformin, the rebirth of a biguanide: Mechanism of action and place in the prevention and treatment of insulin resistance. *Exp Clin Endocrinol Diabetes.* 2001;109(Suppl. 2):S259–64.

157. Hundal RS, Inzucchi SE. Metformin: New understandings, new uses. *Drugs.* 2003;63(18):1879–94.

158. Bestermann W, Houston MC, Basile J, Egan B, Ferrario CM, Lackland D, et al. Addressing the global cardiovascular risk of hypertension, dyslipidemia, diabetes mellitus, and the metabolic syndrome in the southeastern United States, part II: Treatment recommendations for management of the global cardiovascular risk of hypertension, dyslipidemia, diabetes mellitus, and the metabolic syndrome. *Am J Med Sci.* 2005;329(6):292–305.

159. Knowler WC, Barrett-Connor E, Fowler SE, Hamman RF, Lachin JM, Walker EA, et al. Reduction in the incidence of type 2 diabetes with lifestyle intervention or metformin. *N Engl J Med.* 2002;346(6):393–403.

160. Wilson DM, Abrams SH, Aye T, Lee PD, Lenders C, Lustig RH, et al. Metformin extended release treatment of adolescent obesity: A 48-week randomized, double-blind, placebo-controlled trial with 48-week follow-up. *Arch Pediatr Adolesc Med.* 2010;164(2):116–23.

161. Yanovski JA, Krakoff J, Salaita CG, McDuffie JR, Kozlosky M, Sebring NG, et al. Effects of metformin on body weight and body composition in obese insulin-resistant children: A randomized clinical trial. *Diabetes.* 2011;60(2):477–85.

162. Legro RS. Impact of metformin, oral contraceptives, and lifestyle modification on polycystic ovary syndrome in obese adolescent women: Do we need a new drug? *J Clin Endocrinol Metab.* 2008;93(11):4218–20.

163. Mastorakos G, Koliopoulos C, Deligeoroglou E, Diamanti-Kandarakis E, Creatsas G. Effects of two forms of combined oral contraceptives on carbohydrate metabolism in adolescents with polycystic ovary syndrome. *Fertil Steril.* 2006;85(2):420–7.

164. Hoeger K, Davidson K, Kochman L, Cherry T, Kopin L, Guzick DS. The impact of metformin, oral contraceptives, and lifestyle modification on polycystic ovary syndrome in obese adolescent women in two randomized, placebo-controlled clinical trials. *J Clin Endocrinol Metab.* 2008;93(11):4299–306.

165. Ibanez L, de Zegher F. Ethinylestradiol-drospirenone, flutamide-metformin, or both for adolescents and women with hyperinsulinemic hyperandrogenism: Opposite effects on adipocytokines and body adiposity. *J Clin Endocrinol Metab.* 2004;89(4):1592–7.

166. Bridger T, MacDonald S, Baltzer F, Rodd C. Randomized placebo-controlled trial of metformin for adolescents with polycystic ovary syndrome. *Arch Pediatr Adolesc Med.* 2006;160(3):241–6.

167. Allen HF, Mazzoni C, Heptulla RA, Murray MA, Miller N, Koenigs L, et al. Randomized controlled trial evaluating response to metformin versus standard therapy in the treatment of adolescents with polycystic ovary syndrome. *J Pediatr Endocrinol Metab.* 2005;18(8):761–8.

168. Arslanian SA, Lewy V, Danadian K, Saad R. Metformin therapy in obese adolescents with polycystic ovary syndrome and impaired glucose tolerance: Amelioration of exaggerated adrenal response to adrenocorticotropin with reduction of insulinemia/insulin resistance. *J Clin Endocrinol Metab.* 2002;87(4):1555–9.

169. Klein DJ, Cottingham EM, Sorter M, Barton BA, Morrison JA. A randomized, double-blind, placebo-controlled trial of metformin treatment of weight gain associated with initiation of atypical antipsychotic therapy in children and adolescents. *Am J Psychiatry.* 2006;163(12):2072–9.

170. Bjorkhem-Bergman L, Asplund AB, Lindh JD. Metformin for weight reduction in non-diabetic patients on antipsychotic drugs: A systematic review and meta-analysis. *J Psychopharmacol.* 2011;25(3):299–305.

171. Fu JF, Liang L, Zou CC, Hong F, Wang CL, Wang XM, et al. Prevalence of the metabolic syndrome in Zhejiang Chinese obese children and adolescents and the effect of metformin combined with lifestyle intervention. *Int J Obes (Lond).* 2007;31(1):15–22.

172. Atabek ME, Pirgon O. Use of metformin in obese adolescents with hyperinsulinemia: A 6-month, randomized, double-blind, placebo-controlled clinical trial. *J Pediatr Endocrinol Metab.* 2008;21(4):339–48.

173. Clarson CL, Mahmud FH, Baker JE, Clark HE, McKay WM, Schauteet VD, et al. Metformin in combination with structured lifestyle intervention improved body mass index in obese adolescents, but did not improve insulin resistance. *Endocrine.* 2009;36(1):141–6.

174. Gambineri A, Patton L, De Iasio R, Cantelli B, Cognini GE, Filicori M, et al. Efficacy of octreotide-LAR in dieting women with abdominal obesity and polycystic ovary syndrome. *J Clin Endocrinol Metab.* 2005;90(7):3854–62.

175. Cummings DE, Clement K, Purnell JQ, Vaisse C, Foster KE, Frayo RS, et al. Elevated plasma ghrelin levels in Prader Willi syndrome. *Nat Med.* 2002;8(7):643–4.

176. De Waele K, Ishkanian SL, Bogarin R, Miranda CA, Ghatei MA, Bloom SR, et al. Long-acting octreotide treatment causes a sustained decrease in ghrelin concentrations but does not affect weight, behaviour and appetite in subjects with Prader–Willi syndrome. *Eur J Endocrinol.* 2008;159(4):381–8.

177. Lustig RH, Rose SR, Burghen GA, Velasquez-Mieyer P, Broome DC, Smith K, et al. Hypothalamic obesity caused by cranial insult in children: Altered glucose and insulin dynamics and reversal by a somatostatin agonist. *J Pediatr.* 1999;135(2 Pt 1):162–8.

178. Lustig RH, Hinds PS, Ringwald-Smith K, Christensen RK, Kaste SC, Schreiber RE, et al. Octreotide therapy of pediatric hypothalamic obesity: A double-blind, placebo-controlled trial. *J Clin Endocrinol Metab.* 2003;88(6):2586–92.

179. Lustig RH, Greenway F, Velasquez-Mieyer P, Heimburger D, Schumacher D, Smith D, et al. A multicenter, randomized, double-blind, placebo-controlled, dose-finding trial of a long-acting formulation of octreotide in promoting weight loss in obese adults with insulin hypersecretion. *Int J Obes (Lond).* 2006;30(2):331–41.

180. Dietz J, Schwartz J. Growth hormone alters lipolysis and hormone-sensitive lipase activity in 3T3-F442A adipocytes. *Metabolism.* 1991;40(8):800–6.

181. Wald AB, Uli NK. Pharmacotherapy in pediatric obesity: Current agents and future directions. *Rev Endocr Metab Disord.* 2009;10(3):205–14.

182. Hoybye C, Hilding A, Jacobsson H, Thoren M. Growth hormone treatment improves body composition in adults with Prader–Willi syndrome. *Clin Endocrinol (Oxf).* 2003;58(5):653–61.

183. Carrel AL, Myers SE, Whitman BY, Allen DB. Benefits of long-term GH therapy in Prader–Willi syndrome: A 4-year study. *J Clin Endocrinol Metab.* 2002;87(4):1581–5.

184. Myers SE, Davis A, Whitman BY, Santiago JV, Landt M. Leptin concentrations in Prader–Willi syndrome before and after growth hormone replacement. *Clin Endocrinol (Oxf).* 2000;52(1):101–5.

185. Snel YE, Doerga ME, Brummer RJ, Zelissen PM, Zonderland ML, Koppeschaar HP. Resting metabolic rate, body composition and related hormonal parameters in growth hormone-deficient adults before and after growth hormone replacement therapy. *Eur J Endocrinol.* 1995;133(4):445–50.

186. Gregory JW, Greene SA, Jung RT, Scrimgeour CM, Rennie MJ. Changes in body composition and energy expenditure after six weeks' growth hormone treatment. *Arch Dis Child.* 1991;66(5):598–602.

187. Hoos MB, Westerterp KR, Gerver WJ. Short-term effects of growth hormone on body composition as a predictor of growth. *J Clin Endocrinol Metab.* 2003;88(6):2569–72.

188. Eden Engstrom B, Burman P, Holdstock C, Karlsson FA. Effects of growth hormone (GH) on ghrelin, leptin, and adiponectin in GH-deficient patients. *J Clin Endocrinol Metab.* 2003;88(11):5193–8.

189. Shadid S, Jensen MD. Effects of growth hormone administration in human obesity. *Obes Res.* 2003;11(2):170–5.

190. Bell J, Parker KL, Swinford RD, Hoffman AR, Maneatis T, Lippe B. Long-term safety of recombinant human growth hormone in children. *J Clin Endocrinol Metab.* 2010;95(1):167–77.

191. Lammer C, Weimann E. [Changes in carbohydrate metabolism and insulin resistance in patients with Prader–Willi syndrome (PWS) under growth hormone therapy]. *Wien Med Wochenschr.* 2007;157(3–4):82–8.

192. Hauffa BP, Knaup K, Lehmann N, Neudorf U, Nagel B. Effects of growth hormone therapy on cardiac dimensions in children and adolescents with Prader–Willi syndrome. *Horm Res Paediatr.* 2011;75(1):56–62.

193. Miller J, Silverstein J, Shuster J, Driscoll DJ, Wagner M. Short-term effects of growth hormone on sleep abnormalities in Prader–Willi syndrome. *J Clin Endocrinol Metab.* 2006;91(2):413–7.

194. Festen DA, de Weerd AW, van den Bossche RA, Joosten K, Hoeve H, Hokken-Koelega AC. Sleep-related breathing disorders in prepubertal children with Prader–Willi syndrome and effects of growth hormone treatment. *J Clin Endocrinol Metab.* 2006;91(12):4911–5.

195. Astrup A. Thermogenic drugs as a strategy for treatment of obesity. *Endocrine.* 2000;13(2):207–12.

196. Boozer CN, Daly PA, Homel P, Solomon JL, Blanchard D, Nasser JA, et al. Herbal ephedra/caffeine for weight loss: A 6-month randomized safety and efficacy trial. *Int J Obes Relat Metab Disord.* 2002;26(5):593–604.

197. Greenway FL, Bray GA. Treatment of hypothalamic obesity with caffeine and ephedrine. *Endocr Pract.* 2008;14(6):697–703.

198. Molnar D, Torok K, Erhardt E, Jeges S. Safety and efficacy of treatment with an ephedrine/caffeine mixture: The first double-blind placebo-controlled pilot study in adolescents. *Int J Obes Relat Metab Disord.* 2000;24(12):1573–8.

199. McBride BF, Karapanos AK, Krudysz A, Kluger J, Coleman CI, White CM. Electrocardiographic and hemodynamic effects of a multicomponent dietary supplement containing ephedra and caffeine: A randomized controlled trial. *JAMA.* 2004;291(2):216–21.

31 Surgical Treatment of Adolescent Obesity

Andrew James Beamish and Torsten Olbers

CONTENTS

INTRODUCTION

Today's worsening global obesity pandemic affects a huge number of children and young people, with over 22% of children classed as overweight across the world [1] and almost 17% of children classed as obese in the United States [2]. While public health policy at the local, national, and international levels struggles to battle this crisis, the suffering at an individual level remains very real. For the obese teenager, life-changing and life-shortening comorbidities are highly likely in adulthood and often a reality long before [3]. The therapeutic options available to this vulnerable group are not only limited but often expensive and frequently ineffective. In this context, the emergence of surgical treatments is offering a promising and effective option for the severely obese adolescent. This chapter examines the background to bariatric surgery in adults and its use in adolescents, explores the selection processes, the role of the multidisciplinary team (MDT), pre- and postoperative considerations, and outcomes in this young and emerging field.

HISTORY OF BARIATRIC SURGERY

Surgery is currently a well-established therapeutic intervention for obesity and its comorbidities in adults. Bariatric surgery began in the 1950s with J. Howard Payne's jejunocolic shunt [4]. This radical procedure involved the bypass of the vast majority of the small intestine. While the results were extremely successful in terms of weight loss, the negative effects on individuals were also profound. Patients often experienced major problems, such as diarrhea, dehydration, and gross and potentially life-threatening nutritional deficiencies, alongside myriad other complaints, such as gallstones and hair loss. A majority of patients required reoperation for complete or partial restoration of the intestinal anatomy [4].

To date, the most commonly reported procedure in adolescents is the Roux-en-Y gastric bypass (RYGB) [5]. The first reports of this approach came in 1966, when Edward E. Mason bypassed the majority of the stomach specifically to reduce weight [6]. Mason hypothesized that the powerful weight loss effects observed in patients undergoing gastrectomy for other reasons, such as peptic ulcer or cancer, could be replicated in patients suffering from severe obesity. In his early series, an impressive average weight loss of 44 kg across 1 year was achieved, but at the expense of a mortality in excess of 8% [7].

Building on this foundation, Mason set out to evaluate the early and long-term effects on metabolism and to develop the operation to achieve "safe control of obesity" [6]. Since then, surgical approaches to treat obesity have advanced enormously and, accompanied by advances in medical and anesthetic practice, the safe control of obesity using surgery has been made possible. Thirty-day mortality now lies below 0.1%, despite the presence of multiple comorbidities in many operated patients [8].

Less than a decade after Mason presented the first gastric bypass procedure, reports emerged detailing the results of surgery performed on children and adolescents [9,10]. When treating adolescents, a number of other issues must be considered in addition to the surgical approach. Adolescents' growth and development is often not complete, and surgery confers lasting effects on eating patterns and nutritional intake. The long-term effects on micronutrient status and dependent systems, such as the skeleton, have yet to be documented in this population. However, for vulnerable individuals suffering from severe obesity, the negative impact of obesity is here and now. Where conservative measures are unsuccessful, surgery represents an effective and valid therapeutic option to reverse or improve multiple disease states and risk factors [5].

WHERE DOES SURGERY FIT IN?

Today, nonsurgical interventions predominate in the treatment of adolescent obesity, and the proportion of adolescents undergoing bariatric surgery is very small. Surgery is certainly not appropriate for every obese patient, but represents an essential and unparalleled option for a significant number of adolescents suffering from severe obesity and its comorbidities.

As covered in other chapters of this book, most nonsurgical interventions for childhood obesity are reliant on major lifestyle alterations involving dietary modification and physical activity programs. Surgery is not a first-line treatment for obesity. However, a referral to the specialist bariatric surgical MDT should be considered to evaluate surgical options when conservative measures persistently fail, generally after at least 6–12 months within a formal weight loss program.

PATIENT SELECTION

Selection criteria have been discussed in many papers in recent years and consensus guidelines are emerging, based predominantly on the original National Institutes of Health (NIH) guidelines [11]. However, these guidelines were developed in 1991 for adults with severe obesity and did not consider adolescents. The normal childhood body mass index (BMI) has been shown to increase with age [12]. Epidemiological analysis has determined appropriate global adolescent cutoff points for overweight and obesity, ranging from around 22 and 27 kg/m^2, respectively, at age 13 years, to the standard adult values of 25 and 30 kg/m^2 at age 18 years [12]. A BMI for age greater than the 99th percentile is associated with elevated cardiovascular and metabolic risk [13] and, in adolescence, this group includes all boys and most girls with a BMI exceeding 35 kg/m^2 [13].

The most appropriate candidates for surgery may well be individuals in later adolescence, whose physical development is more advanced compared with earlier in childhood. Therefore, the use of fixed cutoff points for selection is advocated in order to confer an increasingly conservative approach with decreasing age. In this context, the current guidance recommends that adult BMI cutoff points of 35 kg/m^2 with *serious* comorbidity and 40 kg/m^2 with *other* comorbidity are appropriate primary criteria for surgery during adolescence [14] (Figure 31.1). Serious comorbidity is defined as type 2 diabetes mellitus (T2DM), moderate or severe obstructive sleep apnea (OSA; AHI >15 events/hour), pseudotumor cerebri, or severe steatohepatitis. Other comorbidities include mild OSA, hypertension, insulin resistance, glucose intolerance, dyslipidemia, and impaired quality of life or activities of daily living, as well as other conditions (Figure 31.1).

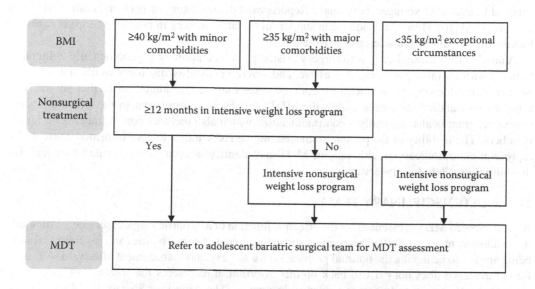

Comorbidity examples

Exceptional circumstances:
- Life-threatening obesity-related comorbidities

Major:
- T2DM
- Moderate-severe OSA
- Benign intracranial hypertension
- Heart failure due to obesity

Minor:
- Impaired fasting glucose
- Impaired glucose tolerance
- Mild OSA
- Hypertension
- Dyslipidemia
- Steatohepatitis
- Panniculitis
- Venous stasis
- GERD
- Urinary incontinence
- Severe psychosocial morbidity
- Impaired ADLs

Exclusion criteria:
- Patient or family/carers not committed to follow up program
- Unable to understand risks/and benefits
- Patient unable to assent/carers unable to consent
- Unstable psychiatric condition
- Ongoing addiction (drugs, medication, alcohol)
- Treatable medical cause of obesity
- Skeletal immaturity (Tanner < IV)

FIGURE 31.1 Inclusion pathway for bariatric surgery. BMI, body mass index; MDT, multidisciplinary team meeting; T2DM, type 2 diabetes mellitus; CV, cardiovascular; OSA, obstructive sleep apnea; GERD, gastroesophageal reflux disease; ADLs, activities of daily living.

It is also largely accepted that surgical candidates should be developmentally mature, having reached Tanner stage IV or V and 95% of estimated growth [15]. An ability to demonstrate both motivation and a mature capacity for decision making, with a full understanding of the potential risks and benefits involved, is also necessary, along with commitment to a lifelong program of follow-up and micronutrient supplementation. Where psychiatric morbidity exists, it should be under formal treatment and be well controlled. Finally, and of crucial importance, the understanding and committed social support of the individual's family or carers, and certainly the absence of abuse or neglect, are essential. Exceptions to the specific criteria exist and debate continues regarding the surgical treatment of younger individuals. Reports exist documenting surgery on children as young as 2 years old [16]. However, evidence in support of bariatric surgery in preadolescence is currently lacking and should be considered experimental.

A number of contraindications to surgery exist, especially among the psychologically vulnerable. Patients with unstable psychotic, depressive, and severe personality disorders would not normally be considered for surgery, although exceptional cases may be considered on formal advice from a psychiatrist and/or consensus within the MDT. An absent commitment to the lifelong postoperative program is also normally a contraindication, which also includes commitment from family members. The inability of the patient to understand the risks and/or to give informed consent also represents contraindications, although the MDT may identify exceptions to this rule where learning disabilities preclude full understanding.

THE MULTIDISCIPLINARY TEAM

An experienced MDT is essential for the effective function of a bariatric surgical service, particularly in the adolescent group. Skilled assessment and management of comorbidities and psychosocial well-being are key to achieving the optimal preparation for surgery and management afterward. Although formal evidence does not exist to back up this assertion, it represents the standard of care and is recommended unanimously across guidance documents. The American Society for Metabolic and Bariatric Surgery (ASMBS) suggests that several key members of the MDT are required [15]. These include a bariatric surgeon, a pediatrician, a dietitian, a mental health specialist, a physical therapist or exercise physiologist, and a dedicated coordinator. The surgeon may be either a bariatric surgeon experienced in pediatric surgery or a pediatric surgeon experienced in bariatric surgery. In fact, it is preferential that both a pediatric surgeon and a bariatric surgeon work together in combination. The pediatrician's specialist expertise will typically be in one or a combination of endocrinology, gastroenterology, nutrition, and adolescence, but they may equally reasonably be an internal medicine specialist or a family practitioner experienced in adolescent medicine. The dietitian should be experienced in working with children and families, and the mental health specialist will typically be a psychiatrist or psychologist with adolescent or pediatric training, specifically experienced in obesity and assessment for obesity surgery. The physical therapist or exercise physiologist should be experienced in providing safe activity programs for severely obese adolescents. Finally, a coordinator must be responsible for coordinating the health-care pathway of each individual adolescent within the program, with particular importance placed on ensuring compliance with follow-up and treatments, such as nutritional supplementation. It is often appropriate for the coordinator to be a core team member who is in direct contact with patients and establishes a relationship of trust. This may be, for example, a nurse specialist or social worker. In addition to the primary team members, support should be available, as required, from specialists in pulmonology, gynecology, endocrinology, infectious diseases, cardiology, sleep disorders, gastroenterology, radiology, psychiatry, and hematology.

DIFFERENT SURGICAL PROCEDURES AVAILABLE

A wide range of bariatric surgical procedures exist today, but most modern reports of bariatric surgery in adolescents describe the use of the RYGB, sleeve gastrectomy (SG), and adjustable gastric band (AGB). Historically, the most commonly used procedure has been the RYGB, although in recent years the use of SG has increased [15]. RYGB was first performed in adolescents in the mid-1970s [9], long preceding SG and AGB. It comes as no surprise, therefore, that the procedure with the greatest evidence base is the RYGB. As suggested by its name, RYGB involves bypassing the stomach by using an intestinal bypass, although no tissue is excised. The majority of the stomach is disconnected from the normal digestive route using a stapling device to leave a small (20–25 mL) gastric pouch in continuity with the esophagus. The jejunum is transected approximately 50–100 cm from the ligament of Treitz, and the distal end (Roux limb) is anastomosed to the gastric pouch, as a gastrojejunal anastomosis. The proximal end (the biliary limb) is attached approximately 80–150 cm distally along the jejunum, as a jejuno-jejunal (JJ) anastomosis. This Roux-en-Y construction means that ingested food passes directly from the esophagus through the small stomach pouch directly into the jejunum, bypassing most of the stomach, all of the duodenum, and the first part of the jejunum. Gastric, pancreatic, and biliary juices flow undiluted through the biliary limb to enter the jejunum at the JJ anastomosis, where juices meet ingested food.

SG involves the excision of the majority of the stomach on its greater curvature side, using a stapling device. The resection line begins approximately 5 cm proximal to the pylorus, proceeding to the angle of His to result in a tube or sleeve-shaped remnant stomach of approximately 25% its original capacity. A calibration tube, or *bougie*, is used to standardize the sleeve size.

The AGB is a synthetic restrictive device applied around the upper stomach to limit the transit of ingested food and therefore the volume that can be ingested. A balloon within the band is inflated with saline via a *port-a-cath* to achieve an adjustable degree of restriction.

There are currently insufficient data to make firm recommendations regarding preferred surgical technique in adolescents. In fact, this debate remains heated even regarding adult patients, and the answer will likely come from adequately powered randomized trials comparing procedures, which in adolescents have not yet emerged. Most bariatric surgeons appear to use the same surgical techniques for adolescents as in adults. The outcomes according to procedure will be discussed later in this chapter.

Proponents of AGB argue its reversibility as a benefit, although its mechanisms of action are more heavily reliant on restriction, compared with the profound gut–brain hormonal effects in RYGB. Surgeons preferring RYGB additionally argue that a long safety record, together with superior long-term weight and comorbidity control and favorable dietary compliance, suggest that this technique should suit adolescents best. SG, a relatively new bariatric technique, has been increasingly used in adolescents in recent years [17], and its short-term weight outcomes appear similar to those of RYGB. An advantage of SG may be a lower risk of long-term nutritional deficiencies, although long-term weight outcome remains unclear. The resection of a large portion of the stomach and the inability to restore normal anatomy after SG are disadvantages of this technique.

PREOPERATIVE WORKUP

A thorough formal overall assessment of the candidate's eligibility should be undertaken. European guidelines [18] suggest that this should include an assessment of general health and nutritional status, a detailed explanation of necessary dietary changes after surgery, and an assessment of patient and family motivation and commitment to fully engage and comply with the lifelong follow-up program. Any existing comorbidities should be optimized with input from appropriate specialists.

Psychological assessment is especially important in the workup for surgery. Adolescents with obesity represent a particularly vulnerable group psychosocially, with exceptionally high prevalence of depressive symptoms, anxiety, and low self-esteem [19]. While these have been demonstrated to improve in many patients, a subgroup representing almost one-fifth of patients experiences ongoing symptoms [19]. It is crucial that full and frank discussions are held in advance of surgery, involving psychologically qualified professionals where necessary, to identify and address any identifiable psychological morbidity. It may be possible to mitigate the impact of mental health issues with close psychological follow-up and support. Some patients may be identified as candidates for cognitive therapies, while others may be identified as unsuitable to undergo surgery at the current time point. It is essential that the patient and family fully understand the benefits, risks, and likely outcomes of surgery, as well as likely limits to its outcomes. Detailed health and nutrition assessment may include pulmonary function, sleep apnea, metabolic and endocrine function, helicobacter testing, body composition, bone density, and indirect calorimetry. A very low-calorie diet for 2 weeks prior to surgery has been shown, in adults, to reduce postoperative complications and improve the perceived difficulty of RYGB [20]. In adolescents, an example program has included a low-calorie diet (800–1200 kcal daily) for 2 to 3 weeks preoperatively [21].

PERIOPERATIVE CARE

Upon successful completion of the low-calorie diet, admission on the day of surgery is appropriate. Treatment should be in a specialist unit, with experience and expertise in providing adolescent bariatric surgical care. Ideally, the environment should be targeted at adolescents, rather than the general pediatric population. On the day of surgery, clinical aspects of management should mirror those adopted locally in adult bariatric surgery. These aspects should be discussed with anesthesiology colleagues and referenced alongside local guidance. Typical modern provisions include consuming clear fluids only from at least 6 h and nil by mouth for at least 2 h before surgery; appropriate thrombosis prophylaxis; and, of course, a final reassuring face-to-face discussion with the patient and his or her relatives to identify and alleviate any worries in advance of surgery.

Following surgery, care should be delivered in a ward environment with specialist experience in adolescent bariatric surgery. AGB, as the least invasive procedure, may be performed as an ambulatory procedure or, more likely, with a single overnight stay for observation. Following SG and RYGB, simple supportive measures, including analgesia and intravenous maintenance fluids, are required during the first 24 postoperative hours, but regular small-volume (20–25 mL) clear oral fluid intake is encouraged from the outset. Appropriate preoperative dietary counseling should allow patients to confidently upscale dietary intake, such that a small-portion soft diet is tolerated before discharge, typically on postoperative day two.

It is common to experience abdominal discomfort and even pain in the first 24–36 h postoperatively, which normally subsides rapidly and should be discussed in advance of surgery. It is not routine to perform a radiological contrast study to confirm adequate passage of fluid. Rather, attentiveness for warning symptoms of a hold-up is necessary. Should individuals regurgitate saliva or experience disproportionate pain levels after swallowing, a contrast study may be indicated. Clinicians should be vigilant for signs and symptoms of early complications, such as tachypnea, tachycardia, elevated oxygen requirement, fever, regurgitation, excessive pain, decreased conscious level, and anxiety. Complications that may be heralded by a combination of these symptoms include bleeding, gastric or intestinal obstruction, gastrointestinal leak, or pulmonary embolus.

Individuals should be well acquainted with a formal plan for obtaining advice and/or medical assessment and assistance in the event of difficulty after discharge. This may be in the form of a specific telephone contact, alongside electronic or paper information sources detailing expected and common symptoms and those symptoms requiring urgent attention. An appropriately staffed rapid-access clinic or suitable place for assessment should be available.

POSTOPERATIVE FOLLOW-UP

Intensive outpatient follow-up within the bariatric program should follow surgery. Regular early contact is important as patients become used to new eating patterns and abilities. A suggested program involves weekly or fortnightly patient visits for the first month, monthly visits up to 6 months, then 3-monthly visits until 2 years postoperatively. It is important to ensure effective and regular communication with the patient's primary care provider, with a clear route of contact for advice and assessment, such that primary care staff members understand and are engaged with the implications of the surgical intervention. This is made more important because of a tendency toward poor follow-up rates in bariatric surgery, as patients' weight and comorbidities, and therefore their immediate need for health care, diminish. The standard for long-term follow-up in the United States is to achieve 75% patients attending at 5 years postoperatively, with all patients prospectively tracked [22]. Additionally, provision for long-term follow-up should plan for transition of care from the adolescent domain to an adult service as patients mature beyond pediatric or adolescent facilities [22].

OUTCOMES

The weight loss and comorbidity improvement resulting from adult obesity is well documented, the most recent meta-analysis incorporating over 160 studies and including 37 randomized trials [8]. This study demonstrated mean BMI reduction at 1 year to be between 11.8 and 13.5 kg/m^2 across the three procedures discussed in this chapter. The increasing body of evidence in adolescents shows similar BMI reductions beyond 6 months of 11.6 kg/m^2 after AGB, 14.1 kg/m^2 after SG, and 16.6 kg/m^2 after RYGB.

An area of particular interest in adult bariatric surgery is the impressive effect on T2DM. The risk of developing T2DM rises sharply with increasing BMI [23]. Furthermore, there is emerging evidence that adolescent-onset T2DM behaves more aggressively than adult-onset T2DM, with earlier failure of first-line therapies and requirement for insulin [24–26]. A mature literature base describes a marked improvement in glucose homeostasis after surgery, offering nondiabetics protection from developing T2DM [27] and inducing remission in 72% of those with T2DM, with the greatest benefit being when the T2DM diagnosis is new [28]. Adolescent studies, while limited thus far, show T2DM resolution in 79%–100% of cases following RYGB, 50%–94% following SG, and 100% after AGB [29].

Bariatric surgery has marked effects on cardiovascular risk factors, not least BMI, which is associated with a 10% increase in the risk of myocardial infarction per standard deviation BMI increase [30]. Overweight and obesity are associated with an increase in the risk of ischemic stroke of 22% and 64%, respectively [31]. Childhood levels of low-density lipoprotein cholesterol (LDL-C) and high-density lipoprotein cholesterol (HDL-C) track into adulthood, and childhood LDL-C independently predicts carotid artery intima-media thickness in adulthood [32,33]. Obesity is associated with chronic, low-grade inflammation, and an elevated high-sensitivity C-reactive protein, even at low levels of ≥3 mg/L, is associated with a greater prevalence of coronary artery lesions [34]. There is growing epidemiological evidence in the adult literature of an association between overweight or obesity and breast, cervical, colorectal, endometrial, esophageal, gallbladder, kidney, liver, ovarian, pancreatic, stomach, and thyroid cancers [35,36]. Reversal of obesity may reduce the incidence of these cancers and long-term follow-up studies are needed to explore this in detail. Female-specific benefits include an increase in fertility and significantly reduced rates of gestational diabetes and eclampsia, with either no increase, or even a reduction, in risks to the neonate [37].

Additional comorbidity improvements have been shown in adolescents following bariatric surgery and are listed in Table 31.1 [5].

CONCERNS

Surgery can never be entirely without risk, yet bariatric procedures have an excellent safety profile in comparison with many other abdominal surgical procedures, such as cholecystectomy and hernia surgery, at least in adults. A number of potential complications require urgent reoperation in the postoperative period, such as anastomotic or staple line leak, bleeding, or bowel obstruction. Across all adult bariatric procedures, the published mortality rate is 0.22%–0.34% [38,39]. There is only one reported perioperative death following bariatric surgery in adolescents, which was a patient with significant cardiovascular comorbidity [40]. The choice of surgical procedure may be

TABLE 31.1

Outcomes of Adolescent Bariatric Surgery by Procedure

Outcome	Adjustable Gastric Band	Sleeve Gastrectomy	Roux-en-Y Gastric Bypass	All Procedures (95% CI)
BMI reduction (kg/m^2)	8.5–11.7	13.0–17.2	13.3–22.5	13.5 (11.9–15.1)
T2DM resolution (%)	80–100	0–68	67–100	0–100
Insulin resistance resolution (%)	44–77	50–96	100	44–100
Hypertension resolution (%)	50–100	69–100	82–100	50–100
Dyslipidemia resolution (%)	35–100	0–58	87–100	0–100
Obstructive sleep apnea resolution (%)	20–100	56–80	100	20–100
PCOS resolution (%)	—	0	100	0–100

Note: CI, confidence interval; BMI, body mass index; T2DM, type 2 diabetes mellitus; CV, cardiovascular; PCOS, polycystic ovarian syndrome.

influenced by such major comorbidity, since the operative time and physiological burden varies between procedures. Indeed, in a small number of eligible individuals the risk of surgery may feasibly outweigh the benefits, even in this young age group.

Adolescents with severe obesity often demonstrate nutritional deficiencies before bariatric surgery, which frequently persist postoperatively [41]. Protein deficiency is the most common macronutritional deficiency, but micronutrient deficiencies are more prevalent, such as trace elements, essential minerals, and both water-soluble and fat-soluble vitamins. Deficiencies may even be promoted by the consequences of surgery, such as small-intestinal bacterial overgrowth, especially in patients with T2DM [41]. RYGB removes the normal sphincter-controlled gastric emptying of digestive contents, permitting the rapid and unrestricted passage of calorie-rich food into the small bowel, which can lead to dumping syndrome. Symptoms include tremors, sweating, palpitation, fatigue, decreased conscious level, and diarrhea [42]. While symptoms are uncomfortable, most patients consider this to be a positive result of surgery as it can usually be controlled by dietary modification and offers a powerful feedback mechanism for avoidance of the wrong foods [43].

Some concern has been raised regarding the potential maternal and fetal health effects of micronutritional deficiencies during preconception and pregnancy. Testing for such deficiencies appears generally underperformed, although their true prevalence in preconception and pregnant women remains unknown [44]. Counseling regarding folic acid and other nutritional supplementation is, therefore, imperative in female adolescents under consideration for bariatric surgery. Iron deficiency anemia is also a risk in girls of reproductive age [45].

The impact of bariatric surgery on the adolescent skeleton is, as yet, unquantified beyond the first 2 years. Although bone mineral density (BMD) and bone mineral content have been shown to decrease within a year following gastric bypass surgery, levels fall from abnormally high values to reach normal or still above-normal levels for age [46]. Counseling, monitoring, and nutrient and mineral supplementation for bone health remain important after bariatric surgery [47]. The long-term skeletal impact is unknown and, therefore, warrants particular attention in follow-up studies, especially in young patients. Again, looking into the long-term implications of surgery in these young people, the required duration of action would be expected to be longer as the age at surgery decreases. It could therefore be expected that the requirement for reoperation at some future stage, with likely greater attendant risk than primary surgery [48], may be greater in this younger population. The implications of this will become more apparent from long-term follow-up studies in the adult population in the coming years, and similar studies in adolescent populations will provide evidence of its true implications.

Anatomical implications of bariatric procedures must also be considered, since they can introduce relative inaccessibility to parts of the gastrointestinal tract. Conventional diagnostic and therapeutic approaches, such as gastroscopy [49] or endoscopic cholangiography, can be made more difficult or impossible. However, necessity has resulted in the development of novel techniques, including computed tomography virtual gastroscopy [48], double-balloon techniques for enteroscopy after RYGB [50], and even prophylactic cholecystectomy [51], which subsequently lost favor following meta-analysis [52]. Additionally, reversal of the RYGB is technically feasible, without significant complication in the short term [53]; however, the gastric excision of SG cannot be reversed.

ADOLESCENT MORBID OBESITY SURGERY STUDY

In Sweden, adolescent bariatric surgery has been investigated within the Adolescent Morbid Obesity Surgery (AMOS) study. This study examines the outcomes of 81 adolescents aged 13–18 years undergoing RYBG, comparing them with matched control adolescents undergoing nonsurgical treatment and matched adult controls undergoing RYGB. Alongside data regarding the effects of surgery discussed previously, which largely mirror the adult experience, some extremely valuable lessons have been learned pertinent to the adolescent population.

The adolescent population suffering with obesity represents a particularly vulnerable psychosocially morbid population, with disorders of mood, anxiety, and eating being particularly prevalent [54]. While the literature is limited regarding the effect of bariatric surgery on psychosocial outcomes, AMOS has demonstrated significant improvements in self-reported anxiety, depression, and self-perception across 2 postoperative years, alongside nonsignificant improvements in anger and disruptive behavior [19]. Services must be designed to actively seek, recognize, and intervene in vulnerable adolescents, as a 2% attempted suicide rate has been reported [21].

There is little evidence regarding compliance with prescribed mineral and vitamin supplements following bariatric surgery, perhaps largely due to the inherent difficulties in its accurate and reliable quantification. Within AMOS, compliance appears to be worse in adolescents than in the adult population, with incidences of rebellion and apathy toward supplementation. An example of the potential importance of this is the issue of bone health, discussed earlier in the concerns section. While AMOS has described an overall decrease in BMD for age, only a small proportion of patients (5%) reached subnormal levels over the first 2 years [55]. It was also seen in this cohort that individuals whose BMD was below normal for age (<−1) at 2 years had all started from a comparatively low baseline level (<0.5) [55]. These individuals may represent an *at-risk* subgroup to target with interventions to maximize compliance with supplementation. While effective interventions to achieve this are lacking thus far, compound tablet supplements have now emerged, permitting an all-in-one tablet to be taken, which may be preferable to taking multiple tablets.

In the adult population, excess skin represents a major psychosocial and physical problem. It was hypothesized that this might be less problematic in adolescents undergoing RYGB, since their younger skin was expected to retain more elasticity and, having been exposed to the stretching of obesity for a shorter duration, it may resume a normal contour more readily. However, the AMOS study has shown this not to be true. The majority of adolescents reported excess skin after bariatric surgery and the proportion desiring body-contouring surgery was at least the same as in an adult comparison group [56]. Objective measurements were significantly correlated with subjectively experienced excess skin [56]. Perhaps most surprisingly, only weak correlations were observed between the change in BMI and objective measurements, subjective experience, and discomfort from excess skin, rendering prediction of excess skin problems very difficult [56]. Therefore, adolescents undergoing bariatric surgery should be informed that there is a substantial likelihood that they will experience discomfort from excess skin following a major weight loss.

SUMMARY AND CONCLUSIONS

Although the literature base is limited at present in comparison with the adult evidence, bariatric surgery appears to offer adolescents unparalleled weight loss, and improvements to health and quality of life, which appear to closely match those reported in adults. The significant potential negative effects must be recognized, mitigated for, and further investigated in long-term outcome studies. Additionally, quantification of the possible benefits to society and health-care budgets is warranted. Surgery most certainly does not represent a stand-alone answer to adolescent obesity, and truly effective prevention and conservative treatment strategies are urgently needed. However, for the adolescent who is suffering from severe obesity and its incumbent wide-ranging health effects today, the likelihood of achieving a normal weight without surgery is very slim indeed. Bariatric surgery appears to offer significant benefits, present and future, while other therapies fail to match its effectiveness and struggle to achieve and maintain significant weight loss.

REFERENCES

1. Ng M, Fleming T, Robinson M, Thomson B, Graetz N, Margono C, et al. Global, regional, and national prevalence of overweight and obesity in children and adults during 1980–2013: A systematic analysis for the Global Burden of Disease Study 2013. *Lancet.* 2014;384(9945):766–81.
2. Ogden CL, Carroll MD, Kit BK, Flegal KM. Prevalence of childhood and adult obesity in the United States, 2011–2012. *JAMA.* 2014;311(8):806–14.
3. Beamish AJ, Olbers T. Bariatric and metabolic surgery in adolescents: A path to decrease adult cardiovascular mortality. *Current Atherosclerosis Reports.* 2015;17(9):53.
4. Payne JH, Dewind LT, Commons RR. Metabolic observations in patients with jejunocolic shunts. *The American Journal of Surgery.* 1963;106:273–89.
5. Beamish AJ, Johansson SE, Olbers T. Bariatric surgery in adolescents: What do we know so far? *Scandinavian Journal of Surgery: SJS: Official Organ for the Finnish Surgical Society and the Scandinavian Surgical Society.* 2015;104(1):24–32.
6. Mason EE, Ito C. Gastric bypass in obesity. *The Surgical Clinics of North America.* 1967;47(6):1345–51.
7. Mason EE, Ito C. Gastric bypass. *Annals of Surgery.* 1969;170(3):329–39.
8. Chang SH, Stoll CR, Song J, Varela JE, Eagon CJ, Colditz GA. The effectiveness and risks of bariatric surgery: An updated systematic review and meta-analysis, 2003–2012. *JAMA Surgery.* 2014;149(3):275–87.
9. Soper RT, Mason EE, Printen KJ, Zellweger H. Gastric bypass for morbid obesity in children and adolescents. *Journal of Pediatric Surgery.* 1975;10(1):51–8.
10. Randolph JG, Weintraub WH, Rigg A. Jejunoileal bypass for morbid obesity in adolescents. *Journal of Pediatric Surgery.* 1974;9(3):341–5.
11. NIH conference. Gastrointestinal surgery for severe obesity: Consensus Development Conference Panel. *Annals of Internal Medicine.* 1991;115(12):956–61.
12. Cole TJ, Bellizzi MC, Flegal KM, Dietz WH. Establishing a standard definition for child overweight and obesity worldwide: International survey. *The BMJ.* 2000;320(7244):1240–3.
13. Freedman DS, Mei Z, Srinivasan SR, Berenson GS, Dietz WH. Cardiovascular risk factors and excess adiposity among overweight children and adolescents: The Bogalusa Heart Study. *The Journal of Pediatrics.* 2007;150(1):12–7.e2.
14. Pratt JS, Lenders CM, Dionne EA, Hoppin AG, Hsu GL, Inge TH, et al. Best practice updates for pediatric/adolescent weight loss surgery. *Obesity.* 2009;17(5):901–10.
15. Michalsky M, Reichard K, Inge T, Pratt J, Lenders C, American Society for Metabolic and Bariatric Surgery. ASMBS pediatric committee best practice guidelines. *Surgery for Obesity and Related Diseases: Official Journal of the American Society for Bariatric Surgery.* 2012;8(1):1–7.
16. Mohaidly MA, Suliman A, Malawi H. Laparoscopic sleeve gastrectomy for a two-and half year old morbidly obese child. *International Journal of Surgery Case Reports.* 2013;4(11):1057–60.
17. Inge TH, Zeller MH, Jenkins TM, Helmrath M, Brandt ML, Michalsky MP, et al. Perioperative outcomes of adolescents undergoing bariatric surgery: The Teen-Longitudinal Assessment of Bariatric Surgery (Teen-LABS) study. *JAMA Pediatrics.* 2014;168(1):47–53.
18. Fried M, Hainer V, Basdevant A, Buchwald H, Deitel M, Finer N, et al. Inter-disciplinary European guidelines on surgery of severe obesity. *International Journal of Obesity.* 2007;31(4):569–77.

19. Jarvholm K, Karlsson J, Olbers T, Peltonen M, Marcus C, Dahlgren J, et al. Two-year trends in psychological outcomes after gastric bypass in adolescents with severe obesity. *Obesity.* 2015;23(10):1966–72.

20. Van Nieuwenhove Y, Dambrauskas Z, Campillo-Soto A, van Dielen F, Wiezer R, Janssen I, et al. Preoperative very low-calorie diet and operative outcome after laparoscopic gastric bypass: A randomized multicenter study. *Archives of Surgery.* 2011;146(11):1300–5.

21. Olbers T, Gronowitz E, Werling M, Marlid S, Flodmark CE, Peltonen M, et al. Two-year outcome of laparoscopic Roux-en-Y gastric bypass in adolescents with severe obesity: Results from a Swedish Nationwide Study (AMOS). *International Journal of Obesity.* 2012;36(11):1388–95.

22. Michalsky M, Kramer RE, Fullmer MA, Polfuss M, Porter R, Ward-Begnoche W, et al. Developing criteria for pediatric/adolescent bariatric surgery programs. *Pediatrics.* 2011;128(Suppl. 2):S65–70.

23. Mokdad AH, Ford ES, Bowman BA, Dietz WH, Vinicor F, Bales VS, et al. Prevalence of obesity, diabetes, and obesity-related health risk factors, 2001. *JAMA.* 2003;289(1):76–9.

24. Beamish AJ, D'Alessio DA, Inge TH. Controversial issues: When the drugs don't work, can surgery provide a different outcome for diabetic adolescents? *Surgery for Obesity and Related Diseases: Official Journal of the American Society for Bariatric Surgery.* 2015;11(4):946–8.

25. Group TS, Zeitler P, Hirst K, Pyle L, Linder B, Copeland K, et al. A clinical trial to maintain glycemic control in youth with type 2 diabetes. *The New England Journal of Medicine.* 2012;366(24):2247–56.

26. Kahn SE, Haffner SM, Heise MA, Herman WH, Holman RR, Jones NP, et al. Glycemic durability of rosiglitazone, metformin, or glyburide monotherapy. *The New England Journal of Medicine.* 2006;355(23):2427–43.

27. Carlsson LM, Peltonen M, Ahlin S, Anveden A, Bouchard C, Carlsson B, et al. Bariatric surgery and prevention of type 2 diabetes in Swedish obese subjects. *The New England Journal of Medicine.* 2012;367(8):695–704.

28. Sjostrom L, Peltonen M, Jacobson P, Ahlin S, Andersson-Assarsson J, Anveden A, et al. Association of bariatric surgery with long-term remission of type 2 diabetes and with microvascular and macrovascular complications. *JAMA.* 2014;311(22):2297–304.

29. Paulus GF, de Vaan LE, Verdam FJ, Bouvy ND, Ambergen TA, van Heurn LW. Bariatric surgery in morbidly obese adolescents: A systematic review and meta-analysis. *Obesity Surgery.* 2015;25(5):860–78.

30. Yusuf S, Hawken S, Ounpuu S, Bautista L, Franzosi MG, Commerford P, et al. Obesity and the risk of myocardial infarction in 27,000 participants from 52 countries: A case-control study. *Lancet.* 2005;366(9497):1640–9.

31. Strazzullo P, D'Elia L, Cairella G, Garbagnati F, Cappuccio FP, Scalfi L. Excess body weight and incidence of stroke: Meta-analysis of prospective studies with 2 million participants. *Stroke: Journal of Cerebral Circulation.* 2010;41(5):e418–26.

32. Raitakari OT, Juonala M, Kahonen M, Taittonen L, Laitinen T, Maki-Torkko N, et al. Cardiovascular risk factors in childhood and carotid artery intima-media thickness in adulthood: The Cardiovascular Risk in Young Finns study. *JAMA.* 2003;290(17):2277–83.

33. Li S, Chen W, Srinivasan SR, Bond MG, Tang R, Urbina EM, et al. Childhood cardiovascular risk factors and carotid vascular changes in adulthood: The Bogalusa Heart Study. *JAMA.* 2003;290(17):2271–6.

34. Zieske AW, Tracy RP, McMahan CA, Herderick EE, Homma S, Malcom GT, et al. Elevated serum C-reactive protein levels and advanced atherosclerosis in youth. *Arteriosclerosis, Thrombosis, and Vascular Biology.* 2005;25(6):1237–43.

35. Calle EE, Kaaks R. Overweight, obesity and cancer: Epidemiological evidence and proposed mechanisms. *Nature Reviews Cancer.* 2004;4(8):579–91.

36. Bhaskaran K, Douglas I, Forbes H, dos-Santos-Silva I, Leon DA, Smeeth L. Body-mass index and risk of 22 specific cancers: A population-based cohort study of 5.24 million UK adults. *Lancet.* 2014;384(9945):755–65.

37. Maggard MA, Yermilov I, Li Z, Maglione M, Newberry S, Suttorp M, et al. Pregnancy and fertility following bariatric surgery: A systematic review. *JAMA: The Journal of the American Medical Association.* 2008;300(19):2286–96.

38. Sjostrom L, Narbro K, Sjostrom CD, Karason K, Larsson B, Wedel H, et al. Effects of bariatric surgery on mortality in Swedish obese subjects. *The New England Journal of Medicine.* 2007;357(8):741–52.

39. Buchwald H, Estok R, Fahrbach K, Banel D, Sledge I. Trends in mortality in bariatric surgery: A systematic review and meta-analysis. *Surgery.* 2007;142(4):621–32; discussion 32–5.

40. Michalsky M, Teich S, Rana A, Teeple E, Cook S, Schuster D. Surgical risks and lessons learned: Mortality following gastric bypass in a severely obese adolescent. *Journal of Pediatric Surgery Case Reports.* 2013;1(9):321–4.

41. Bal BS, Finelli FC, Shope TR, Koch TR. Nutritional deficiencies after bariatric surgery. *Nature Reviews Endocrinology*. 2012;8(9):544–56.

42. Banerjee A, Ding Y, Mikami DJ, Needleman BJ. The role of dumping syndrome in weight loss after gastric bypass surgery. *Surgical Endoscopy*. 2013;27(5):1573–8.

43. Elliot K. Nutritional considerations after bariatric surgery. *Critical Care Nursing Quarterly*. 2003;26(2):133–8.

44. Gadgil MD, Chang HY, Richards TM, Gudzune KA, Huizinga MM, Clark JM, et al. Laboratory testing for and diagnosis of nutritional deficiencies in pregnancy before and after bariatric surgery. *Journal of Women's Health (Larchmt)*. 2014;23(2):129–37.

45. Alvarez-Leite JI. Nutrient deficiencies secondary to bariatric surgery. *Current Opinion in Clinical Nutrition and Metabolic Care*. 2004;7(5):569–75.

46. Coates PS, Fernstrom JD, Fernstrom MH, Schauer PR, Greenspan SL. Gastric bypass surgery for morbid obesity leads to an increase in bone turnover and a decrease in bone mass. *The Journal of Clinical Endocrinology and Metabolism*. 2004;89(3):1061–5.

47. Malinowski SS. Nutritional and metabolic complications of bariatric surgery. *The American Journal of the Medical Sciences*. 2006;331(4):219–25.

48. Brethauer SA, Kothari S, Sudan R, Williams B, English WJ, Brengman M, et al. Systematic review on reoperative bariatric surgery: American Society for Metabolic and Bariatric Surgery Revision Task Force. *Surgery for Obesity and Related Diseases: Official Journal of the American Society for Bariatric Surgery*. 2014;10(5):952–72.

49. Braley SC, Nguyen NT, Wolfe BM. Late gastrointestinal hemorrhage after gastric bypass. *Obesity Surgery*. 2002;12(3):404–7.

50. Koornstra JJ. Double balloon enteroscopy for endoscopic retrograde cholangiopancreaticography after Roux-en-Y reconstruction: Case series and review of the literature. *The Netherlands Journal of Medicine*. 2008;66(7):275–9.

51. Guadalajara H, Sanz Baro R, Pascual I, Blesa I, Rotundo GS, Lopez JM, et al. Is prophylactic cholecystectomy useful in obese patients undergoing gastric bypass? *Obesity Surgery*. 2006;16(7):883–5.

52. Warschkow R, Tarantino I, Ukegjini K, Beutner U, Guller U, Schmied BM, et al. Concomitant cholecystectomy during laparoscopic Roux-en-Y gastric bypass in obese patients is not justified: A meta-analysis. *Obesity Surgery*. 2013;23(3):397–407.

53. Himpens J, Dapri G, Cadiere GB. Laparoscopic conversion of the gastric bypass into a normal anatomy. *Obesity Surgery*. 2006;16(7):908–12.

54. Jarvholm K, Olbers T, Marcus C, Marild S, Gronowitz E, Friberg P, et al. Short-term psychological outcomes in severely obese adolescents after bariatric surgery. *Obesity*. 2012;20(2):318–23.

55. Beamish AJ, Gronowitz E, Olbers T, Flodmark CE, Marcus C, Dahlgren J. Body composition and bone health in adolescents after Roux-en-Y gastric bypass for severe obesity. *Pediatric Obesity*. 2016, doi: 10.1111/ijpo.12134.

56. Staalesen T, Olbers T, Dahlgren J, Fagevik Olsen M, Flodmark CE, Marcus C, et al. Development of excess skin and request for body-contouring surgery in postbariatric adolescents. *Plastic and Reconstructive Surgery*. 2014;134(4):627–36.

32 Physical Activity Interventions for Treatment and Prevention of Childhood Obesity

Bernard Gutin and Scott Owens

CONTENTS

INTRODUCTION

In principle, the strategy for the treatment and prevention of pediatric obesity is straightforward: (1) identify the causes for why some youths become fatter than others, (2) design interventions to counteract these causes, and (3) implement these interventions on a widespread basis. Unfortunately, none of the processes involved is simple. Thus, a 2015 review of determinants of childhood obesity in Europe concluded, "The true causes of the childhood obesity epidemic remain undiscovered, and the ability of research to identify effective prevention and treatment methods is compromised."[1]

One factor that might lead to ineffective preventive interventions is that our theories of the causes of obesity are often based on information that is valid for adults but faulty as applied to growing youths. For example, obese adults can successfully lose weight by creating an energy deficit through dieting, with moderate physical activity playing a supporting role. Thus, it is appropriate in adults to focus treatment interventions on how to help obese people restrict their dietary energy intake. However, for growing children, how to achieve weight loss is not the relevant question. Instead, we need to determine how to structure interventions so they help the youths to build more lean tissue rather than fat tissue, without necessarily restricting weight. In fact, a physical activity intervention that has a favorable effect on percent body fat (%BF) might increase bone and muscle mass to such a degree that the body mass index (BMI) of the active youths increases more than the BMI of the control subjects.[2] To investigate this issue optimally requires the use of modern techniques to measure body composition. From a research perspective, new techniques are increasingly being employed in pediatric studies, allowing us to clarify the effects of physical activity interventions on various aspects of body composition. For example, dual-energy x-ray absorptiometry (DXA) provides data on three body composition compartments: fat mass, fat-free soft tissue, and bone mineral content.[3] In addition, magnetic resonance imaging (MRI) and computed tomography provide information on potentially harmful visceral adipose tissue (VAT).[4]

DESCRIPTIVE STUDIES EXAMINING THE LINK BETWEEN PHYSICAL ACTIVITY AND CHILDHOOD BODY COMPOSITION

Descriptive investigations typically involve relatively large numbers of free-living children and/or youths in whom physical activity and body composition have been assessed and correlated. For example, the Georgia Lifestyles Project examined the associations between adiposity and moderate and vigorous physical activity in a cross-sectional sample of several hundred adolescents in whom time spent in moderate and vigorous physical activity per day was measured objectively with accelerometry.[5] Moderate physical activity was defined as activity that has a metabolic level of three to six multiples of resting metabolic rate (METS); in behavioral terms, this represents slow-to-brisk walking. Vigorous physical activity was defined as an intensity greater than 6 METS, which represents activities at jogging/running intensities. In this sample, the free-living adolescents did ~40 min/day of moderate physical activity and only ~5 min/day of vigorous physical activity. When the relations of moderate and vigorous physical activity to adiposity were analyzed separately in regression models, only vigorous physical activity was a significant predictor of DXA-derived %BF ($p = .001$ for vigorous physical activity; $p = .67$ for moderate physical activity). Subsequent to that study, a number of other projects in Europe and the United States have conducted similar projects with similar results.[6] Thus, there seems to be something about vigorous physical activity that accounts for its inverse relationship to adiposity.

One line of investigation that may provide insight into the especially important role of vigorous physical activity in the development of a healthy body composition concerns its impact on various components of total energy expenditure. Because free-living youths participate in very little vigorous physical activity (i.e., ~5 min/day on average), the direct effect of the vigorous physical activity on energy expenditure would not seem to be an especially likely candidate as an underlying mechanism. Nonetheless, it is worth considering how vigorous physical activity might indirectly influence various aspects of total energy expenditure.

Resting metabolic rate (RMR) is the largest single component of total energy expenditure, and it is therefore noteworthy that vigorous physical activity stimulates the development of fat-free mass (FFM), the body compartment most highly correlated with RMR. Moreover, these findings are consistent with the results of two other lines of investigation: (1) free-living people with greater amounts of FFM tend to ingest more dietary energy;[7] and (2) youths who engage in relatively large amounts of vigorous physical activity tend to be lean at the same time that they ingest more dietary energy than fatter youths.[8,9] Another aspect of energy expenditure is the excess amount seen after the exercise itself is completed—the post-exercise energy expenditure. This is greatest following especially high-intensity exercise.[10–12] Another component of total energy expenditure is the thermic effect of food (TEF)—that is, the increase in metabolic rate that follows a meal. The TEF is especially great following meals with higher amounts of food energy.[13] Moreover, when people engage in some physical activity following a meal, the exercise and food interact, such that the exercise potentiates the TEF, with the TEF appearing to be greater in normal-weight than obese individuals.[14,15] These aspects of energy expenditure are difficult to measure accurately, except in controlled laboratory settings.[15,16] Therefore, they are seldom investigated in large-scale epidemiologic investigations. Nonetheless, taken together, they suggest that there are several pathways through which vigorous physical activity might be especially effective in raising total energy expenditure, thereby helping growing youths to avoid positive energy balance and develop lean bodies.

Another line of thinking, which is not directly based on energy expenditure, concerns the mechanical effects of vigorous physical activity on developing tissues—that is, the differentiation of immature stem cells into fat cells or lean cells. In culture, mesenchymal (bone marrow) stem cells can differentiate into various forms of mature cells; moreover, mechanisms that stimulate deposition of energy and nutrients into lean tissue tend to direct them away from differentiation into fat tissue and vice versa.[17] Studies using mice have shown that daily exposure to mechanical signals, in the form of a vibrating platform, inhibited the development of fat mass while stimulating the development of bone; there were no dietary differences between the experimental and control groups.[18] When the mechanical stimulation was introduced to the rodents at the same time as an obesogenic diet, it prevented the development of obesity; however, the stimulation did not reverse dietary-induced obesity. This suggests that the processes underlying prevention might be different from those involved in obesity treatment. To the degree that the mechanical effects produced by vibration and those produced by vigorous physical activity are similar, this line of research supports the potential efficacy of vigorous physical activity in promoting the development of lean bodies in growing youths.

It is important to emphasize that vigorous physical activity and appropriate diet play complementary roles in child development, in that active youths are able to ingest relatively large amounts of dietary energy and accompanying nutrients without necessarily becoming obese. This is illustrated by several studies showing that leaner youths tend to ingest more dietary energy than fatter youths.[8,9,19] Moreover, a descriptive study of adolescents found that higher levels of bone mass and height were associated with vigorous physical activity, along with relatively high intakes of energy, calcium, and vitamin D.[20]

Another important consideration is that physical activities undertaken in childhood, particularly activities that apply large forces quickly, convey optimal benefits to the development of bone mass.[21] Examples of these activities include jumping, hopping, and tumbling.[22] It also appears that increases in bone strength may be mediated in part by increases in lean mass associated with greater amounts of physical activity.[23]

It is important to point out that although correlations provide valuable information about the relationships between physical activity and body composition, they have an important limitation in that they do not clearly indicate directional causality—that is, whether the correlation of high levels of vigorous physical activity with low levels of adiposity might be due to physical activity influencing adiposity or by adiposity influencing physical activity, or both.[24] Therefore, findings from such studies should be considered as hypothesis generating rather than hypothesis testing. Randomized controlled trials are needed to test hypotheses generated by descriptive studies.

RANDOMIZED CONTROLLED TRIALS EXAMINING THE LINK BETWEEN PHYSICAL ACTIVITY AND CHILDHOOD BODY COMPOSITION

Within the category of randomized trials, an important factor to consider is where the trials fall on the spectrum of *efficacy* to *effectiveness*. At one end of the spectrum, we have trials that are tightly controlled and monitored to ensure that the subjects actually receive the doses of physical activity that are supposedly under investigation. For example, in some adult studies, subjects are brought into a research laboratory in which their individual physical activity prescriptions are supervised to ensure that they receive the exact dose of physical activity specified in the research design. In such projects, subjects may walk on treadmills at their specified physical activity prescriptions in order to determine the *efficacy* of different volumes and intensities of physical activity.[25] Such trials are quite rare, especially in youths, because of the intensity of supervision needed to implement them. Nonetheless, they provide relatively definitive information about what types and amounts of physical activity should be incorporated into trials that go on to test the effectiveness of physical activity recommendations.

Within the pediatric literature, the trials conducted over the last 20 years at the Georgia Prevention Institute of the Medical College of Georgia provide examples of trials that are close to the efficacy end of the spectrum. To ensure that the youths actually receive the prescribed dose of physical activity, they are brought by bus from their schools to a research gymnasium to participate in a program that is offered every school day—that is, five days/week. In one of the early studies, it was found that youths preferred playing games that were modified to keep them active for the entire physical activity period, in contrast to exercising on treadmills or other machines.[26] Thus, subsequent studies used such games to provide the physical activity. The staff-to-subject ratio was quite high, ensuring that the youths participated actively. Moreover, every subject wore a heart rate (HR) monitor every minute of every session so that the intensity of their effort could be estimated. This enabled the investigators to show that the youths who maintained higher HRs during the sessions exhibited greater beneficial changes in the outcome variables.[27] These analyses provided only indirect dose–response information because the youths were not randomly assigned to different intensities. Thus, youths who maintained higher HRs may have been predisposed to enjoy or profit from the higher intensities of physical activity.

As we move further along the efficacy–effectiveness spectrum, the conditions of some of the Georgia trials became closer to "real-world" conditions; that is, they had greater *ecological validity*. For example, in some trials, the youths remained in their regular schools at the close of the school day for the physical activity sessions, rather than being taken by bus to the research gym at the university. Nonetheless, the trials retained a high degree of supervision and HR monitoring, thus remaining toward the midpoint of the efficacy–effectiveness spectrum.

To the degree that the fidelity of the physical activity intervention is well controlled, and sensitive instruments are used to measure body composition, a clear picture of the true efficacy of the physical activity intervention can be obtained. Such information tells us what types of physical activity are appropriate to employ in real-world settings. However, in striving to learn more about the *effectiveness* of physical activity, interventions are typically less controlled, with the result that the distinctions between intervention and control groups in the physical training dose actually received may be less clear, leading to smaller group differences in the outcome variables. In this chapter, we are focusing on efficacy studies, while other chapters in this book discuss other effectiveness trials that have incorporated physical activity into the broader context of school or community-based studies.

To determine the efficacy of different intensities of physical activity, it would be ideal to randomize youths to different physical activity intensities and then supervise them carefully to ensure that they actually carry out the exercise prescriptions. Although the number of such studies is somewhat limited, two recent reviews concluded that vigorous-intensity physical activity is more efficacious than moderate-intensity physical activity for improving the body composition of youths.[6,28] In addition, some indirect evidence of the value of vigorous-intensity physical activity has been provided by trials in which overweight/obese youths participated in vigorous aerobic physical activity interventions, and maintained average HRs greater than 150 bpm; this shows that even overweight youths can profitably maintain high physical activity intensities.[6,27,29–32] Moreover, positive correlations were found between HRs during the training sessions and beneficial changes in body composition.[27] Other recent studies have found similar results.[32–34] Thus, it appears that obese youths can enhance their body composition without dieting by maintaining relatively high physical activity intensities for 40-min periods, undertaken for three to five sessions/week for 4-month intervention periods. This can be viewed as secondary prevention of obesity in the sense that it can prevent overweight/obese youths from going on to become even fatter.

However, in youths who were not preselected as overweight or obese, several projects failed to find that the interventions had a favorable effect on the adiposity of the subjects as measured with skinfolds.[35,36] Although these results cast doubt on the value of physical activity alone as a form of primary prevention, they also led to consideration of another factor: how the exercise dose was administered. Perhaps (1) the intervention sessions needed to be longer than the 40-min periods previously used with the obese youths; (2) the intervention duration needed to be greater than the several-week period typically used; and (3) the fidelity of the intervention needed to be more closely supervised. Another possibility concerned the measurement of the outcomes; new imaging techniques such as DXA and MRI might be more capable of detecting changes in body composition.

Therefore, our Medical College of Georgia group undertook a series of studies in which the doses of physical activity were greater than previously used and the body composition changes were measured with high-technology imaging techniques. The first of these projects involved 8–12-year-old black girls;[37] African American girls were chosen because they were the demographic group in Georgia most likely to become obese and we wanted to investigate physical activity as the primary prevention. We imparted a physical activity dose of 80 min in duration: 25 min of skills development, 35 min of more vigorous physical activity, and 20 min of strength training and stretching. Subjects wore HR monitors, and were closely supervised. The sessions were offered 5 days/week and the intervention lasted for 10 months; average attendance was 54%—that is, slightly more than 2.5 days/week. DXA was used to measure total body composition and MRI was used to measure VAT. The intervention elicited favorable changes in %BF, VAT, and bone mass. Higher HR during the physical activity was associated with greater increases in bone mass and greater decreases in %BF. A follow-up study with black boys elicited similar results, but only in boys attending the physical activity sessions at least 3 days/week.[30]

Recent controlled exercise interventions lend support to the value of vigorous physical activity interventions on measures of body composition in obese youths. In a group of 34 obese adolescent females randomly assigned to 12 weeks of either vigorous- or moderate-intensity interval training, post-training decreases in %BF were significantly greater in the vigorous intensity group than in the moderate intensity group.[32] In another study, 48 overweight children were randomized to six weeks of either vigorous-intensity running, lower-intensity running, or a nonrunning control group. Total distance run per training session was equated between the running groups. Following training, decreases in the sum of skinfolds were significantly greater in the vigorous-intensity running group (−12%) than in the lower intensity running group (−0.5%) or the nonrunning control group (+8.0%).[38]

Studies that have focused directly on bone development have found that the greatest osteogenic effects on the growing skeleton are provided by physical activity that has a high loading magnitude applied at a rapid rate[21]—that is, vigorous physical activity.

Thus, it is clear that vigorous physical activity, without any restriction of dietary energy intake, can have favorable effects in helping both obese and nonobese youths to enhance their body composition. Almost all of the pertinent studies have used physical activity that was essentially aerobic in nature; that is, the activities involved large-muscle physical activity.

Another question for the design of physical activity interventions concerns the potential role of resistance training (RT). Because RT customarily involves taking the working muscles to momentary muscle failure, RT is high in intensity and might be classified as vigorous physical activity; thus, it might be expected to be especially effective in building muscle and bone mass. However, the literature related to this issue is sparse and it is not clear if incorporating RT into physical activity interventions has a positive effect on total body composition. In one recent study, the effects of 3 months of aerobic training versus RT were compared in a group of 45 obese adolescent boys.[39] Total adiposity decreased significantly and similarly in the two groups.

Because of the especially significant role of VAT in cardiometabolic risk, a recent meta-analysis of diet and exercise interventions is noteworthy.[40] The small number of interventions that involved diet alone did not show a significant effect on VAT. However, interventions that focused on exercise alone, or exercise plus diet, showed significant reductions in VAT. This meta-analysis supports the important role of physical activity in enhancing health-related body composition.

CONCLUSIONS

Based on this review of the scientific literature, how can physical activity be most effectively incorporated into interventions designed to treat or prevent pediatric obesity? The first recommendation is to recognize that children are not simply small adults. The biologic growth processes involved in the development of lean and healthy bodies are fundamentally different from the processes involved in adults. Thus, dieting for weight loss, which is appropriate for many adults, should not be the primary focus of preventive interventions in youths. Moreover, control of body weight should not be the primary index to evaluate the success of the interventions. Instead, the interventions should focus on the development of lean tissue at the same time that they prevent excess accretion of fat mass. Because the development of lean mass is energetically expensive, children should be encouraged to ingest substantial amounts of nutrient-dense foods to support healthy growth. The diet composition that is optimal for this development is discussed elsewhere in this volume.

A second recommendation concerns the type of physical activity intervention that would be optimal for youths who are already obese and unfit. With respect to physical activity intensity, a number of studies have shown that such youths can engage in physical activity that elicits HRs greater than 150 bpm without excessive danger of injury. Nonetheless, it is reasonable to be cautious about engaging too abruptly in vigorous physical activity to avoid excessive fatigue and a resulting disinclination to continue in the exercise program.

Many of the descriptive studies reviewed here that concluded that vigorous physical activity was likely to be more beneficial than moderate physical activity used time–motion indices (e.g., accelerometry) to classify physical activity into moderate or vigorous categories. However, such physical activity categorization does not take individual differences in fitness into account. For example, lean/fit youths might find moderate physical activity, such as brisk walking, to elicit HRs of 120 bpm, while obese/unfit youths might reach HRs of 170 bpm while walking. Thus, in keeping with the overload principle, the lean/fit youths would need to incorporate running into their regimens to derive increased benefit, while the obese/unfit youths would be more likely to obtain benefit from a brisk-walking regimen. Regardless of initial fitness level, as fitness improves, the intensity of their regimens can be increased.

With respect to the duration of the physical activity sessions, dose–response studies of obese/unfit youths have shown beneficial body composition changes with regimens of 20–40 min/session, offered five times/week, with the physical activity interventions lasting 4–10 months. However, for youths who begin a physical activity regimen while relatively fit and lean, further improvements in body composition may require that the intervention sessions last longer, perhaps as long as 60–80 min/session.[30,37,41] There is a need for a comprehensive meta-analysis to determine the precise effect of these types of interventions on the body composition/obesity of youths.

A final recommendation is that physical activity efforts involving youths be persistent and continuous in order to retain the beneficial effects. For example, in the 3-year FitKid study, the beneficial effects of after-school physical activity on %BF and cardiorespiratory fitness observed during the first and second school years (when the youths were active in the intervention) were lost over the subsequent summer months (when the intervention was suspended).[42] This phenomenon has been observed by others as well.[43] However, it is noteworthy that over the entire 3 school years of the FitKid intervention, DXA measurements showed that the youths who participated in the after-school program at least 2 days/week showed consistent and significantly greater increases than the control subjects in fat-free soft tissue and bone mass.[2] More longitudinal studies in growing youths are needed to determine the patterns and magnitudes of effect for various aspects of body composition.

These recommendations can be incorporated into various specific activities. In our studies at the Medical College of Georgia, we have found that the youths prefer physical activity that is part of skills and games modified to include vigorous physical activity (e.g., soccer, basketball, dance), rather than exercising on machines that might be found in an adult fitness facility (e.g., treadmills, cycles, rowers). If facilities and leadership for these activities are provided on a widespread basis in clinical settings, schools, and community centers, then they can contribute to the treatment and prevention of pediatric obesity, leading to the improvement of public health into future generations.

REFERENCES

1. Alexander D, Rigby MJ, Di Mattia P, Zscheppang A. Challenges in finding and measuring behavioural determinants of childhood obesity in Europe. *Z Gesundh Wiss*. 2015;23(2):87–94.
2. Gutin B, Yin Z, Johnson M, Barbeau P. Preliminary findings of the effect of a 3-year after-school physical activity intervention on fitness and body fat: The Medical College of Georgia Fitkid Project. *Int J Pediatr Obes*. 2008;3(Suppl. 1):3–9.

3. Gutin B, Litaker M, Islam S, Manos T, Smith C, Treiber F. Body-composition measurement in 9–11-y-old children by dual-energy X-ray absorptiometry, skinfold-thickness measurements, and bioimpedance analysis. *Am J Clin Nutr.* 1996;63(3):287–292.

4. Owens S, Litaker M, Allison J, Riggs S, Ferguson M, Gutin B. Prediction of visceral adipose tissue from simple anthropometric measurements in youths with obesity. *Obes Res.* 1999;7(1):16–22.

5. Gutin B, Yin Z, Humphries MC, Barbeau P. Relations of moderate and vigorous physical activity to fitness and fatness in adolescents. *Am J Clin Nutr.* 2005;81(4):746–750.

6. Owens S, Galloway R, Gutin B. The case for vigorous physical activity in youth. *Am J Lifestyle Med.* 2015.

7. Blundell JE, Caudwell P, Gibbons C, et al. Body composition and appetite: Fat-free mass (but not fat mass or BMI) is positively associated with self-determined meal size and daily energy intake in humans. *Br J Nutr.* 2012;107(3):445–449.

8. Cuenca-Garcia M, Ortega FB, Ruiz JR, et al. More physically active and leaner adolescents have higher energy intake. *J Pediatr.* 2014;164:159–166.

9. Stallmann-Jorgensen IS, Gutin B, Hatfield-Laube JL, Humphries MC, Johnson MH, Barbeau P. General and visceral adiposity in black and white adolescents and their relation with reported physical activity and diet. *Int J Obes (Lond).* 2007;31(4):622–629.

10. Borsheim E, Bahr R. Effect of exercise intensity, duration and mode on post-exercise oxygen consumption. *Sports Med.* 2003;33(14):1037–1060.

11. Brehm BA, Gutin B. Recovery energy expenditure for steady state exercise in runners and nonexercisers. *Med Sci Sports Exerc.* 1986;18(2):205–210.

12. Greer BK, Sirithienthad P, Moffatt RJ, Marcello RT, Panton LB. EPOC comparison between isocaloric bouts of steady-state aerobic, intermittent aerobic, and resistance training. *Res Q Exerc Sport.* 2015;86(2):190–195.

13. Hill JO, Heymsfield SB, McMannus C, 3rd, DiGirolamo M. Meal size and thermic response to food in male subjects as a function of maximum aerobic capacity. *Metabolism.* 1984;33(8):743–749.

14. Segal KR, Gutin B. Thermic effects of food and exercise in lean and obese women. *Metabolism.* 1983;32(6):581–589.

15. Segal KR, Presta E, Gutin B. Thermic effect of food during graded exercise in normal weight and obese men. *Am J Clin Nutr.* 1984;40(5):995–1000.

16. Goran MI, Shewchuk R, Gower BA, Nagy TR, Carpenter WH, Johnson RK. Longitudinal changes in fatness in white children: No effect of childhood energy expenditure. *Am J Clin Nutr.* 1998;67(2):309–316.

17. Muruganandan S, Roman AA, Sinal CJ. Adipocyte differentiation of bone marrow-derived mesenchymal stem cells: Cross talk with the osteoblastogenic program. *Cell Mol Life Sci.* 2009;66(2):236–253.

18. Luu YK, Capilla E, Rosen CJ, et al. Mechanical stimulation of mesenchymal stem cell proliferation and differentiation promotes osteogenesis while preventing dietary-induced obesity. *J Bone Miner Res.* 2009;24(1):50–61.

19. Fulton JE, Dai S, Steffen LM, Grunbaum JA, Shah SM, Labarthe DR. Physical activity, energy intake, sedentary behavior, and adiposity in youth. *Am J Prev Med.* 2009;37(Suppl. 1):S40–49.

20. Gutin B, Stallmann-Jorgensen IS, Le AH, Johnson MH, Dong Y. Relations of diet and physical activity to bone mass and height in black and white adolescents. *Pediatr Rep.* 2011;3(2):e10.

21. Gunter KB, Almstedt HC, Janz KF. Physical activity in childhood may be the key to optimizing lifespan skeletal health. *Exerc Sport Sci Rev.* 2012;40(1):13–21.

22. Janz KF, Thomas DQ, Ford MA, Williams SM. Top 10 research questions related to physical activity and bone health in children and adolescents. *Res Q Exerc Sport.* 2015;86(1):5–12.

23. Janz KF, Gilmore JM, Levy SM, Letuchy EM, Burns TL, Beck TJ. Physical activity and femoral neck bone strength during childhood: The Iowa Bone Development Study. *Bone.* 2007;41(2):216–222.

24. Millward J. Energy balance and obesity: A UK perspective on the gluttony v. sloth debate. *Nutr Res Rev.* 2013;26(2):89–109.

25. Kraus WE, Torgan CF, Duscha BD, et al. Studies of a targeted risk reduction intervention through defined exercise (STRRIDE). *Med Sci Sports Exerc.* 2001;33(10):1774–1784.

26. Gutin B, Riggs S, Ferguson M, Owens S. Description and process evaluation of a physical training program for obese children. *Res Q Exerc Sport.* 1999;70(1):65–69.

27. Barbeau P, Gutin B, Litaker M, Owens S, Riggs S, Okuyama T. Correlates of individual differences in body-composition changes resulting from physical training in obese children. *Am J Clin Nutr.* 1999;69(4):705–711.

28. Parikh T, Stratton G. Influence of intensity of physical activity on adiposity and cardiorespiratory fitness in 5–18 year olds. *Sports Med.* 2011;41(6):477–488.

29. Gutin B, Harris RA, Howe CA, Johnson MH, Zhu H, Dong Y. Cardiometabolic biomarkers in young black girls: Relations to body fatness and aerobic fitness, and effects of a randomized physical activity trial. *Int J Pediatr.* 2011:219268.

30. Howe CA, Harris RA, Gutin B. A 10-month physical activity intervention improves body composition in young black boys. *J Obes.* 2011;2011:358581.

31. Owens S, Gutin B, Allison J, et al. Effect of physical training on total and visceral fat in obese children. *Med Sci Sports Exerc.* 1999;31(1):143–148.

32. Racil G, Ben Ounis O, Hammouda O, et al. Effects of high vs. moderate exercise intensity during interval training on lipids and adiponectin levels in obese young females. *Eur J Appl Physiol.* 2013;113(10):2531–2540.

33. Sayers A, Mattocks C, Deere K, Ness A, Riddoch C, Tobias JH. Habitual levels of vigorous, but not moderate or light, physical activity is positively related to cortical bone mass in adolescents. *J Clin Endocrinol Metab.* 2011;96(5):E793–802.

34. Winther A, Dennison E, Ahmed LA, et al. The Tromso Study: Fit Futures; A study of Norwegian adolescents' lifestyle and bone health. *Arch Osteoporos.* 2014;9(1):185.

35. Tolfrey K, Campbell IG, Batterham AM. Exercise training induced alterations in prepubertal children's lipid-lipoprotein profile. *Med Sci Sports Exerc.* 1998;30(12):1684–1692.

36. Tolfrey K, Jones AM, Campbell IG. Lipid-lipoproteins in children: An exercise dose-response study. *Med Sci Sports Exerc.* 2004;36(3):418–427.

37. Barbeau P, Johnson MH, Howe CA, et al. Ten months of exercise improves general and visceral adiposity, bone, and fitness in black girls. *Obesity (Silver Spring).* 2007;15(8):2077–2085.

38. Lau PW, Wong del P, Ngo JK, Liang Y, Kim CG, Kim HS. Effects of high-intensity intermittent running exercise in overweight children. *Eur J Sport Sci.* 2014;15(2):182–190.

39. Lee S, Bacha F, Hannon T, Kuk JL, Boesch C, Arslanian S. Effects of aerobic versus resistance exercise without caloric restriction on abdominal fat, intrahepatic lipid, and insulin sensitivity in obese adolescent boys: A randomized, controlled trial. *Diabetes.* 2012;61(11):2787–2795.

40. Vissers D, Hens W, Hansen D, Taeymans J. The effect of diet or exercise on visceral adipose tissue in overweight youth. *Med Sci Sports Exerc.* 2016. Published ahead of print: doi:10.1249/ MSS.0000000000000888.

41. Davis CL, Pollock NK, Waller JL, et al. Exercise dose and diabetes risk in overweight and obese children: A randomized controlled trial. *JAMA.* 2012;308(11):1103–1112.

42. Yin Z, Moore JB, Johnson MH, Vernon MM, Gutin B. The impact of a 3-year after-school obesity prevention program in elementary school children. *Child Obes.* 2012;8(1):60–70.

43. Carrel AL, Clark RR, Peterson S, Eickhoff J, Allen DB. School-based fitness changes are lost during the summer vacation. *Arch Pediatr Adolesc Med.* 2007;161(6):561–564.

33 Life Course Approach to the Prevention of Childhood Obesity

Regien Biesma and Mark Hanson

CONTENTS

INTRODUCTION

The concept, called *primordial prevention*, that a condition such as childhood obesity can be prevented by avoiding the development of risk factors in the population raises several questions. First, to what extent do we understand the biological and other drivers or risk factors for obesity? Second, do we have available biomarkers of exposure to such drivers in individuals or groups and/or other means of assessing their susceptibility before the condition becomes manifest? And third, do we have the means of preventing the condition? The concept of such prevention inevitably focuses attention on interventions starting in infancy (as reviewed in Chapter 34), when the trajectory of weight gain appears to be particularly important [1], but such interventions will need to be sustained through childhood if they are to be effective [2]. Other research raises the possibility that maternal body mass index (BMI) at conception or weight gain in pregnancy constitute independent risk factors for childhood obesity [3], suggesting that interventions may need to be started before the child is born. In turn, this leads to the concept that attention needs to be given to the preconception period if the risk of obesity in the next generation is to be minimized.

There are now numerous animal studies showing that parental (both paternal and maternal) obesity, malnutrition (i.e., unbalanced macro- and micronutrient diets), and experimentally induced diabetes mellitus can pass risk of obesity to the offspring [4]. A range of epidemiological studies similarly support the concept of such transgenerational transmission of risk [5]. Translating these concepts into public health initiatives is challenging, as discussed in the last sections of this chapter, and is likely to necessitate a paradigm shift in our thinking about the prevention of noncommunicable diseases (NCDs) and their risk factors such as childhood obesity. These issues are encapsulated in the field of developmental origins of health and disease (DOHaD) [6], a relatively new area of biomedical science. The economic implications of non-communicable diseases are encapsulated in the concept of the passage of health capital from one generation to the next [7], and these are particularly important in low- and middle-income countries (LMICs) and populations undergoing socioeconomic transitions. This chapter describes aspects of the prevention of childhood obesity focusing on processes early in life with some emphasis on LMICs.

LIFE COURSE BIOLOGY: NOT JUST DARWINIAN FITNESS

Biologists are very familiar with the concept of the life cycle, whereby members of a species grow and develop to reproductive competence, reproduce, and then perish. This concept is enshrined in evolutionary biology as "Darwinian fitness," by which beneficial adaptations in individuals promote their survival and fecundity in a given environment, giving them an advantage in passing on their genes to the next generation. While the nineteenth-century concept of the "survival of the fittest" [8] has been used to justify a range of human activities, and the metaphor of evolution is applied to a wide variety of aspects of human life [9], its application to medicine is not so straightforward [10]. The concept of fitness as an individual property is undermined by humanitarian considerations by which humans strive to preserve life, and provide opportunities for reproduction, in members of our species perceived to be weaker, unhealthy, or infertile. On the other hand, we are increasingly exposed to evolutionarily novel environments, offering calorie-dense and unbalanced nutrition, a sedentary lifestyle, 24 h access to entertainment, and exposure to a wide range of environmental toxicants—all of which are challenging our fitness because they can affect us during the phase of the life course when we are growing and commencing reproductive activity. Our evolved biology is simply not matched to these environments [11]. The problem is particularly acute in low-income countries (LIC) as they pass through socioeconomic transitions, leading to dramatic increases in obesity and NCD risk even in young people [12] (Figure 33.1).

In parallel with these changes, human life expectancy has increased dramatically over the last century such that, in, for example, the United States, it now stands at a mean of 76 years for men and 81 years for women, although these figures hide wide variations related to socioeconomic status (SES), both within as well as between populations and in attitudes to perceived longevity that affect behavior [13]. Nonetheless, survival into the postreproductive period means that a more complete life course concept of human health, as opposed to the more restricted life-cycle model, needs to be considered. This is particularly important as some of the factors influencing childhood health and risk of obesity are related to parental behaviors and are passed from generation to generation by a range of social as well as biological processes [14].

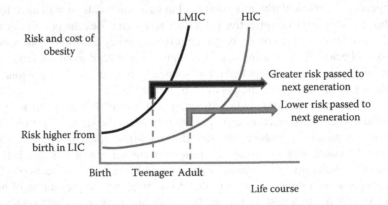

FIGURE 33.1   Risk of obesity is increased from birth in a low-income country (LIC), compared with a high-income country (HIC, gray line) as a result of parental malnutrition, low birth weight, and stunting, and so on. Greater mismatch occurs on the transition to a low-middle income country (LMIC, black line). In addition, teenage pregnancy passes greater risk to the next generation earlier, compared with HIC.

INTERGENERATIONAL PASSAGE OF OBESITY RISK

There is substantial evidence that early-life influences, in particular prenatal environmental conditions such as maternal adiposity, play an important role in the development of obesity in children. Young women are increasingly entering pregnancy with BMIs of more than 30 kg/m², which results in health risks to both the pregnant woman and her infant [15]. As reviewed in other chapters of this book, overweight or obesity, unbalanced diet, and preexisting conditions, such as type 2 diabetes or metabolic syndrome in the mother [16] and also to an extent in the father [17], are associated with greater risk of obesity in the child. These effects are amplified in first pregnancies [18]. In addition, conditions such as gestational diabetes mellitus (GDM) have been thought to be associated with greater risk of obesity in the offspring, although this is still uncertain [16,19]. There are reported ethnic differences in such risk [20] and in the extent to which such risk is passed even by mild diabetes [21].

Considerable research is underway into the mechanisms underlying such risk. The changes in phenotype in the developing individual, for example, in response to maternal malnutrition (either inadequate or excessive) involve epigenetic processes that relate to fat deposition and can be measured at birth [22,23]. The changes in the incidence of obesity between generations have occurred too rapidly to be accounted for purely by genetic predisposition, but nonetheless there are genetic–epigenetic interactions occurring in aspects of such phenomena [24]. It is important to realize, too, that these processes operate within the range of normal diets of the general population, at least in European populations. This is not surprising because fat deposition, at least in the neonate, can in terms of evolutionary biology be seen to be adaptive, providing a source of nutrition in the face of poor maternal care and assisting with the supply of fatty acids essential for brain development [25]. In this context, it is interesting that malnutrition in Indian babies is associated with greater abdominal fat distribution in proportion to body weight in comparison with Caucasian babies [26] and that in the Generation R study faster fetal growth was associated with greater childhood BMI [27]. The effects appear to be sustained across the life course, as in the Hertfordshire cohort low birth weight was related to greater central versus peripheral fat mass in men aged 64–72 years [28]. In a Western population, an imprudent maternal diet before conception and in early pregnancy is associated with greater liver blood flow and less shunting of blood returning from the placenta through the ductus venous in the late gestation fetus [29], a pattern linked to greater adiposity at birth and at age 4 in the child [30]. This emphasizes the importance of the liver in fetal metabolic and body composition development.

LIFE COURSE

A life course approach to disease is not a new concept, and its theoretical basis in terms of critical periods, accumulative damage, and pathway analysis is well established [31]. Taking a life course view of obesity highlights several aspects of the problem that are relevant to the prevention of the condition. The simplest view of the rising risk throughout life (as in Figure 33.1) is that this is due to the accumulation of damage due to lifestyle factors and a declining ability to repair such damage. From this viewpoint, the development of obesity is pathological from the beginning and has little adaptive significance. Moreover, reduction of exposure to factors that produce damage should reduce risk at any point in the life course. Although there is some validity in this concept, it cannot account for the entire trajectory of risk because, although some adult interventions have achieved positive results, others have proved to be disappointing [32–35]. For example, sustained weight loss in volunteers does not reset appetite and satiety control mechanisms even after a year [36], and there is considerable evidence that aspects of appetite, food preference, and taste are established in early life [37].

A second aspect of the life course concept is that components of the trajectory are set during "sensitive" or, if not reversible, "critical" periods of development. There may be some evidence for this in childhood obesity [1], although the precise timing of any sensitive period is not established unequivocally. Some studies conclude that interventions should be focused in the primary school years or before [38], others that the major increase in fat mass occurs in older, teenage, children [39–42].

There is also evidence for gender differences with better cardiovascular risk profiles occurring in girls who changed to normal weight by adolescence than those who remained overweight. However, this was not the case in boys who kept an intermediate risk profile when altering their overweight status as they moved from childhood through adolescence suggesting the importance of intervention strategies during early childhood [43].

Once established, the implication of the critical- or sensitive-period concept is that obesity will occur later in life irrespective of later environment, behavior, and so on. This in *sensu strictu* relates to the use of the term *trajectory*, because the analogy with a ballistic trajectory is that, once set, its path and destination can be predicted. Clearly, this is not true for obesity in adults, which is likely to be a combination of early and later risk factors.

A third way of envisaging the life course model is that a condition "tracks" from childhood into adult life [44,45]. This might be because there is a limited opportunity to reverse the degree of the condition, which is analogous to the trajectory analogy, or because the response to a challenge at any point depends on the responses at the immediately preceding point. There is evidence for tracking of overweight and obesity within the childhood period [43,46,47]. This is a model of path dependency, for example, the response to risk at any point in time is not simply dependent on the level of the risk factors to which an individual is exposed (the ordinate in Figure 33.1) but also on the path taken to reach that point. A range of factors can affect this slope, in other words, the degree of tracking such as SES [48] and ethnicity [45]. There is also evidence for the tracking of lifestyle risk factors such as diet, sedentary activities, and exercise preference [49–52]. The resulting effect on obesity risk can be measured by the slope of the line relating risk to time. For type 2 diabetes, for example, the amplifying effect of low birth weight on the adult risk factors for ill health (diet, BMI, smoking, alcohol consumption) has been shown [53]. This is important as it reveals the importance of physiological testing of responses to small changes in risk, or to short interventions, in establishing where an individual lies on a particular risk trajectory. Advancing this field through the use of early biomarkers of later risk is, therefore, important [54].

CHILDHOOD OBESITY IN THE TRANSITION FROM HIGH-TO LOW- AND MIDDLE-INCOME COUNTRIES

Since the 1950s, economic development and major societal changes, such as modernization, individualization, and urbanization, changed lifestyles in high-income countries (HICs) [55]. These societal changes led to big increases in food availability and variety, as well as changes in the culture of food, such as flexible-eating patterns, solo eating instead of family meals, eating while watching TV, restaurant eating, irregular eating, and snacking [56]. In addition, there were significant changes in the way physical activity was incorporated into daily life. The so-called baby boomer cohort were the first generation to be exposed *en masse* to obesogenic risk factors and global marketing of foods as they entered adulthood, and this is likely to have contributed to obesity in the next generation. By the 1980s, the prevalence of obesity increased rapidly in both adults and children in HICs [57,58]. The overall mean BMI values in children increased and the heaviest children became even heavier [59]. Initially, obesity was mainly a problem among higher-SES children who had greater access to energy-dense diets [60,61]. However, since 2000 this trend has reversed in HICs and childhood obesity has become much more prevalent·in deprived population groups [62]. For example, in the United States, racial/ethnic and SES-related disparities in childhood obesity had not changed from 2001 to 2010 [63]. In Europe, similar trends and patterns of social inequality in childhood obesity can be observed and are often grounded in parental risk factors [64]. For example, young low-SES mothers are less likely to breast-feed and, if they do, do so for a shorter

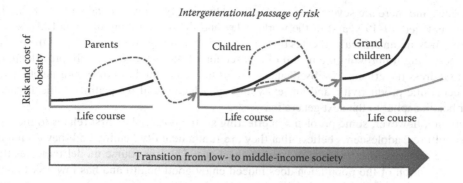

FIGURE 33.2 Transition from low-income country (LIC) to middle-income country (MIC) increases the risk and the cost of obesity in subsequent generations through effects on prenatal and child development. This effect is amplified in successive generations (black lines moving from left to right). Timely intervention, for example in adolescence, not only reduces risk in that generation but also passes reduced risk to the next generation (gray lines).

duration, while they are more likely to start early use of infant formula and cow's milk consumption [65]. These mothers are more likely to be overweight and obese and less likely to adhere to lifestyle guidelines. This all implies a vicious cycle of "obesity begetting obesity": a girl born to an overweight or obese low-SES mother is very likely herself to enter her first pregnancy being overweight or obese.

What happened in HICs in one generation (starting with greater affluence and urbanization in the 1950s) is now happening at a much faster rate in LMICs with much steeper and shorter trajectories (Figure 33.2) while the switch from rich to poor has already happened [66,67]. In contrast to the orderly transition of problems of undernutrition to problems of overnutrition in HICs, the distribution of childhood malnutrition is shifting from a predominance of undernutrition to a dual burden of under- and overnutrition [66]. This phenomenon is particularly seen in transition economies, where prevalence rates of obesity exceeding 15% in children and adolescents are common, such as Mexico (42%), Brazil (22%), India (22%), and Argentina (19%) [68]. Obesity may co-occur with stunting or anemia due to shared underlying determinants or physiological links, emphasizing the importance of the mismatch concept, and poses a novel public-health challenge [12]. In addition, LMICS are faced with a rapidly growing chronic NCD burden and continual high rates of infectious diseases [69,70]. These challenges may interact as some infections increase the risk of certain chronic diseases and vice versa. For example, diabetes has been associated with a threefold increased risk of tuberculosis, and both HIV and tuberculosis have been linked to an increased risk of developing diabetes; coincident HIV, tuberculosis, and diabetes are reported to worsen outcomes [70].

WHEN MIGHT BE THE BEST TIME TO START INTERVENTIONS?

Juonala et al. (2011) have reported that obese children who are able to become nonobese adults have no greater risk of cardiometabolic disease than adults who have never been obese [71]. However, within childhood, it is not certain how long the critical period is when it may be possible to reverse the risk extends, and there are methodological problems with the existing studies. The safest conclusion is conservative, viz. that interventions should start early and be maintained: this was one of the conclusions reached in the World Health Organization (WHO) ECHO final report [72].

A life course approach, targeting the developmental components of obesity risk, is crucial to curbing the obesity epidemic in both HICs and LMICs. Perhaps the most effective strategy would be to target the preconception period to improve prospective parents' body composition and lifestyle, preferably resulting in women with a healthy prepregnancy BMI, lower gestational weight gain, and postpartum weight retention before conception [73]. In many societies, this means targeting adolescents, and there are several reasons for this. One simply concerns scale: there are 1.2 billion adolescents (aged 10–19 years) in the world today and the demography of some LMICs, such as much of sub-Saharan Africa, indicates that this age group already comprises 25% of the population and is increasing. Improving the health of this section of the population might provide an opportunity to redress the effects of a disadvantaged start to life [74] and improve their health and well-being, economic productivity, and longevity. It may reduce social inequalities in health and pass greater health capital to the next generation.

There are, however, some problems in effecting such a policy. The first relates to the fact that in most cultures, adolescents believe that they are fundamentally healthy and they do not access health-care services for screening or routine checkups. The life course model indicates that the adolescent section of the population does indeed enjoy good health and has low risk in absolute terms, but that nonetheless a substantial proportion of people at this age are on a steep trajectory of risk. Unfortunately, many adolescents discount future health against shorter-term goals, and this is particularly true of those of lower socioeconomic and educational status in migrant and displaced groups [75]. A high proportion of pregnancies in this age group are unplanned, and adolescent girls may not access health care until late in the first trimester, by which time it is too late to promote healthy development of the embryo [76]. Moreover, many women who have unhealthy lifestyles do not change their behaviour when they are pregnant [77]. In both HICs and LMICs there is a substantial gap in the provision of health care between contraception and antenatal services [78,79].

OPPORTUNITIES FOR GLOBAL ACTION

There is an urgent need to address the problem of obesity in young people. The need is unlikely to be met through the formal educational system in many societies, although new methods of engaging adolescents and younger children in science literacy and investigative schemes, both in and out of school, offer promise [80–82]. Cost–benefit analyses of a range of interventions in younger and older children have been conducted [83], making an economic case for investment in this area.

The launch of the Sustainable Development Goals (SDGs) in September 2015 marks a new era in global health. While the foregoing Millennium Development Goals (MDGs) have not been completely met, there has been substantial progress in maternal and child health even though globally malnutrition and preexisting conditions, such as obesity, still account for nearly 45% of deaths of children under 5 years and more than 25% of maternal deaths, respectively [84,85]. We are moving into an era when the well-being and quality of life of those whose lives have been saved is a critical issue for humanitarian and equality as well as economic reasons. Unlike the MDGs, the SDGs have a focus on NCDs. For example, SDG 3.4 states: "By 2030, reduce by one third premature mortality from non-communicable diseases through prevention and treatment and promote mental health and wellbeing." There is also a clear focus on adolescents and prospective mothers, with SDG 2.2 stating: "By 2030 end all forms of malnutrition and address the nutritional needs of adolescent girls, pregnant and lactating women" [84].

The importance of the shift in emphasis is even clearer in the new Global Strategy for Women's, Children's and Adolescents' Health launched under the United Nations Secretary-General's Every Woman Every Child initiative [86]. The Global Strategy explicitly mentions adolescents and young people as one of their key target groups, also referring to the "SDG Generation," and alludes to the economic benefits of this approach, in particular for sub-Saharan Africa. The WHO ECHO Commission was referred to in the last section. Other initiatives that have focused on a more holistic life course approach are the International Federation of Gynecology and Obstetrics (FIGO) Recommendations on Adolescent, Preconception and Maternal Nutrition [87], the Agency for Healthcare Research and Quality [88], the Doha Declaration of the World Innovation Summit for Health [89], United Nations Educational, Scientific and Cultural Organization (UNESCO) [90], and the National Institute for Health and Care Excellence [91].

CONCLUSIONS

Over the past 50 years, the effects of global transition and socioeconomic development have resulted in an increased exposure to the obesogenic environment, an evolutionary novel environment to which human populations were not previously exposed and to which they have not adapted. Initially, this transition happened only in affluent groups in HICs but in the past decades this pattern has reversed, rapidly affecting the poor in both developed and developing countries. As a result, the worldwide prevalence of childhood obesity has increased at an alarming rate while the onset of NCDs is now occurring much earlier in life [92,93]. A major concern in this scenario is the transmission of the risk of obesity to successive generations, in particular in LMICs where both over- and undernutrition fuels the epidemic. To reverse this trend in childhood obesity, interventions must therefore start very early in life, preferably before conception, and be sustained in a variety of ways thereafter. The life course approach of targeting adolescents and young people was recently recognized in global strategies as both a necessary and a cost-effective investment. Primordial prevention of childhood obesity may offer the best value for money and has the potential to minimize exposure to early-life risk factors in the next generation.

ACKNOWLEDGMENTS

MAH is supported by the British Heart Foundation.

REFERENCES

1. Taveras EM, Rifas-Shiman SL, Sherry B, Oken E, Haines J, Kleinman K, et al. Crossing growth percentiles in infancy and risk of obesity in childhood. *Archives of Pediatrics and Adolescent Medicine*. 2011;165(11):993–8.
2. Wen LM, Baur LA, Simpson JM, Xu H, Hayes AJ, Hardy LL, et al. Sustainability of effects of an early childhood obesity prevention trial over time: A further 3-year follow-up of the healthy beginnings trial. *JAMA Pediatrics*. 2015;169(6):543–51.
3. Poston L. Maternal obesity, gestational weight gain and diet as determinants of offspring long term health. *Best Practice and Research Clinical Endocrinology and Metabolism*. 2012;26(5):627–39.
4. Li M, Sloboda DM, Vickers MH. Maternal obesity and developmental programming of metabolic disorders in offspring: Evidence from animal models. *Experimental Diabetes Research*. 2011;2011:592408.
5. Eriksson JG, Sandboge S, Salonen MK, Kajantie E, Osmond C. Long-term consequences of maternal overweight in pregnancy on offspring later health: Findings from the Helsinki Birth Cohort Study. *Annals of Medicine*. 2014;46(6):434–8.
6. DOHaD. International society. www.dohadsoc.org. Accessed July 1, 2016.
7. Hanson MA, Gluckman PD. Developmental origins of health and disease—Global public health implications. *Best Practice and Research Clinical Obstetrics and Gynaecology*. 2015;29(1):24–31.
8. Claeys G. The "survival of the fittest" and the origins of social darwinism. *Journal of the History of Ideas*. 2000;61(2):223–40.
9. Ridley M. *The Evolution of Everything: How Ideas Emerge*. London: HarperCollins Publishers, 2015.
10. Gluckman PD, Beedle A, Hanson MA. *Principles of Evolutionary Medicine*. Oxford: Oxford University Press, 2009.
11. Gluckman P, Hanson M. *Mismatch: Why Our World No Longer Fits Our Bodies*. Oxford: Oxford University Press, 2006.
12. Tzioumis E, Adair LS. Childhood dual burden of under- and overnutrition in low- and middle-income countries: A critical review. *Food and Nutrition Bulletin*. 2014;35(2):230–43.
13. Pepper GV, Nettle D. Perceived extrinsic mortality risk and reported effort in looking after health: Testing a behavioral ecological prediction. *Human Nature*. 2014;25(3):378–92.
14. Parks EP, Kumanyika S, Moore RH, Stettler N, Wrotniak BH, Kazak A. Influence of stress in parents on child obesity and related behaviors. *Pediatrics*. 2012;130(5):e1096–104.
15. Herring SJ, Rose MZ, Skouteris H, Oken E. Optimizing weight gain in pregnancy to prevent obesity in women and children. *Diabetes, Obesity and Metabolism*. 2012;14(3):195–203.
16. Kim SY, England JL, Sharma JA, Njoroge T. Gestational diabetes mellitus and risk of childhood overweight and obesity in offspring: A systematic review. *Experimental Diabetes Research*. 2011;2011:541308.

17. Gaillard R, Steegers EA, Duijts L, Felix JF, Hofman A, Franco OH, et al. Childhood cardiometabolic outcomes of maternal obesity during pregnancy: The Generation R Study. *Hypertension.* 2014;63(4):683–91.

18. Reynolds RM, Osmond C, Phillips DI, Godfrey KM. Maternal BMI, parity, and pregnancy weight gain: Influences on offspring adiposity in young adulthood. *The Journal of Clinical Endocrinology and Metabolism.* 2010;95(12):5365–9.

19. Maftei O, Whitrow MJ, Davies MJ, Giles LC, Owens JA, Moore VM. Maternal body size prior to pregnancy, gestational diabetes and weight gain: Associations with insulin resistance in children at 9–10 years. *Diabetic Medicine: A Journal of the British Diabetic Association.* 2015;32(2):174–80.

20. Xiang AH, Black MH, Li BH, Martinez MP, Sacks DA, Lawrence JM, et al. Racial and ethnic disparities in extremes of fetal growth after gestational diabetes mellitus. *Diabetologia.* 2015;58(2):272–81.

21. Landon MB, Rice MM, Varner MW, Casey BM, Reddy UM, Wapner RJ, et al. Mild gestational diabetes mellitus and long-term child health. *Diabetes Care.* 2015;38(3):445–52.

22. Godfrey KM, Sheppard A, Gluckman PD, Lillycrop KA, Burdge GC, McLean C, et al. Epigenetic gene promoter methylation at birth is associated with child's later adiposity. *Diabetes.* 2011;60(5):1528–34.

23. Richmond RC, Timpson NJ, Sorensen T. Exploring possible epigenetic mediation of early-life environmental exposures on adiposity and obesity development. *International Journal of Epidemiology.* 2015;44(4):1191–8.

24. Teh AL, Pan H, Chen L, Ong ML, Dogra S, Wong J, et al. The effect of genotype and in utero environment on interindividual variation in neonate DNA methylomes. *Genome Research.* 2014;24(7):1064–74.

25. Kuzawa CW, Chugani HT, Grossman LI, Lipovich L, Muzik O, Hof PR, et al. Metabolic costs and evolutionary implications of human brain development. *Proceedings of the National Academy of Sciences of the United States of America.* 2014;111(36):13010–5.

26. Yajnik CS, Fall CH, Coyaji KJ, Hirve SS, Rao S, Barker DJ, et al. Neonatal anthropometry: The thin-fat Indian baby—The Pune Maternal Nutrition Study. *International Journal of Obesity and Related Metabolic Disorders: Journal of the International Association for the Study of Obesity.* 2003;27(2):173–80.

27. Gishti O, Gaillard R, Manniesing R, Abrahamse-Berkeveld M, van der Beek EM, Heppe DH, et al. Fetal and infant growth patterns associated with total and abdominal fat distribution in school-age children. *The Journal of Clinical Endocrinology and Metabolism.* 2014;99(7):2557–66.

28. Kensara OA, Wootton SA, Phillips DI, Patel M, Jackson AA, Elia M, et al. Fetal programming of body composition: Relation between birth weight and body composition measured with dual-energy X-ray absorptiometry and anthropometric methods in older Englishmen. *The American Journal of Clinical Nutrition.* 2005;82(5):980–7.

29. Haugen G, Hanson M, Kiserud T, Crozier S, Inskip H, Godfrey KM. Fetal liver-sparing cardiovascular adaptations linked to mother's slimness and diet. *Circulation Research.* 2005;96(1):12–4.

30. Godfrey KM, Haugen G, Kiserud T, Inskip HM, Cooper C, Harvey NC, et al. Fetal liver blood flow distribution: Role in human developmental strategy to prioritize fat deposition versus brain development. *PloS One.* 2012;7(8):e41759.

31. Burton-Jeangros C, Cullati S, Sacker A, Blane D. *A Life Course Perspective on Health Trajectories and Transitions.* London: Springer, 2015.

32. Picot J, Jones J, Colquitt JL, Gospodarevskaya E, Loveman E, Baxter L, et al. The clinical effectiveness and cost-effectiveness of bariatric (weight loss) surgery for obesity: A systematic review and economic evaluation. *Health Technology Assessment (Winchester, England).* 2009;13(41):1–190, 215–357, iii–iv.

33. Loveman E, Frampton GK, Shepherd J, Picot J, Cooper K, Bryant J, et al. The clinical effectiveness and cost-effectiveness of long-term weight management schemes for adults: A systematic review. *Health Technology Assessment.* 2011;15(2):1–182.

34. Ara R, Blake L, Gray L, Hernandez M, Crowther M, Dunkley A, et al. What is the clinical effectiveness and cost-effectiveness of using drugs in treating obese patients in primary care? A systematic review. *Health Technology Assessment.* 2012;16(5):iii–xiv, 1–195.

35. Mann T, Tomiyama AJ, Ward A. Promoting public health in the context of the "obesity epidemic": False starts and promising new directions. *Perspectives on Psychological Science: A Journal of the Association for Psychological Science.* 2015;10(6):706–10.

36. Sumithran P, Prendergast LA, Delbridge E, Purcell K, Shulkes A, Kriketos A, et al. Long-term persistence of hormonal adaptations to weight loss. *The New England Journal of Medicine.* 2011;365(17):1597–604.

37. Mennella JA. Ontogeny of taste preferences: Basic biology and implications for health. *The American Journal of Clinical Nutrition.* 2014;99(3):704S–11S.

38. Gardner DS, Hosking J, Metcalf BS, Jeffery AN, Voss LD, Wilkin TJ. Contribution of early weight gain to childhood overweight and metabolic health: A longitudinal study (EarlyBird 36). *Pediatrics.* 2009;123(1):e67–73.

39. Hughes AR, Sherriff A, Lawlor DA, Ness AR, Reilly JJ. Timing of excess weight gain in the Avon Longitudinal Study of Parents and Children (ALSPAC). *Pediatrics.* 2011;127(3):e730–6.

40. Datar A, Shier V, Sturm R. Changes in body mass during elementary and middle school in a national cohort of kindergarteners. *Pediatrics.* 2011;128(6):e1411–7.

41. Flegal KM, Troiano RP. Changes in the distribution of body mass index of adults and children in the US population. *International Journal of Obesity and Related Metabolic Disorders: Journal of the International Association for the Study of Obesity.* 2000;24(7):807–18.

42. Kimm SY, Barton BA, Obarzanek E, McMahon RP, Kronsberg SS, Waclawiw MA, et al. Obesity development during adolescence in a biracial cohort: The NHLBI Growth and Health Study. *Pediatrics.* 2002;110(5):e54.

43. Lawlor DA, Benfield L, Logue J, Tilling K, Howe LD, Fraser A, et al. Association between general and central adiposity in childhood, and change in these, with cardiovascular risk factors in adolescence: Prospective cohort study. *BMJ.* 2010;341:c6224.

44. Singh AS, Mulder C, Twisk JW, van Mechelen W, Chinapaw MJ. Tracking of childhood overweight into adulthood: A systematic review of the literature. *Obesity Reviews: An Official Journal of the International Association for the Study of Obesity.* 2008;9(5):474–88.

45. Howe LD. Trajectories and transitions in childhood and adolescent obesity. In al B-Je, ed. *A Life Course Perspective on Health Trajectories and Transitions.* London: Springer, pp. 19–37, 2015.

46. Wright CM, Emmett PM, Ness AR, Reilly JJ, Sherriff A. Tracking of obesity and body fatness through mid-childhood. *Archives of Disease in Childhood.* 2010;95(8):612–7.

47. Reilly JJ, Bonataki M, Leary SD, Wells JC, Davey-Smith G, Emmett P, et al. Progression from childhood overweight to adolescent obesity in a large contemporary cohort. *International Journal of Pediatric Obesity: IJPO—An Official Journal of the International Association for the Study of Obesity.* 2011;6(2–2):e138–43.

48. HSCIC. English indices of deprivation. www.gov.uk/government/collections/english-indices-of-deprivation. Health and Social Care Information Centre (HSCIC). Accessed July 1, 2016.

49. Pearson N, Salmon J, Campbell K, Crawford D, Timperio A. Tracking of children's body-mass index, television viewing and dietary intake over five-years. *Preventive Medicine.* 2011;53(4–5):268–70.

50. Jones RA, Hinkley T, Okely AD, Salmon J. Tracking physical activity and sedentary behavior in childhood: A systematic review. *American Journal of Preventive Medicine.* 2013;44(6):651–8.

51. Biddle SJ, Pearson N, Ross GM, Braithwaite R. Tracking of sedentary behaviours of young people: A systematic review. *Preventive Medicine.* 2010;51(5):345–51.

52. Telama R. Tracking of physical activity from childhood to adulthood: A review. *Obesity Facts.* 2009;2(3):187–95.

53. Li Y, Ley SH, Tobias DK, Chiuve SE, VanderWeele TJ, Rich-Edwards JW, et al. Birth weight and later life adherence to unhealthy lifestyles in predicting type 2 diabetes: Prospective cohort study. *British Medical Journal.* 2015;351:h3672.

54. Hanson MA, Costello PC. Epigenetic biomarkers and global health. In Burdge GC, ed. *Nutrition, Epigenetics and Health.* London: World Scientific, In press.

55. Buckley J. Baby boomers, obesity, and social change. *Obesity Research and Clinical Practice.* 2008;2(2):71–142.

56. Offer A. *The Challenge of Affluence: Self-Control and Well-Being in the United States and Britain since 1950.* Oxford: Oxford University Press, 2006.

57. Kim J, Peterson KE, Scanlon KS, Fitzmaurice GM, Must A, Oken E, et al. Trends in overweight from 1980 through 2001 among preschool-aged children enrolled in a health maintenance organization. *Obesity (Silver Spring).* 2006;14(7):1107–12.

58. Ng M, Fleming T, Robinson M, Thomson B, Graetz N, Margono C, et al. Global, regional, and national prevalence of overweight and obesity in children and adults during 1980–2013: A systematic analysis for the Global Burden of Disease Study 2013. *Lancet.* 2014;384(9945):766–81.

59. Skinner AC, Skelton JA. Prevalence and trends in obesity and severe obesity among children in the United States, 1999–2012. *JAMA Pediatrics.* 2014;168(6):561–6.

60. Wang Y, Lim H. The global childhood obesity epidemic and the association between socio-economic status and childhood obesity. *International Review of Psychiatry (Abingdon, England).* 2012;24(3):176–88.

61. Singh GK, Kogan MD, van Dyck PC. A multilevel analysis of state and regional disparities in childhood and adolescent obesity in the United States. *Journal of Community Health.* 2008;33(2):90–102.

62. Brunt H, Lester N, Davies G, Williams R. Childhood overweight and obesity: Is the gap closing the wrong way? *Journal of Public Health.* 2008;30(2):145–52.

63. Rossen LM, Schoendorf KC. Measuring health disparities: Trends in racial-ethnic and socioeconomic disparities in obesity among 2- to 18-year old youth in the United States, 2001–2010. *Annals of Epidemiology.* 2012;22(10):698–704.

64. Monasta L, Batty GD, Macaluso A, Ronfani L, Lutje V, Bavcar A, et al. Interventions for the prevention of overweight and obesity in preschool children: A systematic review of randomized controlled trials. *Obesity Reviews.* 2011;12(5):e107–18.

65. Puhl RM, Luedicke J, Depierre JA. Parental concerns about weight-based victimization in youth. *Childhood Obesity (Print).* 2013;9(6):540–8.

66. Haddad L, Cameron L, Barnett I. The double burden of malnutrition in SE Asia and the Pacific: Priorities, policies and politics. *Health Policy and Planning.* 2015;30(9):1193–206.

67. Popkin BM, Adair LS, Ng SW. Global nutrition transition and the pandemic of obesity in developing countries. *Nutrition Reviews.* 2012;70(1):3–21.

68. Gupta N, Goel K, Shah P, Misra A. Childhood obesity in developing countries: Epidemiology, determinants, and prevention. *Endocrine Reviews.* 2012;33(1):48–70.

69. Young F, Critchley JA, Johnstone LK, Unwin NC. A review of co-morbidity between infectious and chronic disease in Sub Saharan Africa: TB and diabetes mellitus, HIV and metabolic syndrome, and the impact of globalization. *Globalization and Health.* 2009;5:9.

70. Beaglehole R, Bonita R, Horton R, Adams C, Alleyne G, Asaria P, et al. Priority actions for the non-communicable disease crisis. *Lancet.* 2011;377(9775):1438–47.

71. Juonala M, Magnussen CG, Berenson GS, Venn A, Burns TL, Sabin MA, et al. Childhood adiposity, adult adiposity, and cardiovascular risk factors. *The New England Journal of Medicine.* 2011;365(20):1876–85.

72. WHO. Final report of the commission on ending childhood obesity. http://apps.who.int/iris/bitstr eam/10665/204176/1/9789241510066_eng.pdf. Accessed July 1, 2016.

73. Hanson MA, Gluckman PD, Ma RC, Matzen P, Biesma RG. Early life opportunities for prevention of diabetes in low and middle income countries. *BMC Public Health.* 2012;12:1025.

74. Viner RM, Ozer EM, Denny S, Marmot M, Resnick M, Fatusi A, et al. Adolescence and the social determinants of health. *Lancet.* 2012;379(9826):1641–52.

75. McLennan AK, Jayaweera H. Non-communicable diseases and risk factors in migrants from South Asian countries. Oxford: COMPASS, University of Oxford, 2014.

76. Leary C, Leese HJ, Sturmey RG. Human embryos from overweight and obese women display phenotypic and metabolic abnormalities. *Human Reproduction.* 2015;30(1):122–32.

77. Inskip HM, Crozier SR, Godfrey KM, Borland SE, Cooper C, Robinson SM, et al. Women's compliance with nutrition and lifestyle recommendations before pregnancy: General population cohort study. *British Medical Journal.* 2009;338:b481.

78. Shawe J, Delbaere I, Ekstrand M, Hegaard HK, Larsson M, Mastroiacovo P, et al. Preconception care policy, guidelines, recommendations and services across six European countries: Belgium (Flanders), Denmark, Italy, the Netherlands, Sweden and the United Kingdom. *The European Journal of Contraception and Reproductive Health Care: The Official Journal of the European Society of Contraception.* 2015;20(2):77–87.

79. Davies SC. Annual report of the Chief Medical Officer, 2014, the health of the 51%: women. 2015.

80. Llargues E, Franco R, Recasens A, Nadal A, Vila M, Perez MJ, et al. Assessment of a school-based intervention in eating habits and physical activity in school children: The AVall study. *Journal of Epidemiology and Community Health.* 2011;65(10):896–901.

81. Bay JL, Mora HA, Sloboda DM, Morton SM, Vickers MH, Gluckman PD. Adolescent understanding of DOHaD concepts: A school-based intervention to support knowledge translation and behaviour change. *Journal of Developmental Origins of Health and Disease.* 2012;3(6):469–82.

82. Grace M, Woods-Townsend K, Griffiths J, Godfrey K, Hanson M, Galloway I, et al. Developing teenagers' views on their health and the health of their future children. *Health Education.* 2012;112(6):543–59.

83. Gortmaker SL, Long MW, Resch SC, Ward ZJ, Cradock AL, Barrett JL, et al. Cost effectiveness of childhood obesity interventions: Evidence and methods for CHOICES. *American Journal of Preventive Medicine.* 2015;49(1):102–11.

84. United Nations. Sustainable development goals. https://sustainabledevelopment.un.org/sdgs. Accessed July 1, 2016.

85. Black RE, Victora CG, Walker SP, Bhutta ZA, Christian P, de Onis M, et al. Maternal and child undernutrition and overweight in low-income and middle-income countries. *Lancet.* 2013;382(9890):427–51.

86. Nations U. The global strategy for women's, children's and adolescents' health (2016–2030). 2015. http://globalstrategy.everywomaneverychild.org/.

87. Hanson MA, Bardsley A, De-Regil LM, Moore SE, Oken E, Poston L, et al. The International Federation of Gynecology and Obstetrics (FIGO) recommendations on adolescent, preconception, and maternal nutrition: "Think Nutrition First." *International Journal of Gynaecology and Obstetrics: The Official Organ of the International Federation of Gynaecology and Obstetrics.* 2015;131 Suppl 4:S213.

88. Wang Y, Wu Y, Wilson RF, Bleich S, Cheskin L, Weston C, et al. *Childhood Obesity Prevention Programs: Comparative Effectiveness Review and Meta-Analysis.* Rockville, MD: Agency for Healthcare Research and Quality, 2013.

89. World Innovation Summit for Health (WISH). Strategic action to combat the obesity epidemic. http://www.wish-qatar.org/app/media/383. Accessed July 1, 2016.

90. UNESCO. *Quality Physical Education: Guidelines for Policy-Markers.* 2015.

91. The National Health Institute for Health and Care Excellence (NICE). Weight management: Lifestyle services for overweight or obese children and young people. https://www.nice.org.uk/guidance/ph47/chapter/1-recommendations. Accessed July 1, 2016.

92. Han JC, Lawlor DA, Kimm SY. Childhood obesity. *Lancet.* 2010;375(9727):1737–48.

93. Berends LM, Ozanne SE. Early determinants of type-2 diabetes. *Best Practice and Research Clinical Endocrinology and Metabolism.* 2012;26(5):569–80.

34 Early-Life Interventions for Childhood Obesity Prevention

Paige K. Berger and Leann L. Birch

CONTENTS

INTRODUCTION

The obesity epidemic has affected individuals across the life span. It is of particular concern in early life, as 20% of children are already overweight and obese before they enter school, with higher rates among low-income children, and African American and Hispanic children [1,2]. The first years of life are a period of dramatic growth and developmental change, and early-life growth patterns, particularly more rapid weight gain during infancy and early childhood, predict increased risk for obesity later in life [3,4]. Rapid weight gain in infancy has also been associated with increased risk for hypertension [5], coronary heart disease [6], and type 2 diabetes mellitus [7]. Because rapid growth trajectories in early life increase risk for obesity and related comorbidities later in the life span, prevention of rapid weight gain is an obvious target for early intervention. However, at present, there is limited evidence on how to do this [1].

In infancy, as in later life, dietary intake is a key determinant of energy balance and weight gain. Unlike adults, who are able to make their own dietary choices, infants and young children are dependent on parents or other caregivers to provide developmentally appropriate foods that support healthy growth. With respect to factors affecting weight gain, parents control the timing and duration of feedings, as well as the quality and quantity of foods offered to the child [8]. Caregivers also structure children's opportunities for other activities that can also affect energy balance and early growth, including sleep and active play [9,10]. All aspects of caregiving that can affect growth and energy balance are potential targets for early interventions to prevent rapid weight gain and reduce obesity risk.

This chapter will address interventions for obesity prevention during the first two years of postnatal life. The first section will highlight emerging evidence for opportunities to promote normative growth in infancy by influencing infant sleep and nutrition and feeding behaviors, and by the regulation of emotion. This is followed by a discussion of some of the recently completed and ongoing randomized controlled trials that involve multicomponent behavioral interventions in the first 24 months of life.

Emerging Evidence for Modifiable Risk Factors in Early Obesity Prevention

Sleep

Shorter sleep duration has been recognized as a factor in the development of obesity. There is an inverse association between shorter sleep duration and higher weight status that has been noted among adults, infants and children [11]. In the first weeks of life, infants spend the majority of their time sleeping, and typically wake every few hours to feed. Shorter sleep duration is therefore related to a higher frequency of feeding in early infancy, which can increase energy intake and growth [12]. Sleep duration also affects several hormones responsible for appetite regulation, and individuals with curtailed sleep duration have lower levels of leptin, a satiety signal, and higher levels of ghrelin, a hunger signal [13]. Moreover, shorter sleep duration may decrease energy expenditure by producing fatigue and low activity levels [14].

Observational studies provide most of the data on the association between shorter sleep duration and weight status in childhood. For example, Locard and colleagues first reported that 5-year-olds who slept less than 11 h/day were at significant risk of overweight [15]. Since that time, studies have demonstrated that shorter sleep duration in early childhood, between the ages of 3 and 5 years, predicts overweight in later childhood [1,16]. However, less is known about the association between shorter sleep duration and overweight or weight gain in infancy. Some studies have shown that shorter sleep duration is associated with body size in the first few months of life [17], and less than 12 h of sleep per day predicts overweight and obesity in early childhood [18]. Other studies, however, have reported null findings [19]. The potential for reverse causation also complicates matters, as it is possible that larger infants take larger feedings, which lead to increased sleep duration. While this relationship requires further study, shorter sleep duration has been recognized as a modifiable risk factor for obesity.

Randomized controlled trials have shown that interventions can be effective in prolonging sleep duration in infancy [3,12]. For example, parents and caregivers instructed on techniques to soothe breast-fed infants significantly increased hours of nocturnal sleep [12]. This is important, as sleep patterns are developing within the first few months of life, and strategies that improve infant sleep duration may prevent short- and long-term risk of both sleep problems [20] and obesity [21]. However, only a few studies have examined the impact of such interventions on growth patterns and weight status in the first 2 years of life [3,12]. Early-life sleep interventions hold promise, but there is a need for additional research.

Nutrition and Feeding Behaviors

Breast-feeding promotion is a popular strategy for the prevention of childhood obesity during infancy [11], and the links between breast-feeding and childhood obesity are reviewed in Chapter 11. Breast-feeding and human milk are considered the normative standards of nutrition in the first few months of life. Indeed, the American Academy of Pediatrics advocates exclusive breast-feeding for the first 6 months after birth because of several protective effects [22]. First, breast-feeding encourages self-regulation by the infant who is able to adjust milk intake to match energy needs, which has long-term behavioral effects [23]. Second, human milk contains nutritive and nonnutritive components that best meet the requirements of infant growth [24,25]. There is also emerging evidence that breast-feeding establishes healthy gut microbiota that affect metabolism [23]. Breast-fed infants also gain weight more slowly than formula-fed infants, and this early-life growth pattern is recognized as protective against obesity [26,27]. However, randomized controlled trials that have been shown to improve breast-feeding duration and exclusivity have not examined the effects on risk for obesity [10,28]. Indeed, the only randomized controlled trial that examined breast-feeding promotion and obesity risk found no association [28]. Because of the limited number of early-life interventions with growth outcomes, and the potential for confounding factors inherent in a woman's decision to breast-feed that may also predict weight status (e.g., socioeconomic status), clear evidence that breast-feeding reduces the risk of childhood obesity is currently lacking [11]. That being said, there is more definitive evidence that formula feeding increases the risk of childhood obesity [29], and though this may be tempered by formula composition [30], it suggests that breast-feeding may be the better alternative for its prevention.

The timing of solid food introduction has also been proposed as an opportunity for the early prevention of childhood obesity, although the findings are inconsistent [11,31]. It is recommended that the introduction of solids does not occur prior to ages 4–6 months, at which time solids may be added to the diet, along with continued breast-feeding or formula until at least age 12 months [22]. However, introducing solids prior to the recommendation is still a common practice among parents and caregivers that increases the risk of obesity [31]. While the underlying mechanism has not been established, it has been postulated that the early introduction of solids is associated with increased energy intake, as infants may not modify milk consumption when solids are also on the table. Evidence from observational studies indicated that earlier introduction of solids was associated with rapid weight gain in the first few months of life [32,33]. Earlier introduction of solids also predicts overweight and obesity at age 10 years [34], though findings over the long term are inconsistent [35]. Only one randomized controlled trial has investigated whether the timing of solids affects growth in infancy. Mehta and colleagues found that infants assigned to early (i.e., 3 months) versus late (i.e., 6 months) introduction of solids did not differ in weight gain by age 12 months [36]. In a recent longitudinal study, Vail and colleagues provided evidence for reverse causation, showing that heavier infants tend to be introduced to solid foods at an earlier age [31]. Additional research is needed, as strategies to delay the introduction of solids have been shown to be effective and may be a safeguard against childhood obesity [3,12].

The development of flavor preferences in infancy has garnered attention as it relates to weight status in childhood [1,11]. Infants have several innate responses that affect their acceptance of new foods, including a preference for sweet and salty tastes and a tendency to reject new, unfamiliar foods, especially foods that are neither sweet nor salty tasting. These predispositions may tip the scale toward greater intake of energy-dense foods (e.g., french fries, sugar-sweetened beverages) versus nutrient-dense foods (e.g., pureed vegetables, meats) in infancy; eating behaviors that have been shown to persist through childhood and increase the risk of obesity [37]. Fortunately, eating behaviors are malleable, and the first 24 months of life are an opportune time to promote acceptance of foods typical of a healthy diet [8]. For example, Birch and colleagues found that the neophobic response to new and unfamiliar foods is modified by repeated opportunities to taste them [12,38,39]. This practice was shown to increase intake of green beans, squash, and other vegetables in infants over the period of 1 week [12]. While repeated exposure has been shown to be efficacious in promoting food acceptance, few randomized controlled trials have examined how this affects growth patterns in infancy and risk of obesity in childhood.

Regulation of Distress, Temperament, and Emotion

Infants "come equipped" with different temperaments, or predispositions, to behave in a particular way. Temperament is determined through a balance in reactivity (ease of arousal) and self-regulation (control of arousal). High reactivity has been shown to predict weight gain and may be a risk factor of obesity, while high self-regulation has been shown to predict a lower weight status and may be a protective factor against obesity [40,41]. It follows that an infant with high reactivity and low self-regulation, or an infant with a negative temperament, may be more susceptible to rapid weight gain. This is because a negative infant is by definition prone to react with more negative affect and more frequent expressions of distress, and parents and caregivers are more likely to use feeding as a first response to fussiness [12,42]. "Feeding to soothe" an infant with high reactivity and low self-regulation increases opportunities for intake. It has been associated with energy imbalance and subsequent obesity [42]. Indeed, Stifter and colleagues found that feeding to soothe was a common practice among mothers of infants who were higher in negativity, and these infants were heavier in the first few months of life [42].

Because feeding to soothe can occur in the absence of hunger, it is possible that through their experience with feeding to soothe, the infant may learn to eat, not only in response to hunger, but to alleviate negative emotions. Particularly for highly reactive, negative infants, if caregivers respond indiscriminately to crying, fussing, and other expressions of distress with feeding, then the infant may learn to eat to reduce emotional distress. Studies suggest that the use of feeding in response to infants' emotions, or to manage their behaviors, can have long-term effects on eating behaviors and weight status. For example, Blissett and colleagues found that children ages 3–5 years whose mothers frequently used food to regulate emotions (e.g., cookies), ate more sweet and palatable foods than children whose mothers used this practice infrequently. This relationship was exaggerated in response to negative emotions [43]. Moreover, Boggiano and colleagues recently found that adolescents who reported eating sweet and palatable foods to reduce negative feelings had an increased risk of weight gain over 2 years [44]. Taken together, these findings suggest that parent regulation of infant emotion through the use of feeding to soothe may lead to eating behaviors over the short and long term that increase obesity risk.

While it is possible that temperamental negativity can increase the risk for overfeeding through the use of feeding to soothe, it turns out that the caregiver's response to infant negativity is key; results of one recent study indicated that negativity was only associated with higher weight status if mothers reported using higher levels of feeding to soothe, as infants high in negativity whose mothers used lower levels of feeding to soothe had normal weight status [45]. Taken together, these findings suggest the potential efficacy of interventions that target parenting and feeding practices, particularly the use of responsive parenting.

EXAMPLES OF MULTICOMPONENT INTERVENTIONS FOR EARLY OBESITY PREVENTION

The preceding section of this chapter highlighted potential opportunities for the prevention of childhood obesity during infancy. Sleeping, feeding, and coping with distress are core components of infant life that develop dramatically in the first few years after birth [1,11]. These behaviors have been targeted in early interventions to promote normative growth in infancy, an important determinant of obesity in childhood and beyond. Over the last few years, the first randomized controlled trials have been conducted, designed to build upon the evidence presented in the previous section of this chapter. Most have been multicomponent interventions, focusing on factors hypothesized to prevent excessive growth in the first 12–24 months. The rationale for multicomponent interventions is that the multifaceted nature of obesity requires a multifaceted approach for prevention. Though preliminary findings suggest that multicomponent behavioral interventions for parents and their infants hold promise, data are not consistent [12]. Discrepant findings may be related to differences in the intervention components included, intervention dose, barriers to implementation, lack of a theoretical framework or preliminary data to inform study design, and lack of valid and reliable measures of parent–infant behavior hypothesized to mediate the intervention effects [11]. Nevertheless, an evaluation of multicomponent behavioral interventions to date shows the progress that is being made toward obesity prevention in early life and guides future studies for parents and their infants.

Paul and colleagues conducted a multicomponent behavioral intervention to promote healthy infant growth in the first 12 months through improved sleeping and feeding [12]. In the Sleeping and Intake Methods Taught to Infants and Mothers Early in Life (SLIMTIME) study, mother–infant dyads were randomized to one of four treatments delivered at two nurse home visits: "Soothe/Sleep," "Introduction to Solids," "Soothe/Sleep" plus "Introduction to Solids," and control. The "Soothe/Sleep" intervention taught parents to discriminate between sources of infant distress. They learned alternative soothing techniques to reduce the use of feeding for nonhunger-related fussiness and increase infant sleep duration. The "Introduction to Solids" intervention taught parents to delay the introduction of solids and how to promote acceptance of new solid foods through repeated exposure. The study found that infants who received both interventions, designed to affect feeding, sleeping, and soothing, had lower weight-for-length percentiles, a measure used to monitor normal infant growth, than did those receiving neither or only one intervention component. In addition, results from a second randomized trial by the same researchers who also used nurse home visits to deliver interventions has shown positive effects on infant growth, with infants in the parenting intervention growing less rapidly from birth to 6 months relative to control [46]. Taken together, these findings suggest that multicomponent behavioral interventions may have potential for long-term obesity prevention [12].

Wen and colleagues also conducted a home-based intervention to promote normal growth in the first 24 months through improved feeding [47]. In the Healthy Beginnings Trial, mother–infant dyads were randomized to intervention or control groups. The intervention group received eight nurse home visits to promote breast-feeding, delay introduction of solids, and increase food acceptance. This environment allowed nurses to first monitor parent–infant feeding interactions and then deliver one-on-one consultations. The study found that infants in the intervention group had a lower body mass index (BMI) versus infants in the control group at 2 years. However, a follow-up study revealed that there were no differences between groups 3 years later [47]. This suggests that multicomponent behavioral interventions can show efficacy in promoting healthy infant growth, particularly in the home environment. However, without continued intervention, the effects may not persist into early childhood [47].

While the multicomponent behavioral interventions just described noted effects on parental knowledge, practices, infant behaviors, and infant growth or weight status, several other trials have reported intervention effects on maternal and infant behavior but null findings with respect to weight status and growth. Taveras and colleagues designed a study focused on promoting parenting practices hypothesized to reduce obesity risk, with infant growth as a secondary outcome [3]. In the First Steps for Mommy and Me study, mother–infant dyads who were assigned to an intervention with motivational interviewing during well-child clinic visits, counseling with a health educator, and monthly parenting workshops reported later introduction of solids and larger increases in sleep duration compared with the control group. However, there were no differences between intervention and control infants in weight-for-length z-scores at 6 months [3]. In another intervention trial, Campbell and colleagues conducted a study to enhance parenting practices that focused on infant feeding and activity and included infant growth as a secondary outcome [48]. In the Infant Feeding Activity and Nutrition Trial (InFANT), mother–infant dyads who participated in dietitian-delivered education sessions on feeding style, timing of solid food introduction, and management of food rejection reported modest improvements in dietary behaviors of infants, but no differences in BMI z-scores compared with the control group at 20 months [48].

A recent study by Russell and colleagues was aimed at promoting healthy growth in the first year through improved feeding [49]. In the Greenlight study, mother–infant dyads were randomized to receive low-literacy materials covering six core topics at well-child clinic visits: satiety cues, sweetened beverages, delayed introduction of solids, portion sizes, nonsedentary activity, and breast-feeding. Preliminary findings suggest that while the intervention was effective in promoting parent acceptance of feeding behaviors that might prevent obesity, it did not result in significant differences between treatment and control in infant growth or weight status [49].

Finally, Daniels and colleagues recently completed an intervention using parent education and peer support to optimize feeding practices and food preferences for obesity prevention in infancy [50]. In the NOURISH trial, mother–infant dyads were randomized to two intervention modules timed around the introduction of solids and the emergence of autonomy and independence. In these modules, a dietitian and psychologist addressed topics including neophobia, portion control, timing of snacks, and hunger/satiety cues, and parents were instructed to help develop self-regulation in infants. The study found that infants in the intervention group had lower BMI z-scores and less rapid weight gain compared with infants in the control group from birth to 14 months. However, there were no differences between groups at age 2 years or at age 5 years [50]. There was, however, a nonsignificant trend toward lower BMI z-scores for infants in the intervention group [50].

Because multicomponent behavioral interventions to date have reported mixed findings, additional research is needed to identify efficacious interventions. A publication summarizing the proceedings of a National Institutes of Health Workshop on the Prevention of Obesity in Infancy [11] acknowledged the opportunities for intervention during the period from birth to 24 months, but concluded that there is little evidence for how to prevent obesity during this early period. A pressing research priority is to improve measures of parent and infant behavior, infant growth, weight gain, and body composition. Such measures are essential to providing evidence that will aid in determining which interventions impact early growth and thereby reduce obesity risk. Nonetheless, the committee determined that future interventions that address these challenges and develop parenting behaviors to promote establishing routines, healthy sleep patterns, and appropriate feeding practices have potential for obesity prevention [11].

CONCLUSION

Infancy is a critical period of development and a time of both opportunity and vulnerability for risk of obesity. Infants experience rapid changes in weight and growth outcomes in the first few months of life that may put them on a fast track toward overweight and obesity in the first few years. The link between rapid weight gain in infancy and later obesity risk is well established, but little is known about the mechanisms underlying this association, and this limits our ability to develop efficacious interventions. A lack of validated measures of potential mediators and moderators of the relation between early environmental exposures, particularly parental and infant behaviors, and weight outcomes in infancy is also a barrier to progress. These rapid changes in growth are paralleled by rapid changes in behavior, which may ultimately affect weight status. Multicomponent behavioral interventions in the first 24 months show promise in reducing early obesity risk. However, a great deal of additional evidence is needed to develop effective, resource-efficient interventions that are scalable and appropriate for high-risk, underserved populations. Because infant behaviors surrounding feeding, sleeping, and coping with distress are both malleable and putative contributors to early rapid weight gain, interventions that teach parenting and feeding practices may prevent obesity while also promoting positive behavioral outcomes, including responsive parenting, increased infant sleep duration, self-regulation, and infant dietary patterns, more consistent with current guidance.

REFERENCES

1. Paul IM, Bartok CJ, Downs DS, Stifter CA, Ventura AK, Birch LL. Opportunities for the primary prevention of obesity during infancy. *Adv Pediatr.* 2009;56:107–33.
2. Ogden CL, Carroll MD, Kit BK, Flegal KM. Prevalence of childhood and adult obesity in the United States, 2011–2012. *JAMA.* 2014;311(8):806–14.
3. Taveras EM, Blackburn K, Gillman MW, Haines J, McDonald J, Price S, et al. First steps for mommy and me: A pilot intervention to improve nutrition and physical activity behaviors of postpartum mothers and their infants. *Matern Child Health J.* 2011;15(8):1217–27.
4. Baird J, Fisher D, Lucas P, Kleijnen J, Roberts H, Law C. Being big or growing fast: Systematic review of size and growth in infancy and later obesity. *BMJ.* 2005;331(7522):929.
5. Huxley RR, Shiell AW, Law CM. The role of size at birth and postnatal catch-up growth in determining systolic blood pressure: A systematic review of the literature. *J Hypertens.* 2000;18(7):815–31.
6. Barker DJ, Osmond C, Forsen TJ, Kajantie E, Eriksson JG. Trajectories of growth among children who have coronary events as adults. *N Engl J Med.* 2005;353(17):1802–9.
7. Bhargava SK, Sachdev HS, Fall CH, Osmond C, Lakshmy R, Barker DJ, et al. Relation of serial changes in childhood body-mass index to impaired glucose tolerance in young adulthood. *N Engl J Med.* 2004;350(9):865–75.
8. Birch LL, Doub AE. Learning to eat: Birth to age 2 y. *Am J Clin Nutr.* 2014;99(3):723 S–8 S.
9. Pinilla T, Birch LL. Help me make it through the night: Behavioral entrainment of breast-fed infants' sleep patterns. *Pediatrics.* 1993;91(2):436–44.

10. Wen LM, Baur LA, Simpson JM, Rissel C, Flood VM. Effectiveness of an early intervention on infant feeding practices and "tummy time": A randomized controlled trial. *Arch Pediatr Adolesc Med.* 2011;165(8):701–7.

11. Lumeng JC, Taveras EM, Birch L, Yanovski SZ. Prevention of obesity in infancy and early childhood: A National Institutes of Health workshop. *JAMA Pediatr.* 2015;169(5):484–90.

12. Paul IM, Savage JS, Anzman SL, Beiler JS, Marini ME, Stokes JL, et al. Preventing obesity during infancy: A pilot study. *Obesity (Silver Spring).* 2011;19(2):353–61.

13. Boeke CE, Storfer-Isser A, Redline S, Taveras EM. Childhood sleep duration and quality in relation to leptin concentration in two cohort studies. *Sleep.* 2014;37(3):613–20.

14. Chen X, Beydoun MA, Wang Y. Is sleep duration associated with childhood obesity? A systematic review and meta-analysis. *Obesity (Silver Spring).* 2008;16(2):265–74.

15. Locard E, Mamelle N, Billette A, Miginiac M, Munoz F, Rey S. Risk factors of obesity in a five year old population: Parental versus environmental factors. *Int J Obes Relat Metab Disord.* 1992;16(10):721–9.

16. Agras WS, Hammer LD, McNicholas F, Kraemer HC. Risk factors for childhood overweight: A prospective study from birth to 9.5 years. *J Pediatr.* 2004;145(1):20–5.

17. Tikotzky L, DE M G, Har-Toov J, Dollberg S, Bar-Haim Y, Sadeh A. Sleep and physical growth in infants during the first 6 months. *J Sleep Res.* 2010;19(1 Pt 1):103–10.

18. Taveras EM, Rifas-Shiman SL, Oken E, Gunderson EP, Gillman MW. Short sleep duration in infancy and risk of childhood overweight. *Arch Pediatr Adolesc Med.* 2008;162(4):305–11.

19. Klingenberg L, Christensen LB, Hjorth MF, Zangenberg S, Chaput JP, Sjodin A, et al. No relation between sleep duration and adiposity indicators in 9–36 months old children: The SKOT cohort. *Pediatr Obes.* 2013;8(1):e14–8.

20. Mindell JA, Du Mond CE, Sadeh A, Telofski LS, Kulkarni N, Gunn E. Long-term efficacy of an internet-based intervention for infant and toddler sleep disturbances: One year follow-up. *J Clin Sleep Med.* 2011;7(5):507–11.

21. Parmelee AH, Jr., Wenner WH, Schulz HR. Infant sleep patterns: From birth to 16 weeks of age. *J Pediatr.* 1964;65:576–82.

22. Eidelman AI. Breastfeeding and the use of human milk: An analysis of the American Academy of Pediatrics 2012 Breastfeeding Policy Statement. *Breastfeed Med.* 2012;7(5):323–4.

23. Thompson AL. Developmental origins of obesity: Early feeding environments, infant growth, and the intestinal microbiome. *Am J Hum Biol.* 2012;24(3):350–60.

24. Koletzko B, von Kries R, Closa R, Escribano J, Scaglioni S, Giovannini M, et al. Lower protein in infant formula is associated with lower weight up to age 2 y: A randomized clinical trial. *Am J Clin Nutr.* 2009;89(6):1836–45.

25. Savino F, Fissore MF, Grassino EC, Nanni GE, Oggero R, Silvestro L. Ghrelin, leptin and IGF-I levels in breast-fed and formula-fed infants in the first years of life. *Acta Paediatr.* 2005;94(5):531–7.

26. Dewey KG. Nutrition, growth, and complementary feeding of the breastfed infant. *Pediatr Clin North Am.* 2001;48(1):87–104.

27. Singhal A, Lanigan J. Breastfeeding, early growth and later obesity. *Obes Rev.* 2007;8 Suppl 1:51–4.

28. Martin RM, Patel R, Kramer MS, Guthrie L, Vilchuck K, Bogdanovich N, et al. Effects of promoting longer-term and exclusive breastfeeding on adiposity and insulin-like growth factor-I at age 11.5 years: A randomized trial. *JAMA.* 2013;309(10):1005–13.

29. Kramer MS, Guo T, Platt RW, Vanilovich I, Sevkovskaya Z, Dzikovich I, et al. Feeding effects on growth during infancy. *J Pediatr.* 2004;145(5):600–5.

30. Mennella JA, Ventura AK, Beauchamp GK. Differential growth patterns among healthy infants fed protein hydrolysate or cow-milk formulas. *Pediatrics.* 2011;127(1):110–8.

31. Vail B, Prentice P, Dunger DB, Hughes IA, Acerini CL, Ong KK. Age at weaning and infant growth: Primary analysis and systematic review. *J Pediatr.* 2015;167(2):317–24.e1.

32. Ong KK, Emmett PM, Noble S, Ness A, Dunger DB, Team AS. Dietary energy intake at the age of 4 months predicts postnatal weight gain and childhood body mass index. *Pediatrics.* 2006;117(3):e503–8.

33. Shukla A, Forsyth HA, Anderson CM, Marwah SM. Infantile overnutrition in the first year of life: A field study in Dudley, Worcestershire. *Br Med J.* 1972;4(5839):507–15.

34. Seach KA, Dharmage SC, Lowe AJ, Dixon JB. Delayed introduction of solid feeding reduces child overweight and obesity at 10 years. *Int J Obes (Lond).* 2010;34(10):1475–9.

35. Gillman MW, Rifas-Shiman SL, Camargo CA, Jr., Berkey CS, Frazier AL, Rockett HR, et al. Risk of overweight among adolescents who were breastfed as infants. *JAMA.* 2001;285(19):2461–7.

36. Mehta KC, Specker BL, Bartholmey S, Giddens J, Ho ML. Trial on timing of introduction to solids and food type on infant growth. *Pediatrics.* 1998;102(3 Pt 1):569–73.

37. Beauchamp GK, Mennella JA. Early flavor learning and its impact on later feeding behavior. *J Pediatr Gastroenterol Nutr.* 2009;48 Suppl 1:S25–30.

38. Birch LL, Marlin DW. I don't like it; I never tried it: Effects of exposure on two-year-old children's food preferences. *Appetite.* 1982;3(4):353–60.

39. Birch LL, Gunder L, Grimm-Thomas K, Laing DG. Infants' consumption of a new food enhances acceptance of similar foods. *Appetite.* 1998;30(3):283–95.

40. Darlington AS, Wright CM. The influence of temperament on weight gain in early infancy. *J Dev Behav Pediatr.* 2006;27(4):329–35.

41. Anzman SL, Birch LL. Low inhibitory control and restrictive feeding practices predict weight outcomes. *J Pediatr.* 2009;155(5):651–6.

42. Stifter CA, Anzman-Frasca S, Birch LL, Voegtline K. Parent use of food to soothe infant/toddler distress and child weight status: An exploratory study. *Appetite.* 2011;57(3):693–9.

43. Blissett J, Haycraft E, Farrow C. Inducing preschool children's emotional eating: Relations with parental feeding practices. *Am J Clin Nutr.* 2010;92(2):359–65.

44. Boggiano MM, Wenger LE, Turan B, Tatum MM, Morgan PR, Sylvester MD. Eating tasty food to cope: Longitudinal association with BMI. *Appetite.* 2015;87:365–70.

45. Savage JS, Birch LL, Marini M, Anzman-Frasca S, Paul IM. Effect of the INSIGHT responsive parenting intervention on rapid infant weight gain and overweight status at age 1 year: A randomized clinical trial. *JAMA Pediatr.* 2016;170(8):742–9. doi:10.1001/jamapediatrics.2016.0445.

46. Savage J, Paul I, Marini M, Anzman-Frasca S, Beiler J, Birch L, eds. Parenting intervention reduces infant rapid weight gain. *Pediatr Acad Soc.* 2015.

47. Wen LM, Baur LA, Simpson JM, Xu H, Hayes AJ, Hardy LL, et al. Sustainability of effects of an early childhood obesity prevention trial over time: A further 3-year follow-up of the healthy beginnings trial. *JAMA Pediatr.* 2015;169(6):543–51.

48. Campbell KJ, Lioret S, McNaughton SA, Crawford DA, Salmon J, Ball K, et al. A parent-focused intervention to reduce infant obesity risk behaviors: A randomized trial. *Pediatrics.* 2013;131(4):652–60.

49. Russell L, Perrin EM, Yin HS, Delamater AM, Bronaugh A, Bian A, et al., eds. Greenlight: A randomized trial adressing health literacy and communication to prevent pediatric obesity. *Pediatr Acad Soc.* 2015.

50. Daniels LA, Mallan KM, Nicholson JM, Thorpe K, Nambiar S, Mauch CE, et al. An early feeding practices intervention for obesity prevention. *Pediatrics.* 2015;136(1):e40–9.

35 Home/Family-Based Strategies for Prevention of Obesity in Infancy and Early Childhood

Sarah-Jeanne Salvy and Kayla de la Haye

CONTENTS

INTRODUCTION

Although a recent nationally representative study found a decline in obesity in 2- to 5-year-old children, this was not true for low-income and minority children [1]. In fact, 40% of low-income children enrolled in federally funded programs are already overweight or obese by age 5 [2]. This failure to effectively prevent the onset of obesity among at-risk children will only intensify and perpetuate health disparities, because once established, obesity is hard to reverse [3], and overweight youth have a 70% chance of becoming obese adults [4]. The stability of obesity across the life span, and the physical, psychosocial, and financial costs related to obesity for individuals and the larger society [5], raise the impetus to correct weight trajectories among at-risk children *before they become overweight or obese*. Unfortunately, extant childhood obesity interventions and prevention efforts have had limited success, especially among underserved children whose families are low income and of color.

In this chapter, we critically appraise existing family- or home-based obesity interventions and prevention programs, and highlight the key components of these efforts that we believe are essential in achieving positive outcomes in children; particularly children most at risk for obesity. Further, we present an innovative, sustainable, scalable, and potentially cost-effective model of delivery for obesity prevention initiated in infancy that we call *COPE* (Childhood Obesity Prevention @ homE/

Contrarrestar Obesidad: Programa para niños En casa). This collaboration emerged in response to the unmet needs and resources available to address the increasing prevalence of obesity among children enrolled in federally funded programs.

OBESITY PREVENTION PROGRAMS SHOULD TARGET THE FAMILY AND THE HOME ENVIRONMENT

Although the clustering of overweight and obesity in families is partially explained by shared genetics, familial behaviors and shared environments largely determine the expression and maintenance of obesogenic behaviors [6,7]. Thus, targeting the family and home environment is likely to impact the expression of obesity among families with and without genetic risk [8]. As a primary source of socialization for children, families, and in particular parents, have the opportunity to make certain foods and activities available, model and reinforce healthier food options and physical activity habits, and implement certain parenting practices. Because eating and physical activity habits established in these early years track into adulthood, early family influences have a lasting impact on children's health [9,10].

Much research has been conducted on the advantages of modifying the family environment to "treat" obesity [11], as reviewed for example in Chapters 15 and 29. Family-based obesity interventions concurrently target parents (typically mothers) and children and focus on the adoption of a lifelong, healthy lifestyle to improve nutrition, physical activity, and psychosocial health [11–13]. The curriculum combines lifestyle and cognitive-behavioral techniques to improve nutrition, physical activity, and overall psychosocial health. Parents are taught multiple skills such as how to structure the family environment to support healthy behaviors, parenting practices conducive to children's healthy changes, how to model healthy behaviors for their children, and how to problem solve in the face of challenges. Short and long-term studies have shown that targeting parents as active participants improves child weight trajectories over a 5- and 10-year follow-up, as well as the youth's health-related risk factors, energy intake, and psychosocial functioning [11]. Although the family-centered model has been shown to be efficacious for weight loss in parents and children [14,15], the ability of this model to *prevent* the development of childhood obesity (as opposed to treating children who are already overweight or obese) is not clear. In fact, including parents and family members is less common for programs focused on preventing the onset of obesity (as opposed to "treating" obesity). Only 40% of childhood obesity prevention programs include a family component and only 5% explicitly target behavioral change among multiple family members [16].

In theory, the application of family-based approaches for obesity prevention appears to be promising; however, the question of *treatment* (weight loss) versus *prevention* (averting excessive weight gain) brings the issue of intervention timing. The vast majority of family-based obesity interventions have focused on school-age children when youth are already overweight or obese. This is unfortunate as there is now clear evidence that rapid weight gain as early as in the first 4–6 months of life is already associated with greater odds of child overweight or obesity later in childhood and adolescence [17–19].

OBESITY PREVENTION EFFORTS SHOULD BE INITIATED IN INFANCY AND EARLY CHILDHOOD

As reviewed in preceding chapters, early childhood is clearly a pivotal time for the formation of lifelong eating and physical activity habits [e.g., 9,10,20–24] and for the intergenerational transmission of obesity, yet controlled trials focusing on weight management or obesity prevention for children under the age of 5 years of age are scarce [25]. A small number of obesity interventions and prevention programs targeting infancy and early childhood have had some level of success in decreasing or preventing obesity, as reviewed in Chapter 34 [26–30]. However, the impact and sustainability of these programs have been limited by their short duration (<6 months) and low dosage. The short duration of these interventions is problematic for the maintenance of healthy changes. Even when maintenance is directly addressed or planned as part of the intervention, the maintenance phase rarely (if ever) exceeds a few weekly 1 h sessions, which is doubtfully sufficient to ensure mastery of learned skills into lifelong healthy habits. Furthermore, the duration of existing efforts is not sufficient to cover the key developmental periods and nutritional transitions during and beyond early infancy, which are critical for obesity development [31].

EMBEDDING OBESITY PREVENTION EFFORTS INTO EXISTING HOME-BASED SERVICE SYSTEMS TO PROMOTE SUSTAINABILITY, SCALABILITY, AND COST EFFECTIVENESS

Few childhood obesity interventions and prevention efforts have been integrated into existing service delivery systems, creating significant barriers in their reach and impact. Existing programs typically require the parent and the child to attend intervention sessions outside their general daily routines (e.g., evening educational classes in outpatient clinics). As a result, less than 50% of families involved in obesity interventions complete follow-up visits, and attrition is especially problematic for low-income families and for those who live in remote areas [32–34]. The high rates of attrition, in both the initial intervention implementation and during the maintenance phase, seriously limit the impact of these efforts in achieving clinically significant long-term outcomes, particularly among at-risk children and their families [32,33]. Not only does the outpatient model impose a considerable burden on families, which likely interferes with treatment adherence, but it can also be argued that this modality is not optimal for the generalization of behavior change to the family's natural environment.

A related limitation of current obesity interventions and prevention delivery models in specialized clinics or other medical settings pertains to the limited scope of these existing obesity efforts. Over the last decades, there has been a burgeoning of new programs tackling obesity management or the development of obesity risks. Unfortunately, the narrow focus on obesity makes it difficult to simultaneously address barriers such as a lack of access to resources and culturally competent services, poverty, unemployment, housing instability, food insecurity, family conflict and violence, and neighborhood characteristics—all of which profoundly affect the ability of at-risk families to engage in these programs and adhere to lifestyle changes. A more holistic approach to obesity prevention, which simultaneously addresses these barriers, could be adopted by embedding efforts into existing, comprehensive service delivery systems that target families. This is likely to be critical to developing effective and sustainable family-centered programs in real-world settings.

HOME VISITATION PROGRAMS: AN UNTAPPED OPPORTUNITY FOR PREVENTING CHILDHOOD OBESITY

Ideally, obesity initiatives should be (1) focused on the child's ecological niche (family and home environment) to shape children's health trajectories and promote generalizability and sustainability; (2) initiated in infancy and early childhood, when key eating and physical activity habits develop; and (3) embedded in existing service systems for an extended period of time to promote the consolidation of healthy habits for life among diverse families. Developing a nationwide obesity prevention program that provides in-home services to at-risk infants and their families for a sustained period of time, and which is effectively tailored for diverse families, would be cost prohibitive *unless* these services are integrated into an effective and sustainable service-delivery system.

Fortunately, home visitation programs (HVPs) already provide comprehensive home-based support, education, assessment, community linkage, referral, and advocacy to more than 500,000 low-income, underserved, at-risk children and their families in the United States annually. HVPs have been in place for more than 40 years and currently have $1.5 billion annual investment from the Affordable Care Act [35], which speaks to the sustainability of the services provided. The free and voluntary weekly home visits begin during pregnancy, or shortly after birth, and continue until the child reaches 2–5 years of age. HVP sites/chapters are housed and overseen by accredited community health organizations or agencies. Locally hired home visitors provide services tailored for the cultural and linguistic needs of their constituents. HVPs are embedded in a comprehensive system of child and maternal health services designed to promote optimal child development and prevent adverse outcomes, including child abuse and neglect, academic underachievement, psychological maladjustment, and antisocial behavior [36–38]. Randomized controlled trials (RCTs) show that high-quality HVPs effectively improve children's physical and psychosocial health, such as birth outcomes, breast-feeding, immunization rates, and overall cognitive and social development [36–38]. Despite the success of HVPs in improving the outcomes of at-risk children, there has been no explicit and systematic effort to target childhood obesity as part of these services. This is surprising as the HVP structure, with its strong partnership with WIC (women, infants, and children) programs, provides an ideal model for scalable and sustainable obesity prevention among underserved children:

1. The provision of in-home services removes barriers to accessing the program (e.g., transportation, childcare), promotes the generalization of skills to the home environment, and enables ethnically and racially diverse families to access culturally competent health services.
2. HVPs have existing partnerships with WIC programs nationwide.
3. The programs already address many barriers to healthy lifestyles such as unemployment, family conflict and violence, housing instability, and neighborhood characteristics.
4. The extensive time frame for service delivery (3–5 years) makes it possible for home visitors to transfer and reinforce health knowledge, skills and new behaviors, and to help families develop social and community networks promoting sustainability of health outcomes.
5. The widespread presence of HVPs across the United States, and established infrastructures in many urban and rural areas, are critical for the scalability of services across the United States.

COPE: Childhood Obesity Prevention @ homE/Contrarrestar
Obesidad: Programa para niños En casa

COPE is a collaboration, which emerged in response to both the limitations of existing childhood obesity prevention initiatives outlined in the last sections and the unmet needs and resources voiced by HVPs to address the increasing prevalence of obesity among children in their programs. Consistent with a capacity-building approach, COPE aims to extend the mission and capabilities of HVPs in delivering established nutrition guidelines and physical activity recommendations using an engaging, culturally sensitive, and community-forming model of delivery. It is important to note that COPE does not target weight loss; rather it focuses on the promotion of healthy behaviors in all HVP children and their families, regardless of weight status, and ultimately the prevention of the development of obesity in early childhood.

COPE Curriculum Content

Nutrition
The curriculum promotes foods that support children's healthy development:

1. *Increase/promote intake of vegetables and fruits* (≥5 servings/day of fruits and vegetables). Parents/mothers are given age-appropriate recipes and strategies to increase children's fruit and vegetable intake.

2. *Limiting intake of high-fat and high-sugar foods.* Mothers learn to modify their families' favorite foods and recipes to decrease fat and sugar content.
3. *Eliminate sugar-sweetened beverage intake,* including information and activities on sugar content of popular sweetened beverages, long-term effects of high sugar consumption, importance of drinking water, and impact of advertising [39].
4. *Appropriate portion sizes for infants and preschoolers.* Parents are taught to offer small portions, to follow a meal and snack schedule, and to help their children understand when they are satiated.

Physical Activity

Although there is no unequivocally accepted guidelines for the number of minutes young children (2–5 years of age) should be active each day [40], the US Department of Health and Human Services (DHHS) has summarized consensus recommendations among the National Association for Sport and Physical Education, the American College of Sports Medicine, and the National Institutes of Health that include (1) accumulate at least 60 min of *structured* physical activity each day (>3 years old); (2) engage in at least 60 min, and up to several hours, of *unstructured* physical activity each day; and (3) avoid being sedentary for more than 60 min at a time, except when sleeping. The American Academy of Pediatrics Expert Committee report for clinicians further suggests limiting screen time to a maximum of 2 h per day for children 2 years of age and older and removing televisions and other screens from children's primary sleeping area [12]. These guidelines are consistent with the US Department of Agriculture (USDA) recommendations that "Children ages 2–5 years should play actively several times each day [...] and that physical activities for young children should be developmentally appropriate, fun, and offer variety" [40].

The COPE intervention manual is premised on these guidelines and teaches parents to make activity and play a daily habit for their children and entire family by exploiting lifestyle activities (e.g., taking the stairs, walking to the shop). Home visitors are trained to help parents design activities around their local environment, schedule, and preferences, and to optimize their use of safe indoor and outdoor spaces that are suitable for structured and unstructured activities with children. Parents are provided with information about resources and free group activities conducive to physical activity (e.g., parks, walking clubs, outings) and classes they can take with their children and with other HVP families. The curriculum emphasizes the importance of parents coengaging in activities with their children to set a good example through modeling and to provide opportunities for their children to be physically active.

Developmental Considerations: Neophobia and Food-Related Tantrums

Young children are highly neophobic and resist trying new foods, which can be a barrier to their acceptance of healthy foods such as fruits and vegetables. Research has shown that parents typically present a rejected food 3–5 times before deciding that their child does not like the food, although 10–15 exposures is actually necessary to overcome food rejection by young children [41]. Similar to the approach used in the LAUNCH intervention [42], COPE includes behavioral strategies and activities to help parents address neophobia and increase children's acceptance of novel foods: that is, repeated presentations and multisensory exposures (i.e., smell, touch, taste) of foods [43,44], gradual texture shaping, parents/caregivers modeling, and involvement of children in the selection and the preparation of new foods. Tantrums around eating can also be a barrier for healthy food consumption, and persistent tantrums around meals and food at age 3 has been found to predict obesity at age 5 [45]. COPE further targets strategies for mealtime behaviors [46] including redirection, extinction/planned ignoring, positive reinforcement of appropriate behaviors, scheduling of meals and snacks, and avoiding using food as reward or to soothe.

FORMAT OF THE EDUCATION DELIVERED TO FAMILIES

Through our formative work and pilot research it became clear that didactic and experiential approaches were needed to effectively reach, engage, and mobilize families.

Didactic Individualized Education

The didactic strategy focuses on in-home individualized coaching to help mothers implement changes in their natural environment. A strong emphasis is placed on *gradual goal setting* in which mothers set objectives for their children's weekly activity and diet (e.g., decreasing by "x" the number of sugar-sweetened beverages; trying "x" new vegetables this week) and on *parent modeling* healthy behaviors (i.e., parent coengaging in healthy behaviors with their children). Parents are also taught *behavior management and cognitive-behavioral strategies* to change their home environment. For example, mothers receive individual shaping to gradually eliminate high–energy dense foods from the home environment and prevent mindless eating. Parents also work on modifying their home to make it more conducive to making choices that support exercising, such as removing computers and televisions from sleeping areas [12].

Social and Experiential Activities

These activities were developed based on families' desire to engage in experiential/hands-on activities and strategies (e.g., concrete demonstrations, activities, and practices) to develop practical skills that generalize to their everyday life. They also requested *social activities* centered on health behaviors. The social and experiential activities that we created (Table 35.1) are similar to those delivered as part of the National Institute of Food and Agriculture's Expanded Food and Nutrition Education Program [47]. These activities aim to promote the development of supportive, healthy social networks and communities to reinforce healthy changes and assist long-term sustainability.

CONCLUSION

In fiscal year 2009–2010, 46 states and the District of Columbia made $1.5 billion available for early childhood HVPs, with most states investing in at least two programs [48]. Investment in these services remains strong, with the Affordable Care Act allocating $1.5 billion for states to invest in these programs [35]. Given that 40% of children enrolled in federally funded programs are overweight or obese by the age of 5, it is expected that the Health Resources and Services Administration, Maternal, Infant and Early Childhood Home Visiting (HRSA MIECHV) program will mandate HVPs to address childhood obesity as a part of their services. COPE provides an innovative,

---

TABLE 35.1
Summary of COPE Activities

Activities	Description
Communal cooking	These gatherings aim to teach parents how to cook healthy meals with the foods they receive from WIC/food bank, and advance meal preparation to promote healthy home cooking and decrease reliance on fast food. The gatherings are led by our HVP *Culinary Program Coordinator,* and take place in the Wellness Homes operated by our Healthy Families America home visitation partner Antelope Partners for Health (AVPH). These homes were given to AVPH by the city of Lancaster to promote preventive care and education to underserved families. These homes have Wi-Fi and a fully equipped kitchen.
Community gardening	A Mariposa master gardener teaches children and parents gardening techniques such as soil preparation and irrigation; planting, growing and harvesting fruits and vegetables. The classes include USDA/MyPlate activities targeting healthy meals and snacks. The gardens are located on Wellness Homes' grounds. Families are encouraged to tend the gardens with other local families.
Food management	These classes/tours are designed to improve food resource management practices such as purchasing; selecting, or otherwise obtaining, preparing, and storing foods to increase sustained availability of healthy foods throughout the month. This material is delivered during tours at local farmers markets and grocery stores.
Mobile food demos	Mobile cooking demonstrations hosted in neighborhood farmers, markets.

---

scalable, sustainable, and potentially cost-effective approach to existing gaps. Once home visitors are trained to implement COPE, the material is delivered as part of the weekly home visits. This delivery model is designed to reach families who have historically faced disparities in services in order to improve the children's health and reduce the financial burdens for society as a whole.

REFERENCES

1. Ogden CL, Carroll MD, Flegal KM. Prevalence of obesity in the United States. *JAMA*. 2014;312:189–90.
2. Wojcicki JM, Heyman MB. Let's Move: Childhood obesity prevention from pregnancy and infancy onward. *N Engl J Med*. 2010;362:1457–9.
3. Oude Luttikhuis H, Baur L, Jansen H, Shrewsbury VA, O'Malley C, Stolk RP, et al. Interventions for treating obesity in children. *Cochrane Database Syst Rev*. 2009:CD001872.
4. Singh AS, Mulder C, Twisk JW, van Mechelen W, Chinapaw MJ. Tracking of childhood overweight into adulthood: A systematic review of the literature. *Obes Rev*. 2008;9(5):474–88.
5. Committee on Accelerating Progress in Obesity Prevention Institute of Medicine. Accelerating progress in obesity prevention: Solving the weight of the nation. Washington, DC, 2012.
6. Hebebrand J, Hinney A. Environmental and genetic risk factors in obesity. *Child Adolesc Psychiatr Clin N Am*. 2009;18:83–94.
7. Contaldo F, Pasanisi F. Obesity epidemics: Secular trend or globalization consequence? Beyond the interaction between genetic and environmental factors. *Clin Nutr*. 2004;23:289–91.
8. de Silva-Sanigorski AM, Waters E, Calache H, Smith M, Gold L, Gussy M, et al. Splash!: A prospective birth cohort study of the impact of environmental, social and family-level influences on child oral health and obesity related risk factors and outcomes. *BMC Public Health*. 2011;11:505.
9. Birch LL, Davison KK. Family environmental factors influencing the developing behavioral controls of food intake and childhood overweight. *Pediatr Clin North Am*. 2001;48:893–907.
10. Spruijt-Metz D, Li C, Cohen E, Birch L, Goran M. Longitudinal influence of mother's child-feeding practices on adiposity in children. *J Pediatr*. 2006;148:314–20.
11. Epstein LH, Paluch RA, Roemmich JN, Beecher MD. Family-based obesity treatment, then and now: Twenty-five years of pediatric obesity treatment. *Health Psychol*. 2007;26:381–91.
12. Barlow SE. Expert committee recommendations regarding the prevention, assessment, and treatment of child and adolescent overweight and obesity: Summary report. *Pediatrics*. 2007;120 (Suppl 4):s164–92.
13. Lau DC, Obesity Canada Clinical Practice Guidelines Steering C, Expert P. Synopsis of the 2006 Canadian clinical practice guidelines on the management and prevention of obesity in adults and children. *CMAJ*. 2007;176:1103–6.
14. Savoye M, Nowicka P, Shaw M, Yu S, Dziura J, Chavent G, et al. Long-term results of an obesity program in an ethnically diverse pediatric population. *Pediatrics*. 2011;127:402–10.
15. Ball GDC, Mackenzie KA, Newton MS, Alloway CA, Slack JM, Plotnikoff RC, et al. One-on-one lifestyle coaching for managing adolescent obesity: Experience from a real-world, clinical setting. *Paediatr Child Health*. 2011;16:346–55.
16. Stice E, Shaw H, Marti CN. A meta-analytic review of obesity prevention programs for children and adolescents: The skinny on interventions that work. *Psychol Bull*. 2006;132:667–91.
17. Ong KK, Loos RJ. Rapid infancy weight gain and subsequent obesity: Systematic reviews and hopeful suggestions. *Acta Paediatr*. 2006;95:904–8.
18. Stettler N, Baumann M. Excess weight gain in the first 18 months of life is associated with later childhood overweight, obesity and greater arterial wall thickness. *Evid Based Nurs*. 2014;17:85.
19. Taveras EM, Rifas-Shiman SL, Sherry B, Oken E, Haines J, Kleinman K, et al. Crossing growth percentiles in infancy and risk of obesity in childhood. *Arch Pediatr Adolesc Med*. 2011;165:993–8.
20. Rollins BY, Loken E, Savage JS, Birch LL. Maternal controlling feeding practices and girls' inhibitory control interact to predict changes in BMI and eating in the absence of hunger from 5 to 7 y. *Am J Clin Nutr*. 2014;99:249–57.
21. Park S, Li R, Birch L. Mothers' child-feeding practices are associated with children's sugar-sweetened beverage intake. *J Nutr*. 2015;145:806–12.
22. Eriksson B, Henriksson H, Lof M, Hannestad U, Forsum E. Body-composition development during early childhood and energy expenditure in response to physical activity in 1.5-y-old children. *Am J Clin Nutr*. 2012;96:567–73.
23. Hinkley T, Teychenne M, Downing KL, Ball K, Salmon J, Hesketh KD. Early childhood physical activity, sedentary behaviors and psychosocial well-being: A systematic review. *Prev Med*. 2014;62:182–92.

24. Telama R, Yang X, Leskinen E, Kankaanpaa A, Hirvensalo M, Tammelin T, et al. Tracking of physical activity from early childhood through youth into adulthood. *Med Sci Sports Exerc*. 2014;46:955–62.

25. Bond M, Wyatt K, Lloyd J, Welch K, Taylor R. Systematic review of the effectiveness and cost-effectiveness of weight management schemes for the under fives: A short report. *Health Technol Assess*. 2009;13:1–75, iii.

26. Campbell KJ, Lioret S, McNaughton SA, Crawford DA, Salmon J, Ball K, et al. A parent-focused intervention to reduce infant obesity risk behaviors: A randomized trial. *Pediatrics*. 2013;131:652–60.

27. Daniels LA, Mallan KM, Battistutta D, Nicholson JM, Perry R, Magarey A. Evaluation of an intervention to promote protective infant feeding practices to prevent childhood obesity: Outcomes of the NOURISH RCT at 14 months of age and 6 months post the first of two intervention modules. *Int J Obes (Lond)*. 2012;36:1292–8.

28. Lioret S, Campbell KJ, Crawford D, Spence AC, Hesketh K, McNaughton SA. A parent focused child obesity prevention intervention improves some mother obesity risk behaviors: The Melbourne infant program. *Int J Behav Nutr Phys Act*. 2012;9:100.

29. Paul IM, Savage JS, Anzman SL, Beiler JS, Marini ME, Stokes JL, et al. Preventing obesity during infancy: A pilot study. *Obesity (Silver Spring)*. 2011;19:353–61.

30. Taveras EM, Gortmaker SL, Hohman KH, Horan CM, Kleinman KP, Mitchell K, et al. Randomized controlled trial to improve primary care to prevent and manage childhood obesity: The High Five for Kids study. *Arch Pediatr Adolesc Med*. 2011;165:714–22.

31. Dietz WH. Critical periods in childhood for the development of obesity. *Am J Clin Nutr*. 1994;59:955–9.

32. Zeller M, Kirk S, Claytor R, Khoury P, Grieme J, Santangelo M, et al. Predictors of attrition from a pediatric weight management program. *J Pediatr*. 2004;144:466–70.

33. Skelton JA, Beech BM. Attrition in paediatric weight management: A review of the literature and new directions. *Obes Rev*. 2011;12: 273–81.

34. Irby MB, Boles KA, Jordan C, Skelton JA. TeleFIT: Adapting a multidisciplinary, tertiary-care pediatric obesity clinic to rural populations. *Telemed J E Health*. 2012;18:247–9.

35. Thompson DK, Clark MJ, Howland LC, Mueller MR. The Patient Protection and Affordable Care Act of 2010 (PL 111–148): An analysis of maternal-child health home visitation. *Polic Polit Nurs Pract*. 2011;12:175–85.

36. Tschudy MM, Platt RE, Serwint JR. Extending the medical home into the community: A newborn home visitation program for pediatric residents. *Acad Pediatr*. 2013;13:443–50.

37. Wakefield MK, Sheldon GH. Special supplement on the Maternal, Infant, and Early Childhood Home Visiting (MIECHV) program. Foreword. *Pediatrics*. 2013;132 Suppl 2:S57–8.

38. U.S. Department of Health and Human Services Health Resources and Services Administration for Children & Families. The Maternal, Infant, and Early Childhood Home Visiting Program–partnering with parents to help children succeed. Washington, DC, 2015.

39. Ebbeling CB, Feldman HA, Chomitz VR, Antonelli TA, Gortmaker SL, Osganian SK, et al. A randomized trial of sugar-sweetened beverages and adolescent body weight. *N Engl J Med*. 2012;367:1407–16.

40. United States Department of Agriculture. How much physical activity is needed? http://choosemyplate.gov/physical-activity/amount.html.

41. Pliner P, Salvy SJ. Food neophobia in humans. In Shepherd R, Raats M, eds. *Psychology of Food Choice*. CABI Publishing, 2006.

42. Stark LJ, Clifford LM, Towner EK, Filigno SS, Zion C, Bolling C, et al. A pilot randomized controlled trial of a behavioral family-based intervention with and without home visits to decrease obesity in pre-schoolers. *J Pediatr Psychol*. 2014;39:1001–12.

43. Wardle J, Cooke LJ, Gibson EL, Sapochnik M, Sheiham A, Lawson M. Increasing children's acceptance of vegetables; a randomized trial of parent-led exposure. *Appetite*. 2003;40:155–62.

44. Wardle J, Herrera ML, Cooke L, Gibson EL. Modifying children's food preferences: The effects of exposure and reward on acceptance of an unfamiliar vegetable. *Eur J Clin Nutr*. 2003;57:341–8.

45. Agras WS, Hammer LD, McNicholas F, Kraemer HC. Risk factors for childhood overweight: A prospective study from birth to 9.5 years. *J Pediatr*. 2004;145:20–5.

46. Linscheid TR. Behavioral treatments for pediatric feeding disorders. *Behav Modif*. 2006;30:6–23.

47. U.S Department of Agriculture NIFA Program Leadership. Expanded Food and Nutrition Education Program Policies. 2013. http://www.nifa.usda.gov/nea/food/efnep/pdf/program-policy.pdf.

48. Pew Center. States and the new federal home visiting initiative 2010. http://www.pewstates.org/research/reports/states-and-the-new-federal-home-visiting-initiative-85899377168?p=3.

36 Community and School-Based Interventions for Childhood Obesity

Noe C. Crespo and John P. Elder

CONTENTS

INTRODUCTION

Over the past 20 years, the socioecological model (SEM) [1] has emerged as the dominant and guiding framework for the development, implementation, and evaluation of community-based health promotion efforts. The SEM identifies the independent and interactive effects of factors at multiple levels that influence individual and population health. These factors range from individual-level factors (e.g., knowledge and behavior), interpersonal factors (e.g., family, peers), organizational factors (e.g., schools and work sites), environmental factors (e.g., built environment and social environment), and policy factors (e.g., health policy) [2]. The SEM has also been adapted to study several chronic diseases (e.g., cancer, type 2 diabetes, heart disease, obesity) [3–5], several health behaviors (e.g., cancer screening, physical activity, and nutrition) [6–9], and for use in specific population subgroups such as Latinos [10]. The wide use of the SEM has helped to identify opportunities to revert the current obesogenic environments and to identify areas where greater efforts are needed to create healthier communities [5].

As reviewed in several of the preceding chapters of this book, childhood obesity is the result of a constellation of factors that influence daily choices and opportunities for children to eat healthy and engage in regular physical activity [11,12]. Characteristics of the community environment such as the presence and proximity of parks, street connectivity, presence and proximity to grocery stores, neighborhood safety, and access to effective health promotion programs and resources can also influence children's energy balance [12], as reviewed in Chapter 1. The home environment has a particularly strong influence on children's health behaviors given the important role of the parent in modeling and supporting children's health behaviors (e.g., parent monitoring of children's eating behaviors and logistic support for physical activity) [13,14], as reviewed, for example, in Chapter 15. The aim of this chapter is to review notable school- and community-based childhood obesity prevention studies and some of the key factors that led to their success. Two specific studies are described in more detail in order to draw attention to the contextual and qualitative aspects of these efforts that may not otherwise be included in published scientific articles. This contextual information may provide greater insights for practitioners and researchers who work within schools and other community organizations to combat childhood obesity.

SCHOOL-BASED INTERVENTIONS

Schools play an important role in children's lives and well-being. Schools provide children, not only with an important learning environment, but also with direct and impactful opportunities to establish healthy eating and physical activity habits. Not surprisingly, schools have been the predominant setting for implementing behavioral, environmental, and policy interventions aimed at preventing and reducing childhood obesity [15,16,17,18]. There are several examples of effective short-term and long-term school-based interventions. Specifically, school-based nutrition and physical activity curricula that are incorporated into existing curricula show significant effects on child obesity. The Planet Health program, for example, was a school-based nutrition and physical activity curriculum that showed significant reductions in the prevalence of obesity among girls and reductions in television viewing time compared with children in control schools [19]. Another school-based curriculum implemented in San Jose, California, resulted in significant reductions in children's body mass index (BMI) and television viewing time [20]. Children who attend schools that participate in a coordinated program that incorporates school-based healthy eating recommendations demonstrate lower rates of obesity compared with children who attend schools without nutrition programs [21]. Beyond obesity outcomes, several school-based studies also demonstrate important improvements in children's eating and physical activity behaviors. A large systematic, multisite trial (CATCH) resulted in significant increases in children's physical activity and reductions in fat intake [22], and several of these outcomes were maintained over 3 years [23]. The TAAG school-based study also demonstrated significant improvements in girls' physical activity [24]. Despite these successes, several review studies show mixed or inconclusive findings stemming from school-based efforts [25,26]. It appears that the success of these efforts are dependent on the level of "reach," "penetration," and "adoption" of such programs within the school system; in other words, the level of institutionalization. Institutionalization of school-based programs and policies requires the full buy in and participation from parents and school personnel (e.g., administrators, teachers, and staff). Programs and strategies must also be tailored to the contextual factors (e.g., language, cultural norms) relevant to the target population and community setting [27]. Programs that tailor messages and strategies to the gender and age of children are more successful at changing children's behaviors given that social norms and social influences differ between boys and girls, and these social influences change as children age [26,28]. Thus, the success of each school-based study is largely dependent on the specific contextual factors where the intervention took place. To this end, researchers and practitioners are urged to share and publish more contextual information stemming from community interventions in order to better understand the factors that contribute to their success. In the following sections, we describe the implementation and evaluation of two multilevel school- and community-based childhood obesity prevention interventions among Latino families and describe the lessons learned and the important contextual factors that influenced successful outcomes.

The *Aventuras Para Niños* (APN) study was a unique and ambitious project designed to evaluate the independent and interactive effects of interventions occurring in the micro- and macroenvironments that were aimed at preventing and controlling childhood obesity among Latino children [14,29]. The intervention targeted the microenvironment, operationalized as the composite of the home environment, parental, and family influence. The macroenvironment intervention targeted physical, environmental, and policy changes within elementary schools, local restaurants, parks, and grocery stores in the communities where children (K-2nd grade) resided (South Bay, San Diego, CA). A total of 808 families and 13 schools were enrolled into the study. One of the first challenges to conducting large-scale community interventions is to successfully enroll the target population. APN recruitment efforts first focused on obtaining the buy in, approval, and participation of school principals, administrators, and other key stakeholders. This was accomplished through a series of meetings with school administrators and by engaging in discussions that emphasized the positive role that schools play in their students' lives and the benefits of engaging in a mutually beneficial collaboration with the project team. Thus, a critical step for a successful community project is to establish a meaningful and mutually beneficial partnership between community organizations and the research team. Another important challenge in community-based health promotion research is to establish and maintain the trust between the practitioner/researcher and the community residents. Toward this goal, APN identified and hired eight community-health workers (also known as lay health advisors or *promotoras*) to work with the project team and serve as the communication bridge between the research team and the community residents. The work of *promotoras* has been identified as a key contributor to the success of many community-based studies, especially among diverse populations [30]. *Promotoras* can serve different roles depending on the goals of the project and skills/experience of the *promotora*. In APN, *promotoras* were paid project members who were also members of the target community. The *promotoras* were mothers of children who attended the intervention schools, lived in the target community, and were also demographically similar to the target population. The *promotoras* are able to offer unique insights about how to best implement meaningful and culturally appropriate changes in the target community given that they have firsthand knowledge of the cultural factors that can facilitate or impede change. *Promotoras* also have a unique understanding of the formal and informal social networks that can be leveraged to achieve the desired outcomes. This approach is particularly important when targeting communities that have historically experienced adversity (e.g., discrimination) that has led to systemic mistrust of state institutions and organizations. The *promotoras* in APN played an important role in both establishing trust and engaging community residents and leaders in project activities.

APN implemented several school-level strategies with mixed results. The most successful school-based strategies of APN were the "Start with Salad" cafeteria intervention and the "Peaceful Playground" intervention [31]. Start with Salad was a cafeteria intervention designed to reinforce children for eating a salad item from their plate prior to eating any other item. Adult volunteers (usually cafeteria staff or *promotoras*) monitored children's behaviors during lunchtime to ensure their safety and to help with the flow of students through the lunch line. These adult volunteers were trained by APN staff to monitor, identify, and reward children who consumed vegetables prior to any other item on their plate. Rewards were given to children in the form of stickers, which were placed on the child's shirt/blouse, and verbal praise was given from the adult. Start with Salad was successful because it was easy to implement in all schools and was well received by the cafeteria staff and children. Peaceful Playgrounds was an effective school environmental intervention designed to encourage children to move more during recess time [32]. After several planning meetings with school administrators and parents, APN received approval to paint all intervention school playgrounds using the Peaceful Playgrounds stencils and artwork. Adult volunteers painted the surface of these playgrounds according to the Peaceful Playgrounds designs. Children showed an immediate positive reaction toward these new surfaces and began to play in and around these surfaces. These two school-based interventions highlight the positive and successful social and physical environmental changes that can occur quickly within schools. However, not all school intervention activities were successful. For example, the "Take 10!" classroom intervention did not appear to be successful because it detracted from academic activities and it was difficult for teachers to manage physical activities in small classroom spaces with 30 or more children per class [33]. Teachers prioritized classroom control over activities during instructional time, and only one teacher in a total of six schools maintained the effort for more than a week. Another strategy that was not successful was the "Walking School Bus," which was designed to increase children's active commuting to school [34]. Mothers were asked to help escort their own and neighbors' children to school; however, they were intimidated by the responsibility of keeping multiple children safe on busy streets and therefore none volunteered. These challenges highlight the need to test and refine multiple strategies and to allow for community residents to self-select the strategies that work best for them.

In line with the SEM, APN also targeted improvements in local parks in order to encourage greater use of those parks and increase physical activity opportunities for children. APN also implemented environmental prompts and incentive strategies within elementary schools, local restaurants, and grocery stores to encourage healthy eating and purchasing of healthier options. APN project staff worked with the community *promotoras* on each of these efforts. One major success came directly from the work of the *promotoras*. Over the course of the 3-year study, *promotoras* received regular training in advocacy efforts from APN staff. The *promotoras* identified that local parks needed major renovations in order to make them safer and more appealing for community residents. APN worked with the *promotoras* to formulate an action plan that included obtaining signatures of support from community residents and advocating for these park improvements at city council meetings. The *promotoras* took photos of the poor conditions of the parks and presented these photos during city council meetings and they voiced their concerns over the conditions of parks. These efforts led to the city council's approval of almost half a million dollars to be used to renovate and upgrade one of the largest parks in the community. This success highlights the tremendous potential that is harnessed when working directly with community residents to achieve long-term environmental changes. More importantly, this underscores the importance of supporting and empowering community residents to take the lead in advocating for changes that are meaningful to their families and their own community. The restaurant intervention consisted of targeting locally owned restaurants and promoting changes in their children's menu so that menu options were healthier. The *promotoras* identified several local restaurants and met with the restaurant owners. Over half of the 112 restaurants that were approached agreed to create and/or modify a healthy menu for children. In order to reduce barriers toward implementation, the *promotoras* worked with the restaurant owners to identify simple modifications to their existing menus, and the APN project provided restaurant owners with newly printed children's menus that included healthier options. These new menus also displayed the APN project logo to highlight the project's endorsement of the healthier menu options. In addition, these restaurants were featured in the school newsletters, which promoted the restaurant and their new healthier menus. The grocery store intervention consisted in the development and implementation of a frequent produce buyer program. The program was designed to increase the purchasing of fruits and vegetables through a frequent-buyer card in which the shopper earned a free pound of produce after nine separate purchases of produce. Few grocery stores agreed to participate in this program and as a result very few (<4%) families used the frequent-buyer cards. These examples, of varying success, provide insights into the complexities and the opportunities that arise when working in partnership with community organizations. One major challenge to school-based efforts has been the limited carryover of physical activity and healthy dietary behaviors beyond the school grounds and school time. This necessitates expanding efforts to include other community settings where children can be physically active and eat healthy (e.g., parks and recreation centers).

COMMUNITY-BASED INTERVENTIONS

Many modern urban cities have designated community spaces (e.g., parks) where children and adults can participant in leisure-time physical activity. Children who live in close proximity to parks, walking trails, and recreational facilities also use those facilities more often, engage in more physical activity, and have lower obesity rates [35]. Unfortunately, the distribution and quality of green spaces are not equally distributed across communities. Both the density and quality of parks is much lower within minority and low-income communities compared with more affluent communities [36]. Thus, the equitable distribution of parks and recreational facilities remains an important goal to achieve. Barriers to accessing parks and recreation centers and participating in physical activity within these spaces include lack of awareness that these facilities exist and of the programs they offer, living far from those facilities, having safety concerns, and lack of free age- and culturally appropriate programs [36]. To overcome some of these challenges, many cities have improved and expanded signage in order to inform residents of the location and the programs offered in local community centers [37]. Cities such as Phoenix, AZ have redesigned bicycle and walking paths, implemented the GRID Bike Share Program, and improved street safety features so that residents can more easily walk and/or bike to various locations. Other cities have reduced fencing around parks so that parks are more inviting and accessible, and have worked with local parent groups to increase adult supervision in parks in order to address safety concerns. Improvements in park quality and increasing the number of parks in a neighborhood also increase the value of the homes in those communities [38]. It is therefore mutually beneficial for private organizations, such as real estate agencies, to work with city parks and recreation departments to improve parks and recreational facilities. Shared use agreements between schools and local parks also provide expanded opportunities for children to engage in physical activity after school. These examples highlight the need to further expand collaborations between parks and recreation departments and other public/private organizations in order to improve access to, and use of, community spaces that promote physical activity for all children. Recreation centers also play an important role in children's dietary behaviors. Recreation centers can influence access to healthier food options through items sold in vending machines and via the foods sold in sponsored events. In addition, recreation centers often provide children with meals as part of summer and after-school programs. This represents an important opportunity to influence the dietary quality of the foods that children are provided as part of these programs. Parks and recreation departments can work with local food retailers and distributors, local farms, and farmers market organizations to increase access to healthy and affordable foods within and around community centers. Despite the potential of recreation centers to impact the health of children, there are currently very few programs or initiatives that specifically target recreation centers for the implementation and evaluation of health promotion programs to increase children's physical activity [39,40]. Next, we will describe the implementation and evaluation of a large citywide childhood obesity prevention intervention delivered in recreation centers.

The MOVE/me Muevo project was developed using a multilevel approach to target children's physical activity, dietary behaviors, and child BMI [41]. The study enrolled 30 recreation centers in San Diego, CA and 541 families who lived within 2 miles of one of the recreation centers identified. Fifteen recreation centers, and the corresponding families who lived near the recreation centers, were randomly assigned to receive the intervention and the other fifteen served as a comparison group. Project team members met with center directors and administrators to identify recreation-level outcomes and develop an action plan to achieve those outcomes. Recreation center administrators identified that increasing the use of facilities and programs were the top priorities. To achieve these outcomes, the study team designated one team member to work directly with each center director to develop specific strategies that would improve the center's visibility and attendance by community residents. These strategies included improving signage placement and information about programs within and immediately around the community centers, improving customer service via staff trainings, and identifying ways to expand program offerings to children and families. In addition, center directors were encouraged to identify policies that would increase healthier food options within the recreation centers and in sponsored events. For example, vending machine contracts were evaluated to identify changes that would improve the proportion of healthy snacks and beverage offerings. Two health coaches also worked directly with families in order to promote greater use and participation in programs offered in the recreation centers. Over the course of the 2-year intervention, several family workshops were held at the community centers in order to increase families' exposure to the recreation centers and to implement interactive education activities related to healthy eating and physical activity. Similar to the APN study described earlier, important and sustainable macrolevel outcomes were achieved over the 2-year study. The existing city's vending machine contract was evaluated and changes were made to the contract to explicitly require that at least 50% of the items in all vending machines meet healthy standards for snacks and drinks. Also, center directors enacted new policies that required that healthy options be offered during special events such as during staff meetings. Center informational brochures were also modified to include healthy-living tips related to physical activity and healthy eating. Lastly, the Parks and Recreation Department decided to offer yearly trainings for their staff who wanted to obtain specialized certifications (e.g., group fitness instructor). Similar to the APN study, these findings again highlight the importance of working with administrators and empowering them to advocate for systemic changes that can lead to long-term macrolevel changes in community environments that can, in turn, influence children's physical activity and dietary behaviors.

SPECIAL CONSIDERATIONS AND RECOMMENDATIONS

The current trends in childhood obesity have resulted in greater efforts to understand the environmental (proximal and distal) and social factors that support an obesogenic environment. Several school-based programs and strategies have shown promise to reduce or taper childhood obesity [19,20]. However, there are equally several studies that have not been able to do so [25,26,29]. It is clear that interorganizational collaborations and coalitions provide the best opportunities to leverage resources and expertise across multiple community settings and that schools cannot undertake the challenges of combating childhood obesity alone [42]. The list of potential collaborators includes the YMCA, Boys & Girls Clubs, recreation centers, faith-based organizations, community clinics, and private businesses. For example, the Athletes for Life (AFL) project located in Phoenix, AZ, is a sustainable collaboration between Arizona State University and the City of Phoenix Parks and Recreation Department [43]. Through this collaboration, community residents have access to a free, culturally appropriate, and efficacious fitness and nutrition education program. Data support that recreation centers and other recreational facilities can positively influence children's behaviors [41], yet there are still few studies to allow for the development of specific evidence-based recommendations. Important sources of information that are often overlooked or underreported in published studies are the contextual factors and macrolevel changes that can take place during community-based interventions (e.g., environmental and policy changes). These effects may be overlooked or underreported because they may not result in immediate or observable changes in child BMI. For example, the APN study described earlier did not demonstrate significant intervention effects on child BMI despite an intensive family- and school-based approach [29]. However, important improvements were made to a local park due to the advocacy efforts of *promotoras*. It is conceivable that those park improvements would stimulate greater park use and thus more physical activity among community residents living near the park. Similarly, the MOVE/me Muevo study did not show an overall effect on child BMI, but it did show a positive moderating effect on girls' BMI [41]. The MOVE/me Muevo study also resulted in important policy and recreation-level changes that may influence community resident's physical activity and dietary behaviors. These two examples (APN and MOVE/me Muevo) serve as case studies that highlight a possible mismatch between the intervention approach (i.e., community based) and the targeted outcome (i.e., child BMI). Specifically, community-based approaches may result in several important macrolevel outcomes (e.g., policy changes, structural changes, economic improvements) as a function of the levels being targeted (i.e., organizational and environmental). Yet, these macrolevel changes may lead to relatively modest, but potentially long-term, effects on children's physical activity and dietary behaviors, which may or may not lead to observable or immediate changes in child BMI. Thus, we encourage researchers and practitioners who work in community settings to consider refocusing expectations away from individual-level outcomes, such as BMI, to focusing on designing and evaluating broader and macrolevel outcomes, such as changes in policies and environmental (social and built environment) factors that contribute to changing the current obesogenic environments. Special considerations should also be given to designing and implementing programs and strategies that contribute to increasing health equality and access to health-enhancing resources for all children and residents.

REFERENCES

1. Bronfenbrenner, U. 1994. Ecological models of human development. In *International Encyclopedia of Education*, Vol. 3, 2nd ed. Oxford: Elsevier.
2. McLeroy, K., Bibeau, D., Steckler, A., Glanz, K. 1988. An ecological perspective on health promotion programs. *Health Education Quarterly*, 15:351–377.

3. Colorectal Cancer Control Program (CRCCP). Social ecological model. Division of Cancer Prevention and Control, Centers for Disease Control and Prevention. October 27, 2015. Available at http://www.cdc.gov/cancer/crccp/sem.htm.

4. Whittemore, R., Melkus, G.D., Grey, M. 2004. Applying the social ecological theory to type 2 diabetes prevention and management. *Journal of Community Health Nursing*, 21(2):87–99.

5. Swinburn, B., Egger, G., Raza, F. 1999. Dissecting obesogenic environments: The development and application of the framework for identifying and prioritizing environmental interventions for obesity. *Preventive Medicine*, 29:563–570.

6. Sorensen, G., Emmons, K., Hunt, M.K., Barbeau, E., Goldman, R., Peterson, K., Kuntz, K., Stoddard, A., Berkman, L. 2003. Model for incorporating social context in health behavior interventions: Applications for cancer prevention for working-class, multiethnic populations. *Preventive Medicine*, 37(3):188–197.

7. Gregson, J., Foerste, S., Orr, R., Jones, L., Benedict, J., Clarke, B., Hersey, J., Lewis, J., Zotz, K. 2001. System, environmental, and policy changes: Using the social-ecological model as a framework for evaluating nutrition education and social marketing programs with low-income audiences. *Journal of Nutrition Education*, 33(1):S4–S15.

8. Sallis, J.F., Owen, N., Fisher, E.B. 2008. Ecological models of health behavior. In Glanz, K., Rimer, B.K., Viswanath, K. eds., *Health Behavior and Health Education: Theory, Research and Practice*, 4th ed. San Francisco, CA: Jossey-Bass.

9. Spence, J.C., Lee, R.E. 2003. Toward a comprehensive model of physical activity. *Psychology of Sport and Exercise*, 4(1):7–24.

10. Elder, J.P., Ayala, G.X., Parra-Medina, D., Talavera, G.A. 2009. Health communication in the Latino community: Issues and approaches. *Annual Review of Public Health*, 30:227–251.

11. Story, M., Kaphingst, K.M., Robinson-O'Brien, R., Glanz, K. 2008. Creating healthy food and eating environments: Policy and environmental approaches. *Annual Review of Public Health*, 29:253–272.

12. Huang, T.T., Drewnowski, A., Kumanyika, S.K., Glass, T.A. 2009. A systems-oriented multilevel framework for addressing obesity in the 21st century. *Preventing Chronic Disease*, 6(3):A82.

13. Lindsay, A.C., Sussner, K.M., Kim, J., Gortmaker, S. 2006. The role of parents in preventing childhood obesity. *The Future of Children*, 16(1):169–186.

14. Ayala, G.X., Elder, J.P., Campbell, N.R., Arredondo, E., Baquero, B., Crespo, N.C., Slymen, D.J. 2010. Longitudinal intervention effects on parenting of the Aventuras para Niños study. *American Journal of Preventive Medicine*, 38(2):154–162.

15. Doak, C.M., Visscher, T.L.S., Renders, C.M., Seidell, J.C. 2006. The prevention of overweight and obesity in children and adolescents: A review of interventions and programmes. *Obesity Reviews*, 7:111–136.

16. Dunton, G.F., Kaplan, J., Wolch, J., Jerrett, M., Reynolds, K.D. 2009. Physical environmental correlates of childhood obesity: A systematic review. *Obesity Reviews*, 10:393–402.

17. Holub, C.K., Elder, J.P., Arredondo, E.M., Barquera, S., Eisenberg, C.M., Sanchez, L.M., Rivera, J., Lobelo, F., Simoes, E.J. 2013. Obesity control in Latin American and U.S. Latinos: A systematic review. *American Journal of Preventive Medicine*, 44(5):529–537.

18. DeMattia, L., Denney, S.L. 2008. Childhood obesity prevention: Successful community-based efforts. *The Annals of the American Academy of Political and Social Science*. 615(1):83–99.

19. Gortmaker, S.L., Peterson, K., Wiecha, J., Sobol, A.M., Dixit, S., Fox, M.K., Laird, N. 1999. Reducing obesity via a school-based interdisciplinary intervention among youth: Planet Health. *Archives of Pediatric Adolescent Medicine*, 153(4):409–418.

20. Robinson, T.N. 1999. Reducing children's television viewing to prevent obesity: A randomized controlled trial. *JAMA*, 282(16):1561–1567.

21. Veugelers, P.J., Fitzgerald, A.L. 2004. Effectiveness of school programs in preventing childhood obesity: A multilevel comparison. *American Journal of Public Health*, 95:432–435.

22. Luepker, R.V., Perry, C.L., McKinlay, S.M., Nader, P.R., Parcel, G.S., Stone, E.J., Webber, L.S., et al. 1996. Outcomes of a field trial to improve children's dietary patterns and physical activity: The Child and Adolescent Trial for Cardiovascular Health—CATCH collaborative group. *JAMA*, 13(10):768–776.

23. Nader, P.R., Stone, E.J., Lytle, L.A., Perry, C.L., Osganiana, S.K., Kelder, S., Webber, L.S., et al. 1999. Three-year maintenance of improved diet and physical activity: The CATCH cohort—Child and Adolescent Trial for Cardiovascular Health. *Archives of Pediatric and Adolescent Medicine*, 153(7):695–704.

24. Webber, L.S., Catellier, D.J., Lytle, L.A., Murray, D.M., Pratt, C.A., Young, D.R., Elder, J.P., Lohman, T.G., Stevens, J., Jobe, J.B., Pate, R.R. 2008. Promoting physical activity in middle school girls: Trial of activity for adolescent girls. *American Journal of Preventive Medicine*, 34(3):173–184.

25. Gonzalez-Suarez, C., Worley, A., Grimmer-Somers, K., Dones, V. 2009. School-based interventions on childhood obesity: A meta-analysis. *American Journal of Preventive Medicine*, 37(5):418–427.

26. Brown, T., Summerbell, C. 2009. Systematic review of school-based interventions that focus on changing dietary intake and physical activity levels to prevent childhood obesity: An update to the obesity guidance produced by the National Institute for Health and Clinical Excellence. *Obesity Reviews*, 10:110–141.

27. Caprio, S., Daniels, S.R., Drewnowski, A., Kaufman, F.R., Painkas, L.A., Rosenbloom, A.L., Schwimmer, J.B. 2008. Influence of race, ethnicity, and culture on childhood obesity: Implications for prevention and treatment—A consensus statement of Shaping American's Health and the Obesity Society. *Diabetes Care*, 31(11):2211–2221.

28. Kropski, J.A., Kecklery, P.H., Jensen, G.L. 2008. School-based obesity prevention programs: An evidence-based review. *Obesity*, 16:1009–1018.

29. Crespo, N.C., Elder, J.P., Ayala, G.X., Slymen, D.J., Campbell, N.R., Sallis, J.F., McKenzie, T.L., Baquero, B., Arredondo, E.M. 2012. Results of a multi-level intervention to prevent and control childhood obesity among Latino children: The Aventuras Para Niños Study. *Annals of Behavioral Medicine*, 43(1):84–100.

30. Ayala, G.X., Vaz, L., Earp, J.A., Elder, J.P., Cherrington, A. 2010. Outcome effectiveness of the lay health advisor model among Latinos in the United States: An examination by role. *Health Education Research*, 25(5):815–840.

31. Stratton, G., Mullan, E. 2005. The effect of multicolor playground markings on children's physical activity level during recess. *Preventive Medicine*, 41(5):828–833.

32. Ridgers, N.D., Stratton, G., Fairclough, S.J., Twisk, J.W.R. 2007. Long-term effects of a playground markings and physical structures on children's recess physical activity levels. *Preventive Medicine*, 44:393–397.

33. Stewart, J.A., Dennison, D.A., Kohl, H.W., Doyle, J.A. 2004. Exercise level and energy expenditure in the Take 10! in-class physical activity program. *Journal of School Health*, 74(10):397–400.

34. Lee, M.C., Orenstein, M.R., Richardson, M.J. 2008. Systematic review of active commuting to school and children's physical activity and weight. *Journal of Physical Activity and Health*, 5(6):930–949.

35. Blanck, H.M., Allen, D., Bashir, Z., Gordon, N., Goodman, A., Merriam, D., Rutt, C. 2012. Let's go to the park today: The role of parks in obesity prevention and improving the public's health. *Childhood Obesity*, 8(5):423–428.

36. Dai, D. 2011. Racial/ethnic and socioeconomic disparities in urban green space accessibility: Where to intervene? *Landscape and Urban Planning*, 102(4):234–244.

37. National Recreation and Park Association. CDC ACHIEVE healthy communities initiative. http://www.cdc.gov/nccdphp/dch/programs/healthycommunitiesprogram/communities/achieve/. Accessed December 10, 2015.

38. Active Living Research. 2010. *The Economic Benefits of Open Space, Recreation Facilities and Walkable Community Design*. Available at http://activelivingresearch.org/files/Synthesis_Shoup-Ewing_March2010_0.pdf. Accessed December 10, 2015.

39. Moody, J.S., Prochaska, J.J., Sallis, J.F., McKenzie, T.L., Brown, M., Conway, T.L. 2004. Viability of parks and recreation centers as sites for youth physical activity promotion. *Health Promotion Practice*, 5(4):438–443.

40. Foltz, J.L., May, A.L., Belay, B., Nihiser, A.J., Dooyema, C.A., Blanck, H.M. 2012. Population-level intervention strategies and examples of obesity prevention in children. *Annual Review of Nutrition*, 32:391–415.

41. Elder, J.P., Crespo, N.C., Corder, K., Ayala, G.X., Slymen, D.J., Lopez, N.V., Moody, J.S., McKenzie, T.L. 2014. Childhood obesity prevention and control in city recreation centres and family homes: The MOVE/me Muevo Project. *Pediatric Obesity*, 9:218–231.

42. Peterson, K.E., Fox, M.K. 2007. Addressing the epidemic of childhood obesity through school-based interventions: What has been done and where do we go from here? *Journal of Law, Medicine and Ethics*, 35(1):113–130.

43. Crespo, N.C., Chavez, A., Vega-López, S., Ray, F., Tarango, T., Todd, M., Huberty, J., Shaibi, G. 2015. A community-based program improves body composition and cardiovascular fitness among underserved children: The Athletes for Life study. *Oral Presentation. American Public Health Association*.

37 Targeting Reduction in Consumption of Added Sugars for Addressing Childhood Obesity
Translating Research to Clinical Practice

Cara B. Ebbeling and Melissa Gallagher Landry

CONTENTS

INTRODUCTION

Recommendations to reduce dietary sugar have been part of efforts to promote public health[1] and weight loss[2] over the last 4 decades and thus are not novel. However, in recent years, recommendations have become more comprehensive and explicit. The first national nutrition guidelines, released in 1977 as *Dietary Goals for the United States*, included the recommendation to reduce the consumption of "refined and processed sugars and foods high in such sugars."[1] The *2015–2020 Dietary Guidelines for Americans* advocate limiting consumption of added sugars, as defined in the next section, to less than 10% of daily energy (calorie) intake.[3] However, a wide variety of sugary foods is readily available on the shelves of grocery stores, and children in the United States consume just over 85 g (more than 20 teaspoons) of added sugars per day, on average, equating to more than 15% of daily energy intake.[4]

TABLE 37.1

Vignette: Data from Nutrition Assessment (with Potential Relevance to Dietary Intake of Added Sugars)

Patient and Family History

Julia is a 7-year-old Hispanic female living with her single mother and grandmother. Julia's mother has a high-school education and works full time. She has a family medical history of obesity, type 2 diabetes mellitus, and depression.

Anthropometric Data

Height: 133.4 cm (84th percentile, z-score = +1.01), *Weight*: 52.7 kg (99th percentile, z-score = +2.89), *BMI*: 29.6 kg/m² (99th percentile, z-score = +2.64)

Patient BMI trend >95th percentile from age 2 according to electronic medical record

Biochemical Data

Hyperinsulinism

Physical Examination and Medical History

+Acanthosis nigricans (neck), constipation

Food- and Nutrition-Related Data

Meals: Receives free breakfast and lunch at school. Eats dinner at the table with family.

Snacks: Offered midmorning and after school. Snacking is significant for grain-based desserts (though Julia will eat vegetables and whole fruits).

Beverages: 24+ oz. SSBs (100% fruit juice, fruit drink, chocolate milk)
- 8 oz. of homemade juice with Metamucil in the morning, 8 oz. of homemade juice with dinner.
- 4 oz. carton of chocolate milk with lunch.
- 4 oz. juice box for afternoon snack. Julia often asks for more if feeling bored.
- No soda and water occasionally, but Julia states preferring the taste of juice.

Desserts: Cookies and grain-based fruit bars for afternoon and evening snacks.

Beliefs and Attitudes: Grandmother does not like telling Julia "no" when she asks for juice and snack foods. Mother believes that consuming 100% fruit juices (particularly homemade) is important for healthy growth and should be part of Julia's childhood experience.

This chapter provides a reference for clinicians who counsel children and families on weight control, highlighting key research on reducing sugar consumption and considering pragmatic intervention strategies. A vignette is presented in Table 37.1 to set the stage for addressing clinically relevant questions pertaining to dietary sugar. At the end of the chapter, an approach to developing evidence-based care plans to reduce intake of added sugars is exemplified using the vignette.

WHAT IS DIETARY SUGAR?

From a biochemical perspective, the term *sugar* encompasses monosaccharides (glucose, fructose, galactose) and disaccharides comprising two monosaccharides linked by a glycosidic bond (sucrose: glucose–fructose, lactose: glucose–galactose, maltose: glucose–glucose). For the *2015–2020 Dietary Guidelines*,[3] the US Department of Health and Human Services and the Department of Agriculture defined *added sugars* as "sugars that are either added during the processing of foods, or are packaged as such, and include sugars (free, mono- and disaccharides), syrups, naturally occurring sugars that are isolated from a whole food and concentrated so that sugar is the primary component (e.g., fruit juice concentrates), and other caloric sweeteners." This is consistent with the definition put forth by the Food and Drug Administration (FDA) when it proposed to include added sugars on the revised *nutrition facts* panel of labels.[5] The World Health Organization (WHO) defines *free sugars* as "monosaccharides and disaccharides added to foods and beverages by the manufacturer, cook or consumer, and sugars naturally present in honey, syrups, fruit juices and fruit juice concentrates."[6] The WHO strongly recommends limiting intake of free sugars to less than 10% of daily energy intake, consistent with the *Dietary Guidelines*, and further suggests a threshold of 5%.[6] Although generally analogous, the definition of *added sugars* is less explicit than the definition of *free sugars* for fruit juices. We use the term *added sugars* throughout this chapter, to be consistent with the *Dietary Guidelines*, but agree with the explicit recommendation to limit consumption of fruit juice.

The sugars consumed most frequently in the United States are refined beet or cane sugar (sucrose) and high-fructose corn syrup (HFCS). Sucrose and HFCS are similar in sweetness[7] and have the same energy content. While sucrose contains 50% fructose and 50% glucose as a disaccharide, HFCS contains free fructose and free glucose. The two forms of HFCS used by the food industry are HFCS-55 (55% fructose, 42% glucose, 3% hydrolyzable polymers of glucose) in sugar-sweetened beverages (SSBs) and HFCS-42 (42% fructose, 53% glucose, 5% hydrolyzable polymers of glucose) in solid foods. Although, some studies of measured sugar composition indicate higher levels of fructose in beverages made with HFCS.[8,9] The glycosidic bond in sucrose is hydrolyzed by the enzyme sucrase in the brush border of the small intestine, yielding free fructose and free glucose for absorption. As such, while metabolic pathways for glucose and fructose are different, absorption of glucose or fructose is the same whether consumed as sucrose or HFCS. Interventions aimed at decreasing the consumption of added sugars should focus on the sum total of sucrose and HFCS.

WHY IS DIETARY SUGAR AN IMPORTANT CONSIDERATION FOR WEIGHT CONTROL?

The importance of limiting dietary sugar across the life span is underscored by data from observational studies indicating a direct relationship between the consumption of added sugars and risk for obesity,[10] nonalcoholic fatty liver disease,[11] type 2 diabetes mellitus,[12] coronary heart disease,[13] and periodontal disease[14]. Studies also provide insights regarding the influence of early-life experiences with sweet taste on the propensity to consume diets high in added sugars.[15] However, while most public health advocates and clinicians agree that dietary recommendations to reduce the consumption of added sugars may be effective for weight control and reducing the risk for chronic disease, the rationale for such recommendations is a topic of debate.[16–18] With the consensus that added sugars are highly palatable sources of energy, the debate addresses the unique effects of added sugars, compared with other sources of energy, on metabolism. Representing one extreme of the debate, some argue that any adverse outcomes from consuming added sugars are largely a consequence of high-energy content.[17] This perspective arguably may be influenced by ties with the beverage industry. Others have interpreted the published literature differently when considering the metabolic effects of glucose and fructose, the unique effects of consuming sugar in liquid versus solid form, and the hedonic appeal of added sugars.

METABOLIC EFFECTS OF GLUCOSE AND FRUCTOSE

Glucose and fructose have the same number of carbon, hydrogen, and oxygen molecules ($C_6H_{12}O_6$) but different chemical structures and thus are metabolized differently. Each is absorbed into the portal circulation. A substantial portion of glucose passes through the liver and enters the systemic circulation, while most fructose is metabolized in the liver. Glucose triggers insulin release from the β cells of the pancreas, promoting hepatic glycogenesis and glucose uptake by skeletal muscle, adipose tissue, and other tissues throughout the body. When sugar is consumed in large amounts, postprandial hyperglycemia causes an exuberant insulin response and a marked increase in circulating insulin relative to glucagon. This hormonal milieu causes a drop in blood glucose below fasting levels, limited fuel availability, increased hunger, overeating, and ultimately weight gain.[19] The same cascade of events occurs following the consumption of starch, particularly from refined sources, which is quickly metabolized to glucose.[19] In contrast to glucose, fructose does not stimulate insulin secretion from the pancreas and requires energy in the form of adenosine triphosphate (ATP) for metabolism. Fructose metabolism is not regulated by hepatic energy stores. When sugar is consumed in large amounts, rapid absorption of fructose may overwhelm metabolic pathways leading to *de novo* lipogenesis and increased uric acid.[20,21] Hepatic fructose metabolism has been implicated with cardiometabolic risk factors including hepatic steatosis, excess visceral adiposity, dyslipidemia, insulin resistance (hepatic and systemic), inflammation, hypertension, and endothelial dysfunction.[18,20,22]

The rate of absorption of fructose from added sugars compared with natural sources, most notably whole fruits, warrants comment. While fructose from added sugars is absorbed rapidly and has the potential to overwhelm hepatic metabolism when consumed in large amounts, fructose from fruits is absorbed more slowly and does not seem to have the same adverse effects.[18] Slower absorption may be attributed to the integrity of the cellular structure and fiber content of whole fruits. Data from prospective cohort studies suggest that consuming whole fruit protects against cardiometabolic risk, while consuming fruit juice increases risk.[23,24]

UNIQUE EFFECTS OF CONSUMING SUGAR IN LIQUID VERSUS SOLID FORM

Sugar-sweetened carbonated beverages and fruit juices contain approximately 150 kcal per conventional 12 oz. can and 80 kcal per 6 oz. glass, respectively, but often are available in amounts much larger than conventional serving sizes. Several studies indicate imprecise dietary energy compensation following consumption of sugar in liquid form. Compared with solid foods containing the same amount of sugar, beverages require less oral processing (jaw and tongue movements to prepare food for swallowing), have shorter gastric emptying and gastrointestinal transit times, and may attenuate satiety signals and cognitive perceptions of energy intake.[25] As such, children who consume SSBs may not compensate by decreasing other dietary sources of energy, leading to positive energy balance and weight gain. In a study of children aged 7–11 years who were randomly assigned to drink either a sugar-sweetened or sugar-free beverage, de Ruyter et al.[26] found no difference in satiety at 15 minutes following the consumption of a single 250 mL (8.5 oz.) serving. Children who consumed the SSB daily for 18 months accumulated more body fat than their counterparts who consumed the sugar-free beverage, suggesting imprecise compensation.[27]

HEDONIC APPEAL OF ADDED SUGARS

Humans have an innate desire for sweet foods and beverages from birth.[15] Detection of sweet taste activates pleasure centers of the brain associated with reward and triggers strong hedonic responses. A preference for intense sweetness is particularly high in children and declines to adult levels during adolescence.[28] Nevertheless, habitual sensory experiences early in life can modify preference and may have chronic effects on eating patterns and body weight. In a cross-sectional study, Pepino and Mennella[29] observed that children aged 6–10 years who were routinely exposed to sugar water during infancy, compared with those who were not, preferred solutions with higher concentrations of sucrose. Liem and de Graaf[30] reported that repeated exposure to a sucrose-sweetened beverage for 8 days enhanced preference for the beverage in primary-school children.

Research is needed to determine how early-life experiences and availability of sweetened foods interact to influence food preferences, energy consumption, and body weight over the life span. In a small prospective study, Weijs et al.[31] found that the consumption of SSBs during infancy increased the risk of overweight at 8 years of age, independent of self-reported energy intake at the follow-up assessment. Ventura and Mennella[15] point out that repeated exposure to sweet foods or beverages probably does not augment the hedonic response to the sensation of sweetness in general; rather, the context of repeated exposure likely is more important, as children develop expectations regarding the sweetness intensity of familiar foods and beverages in habitual circumstances. Using state-of-the-art methodology (functional magnetic resonance imaging) to evaluate neural responsivity, Burger and Stice[32] noted the activation of taste and reward regions of the brain in adolescents following the consumption of a branded soft drink containing 17 g (just over 4 teaspoons) of sugar in

150 mL (5 oz.). For those who were regular consumers, simply seeing the brand logo activated a region of the brain thought to encode salience or attention to cues.

WHAT ARE THE PRIMARY FOOD SOURCES OF ADDED SUGARS IN THE DIETS OF CHILDREN?

Based on data from the National Health and Nutrition Examination Survey (NHANES), the primary food sources of added sugars for children and adolescents include soda (and energy and sports drinks), fruit drinks, candy, grain- and dairy-based desserts, ready-to-eat cereals, and syrups/toppings.[33] Approximately 65%–70% of added sugars come from foods and beverages purchased at supermarkets or grocery stores as opposed to quick-service restaurants (including pizza takeout/delivery), full-service restaurants, schools, and other places (e.g., vending machines).[33] More calories from added sugars are consumed at home than away from home.[34] Data from a national cross-sectional study of schoolchildren indicate that the consumption of SSBs at home contributes the greatest proportion of calories from added sugars.[35]

WHAT ARE CURRENT RECOMMENDATIONS FOR SUGAR INTAKE?

Previous editions of the *Dietary Guidelines for Americans* included warnings on the adverse health effects of consuming excessive amounts of added sugars with no recommendation for an upper limit. For the first time, the 8th edition of the *Dietary Guidelines* includes a specific recommendation to limit the consumption of added sugars to less than 10% of daily energy intake.[3] The WHO strongly recommends limiting the intake of free sugars to less than 10%, and further suggests a threshold less than 5% of daily energy intake.[6]

WHAT INTERVENTIONS ARE EFFICACIOUS FOR DECREASING SUGAR INTAKE AND PROMOTING WEIGHT LOSS AMONG CHILDREN AND ADOLESCENTS?

A variety of comprehensive obesity interventions have included recommendations to reduce the consumption of added sugars, frequently in combination with messages to increase fruit and vegetable consumption and physical activity and decrease sedentary time.[36] In most intervention studies with a primary focus on reducing the consumption of added sugars, researchers have designated SSBs as a specific target. Interventions include public health initiatives, educational programs in schools, and alterations in beverage availability either at school or home. The impact and outcomes of these public health or research interventions provide insights on preventing and treating obesity in a clinical context.

PUBLIC-HEALTH INITIATIVES

Media campaigns typically do not lead to changes in behavior directly but can increase awareness, alter attitudes and perceptions, and, thus, enhance motivation and intention to change.[37] Boles et al.[37] evaluated the impact of a campaign involving mass media (messaging via web, television, billboards, and transit) and implemented over a calendar year to educate residents of Portland, Oregon, about SSBs. Adults who were aware of the campaign agreed that excess sugar intake causes health problems and reported the intention to decrease the amounts of SSBs that they offered to children. Jordan et al.[38] explored the impact of public service announcements on the intention to reduce child consumption of SSBs in a national sample of parents with children aged 3–17 years. Perceived argument strength among parents was related to the intention to reduce child consumption, with announcements designed to convey messages of fear (e.g., "Are you pouring on the pounds?" with information about negative health outcomes) or nurturance (e.g., "Know where the sugar is hiding," focusing on boxed school lunches) deemed stronger than those that incorporated humor (e.g., "Soda might give you a temporary lift, but it can also make you crash," with adolescents "crashing" their heads in various school settings).

The multifaceted approach taken in New York City to reduce the consumption of SSBs[39] has been well publicized in the lay press. In addition to mass-media educational campaigns, this approach included nutritional standards for beverages (applied in schools, early child-care centers, and camps) and policy changes such as calorie counts on menu boards. A 27% decrease in the consumption of SSBs among high-school students from 2007 to 2013 was attributed to these public health initiatives.[39] Proposals to cap the size of containers used to serve SSBs in food service establishments, tax SSBs, and eliminate SSBs as allowable purchases through the Supplemental Nutrition Assistance Program were rejected but nevertheless may have enhanced awareness of the deleterious effects of consuming SSBs on body weight and the risk for other chronic diseases.

EDUCATIONAL PROGRAMS IN SCHOOLS

Several studies indicate that educational programs can lead to decreases in the consumption of SSBs,[40] and a couple of studies suggest that changes in consumption may have beneficial effects on body weight.[41,42] James et al.[41] conducted a school-based cluster randomized trial in England with 644 students aged 7–11 years. During four classes, a researcher with assistance from teachers encouraged reduced consumption of all "fizzy" beverages and increased consumption of water. Activities included taste testing of fruit to expose students to natural sweetness, a demonstration on how sweetened carbonated soda can adversely affect dentition, and producing songs and art around the message to "ditch the fizz." Over 1 year, the prevalence of obesity decreased by 0.2% among children who received the educational program and increased by 7.5% in the control group, although change in body mass index (BMI) was not different between groups. The group difference in prevalence observed at 1 year was not sustained at 3 years.[43] Sichieri et al.[42] conducted a cluster randomized trial in Brazil with 1140 students aged 9–12 years. They provided education and encouragement to reduce the consumption of SSBs and increase the consumption of water using classroom activities (similar to those implemented by James et al.[41]) during 10 sessions, banners displayed in the school, and water bottles portraying the campaign logo. Over one academic year, BMI decreased among overweight girls in the intervention compared with the control group, but the group effect was not significant in the full cohort.

ALTERATIONS IN BEVERAGE AVAILABILITY

Interventions that alter beverage availability arguably hold the most promise for preventing or treating obesity.

De Ruyter et al.[27] randomly assigned 641 schoolchildren, aged 4–11 years, to receive a sugar-free beverage, artificially sweetened with sucralose and acesulfame potassium, or an SSB containing 26 g of sucrose and 104 kcal. The trial was conducted using a double-blind design. The two beverages had the same level of sweetness and were packaged in indistinguishable cans. Researchers instructed children to drink one can (250 mL, 8.5 oz.) per day. Among 477 children who completed the 18-month study, the increase in BMI z-score was smaller for the group consuming the sugar-free beverage compared with the SSB (0.02 vs. 0.15 units). Likewise, weight (6.33 vs. 7.30 kg) and fat mass (1.02 vs. 1.57 kg) increased less in the group consuming the sugar-free beverage.

Ebbeling et al.[44] randomly assigned 224 overweight and obese adolescents who habitually consumed SSBs to intervention and control groups for 2 years. Participants in the intervention group received home deliveries of noncaloric beverages, as a strategy to displace SSBs, for 1 year. They were offered a menu of options that included water and artificially sweetened ("diet") beverages. Registered dietitians conducted monthly motivational telephone calls with parents, focusing on modeling healthful beverage consumption and stimulus control (removing SSBs from the home) and educational sessions with participants. During educational sessions, dietitians encouraged participants to "think before you drink" and provided information to increase awareness regarding the amounts of sugar in beverages; the benefits of drinking unsweetened water; the possible effects of SSBs in promoting excess energy intake, weight gain, tooth decay, hunger, and lethargy; and misleading beverage labels and advertisements. During calls and educational sessions, dietitians highly encouraged the consumption of water, presenting "diet" beverages as an option during the transition from SSBs to water. Consumption of SSBs dropped to almost zero, based on self-report, with the 1-year intervention. Between-group differences for changes in BMI (-0.57 kg/m^2) and body weight (-1.9 kg) were significant, due to smaller increases in the intervention compared with the control group. After an additional 1-year follow-up period, discontinuation of the home deliveries extinguished group effects. Data obtained at 1 year reflect the effects of an active intervention and arguably are more relevant when considering the efficacy of altering beverage availability at home to promote weight loss.

ARE SOME INDIVIDUALS MORE SUSCEPTIBLE TO EFFECTS OF ADDED SUGARS ON BODY WEIGHT?

Some individuals may be particularly susceptible to the adverse effects of added sugars on body weight and may benefit more than others from interventions aimed at reducing added sugars.[44,45] A combination of factors underlying susceptibility may include ethnicity and race,[44,46] genetics,[47] propensity to secrete insulin in response to sugar consumption,[48] and disparities related to socioeconomic status and early-life feeding experiences.[46] For example, Ebbeling et al.[44] observed a significant difference in BMI between the intervention and control groups among Hispanic participants following a 1-year intervention with home deliveries of noncaloric beverages (-1.79 kg/m^2) and also after an additional 1-year follow-up period (-2.35 kg/m^2). The group effect was not significant among non-Hispanic participants. Consistent with this finding, a reanalysis of data from a 19-month prospective observational study of middle-school students[10] also indicated a strong relationship between change in consumption of SSBs and change in BMI among Hispanics ($p = .007$) but no association among non-Hispanics.[44] Effect modification by variables that may underlie susceptibility warrants additional research.

DEVELOPING EVIDENCE-BASED CARE PLANS TO REDUCE INTAKE OF ADDED SUGARS

Effective dietary interventions for preventing and treating obesity provide a scaffold for sequential changes in diet over time to eventually reach optimal intake. The order and time course of changes established collaboratively between individual patients and health-care providers in clinical settings are based on the unique needs and capacities of families. Often, devising care plans to reduce the intake of sugary foods and particularly beverages is a good place to start regardless of stance in the aforementioned debate. Although most studies of interventions aimed at reducing the consumption of added sugars for weight control have targeted SSBs *per se*, counseling patients to reduce their intake of added sugars from all sources is prudent based on the metabolic effects of glucose and fructose from refined sources and also the possibility of compromised micronutrient intake when foods containing added sugars displace more healthful options.[49]

A reasonable approach to developing dietary-care plans targeting reduction in added sugars, based on evidence when available, includes a nutrition assessment, clear messages to reduce or eliminate the intake of target foods and beverages identified in the assessment, relevant education to foster behavior change consistent with messages, and counseling on modifiable factors associated with the intake of added sugars. Reducing consumption to less than 10% of daily energy intake, as specified in the *Dietary Guidelines* and consistent with the WHO recommendation, is a pragmatic goal. The vignette presented in Table 37.1 captures the type of information that often emerges from a nutrition assessment, with particular attention to the consumption of added sugars, and an intervention pertaining to the vignette is presented in Table 37.2 to exemplify the approach described next.

The following list of target foods and beverages, based on the primary food sources of added sugars in the diets of children and corresponding messages to reduce or eliminate the consumption of these foods, can inform the design of tailored care plans.

- *Beverages.* Drink few or no regular sodas, sports drinks, energy drinks, and fruit drinks. Limit 100% fruit juice to no more than 4 oz. per day for children aged 1–6 years and no more than 8 oz. per day for children aged 7 years and older, consistent with lower limits specified by the American Academy of Pediatrics.[50] Choose water, minimally sweetened beverages (no more than 1 g added sugar per oz.), and unsweetened milk according to general recommendations.[3] (Regarding artificially sweetened beverages, while typically considered safe alternatives to SSBs,[51] additional research is needed to evaluate the possible adverse effects of high sweetness intensity on taste preferences and body weight.[52])
- *Candy and grain- and dairy-based desserts.* Limit candy and desserts with added sugars. Encourage replacement of candy and desserts with vegetables (no added sugars), whole fruits (natural sugar that is more slowly absorbed compared with added sugars), and whole grains (starch that breaks down to glucose more slowly than starch from refined products) that are more abundant in micronutrients.

TABLE 37.2

Back to Vignette: Intervention for Reducing Intake of Added Sugars (Based on Assessment in Table 37.1)

Messages to Reduce or Eliminate Intake of Target Foods and Beverages

Beverages: Drink water and plain milk. Limit 100% fruit juice to no more than 8 oz. per day. Eliminate fruit drinks.
Desserts: Limit dessert intake. Replace with vegetables, fruits, and whole grains.

Relevant Education to Foster Behavior Change Consistent with Messages

Build Awareness to Increase Importance and Enhance Motivation for Change: Link between the consumption of sugar, insulin secretion, acanthosis nigricans, and risk for type 2 diabetes mellitus. Importance of whole fruits, vegetables, and whole grains for relieving constipation.
Develop Knowledge and Skills to Operationalize Messages: Based on estimated daily energy intake of 1640 kcal, prescribe upper limit of ~40 g per day of added sugars: (1640 × 0.10)/4. Support label reading to identify sources and calculate grams of added sugars. Use visuals (e.g., sugar cubes) to enhance knowledge regarding sources of added sugars and motivation for behavior change. Review age-appropriate portion sizes.

Counseling on Modifiable Factors Associated with Intake of Added Sugars

Beliefs and Attitudes: Explore family beliefs around the importance of consuming juice during childhood and use appropriate counseling strategies to adjust misconceptions. Assess alterations in beliefs and attitudes as a result of education and counseling.
Access to Foods and Beverages: Replace juice and grain-based desserts from the home with vegetables, whole fruits, and whole grains to limit opportunities for consuming target foods and beverages and increase the likelihood of consuming more healthful options. Consider ways to improve selections at school breakfast and lunch to further reduce intake of added sugars.
Eating in Response to Boredom: Explore appropriate parental responses to Julia's boredom and support parental limit setting of juice intake in the afternoon.

- *Ready-to-eat cereals and other packaged foods.* Limit cereals and other packaged foods with added sugars. Choose products with less or no added sugars. Choose vegetables, whole fruits, and whole grains without added sugars more often.
- *Table sugar and syrups/toppings.* Avoid adding sugar to foods and beverages during preparation and at the table.

SUMMARY AND CONCLUSIONS

Educational strategies and materials can be designed to build awareness regarding the adverse effects of added sugars on metabolism and risk for chronic disease, enhance motivation for behavior change, and develop knowledge and skills to operationalize messages. Studies of media campaigns and educational strategies used in clinical trials can provide ideas for messaging to build awareness. While added sugars currently are not listed on the Nutrition Facts panel of labels (FDA proposal pending),[5] In May 2016, the FDA finalized plans to list added sugars on the Nutrition Facts panel of labels. Along with providing numerical information, educating patients and families to evaluate total grams of sugar and sources of added sugars in the list of ingredients can be beneficial for assisting patients and families in making food choices. In addition to HFCS, other examples of added sugars include corn syrup, dextrose, evaporated cane juice, fruit juice concentrates, honey, molasses, and syrup. An upper limit for grams of added sugar (10% of daily energy intake) should be estimated for patients: [(total energy in kcal $\times$ 0.10)/(4 g/kcal)]. Visual tools, such as sugar cubes or teaspoons of sugar, can be effective when educating patients and families. Knowing that a bottle (20 oz.) of cola contains more than 16 teaspoons (4 g per teaspoon) or 26 cubes (2.5 g per cube) of sugar is more impactful than knowing that it contains 65 g of sugar.[53] Patients and families may be more likely to avoid consuming products with added sugars if they have guidance in converting abstract (grams of sugar) to concrete (teaspoons or cubes of sugar) information.[53]

Sustained behavior change, leading to weight loss, often does not occur with education alone. Counseling on modifiable factors associated with the consumption of added sugars usually enhances the outcomes of interventions. The following list of factors, although not exhaustive, provides a starting point to explore the unique needs of each patient and family pertaining to reducing the consumption of added sugars: beliefs and attitudes; access to foods and beverages; eating atmospheres and environments; eating away from home; eating outside regular meal and snack times or "grazing;" behavioral responses to food marketing; using foods and beverages containing added sugars as rewards; impulsive intake of added sugars in response to boredom, stress, and other emotions; and the costs of healthful alternatives (particularly in the context of poverty).

REFERENCES

1. U.S. Senate Committee on Nutrition and Human Needs. *Dietary Goals for the United States.* Washington, DC, 1977.
2. Tullis IF. Rational diet construction for mild and grand obesity. *JAMA.* 1973;226(1):70–71.
3. U.S. Department of Health and Human Services and U.S. Department of Agriculture. *2015–2020 Dietary Guidelines for Americans*, 8th Edition. 2015. Available from: http://health.gov/dietaryguidelines/2015/guidelines/
4. Zhang Z, Gillespie C, Welsh JA, Hu FB, Yang Q. Usual intake of added sugars and lipid profiles among the U.S. adolescents: National Health and Nutrition Examination Survey, 2005–2010. *J Adolesc Health.* 2015;56(3):352–359.
5. Department of Health and Human Services. Food and Drug Administration. Proposed definition from FDA in the proposed rule to the revision of the nutrition and supplement facts labels (Docket No. FDA-2012-N-1210). March 2014. Available from: https://www.federalregister.gov/articles/2014/03/03/2014-04387/food-labeling-revision-of-the-nutrition-and-supplement-facts-labels#p-325.
6. World Health Organization. *Guideline: Sugars Intake for Adults and Children.* Geneva: World Health Organization, 2015.

7. White JS. Straight talk about high-fructose corn syrup: What it is and what it ain't. *Am J Clin Nutr.* 2008;88(6):1716S–1721S.

8. Ventura EE, Davis JN, Goran MI. Sugar content of popular sweetened beverages based on objective laboratory analysis: Focus on fructose content. *Obesity (Silver Spring).* 2011;19(4):868–874.

9. Walker RW, Dumke KA, Goran MI. Fructose content in popular beverages made with and without high-fructose corn syrup. *Nutrition.* 2014;30(7–8):928–935.

10. Ludwig DS, Peterson KE, Gortmaker SL. Relation between consumption of sugar-sweetened drinks and childhood obesity: A prospective, observational analysis. *Lancet.* 2001;357(9255):505–508.

11. Ma J, Fox CS, Jacques PF, et al. Sugar-sweetened beverage, diet soda, and fatty liver disease in the Framingham Heart Study cohorts. *J Hepatol.* 2015;63(2):462–469.

12. O'Connor L, Imamura F, Lentjes MA, Khaw KT, Wareham NJ, Forouhi NG. Prospective associations and population impact of sweet beverage intake and type 2 diabetes, and effects of substitutions with alternative beverages. *Diabetologia.* 2015;58(7):1474–1483.

13. Fung TT, Malik V, Rexrode KM, Manson JE, Willett WC, Hu FB. Sweetened beverage consumption and risk of coronary heart disease in women. *Am J Clin Nutr.* 2009;89(4):1037–1042.

14. Lula EC, Ribeiro CC, Hugo FN, Alves CM, Silva AA. Added sugars and periodontal disease in young adults: An analysis of NHANES III data. *Am J Clin Nutr.* 2014;100(4):1182–1187.

15. Ventura AK, Mennella JA. Innate and learned preferences for sweet taste during childhood. *Curr Opin Clin Nutr Metab Care.* 2011;14(4):379–384.

16. Bray GA, Popkin BM. Dietary sugar and body weight: Have we reached a crisis in the epidemic of obesity and diabetes?—Health be damned! Pour on the sugar. *Diabetes Care.* 2014;37(4):950–956.

17. Kahn R, Sievenpiper JL. Dietary sugar and body weight: Have we reached a crisis in the epidemic of obesity and diabetes?—We have, but the pox on sugar is overwrought and overworked. *Diabetes Care.* 2014;37(4):957–962.

18. Ludwig DS. Examining the health effects of fructose. *JAMA.* 2013;310(1):33–34.

19. Ludwig DS. The glycemic index: Physiological mechanisms relating to obesity, diabetes, and cardiovascular disease. *JAMA.* 2002;287(18):2414–2423.

20. Johnson RJ, Nakagawa T, Sanchez-Lozada LG, et al. Sugar, uric acid, and the etiology of diabetes and obesity. *Diabetes.* 2013;62(10):3307–3315.

21. Abdelmalek MF, Lazo M, Horska A, et al. Higher dietary fructose is associated with impaired hepatic adenosine triphosphate homeostasis in obese individuals with type 2 diabetes. *Hepatology.* 2012;56(3):952–960.

22. Bremer AA, Mietus-Snyder M, Lustig RH. Toward a unifying hypothesis of metabolic syndrome. *Pediatrics.* 2012;129(3):557–570.

23. Bazzano LA, Li TY, Joshipura KJ, Hu FB. Intake of fruit, vegetables, and fruit juices and risk of diabetes in women. *Diabetes Care.* 2008;31(7):1311–1317.

24. Wang X, Ouyang Y, Liu J, et al. Fruit and vegetable consumption and mortality from all causes, cardiovascular disease, and cancer: Systematic review and dose-response meta-analysis of prospective cohort studies. *BMJ.* 2014;349:g4490.

25. Cassady BA, Considine RV, Mattes RD. Beverage consumption, appetite, and energy intake: What did you expect? *Am J Clin Nutr.* 2012;95(3):587–593.

26. de Ruyter JC, Katan MB, Kuijper LD, Liem DG, Olthof MR. The effect of sugar-free versus sugar-sweetened beverages on satiety, liking and wanting: An 18 month randomized double-blind trial in children. *PLoS One.* 2013;8(10):e78039.

27. de Ruyter JC, Olthof MR, Seidell JC, Katan MB. A trial of sugar-free or sugar-sweetened beverages and body weight in children. *N Engl J Med.* 2012;367(15):1397–1406.

28. Mennella JA. Ontogeny of taste preferences: Basic biology and implications for health. *Am J Clin Nutr.* 2014;99(3):704S–711S.

29. Pepino MY, Mennella JA. Factors contributing to individual differences in sucrose preference. *Chem Senses.* 2005;30 Suppl 1:i319–320.

30. Liem DG, de Graaf C. Sweet and sour preferences in young children and adults: Role of repeated exposure. *Physiol Behav.* 2004;83(3):421–429.

31. Weijs PJ, Kool LM, van Baar NM, van der Zee SC. High beverage sugar as well as high animal protein intake at infancy may increase overweight risk at 8 years: A prospective longitudinal pilot study. *Nutr J.* 2011;10:95.

32. Burger KS, Stice E. Neural responsivity during soft drink intake, anticipation, and advertisement exposure in habitually consuming youth. *Obesity (Silver Spring).* 2014;22(2):441–450.

33. Drewnowski A, Rehm CD. Consumption of added sugars among US children and adults by food purchase location and food source. *Am J Clin Nutr.* 2014;100(3):901–907.

34. Ervin RB, Kit BK, Carroll MD, Ogden CL. Consumption of added sugar among U.S. children and adolescents, 2005–2008. *NCHS Data Brief.* 2012(87):1–8.

35. Briefel RR, Wilson A, Cabili C, Hedley Dodd A. Reducing calories and added sugars by improving children's beverage choices. *J Acad Nutr Diet.* 2013;113(2):269–275.

36. Foltz JL, May AL, Belay B, Nihiser AJ, Dooyema CA, Blanck HM. Population-level intervention strategies and examples for obesity prevention in children. *Annu Rev Nutr.* 2012;32:391–415.

37. Boles M, Adams A, Gredler A, Manhas S. Ability of a mass media campaign to influence knowledge, attitudes, and behaviors about sugary drinks and obesity. *Prev Med.* 2014;67 Suppl 1:S40–45.

38. Jordan A, Bleakley A, Hennessy M, Vaala S, Glanz K, Strasser AA. Sugar-sweetened beverage-related public service advertisements and their influence on parents. *Am Behav Sci.* 2015;59(14):1847–1865.

39. Kansagra SM, Kennelly MO, Nonas CA, et al. Reducing sugary drink consumption: New York City's approach. *Am J Public Health.* 2015;105(4):e61–64.

40. Avery A, Bostock L, McCullough F. A systematic review investigating interventions that can help reduce consumption of sugar-sweetened beverages in children leading to changes in body fatness. *J Hum Nutr Diet.* 2015;28 Suppl 1:52–64.

41. James J, Thomas P, Cavan D, Kerr D. Preventing childhood obesity by reducing consumption of carbonated drinks: Cluster randomised controlled trial. *BMJ.* 2004;328(7450):1237.

42. Sichieri R, Paula Trotte A, de Souza RA, Veiga GV. School randomised trial on prevention of excessive weight gain by discouraging students from drinking sodas. *Public Health Nutr.* 2009;12(2):197–202.

43. James J, Thomas P, Kerr D. Preventing childhood obesity: Two year follow-up results from the Christchurch obesity prevention programme in schools (CHOPPS). *BMJ.* 2007;335(7623):762.

44. Ebbeling CB, Feldman HA, Chomitz VR, et al. A randomized trial of sugar-sweetened beverages and adolescent body weight. *N Engl J Med.* 2012;367(15):1407–1416.

45. Ebbeling CB, Feldman HA, Osganian SK, Chomitz VR, Ellenbogen SJ, Ludwig DS. Effects of decreasing sugar-sweetened beverage consumption on body weight in adolescents: A randomized, controlled pilot study. *Pediatrics.* 2006;117(3):673–680.

46. Taveras EM, Gillman MW, Kleinman KP, Rich-Edwards JW, Rifas-Shiman SL. Reducing racial/ethnic disparities in childhood obesity: The role of early life risk factors. *JAMA Pediatr.* 2013;167(8):731–738.

47. Qi Q, Chu AY, Kang JH, et al. Sugar-sweetened beverages and genetic risk of obesity. *N Engl J Med.* 2012;367(15):1387–1396.

48. Ebbeling CB, Leidig MM, Feldman HA, Lovesky MM, Ludwig DS. Effects of a low-glycemic load vs low-fat diet in obese young adults: A randomized trial. *JAMA.* 2007;297(19):2092–2102.

49. Gibson S, Boyd A. Associations between added sugars and micronutrient intakes and status: Further analysis of data from the National Diet and Nutrition Survey of Young People aged 4 to 18 years. *Br J Nutr.* 2009;101(1):100–107.

50. Committee on Nutrition. American Academy of Pediatrics: The use and misuse of fruit juice in pediatrics. *Pediatrics.* 2001;107(5):1210–1213.

51. Fitch C, Keim KS. Position of the Academy of Nutrition and Dietetics: Use of nutritive and nonnutritive sweeteners. *J Acad Nutr Diet.* 2012;112(5):739–758.

52. Hampton T. Sugar substitutes linked to weight gain. *JAMA.* 2008;299(18):2137–2138.

53. Adams JM, Hart W, Gilmer L, Lloyd-Richardson EE, Burton KA. Concrete images of the sugar content in sugar-sweetened beverages reduces attraction to and selection of these beverages. *Appetite.* 2014;83:10–18.

38 Lifestyle Interventions for the Prevention of Type 2 Diabetes in Obese Children and Youth

Micah L. Olson and Gabriel Q. Shaibi

CONTENTS

INTRODUCTION

The pediatric obesity epidemic has contributed to the emergence of type 2 diabetes among children and adolescents, as reviewed in Chapter 25. Not only is type 2 diabetes in youth a recent phenomenon, but this phenotype is associated with a rapid onset and aggressive disease course. Unlike this diagnosis in adults, type 2 diabetes can develop within 1 to 4 years in otherwise normoglycemic youth [1]. Youth diagnosed with type 2 diabetes exhibit accelerated microvascular complications [2] and are projected to have a decreased life expectancy [3]. In addition, almost 50% of adolescents with type 2 diabetes are unable to maintain adequate glycemic control and will require insulin therapy within a few years of diagnosis [4].

The discouraging outlook for youth with type 2 diabetes underscores the need for prevention programs. While the most salient and cost-effective approach for diabetes prevention in youth is the primary prevention of obesity, millions of youth are already obese and would be best served by targeted diabetes prevention interventions. Multiple studies in adults have established the effectiveness of lifestyle changes in delaying or preventing the onset of type 2 diabetes in those with prediabetes [5]. The Diabetes Prevention Program demonstrated that an intensive lifestyle program with the goals of 7% weight loss through dietary modification and increased physical activity can prevent or delay the development of type 2 diabetes in those with prediabetes. After an average follow-up of nearly 5 years, those randomized to the intensive lifestyle program arm of the study exhibited a 58% reduction in the incidence of diabetes compared with controls [6].

To date, there are no comprehensive type 2 diabetes prevention studies described in the pediatric literature. In other words, there are no pediatric studies that are designed to directly test whether a lifestyle intervention is effective for preventing the onset of type 2 diabetes. There are a number of reasons for this including the heterogeneity in diabetes risk phenotypes even among obese youth [7], the unknown trajectory and time course of diabetes conversion [1], and the lack of data specifying behavioral and weight loss targets necessary to achieve diabetes risk reduction [8]. In this context, diabetes prevention is conceptually different from weight management. For weight

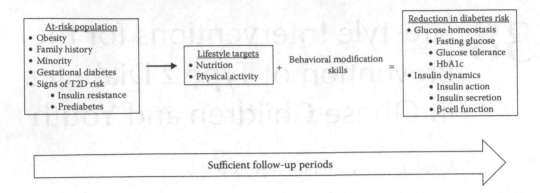

FIGURE 38.1   Conceptual model of diabetes prevention in youths.

management programs, the primary outcome is weight loss (or prevention of weight gain) among obese youth, whereas diabetes prevention programs target high-risk populations (e.g., obese, minority adolescents with a positive family history) where risk stratification is derived from some indicator of glucose homeostasis.

Given these challenges in designing "true" diabetes prevention programs for youth, the majority of pediatric research focuses on the impact of lifestyle interventions on surrogate or proximal measures of diabetes risk factors. These studies manipulate diet and/or physical activity behaviors to induce changes in outcome measures that are either glycemic indictors of diabetes risk (i.e., fasting glucose, 2 h glucose, or HbA1c) or related to the pathophysiology of the disease. From a pathophysiologic perspective, insufficient insulin secretion relative to the degree of insulin resistance contributes to pancreatic β-cell dysfunction leading to the development of impaired glucose homeostasis and eventually type 2 diabetes [9]. Improvements in these glycemic indicators or pathophysiological processes over a sufficient follow-up period could be indicative of reduction in diabetes risk (Figure 38.1).

Although emerging data support the potential efficacy of pharmacological [10] and surgical [11] approaches for reducing diabetes risk factors among obese youth, these studies are beyond the scope of this chapter and are covered in Chapters 30 and 31. The goal of this chapter is to review studies that have examined the associations between the key behavioral targets (diet, physical activity, and their combination) and measures of glycemia (fasting glucose, 2 h glucose, or HbA1c), insulin action (e.g., insulin resistance or insulin sensitivity), or measures of pancreatic β-cell function in populations with an increased risk profile for type 2 diabetes. We will use both observational and interventional studies to support the potential utility of lifestyle intervention to prevent or delay the onset of type 2 diabetes in youth. We will also discuss challenges to and opportunities for the translation of pediatric diabetes prevention programs into real-world settings in order to make the strongest public health impact on this growing epidemic.

NUTRITION AND TYPE 2 DIABETES RISK

Much attention has focused on nutritional factors and type 2 diabetes risk in youth. Macronutrient dietary content (the proportion of calories ingested from carbohydrates, protein, and fat), the makeup of dietary carbohydrates (e.g., glycemic index, fiber, and added sugar), and sugar-sweetened beverage intake have all been studied in relation to risk for type 2 diabetes. We will first review observational studies that evaluate relationships between selected dietary characteristics and markers of glucose homeostasis and later review interventional studies that test whether specific dietary changes can improve risk factors for type 2 diabetes.

OBSERVATIONAL STUDIES LINKING DIETARY PATTERNS WITH TYPE 2 DIABETES RISK FACTORS

A cross-sectional study of 285 healthy adolescents found a significant association between whole grain consumption, body mass index, and insulin sensitivity [12]. The relationship between whole grain consumption and insulin sensitivity was strongest among those adolescents with the highest BMI and suggests that eating whole grains may be protective against the development of type 2 diabetes in youth. Arslanian et al. examined 44 African American and white children and found that a higher dietary fat-to-carbohydrate ratio was associated with significantly lower insulin sensitivity suggesting that higher fat intake is associated with worsening insulin resistance [13]. However, a cross-sectional study of 63 overweight and obese Latino children failed to find any significant associations between macronutrient content and measures of insulin resistance [14]. Despite the lack of association with macronutrient content, higher sugar intake was significantly associated with lower pancreatic β-cell function. In a cross-sectional study of 630 Canadian youth, no associations between macronutrient content and insulin sensitivity or insulin secretion were noted [15]. In a longitudinal analysis of 226 healthy German youth, higher dietary glycemic index in adolescence was prospectively associated with increased insulin resistance over an average follow-up of 12.6 years [16].

As discussed in Chapter 37, dietary intake of sugar-sweetened beverages has received increased attention as a potential causal factor in the current pediatric obesity epidemic [17]. In contrast, the data examining the associations between sugar-sweetened beverage intake and markers of glucose homeostasis in youth are less abundant. Ambrosini et al. prospectively studied 1433 Australian adolescents from age 14 to 17 years but failed to find any significant associations between intake of carbonated drinks or fruit drinks with added sugar and insulin or glucose variables [18]. In a cross-sectional study using NHANES data from 1999 to 2004, sugar-sweetened beverage intake derived from a 24 h recall was associated with greater insulin resistance in girls but not in boys [19]. Similarly, in a study of 630 Canadian children, higher sugar-sweetened beverage intake was associated with measures of insulin resistance among overweight children (BMI ≥ 85th percentile) but not among healthy-weight children [20]. When this cohort was studied prospectively, a higher baseline consumption of added sugars from liquid sources was associated with increased fasting glucose and worsened insulin resistance at 2 years and those with a BMI ≥ 85th percentile were most affected [20].

The inconsistent findings from observational studies make it difficult to draw definitive conclusions regarding the associations between habitual dietary behaviors and type 2 diabetes risk factors in youth. This inconsistency may be attributed to the well-documented challenges in accurately assessing nutrition-related behaviors in youth [21]. Therefore, intervention studies offer a more direct approach to examine whether modifications in dietary patterns can reduce the risk for developing type 2 diabetes.

EFFECTS OF DIETARY INTERVENTIONS ON TYPE 2 DIABETES RISK FACTORS

Dietary interventions are inherently complex due to the interrelatedness of various dietary components (e.g., macronutrient composition and total caloric consumption). In addition, without completely sequestering participants and supplying all consumed meals during the trial, it is difficult to know how compliant participants are with achieving the intended nutritional targets that are being tested. Even with well-developed intervention fidelity plans, researchers are left with some degree of inherent uncertainty in quantifying the degree to which a nutritional behavioral change led to the observed outcome. With these limitations acknowledged, the fundamental importance of diet on the development of type 2 diabetes makes it essential that researchers continue to design and test the effects of various dietary interventions on type 2 diabetes risk among obese youth.

Ebbeling et al. randomized 16 obese adolescents to a reduced-glycemic-load diet or a reduced-fat diet [22]. The reduced-glycemic-load diet was *ad libitum* and targeted a proportion of energy intake between 45% and 50% from carbohydrates and 30%–35% from fat, and participants were counseled to consume low-glycemic foods. The reduced-fat diet was designed to elicit a negative energy balance of 250–500 kcal/day and targeted a proportion of energy intake of 55%–60% from carbohydrates and 25%–30% from fat. Despite the fact that the low-glycemic diet was *ad libitum* and the reduced-fat diet was energy restricted, the reduced-glycemic-load group exhibited a significant decrease in both BMI and fat mass at 12 months compared with the reduced-fat group. In addition, at 12 months the glycemic-load group had a significantly lower increase in insulin resistance compared with the reduced-fat group that was independent of changes in BMI. In a follow-up study of 113 obese Hispanic children, Mirza et al. adapted the dietary intervention to be tailored for Hispanic youth [23]. The intervention lasted 3 months and outcomes were obtained at baseline 3, 12, and 24 months postintervention. Both the low-glycemic diet and low-fat groups exhibited significant decreases in BMI z-score that were sustained at 24 months. However, neither group experienced significant changes in fasting glucose or measures of insulin resistance.

In a similar approach, Krebs et al. randomized 22 severely obese adolescents to a high-protein low-carbohydrate (HPLC) diet or a low-fat (LF) diet [24]. The HPLC diet was restricted to <20 g of carbohydrates per day, but was not given a caloric restriction target. The LF diet was restricted to a calorie goal of 70% of resting energy expenditure and <30% of calories from fat. Both groups experienced a significant reduction in BMI z-score at 13 weeks with the HPLC group achieving a significantly greater decrease in BMI z-score than the LF group. Despite improvements in BMI z-score, no significant changes in glucose tolerance or insulin resistance were observed in either group.

Ramon-Krauel randomized 17 obese 8- to 17-year-old youth with fatty liver to either a low glycemic load diet or a LF diet [25]. The low glycemic load group was counseled to select carbohydrate-containing foods with a low-to-moderate glycemic load and targeted 40% of energy from carbohydrates and 35%–40% from fat. The LF diet targeted 55%–60% of energy from carbohydrates and 20% from fat, with <10% from saturated fat. Both diets were prescribed *ad libitum* and both groups exhibited similar decreases in liver fat, fasting glucose, and insulin resistance at 6 months.

Davis et al. enrolled 16 overweight and obese Latina adolescent females (12–17 years of age) in a 12-week nutrition education intervention focused on decreasing added sugar intake (goal of 10% or less of total daily caloric intake) and increasing dietary fiber (goal of 14 g per 1000 cal) [26]. Despite significant reductions in total calories, grams of carbohydrates, grams of fat, grams of added sugar, and the number of sugar-sweetened beverages, the intervention did not result in any significant changes in insulin sensitivity or insulin secretion. However, there was a trend noted between reductions in added sugar intake and insulin secretion ($p = .075$), suggesting that modest reductions in added sugar intake may reduce diabetes risk profile. In a follow-up trial, 53 overweight and obese Latino adolescents (14–18 years of age) were randomized to one of three groups for 16 weeks: (1) nutrition, (2) nutrition plus strength training, or (3) control [27]. The nutrition education consisted of weekly 1 h classes that focused on the same dietary targets as noted previously. The nutrition plus strength-training group consisted of the nutrition education classes plus a 60 min, twice-per-week, strength-training session. The control group received no intervention between the pre- and postintervention data collection. Both intervention groups achieved a decrease in glucose area under the curve during an oral glucose tolerance test, but there were no other significant intervention effects on BMI, body composition, or measures of insulin sensitivity or β-cell function. There was considerable individual variation in dietary changes within each of the study groups so secondary analyses were performed to compare outcome measures based on reported dietary changes across treatment arms [28]. Those who reported decreases in added sugar intake exhibited significant reductions in insulin area under the curve ($p = .02$) during an oral glucose tolerance test while those who reported increases in fiber intake exhibited reductions in BMI ($p = .01$) and visceral adipose tissue ($p = .03$).

The need for dietary intervention among obese youth aimed at reducing type 2 diabetes risk is evident. Despite a multitude of approaches targeting various aspects of dietary intake, there is insufficient evidence to recommend any one approach. It appears that modulating aspects of macronutrient content may hold promise for improving certain diabetes risk factors. Further studies are needed to identify how changes in dietary patterns and caloric intake contribute to diabetes risk reduction and how to support obese youth and their families to successfully implement these recommended changes.

PHYSICAL ACTIVITY, EXERCISE, AND TYPE 2 DIABETES RISK FACTORS

It has long been established that adults who participate in regular physical activity have lower rates of type 2 diabetes than their sedentary counterparts [29]. Further, the protective effects of physical activity may be independent of weight status and appear to hold in lean, overweight, and obese populations [30]. These observations have led to an increasing body of literature supporting the benefits of exercise training on diabetes risk factors among obese youth. Several reviews [31,32] and a recent meta-analysis [33] have focused on the effects of exercise on insulin action in youth. Collectively, these publications support the efficacy of exercise training (both resistance and aerobic) to improve insulin action in obese youth and suggest that the health improvements are independent of changes in body weight or composition [32].

Bell et al. enrolled 14 obese, hyperinsulinemic normoglycemic youth (9–16 years of age) to participate in 8 weeks (3 days/week for 1 h) of supervised exercise training [34]. The training program included circuits of moderate to vigorous aerobic exercise on a cycle ergometer coupled with resistance exercises using a machine. Compared with baseline, participants exhibited a 12% increase in insulin sensitivity ($p = .02$) as measured by the euglycemic-hyperinsulinemic clamp. This increase was observed in the absence of changes in weight or body composition and supports the concept that exercise alone can improve insulin sensitivity in obese youth. Shaibi et al. randomized 21 obese Latino adolescents 13–17 years of age to either progressive resistance training (twice/week for 16 weeks) or a nonexercise control group [35]. Participants were assessed at baseline and postintervention for insulin sensitivity, insulin secretion, and β-cell function by the frequently sampled intravenous glucose tolerance test. Compared with baseline, resistance-trained youth exhibited a 45% increase in insulin sensitivity while control youth experienced a small, nonsignificant increase. When data were compared across groups, the increase in insulin sensitivity was significantly greater in the intervention compared with controls and was independent of changes in total fat mass or total lean mass. Despite significant increases in insulin sensitivity following resistance training, there were no within- or between-group changes in insulin secretion or β-cell function.

In a series of related studies comparing the effects of aerobic versus resistance exercise on diabetes risk factors in obese youth, Lee et al. found that 3 months of aerobic exercise training (three 60 min sessions/week) led to significant increases in insulin sensitivity in boys and girls [36,37]. Aerobic exercise also led to reductions in total and regional body fat as measured by magnetic resonance imaging. Interestingly, the resistance-training program was only effective at increasing insulin sensitivity and reducing body composition in boys and did not result in diabetes risk reduction in girls. Collectively, these data suggest that sex may moderate the effects of exercise modality (aerobic vs. resistance) on diabetes risk reduction in obese adolescents. An additional important finding from these studies was that both forms of exercise led to reductions in percent body fat but did not result in weight loss.

These studies move the field beyond the conceptual basis for exercise to reduce diabetes risk into the prescriptive model that will be needed to further advance the translation of science into practice. Building on this model, Davis et al. randomized 222 overweight and obese children to receive 13 weeks of low-dose (5 days/week at 20 min/session) or high-dose (5 days/week at 40 min/session) aerobic exercise of similar intensity in order to examine the dose–response effects of exercise on diabetes risk factors in children. In addition to dose–response effects, several key features of this study included (1) the focus on a predominantly prepubertal cohort of children, (2) more than half of the population being an ethnic minority with a family history of type 2 diabetes, and (3) almost 30% of the total sample exhibited prediabetes at baseline. The authors found that both low-dose and high-dose aerobic exercise were equally beneficial for improving measures of insulin sensitivity but that the high-dose exercise was superior to low-dose for improving β-cell function [38]. Despite the beneficial effects of exercise on insulin sensitivity and β-cell function, the prevalence of prediabetes was not changed over the course of the intervention.

Collectively, these studies support the utility of exercise to improve diabetes risk in obese pediatric populations and set the stage for future work to optimize the frequency, intensity, duration, and mode of exercise necessary to elicit beneficial health effects. These data will be instrumental for the translation of research into practice in order to support the concept that exercise is medicine [39].

EFFECTS OF LIFESTYLE INTERVENTIONS ON TYPE 2 DIABETES RISK

Very few randomized controlled trials have described comprehensive lifestyle interventions on type 2 diabetes risk factors in youth. The hallmark features of these comprehensive interventions include nutrition and physical activity components that are supported by evidenced-based behavior change strategies. An exemplar comes from the Yale Bright Bodies weight-management program where Savoye et al. conducted a trial of 209 obese children randomized to the Bright Bodies program or a control group [40]. The intervention group consisted of twice-a-week education sessions for 6 months followed by bimonthly sessions for 6 months. The program was family based and involved nutrition, exercise, and behavior modification. The nutrition counseling focused on better food choices of moderate portion sizes as opposed to a structured meal plan with calorie restriction. The control group consisted of standard weight management clinical visits where youth received general diet and exercise recommendations at baseline and 6 months. At 12 months, fasting estimates of insulin sensitivity significantly improved in the intervention group and worsened in the control group ($p < .001$) while there was no statistically significant change in fasting glucose in either group. Treatment effects were sustained at 2-year follow-up, despite discontinuing the formal intervention after 12 months [41]. A subsample of 23 children who were randomly selected to receive a standard oral glucose tolerance test (OGTT) at the beginning and end of the 12-month study demonstrated significant improvements in markers of insulin sensitivity and glucose tolerance in the intervention group versus the control group [42]. These data led to a follow-up study of the Yale Bright Bodies Healthy Lifestyle Program for obese youth with elevated 2 h glucose levels [43]. Seventy-five obese youth with prediabetes (defined as elevated 2 h glucose levels between 130 and 199 mg/dL) were randomized to a 6-month intensive lifestyle program or standard clinical care. The lifestyle intervention led to significant decreases in 2 h glucose, increases in insulin sensitivity, and greater reversion to normal glucose tolerance compared with the control group. Of note was that both groups experienced increases in weight over the 6 months, but the increase was significantly larger in controls (3.7 kg) compared with intervention youth (0.6 kg) for an overall treatment effect of −3.1 kg ($p = .006$). This series of studies supports the concept that comprehensive diabetes prevention programs can be efficacious for short-term and potentially sustained diabetes risk reduction among high-risk obese youth.

Shaibi et al. examined the impact of a 12-week culturally grounded, community-based lifestyle intervention on insulin sensitivity and glucose tolerance among 15 overweight and obese Latino adolescents aged 14–16 years [44]. The program included weekly nutrition education delivered in groups to families and 3 days/week of moderate-to-vigorous physical activity for youth. A key aspect of the theory-informed intervention was the delivery in the community at a local YMCA by trained community health educators rather than researchers. The program led to significant improvements in both glucose tolerance and insulin sensitivity even in the absence of weight loss. Although the sample size was small, the study supports the translational potential for diabetes prevention interventions to be extended to the community setting for vulnerable and underserved groups of youth at high risk for type 2 diabetes.

These promising studies suggest that comprehensive lifestyle interventions can result in diabetes risk reduction among high-risk obese youth and, contrary to what is known in adults, weight maintenance rather than weight loss may be critical for success. This distinction becomes increasingly important in the context of normal growth trajectories where it may be physiological appropriate for youth to continue to gain weight until final maturation. Therefore, comprehensive diabetes prevention programs leading to reductions in diabetes risk among obese youth are likely the result of improvements in body composition, rather than weight loss *per se*, that are mediated by successful behavior change. Programmatically, this notion has implications for the design, implementation, and evaluation of comprehensive diabetes prevention programs for obese youth where emphasis should be placed on making and sustaining behavior changes and assessing outcomes that are proximal and related to the pathophysiology of type 2 diabetes.

CONCLUSION AND FUTURE DIRECTIONS

Obesity and type 2 diabetes remain challenging public health problems but the available data support the utility of lifestyle intervention for diabetes risk reduction in high-risk obese youth. Both dietary changes and increases in physical activity are essential to diabetes prevention with more research needed to ascertain the optimal dosing of these behavioral targets to result in diabetes prevention. More important than optimizing behavioral changes is the need for a greater understanding of how to operationalize and implement sustained behavioral changes in real-world settings. From a systems perspective, these programs must be developed to address family, social, environmental, and policy factors that influence downstream health behaviors and ultimately diabetes-related health outcomes [45]. This system-level approach is especially important for underserved and vulnerable populations of youth who will likely experience much greater barriers to achieving and maintaining optimal behavioral changes.

REFERENCES

1. Elder DA, Hornung LN, Herbers PM, Prigeon R, Woo JG, D'Alessio DA. Rapid deterioration of insulin secretion in obese adolescents preceding the onset of type 2 diabetes. *J Pediatr.* 2015; 166(3):672–678.
2. TODAY Study Group. Retinopathy in youth with type 2 diabetes participating in the TODAY clinical trial. *Diabetes Care.* 2013; 36(6):1772–1774.
3. Rhodes ET, Prosser LA, Hoerger TJ, Lieu T, Ludwig DS, Laffel LM. Estimated morbidity and mortality in adolescents and young adults diagnosed with type 2 diabetes mellitus. *Diabet Med.* 2012; 29(4):453–463.
4. Group TS, Zeitler P, Hirst K, et al. A clinical trial to maintain glycemic control in youth with type 2 diabetes. *N Engl J Med.* 2012; 366(24):2247–2256.
5. Yoon U, Kwok LL, Magkidis A. Efficacy of lifestyle interventions in reducing diabetes incidence in patients with impaired glucose tolerance: A systematic review of randomized controlled trials. *Metabolism.* 2013; 62(2):303–314.
6. Diabetes Prevention Program Research Group. Reduction in the incidence of type 2 diabetes with lifestyle intervention or metformin. *N Engl J Med.* 2002; 346(6):393–403.
7. Michaliszyn SF, Mari A, Lee S, et al. β-cell function, incretin effect, and incretin hormones in obese youth along the span of glucose tolerance from normal to prediabetes to type 2 diabetes. *Diabetes.* 2014; 63(11):3846–3855.
8. Shaibi GQ, Ryder JR, Kim JY, Barraza E. Exercise for obese youth: Refocusing attention from weight loss to health gains. *Exerc Sport Sci Rev.* 2015; 43(1):41–47.
9. Bacha F, Lee S, Gungor N, Arslanian SA. From pre-diabetes to type 2 diabetes in obese youth: Pathophysiological characteristics along the spectrum of glucose dysregulation. *Diabetes Care.* 2010; 33(10):2225–2231.
10. Yanovski JA, Krakoff J, Salaita CG, et al. Effects of metformin on body weight and body composition in obese insulin-resistant children: A randomized clinical trial. *Diabetes.* 2011; 60(2):477–485.
11. Boza C, Viscido G, Salinas J, Crovari F, Funke R, Perez G. Laparoscopic sleeve gastrectomy in obese adolescents: Results in 51 patients. *Surg Obes Relat Dis.* 2012; 8(2):133–137.
12. Steffen LM, Jacobs DR, Jr., Murtaugh MA, et al. Whole grain intake is associated with lower body mass and greater insulin sensitivity among adolescents. *Am J Epidemiol.* 2003; 158(3):243–250.

13. Arslanian SA, Saad R, Lewy V, Danadian K, Janosky J. Hyperinsulinemia in African-American children: Decreased insulin clearance and increased insulin secretion and its relationship to insulin sensitivity. *Diabetes*. 2002; 51(10):3014–3019.

14. Davis JN, Ventura EE, Weigensberg MJ, et al. The relation of sugar intake to beta cell function in overweight Latino children. *Am J Clin Nutr*. 2005; 82(5):1004–1010.

15. Henderson M, Benedetti A, Gray-Donald K. Dietary composition and its associations with insulin sensitivity and insulin secretion in youth. *Br J Nutr*. 2014; 111(3):527–534.

16. Goletzke J, Herder C, Joslowski G, et al. Habitually higher dietary glycemic index during puberty is prospectively related to increased risk markers of type 2 diabetes in younger adulthood. *Diabetes Care*. 2013; 36(7):1870–1876.

17. Harrington S. The role of sugar-sweetened beverage consumption in adolescent obesity: A review of the literature. *J Sch Nurs*. 2008; 24(1):3–12.

18. Ambrosini GL, Oddy WH, Huang RC, Mori TA, Beilin LJ, Jebb SA. Prospective associations between sugar-sweetened beverage intakes and cardiometabolic risk factors in adolescents. *Am J Clin Nutr*. 2013; 98(2):327–334.

19. Bremer AA, Auinger P, Byrd RS. Relationship between insulin resistance-associated metabolic parameters and anthropometric measurements with sugar-sweetened beverage intake and physical activity levels in US adolescents: Findings from the 1999–2004 National Health and Nutrition Examination Survey. *Arch Pediatr Adolesc Med*. 2009; 163(4):328–335.

20. Wang J. Consumption of added sugars and development of metabolic syndrome components among a sample of youth at risk of obesity. *Appl Physiol Nutr Metab*. 2014; 39(4):512.

21. Collins CE, Watson J, Burrows T. Measuring dietary intake in children and adolescents in the context of overweight and obesity. *Int J Obes (Lond)*. 2010; 34(7):1103–1115.

22. Ebbeling CB, Leidig MM, Sinclair KB, Hangen JP, Ludwig DS. A reduced-glycemic load diet in the treatment of adolescent obesity. *Arch Pediatr Adolesc Med*. 2003; 157(8):773–779.

23. Mirza NM, Palmer MG, Sinclair KB, et al. Effects of a low glycemic load or a low-fat dietary intervention on body weight in obese Hispanic American children and adolescents: A randomized controlled trial. *Am J Clin Nutr*. 2013; 97(2):276–285.

24. Krebs NF, Gao D, Gralla J, Collins JS, Johnson SL. Efficacy and safety of a high protein, low carbohydrate diet for weight loss in severely obese adolescents. *J Pediatr*. 2010; 157(2):252–258.

25. Ramon-Krauel M, Salsberg SL, Ebbeling CB, et al. A low-glycemic-load versus low-fat diet in the treatment of fatty liver in obese children. *Child Obes*. 2013; 9(3):252–260.

26. Davis JN, Ventura EE, Shaibi GQ, et al. Reduction in added sugar intake and improvement in insulin secretion in overweight latina adolescents. *Metab Syndr Relat Disord*. 2007; 5(2):183–193.

27. Davis JN, Kelly LA, Lane CJ, et al. Randomized control trial to improve adiposity and insulin resistance in overweight Latino adolescents. *Obesity*. 2009; 17(8):1542–1548.

28. Ventura E, Davis J, Byrd-Williams C, et al. Reduction in risk factors for type 2 diabetes mellitus in response to a low-sugar, high-fiber dietary intervention in overweight Latino adolescents. *Arch Pediatr Adolesc Med*. 2009; 163(4):320–327.

29. Helmrich SP, Ragland DR, Leung RW, Paffenbarger RS, Jr. Physical activity and reduced occurrence of non-insulin-dependent diabetes mellitus. *N Engl J Med*. 1991; 325(3):147–152.

30. LaMonte MJ, Blair SN, Church TS. Physical activity and diabetes prevention. *J Appl Physiol*. 2005; 99(3):1205–1213.

31. Shaibi GQ, Roberts CK, Goran MI. Exercise and insulin resistance in youth. *Exerc Sport Sci Rev*. 2008; 36(1):5–11.

32. Kim M, Park HN. Does regular exercise without weight loss reduce insulin resistance in children and adolescents? *Int J Endocrinol*. 2013; 2013:1–10.

33. Fedewa MV, Gist NH, Evans EM, Dishman RK. Exercise and insulin resistance in youth: A meta-analysis. *Pediatrics*. 2014; 133(1):e163–e174.

34. Bell LM, Watts K, Siafarikas A, et al. Exercise alone reduces insulin resistance in obese children independently of changes in body composition. *J Clin Endocrinol Metab*. 2007; 92(11):4230–4235.

35. Shaibi GQ, Cruz ML, Ball GD, et al. Effects of resistance training on insulin sensitivity in overweight Latino adolescent males. *Med Sci Sports Exerc*. 2006; 38(7):1208–1215.

36. Lee S, Bacha F, Hannon T, Kuk JL, Boesch C, Arslanian S. Effects of aerobic versus resistance exercise without caloric restriction on abdominal fat, intrahepatic lipid, and insulin sensitivity in obese adolescent boys: A randomized, controlled trial. *Diabetes*. 2012; 61(11):2787–2795.

37. Lee S, Deldin AR, White D, et al. Aerobic exercise but not resistance exercise reduces intrahepatic lipid content and visceral fat and improves insulin sensitivity in obese adolescent girls: A randomized controlled trial. *Am J Physiol Endocrinol Metab.* 2013; 305(10):E1222–E1229.
38. Davis CL, Pollock NK, Waller JL, et al. Exercise dose and diabetes risk in overweight and obese children: A randomized controlled trial. *JAMA.* 2012; 308(11):1103–1112.
39. Sallis R. Exercise is medicine: A call to action for physicians to assess and prescribe exercise. *Phys Sportsmed.* 2015; 43(1):22–26.
40. Savoye M, Shaw M, Dziura J, et al. Effects of a weight management program on body composition and metabolic parameters in overweight children: A randomized controlled trial. *JAMA.* 2007; 297(24):2697–2704.
41. Savoye M, Nowicka P, Shaw M, et al. Long-term results of an obesity program in an ethnically diverse pediatric population. *Pediatrics.* 2011; 127(3):402–410.
42. Shaw M, Savoye M, Cali A, Dziura J, Tamborlane WV, Caprio S. Effect of a successful intensive lifestyle program on insulin sensitivity and glucose tolerance in obese youth. *Diabetes Care.* 2009; 32(1):45–47.
43. Savoye M, Caprio S, Dziura J, et al. Reversal of early abnormalities in glucose metabolism in obese youth: Results of an intensive lifestyle randomized controlled trial. *Diabetes Care.* 2014; 37(2):317–324.
44. Shaibi GQ, Konopken Y, Hoppin E, Keller CS, Ortega R, Castro FG. Effects of a culturally grounded community-based diabetes prevention program for obese Latino adolescents. *Diabetes Educ.* 2012; 38(4):504–512.
45. Hill JO, Galloway JM, Goley A, et al. Scientific statement: Socioecological determinants of prediabetes and type 2 diabetes. *Diabetes Care.* 2013; 36(8):2430–2439.

39 Use of Mobile Health Strategies for the Prevention and Treatment of Childhood Obesity

Cheng K. Fred Wen, Brooke Bell, and Donna Spruijt-Metz

CONTENTS

INTRODUCTION

Modifying key obesity-related behaviors, as outlined in previous chapters, has been a prime focus of pediatric obesity prevention and intervention efforts. In recent years, the incorporation of mobile or wireless health technologies, also known as *mHealth solutions*, into pediatric obesity prevention and intervention studies has rapidly accelerated [1]. The rise of mHealth is partially fueled by the rapid growth in wearable device availability and mobile phone ownership across age groups, geographic regions, and socioeconomic strata. To date, there are an estimated 7 billion mobile phone subscriptions worldwide [2]. In the United States, it is estimated that over 90% of adults and 88% of youth aged 13–17 years own a mobile phone [3]. mHealth technologies have the potential to capture and transmit a wide array of participant data in an accurate and timely fashion. These data range from ubiquitously measured (via sensor) behavioral, biological, and other contextual data (e.g., social interaction and physical location) to self-reported survey questionnaires via ecological momentary assessment (EMA). These temporally dense data are also highly contextualized, taken in the course of daily life, where, when, and how it most matters for understanding and intervening in behavior. With technological innovations that advance both the hardware [4] (i.e., lower power requirement, wireless data transmission, smaller portable sensors) and the software aspects [5] (i.e., increasingly sophisticated algorithms) of mobile devices, mHealth solutions offer clinicians and scientists unprecedented opportunities to understand behaviors and diseases with more clarity and to intervene in complex behaviors and their antecedents in ways that would have been pragmatically impossible to achieve using traditional research methodologies [4].

Deployable and wearable sensors, such as accelerometers, have demonstrated high validity in measuring key obesity-related behaviors [5], including physical activity, time spent in sedentary behavior, sleep patterns, and key risk factors such as blood pressure [6]. Other types of sensors, including deployable and ingestible sensors, can provide highly contextualized and temporally dense data on behaviors. Examples of these sensors include home-deployed sensors that track and transmit speed of gait within the home [7] and medicine-bottle sensors that can track and report on compliance with drug and data collection regiments in real time [8]. Some other key obesity-related behaviors, in particular dietary intake, remain challenging to measure with the current technology. However, progress is being made, for example, through photography and pattern recognition, crowd sourcing, wearable sensors, and other technology-driven mobile solutions [9–12].

In addition to capturing data using wearable and deployable sensors, mobile devices can also facilitate the collection of participants' self-reported data in natural settings multiple times within a day. Experience sampling methods (ESM), such as EMA and other similar methodologies, capitalize on the capability of mobile devices to emit signals (audible, haptic, or embedded in the environment). These signals can be set up to prompt participants for information (1) at random times, (2) at a specific time or within a window of time, (3) in response to specific subjective experiences, or (4) triggered based on sensed events. Self-report and sensor data collected in real or near time and context (location and situation) of events and experiences are considered to be more ecologically valid and may be less prone to recall bias [6].

These and other mHealth solutions can be and have been applied to the prevention and treatment of childhood obesity, and offer four major advantages: (1) improved measurement capabilities and ecological validity, (2) innovative platforms for collecting and displaying data on obesity-related behaviors and their antecedents, (3) the capacity to deliver novel interventions in real time and in context, and (4) the capacity to deliver highly personalized interventions that adapt in an ongoing fashion to each individual's needs. Taken together, these advantages provide the capacity to deliver what has been termed *just-in-time adaptive interventions* or JITAIs [13]. JITAIs are highly personalized mobile interventions that are delivered "just-in-time," that is, when a person is available and in need, for instance after a sensed bout of more than 30 min of inactivity, and anywhere, that is, during the course of a person's everyday life. JITAIs use incoming personal data (from smartphones, sensors, the Internet, etc.) to adapt over time to that specific individual's changing status and circumstances, with the goal to address the individual personalized needs. These highly precise interventions are likely the future of precision behavioral medicine.

While advancements in technologies and research methodologies allow clinicians and researchers to obtain high-resolution data about patients and participants, the use of these data and devices for understanding and changing behavior has been inconsistent across disciplines. The expectations of mHealth currently outshine the efficacy that the current state of evidence supports, leaving many to suspect that mHealth may not meet its expected potential [14]. However, the field is only beginning to understand how to use the temporally dense, highly contextualized data produced by mHealth technologies [15], and current mHealth interventions, particularly in pediatric populations, fail to take full advantage of the intervention capabilities of mHealth technologies [1,5,16]. This chapter will examine the literature on the use of mHealth solutions in preventing and treating pediatric obesity to date and the current technology used for measuring key obesity-related behaviors, describe the current limitations and challenges in using mHealth tools to change behavior, and conclude with suggestions on how researchers and clinicians could take fuller advantage of the sophisticated technologies now available, including implementing research designs that are more suitable to mHealth interventions [13,17,18].

CURRENT STATE OF MHEALTH IN CHILDHOOD OBESITY

Text Messages or Short Message Service

Text messaging, or short message service (SMS), is a commonly used channel for communication among the youth population. The PEW Research Center Teen Relationships Survey study conducted between 2014 and 2015 found that 91% of 13–17-year-old youths who owned a cell phone had engaged in conversations either through instant messaging mobile applications (e.g., WhatsApp and Kik) or SMS in their daily lives [3]. Although 33% of the phone-owning youth reportedly used instant messaging applications (apps) to communicate, SMS has been and continues to be an extensively used communication medium among the youth population [3,19]. Several SMS-based intervention feasibility trials in youth populations have reported that SMS is an acceptable [20–24] and, in some instances, a preferable intervention delivery method compared with other face-to-face or paper-pencil modalities [24,25]. Despite youth's acceptance of and preference for SMS as a medium for communication, the effectiveness of interventions that use SMS as the sole or main intervention modality in pediatric obesity interventions to change adiposity (e.g., body mass index [BMI], BMI z-score, waist circumference, visceral fat, percentage body fat, etc.), metabolic health (e.g., insulin sensitivity), and behavior (e.g., physical activity and dietary intake) has been mixed [1,6,26].

mHealth pediatric obesity prevention and treatment studies published through 2014 were recently systematically reviewed by Turner et al. [1]. Among the 32 unique studies reviewed, eight of them focused on the efficacy of using SMS in changing adiposity, metabolic, and behavioral outcomes. Among these, three studies utilized a randomized controlled trial (RCT) study design to examine the efficacy of using SMS as a weight maintenance intervention condition, in addition to a group-based intervention [27], a face-to-face intervention [28], and other electronic communication methods (i.e., a website) [29]. The three RCT studies sent texts on a weekly [27] or biweekly [28] basis to promote self-reporting and self-monitoring of obesity-related behaviors [27], promote goal setting [28,29], provide tailored suggestions [28,29], and provide reminders for intervention adherence [28,29]. Overall, although one study reported lowered study attrition among participants who received the SMS-based intervention [27], all three studies concluded that the SMS-based approach did not provide additional effects in reducing adiposity, improving metabolic health, or obesity-related behaviors over the other face-to-face intervention modalities [1,27–29]. For the most part, the SMS in these studies was automated "one-size-fits-all," with adaptation to self-reported data on a weekly basis in the more sophisticated studies [27,29]. In one of the two studies that did provide tailored feedback based on the weekly self-monitoring data, higher self-reported physical activity and improved dietary intake were observed among youths who were more compliant [27]. This suggests that using SMS as a channel to disseminate adaptive and personalized feedback may potentially be efficacious in changing obesity-related behaviors in youth. Similar results were found in two of the five pilot studies reported on in the Turner et al. review, as well as in four studies that were identified in an updated search, reported here. These studies used SMS to provide personalized feedback, on a daily basis, based on participants' self-reported baseline characteristics [30] and on self-reported [25,31] and sensor-based [16] data. The studies reported that personalized feedback exhibited preliminary efficacy in reducing time spent in sedentary behavior [25,31], time spent in physical activity [30], and increasing fruit and vegetable consumption [31].

Although the existing evidence may suggest that, overall, SMS-based interventions do not achieve significant improvement in obesity-related clinical and behavioral outcomes among youth [1], these studies represent early mHealth efforts. mHealth technologies are developing at a fast pace, and these early efforts are only beginning to scratch the surface of what can be done in a JITAI. While SMS has been shown to be an acceptable method for communicating with youth populations, guidelines on important experimental design factors, such as the effective dose and content of SMS for specific groups of youth, in time and in context, remain to be established [1,13]. Furthermore, most SMS studies to date have not used streaming data or available sensor technologies (for instance, those offered by the mobile phone) that could inform intervention delivery based on location, behavior patterns, context, time, and previous individual reactions to particular messages, timing, and other associated factors. Only one pilot study in children to date has used streaming data from wearable sensors to inform SMS messages in real time and in context, resulting in declines in time spent in sedentary behavior, as well as increases in physical activity [16]. Emerging evidence demonstrates that SMS with just-in-time, adaptive, and contextualized feedback may promote change in important obesity-related behaviors [16,25,30,31]. SMS may be an optimal channel to promote obesity-related behavior change among youth when participant data are incorporated in an ongoing fashion to inform just-in-time and adaptive delivery.

Interventions Using Mobile Applications

Mobile apps provide a variety of functions beyond offering instant communication; that is, they provide interactive ways to collect and use self-reported data from external devices [32] and other sources such as social networks [33], act as platforms for more sophisticated data visualization [32], and offer the possibility of gamifying interventions [33,34]. Some of these advantageous functions offered by mobile apps have been adopted for the prevention and treatment of pediatric obesity. This is documented both by the increase in health-related "off-the-shelf" apps for pediatric obesity prevention and treatment that are available for a fee [35] and the evidence available on pediatric obesity prevention and intervention efforts using mobile apps [1,16]. While the body of evidence on the use of mobile apps to prevent and treat pediatric obesity continues to grow, the efficacy of using mobile apps to change obesity-related behavior or prevent pediatric obesity is considered preliminarily but moderately effective [1,5].

The mHealth pediatric obesity studies included in the review by Turner et al. [1] used a variety of mobile platforms, such as personal digital assistants (PDA), game consoles, and smartphone apps. These platforms were used mostly to deliver an intervention [33,36–41] or to collect data about obesity-related behaviors (either in conjunction with sensors [32,36–38,40–47] or as a medium for self-monitoring and self-reporting [39,40,48–51]). Although the evidence is preliminary, several pilot intervention studies [33,38–41,52,53] have reported intervention effects in changing obesity-related behaviors. These intervention studies used mobile apps as a channel to provide personalized feedback automated from preset algorithms [39,41,52], participants' social circles [38,40], or virtual avatars in the app [33]. In these and a few more recent studies, personalized feedback was constructed using data captured by wearable sensors [16,33,38,41,52] and self-reported data [39,40]. These approaches were found to be efficacious in modifying obesity-related behavior, including increasing time spent in physical activity [40,41]; reducing time spent in sedentary behavior [16]; improving fruit, vegetable, and breakfast consumption [33,39,52]; and changing psychological antecedents to these behaviors, such as lowering the perceived effort in engaging in physical activity [38]. While these approaches have demonstrated some preliminary efficacy in changing obesity-related behavior, it is clear from the literature that the incorporation of user-centered design throughout the app or sensor development process is important in designing an effective mHealth pediatric obesity prevention or intervention study [1]. Using mobile apps and combinations of apps with sensors for changing obesity-related behavior among youth is often reported as acceptable [1,39,40,50,54] and preferable over the traditional paper-pencil modality [39,48]. Several user studies have reported that app designers need to pay attention to gender-specific preferences [42], and design to enhance motivation to continue using the application [36]. The ideal amount of engagement time with any specific app or mobile intervention has yet to be ascertained [44]. Finally, the measurement accuracy of apps, for instance, using apps to record dietary intake, needs to be improved [55].

While the evidence is limited to published pilot or feasibility trials, preliminary results suggest that interventions using mobile apps are not only acceptable [39,40,42,45,50], but also potentially effective intervention delivery methods that result in modifications of obesity-related behavior [33,39–41] and the associated psychological antecedents [37,56] in youth. Personalized feedback based on data ubiquitously captured by wearable sensors and participants' self-reported data shows potential for modifying obesity-related behaviors [1,52,53]. Incorporation of wearable or other deployable sensors [57] will deepen our understanding of the dynamics of obesity-related behaviors in time and context [15]. This understanding will further aid clinicians and researchers in developing personalized, interactive, contextualized feedback necessary to intervene in obesity-related behaviors in real time using JITAIs [13]. The incorporation of mobile apps and wearable devices/sensors to treat and prevent pediatric obesity is still a nascent field, and user-centered design is an essential step for program development.

Wearable and Deployable Devices/Sensors in mHealth Pediatric Obesity Studies

The use of real-time feedback has enormous potential for changing obesity-related behaviors in pediatric populations [16]. However, outcomes are dependent on feedback that is developed based on accurate and timely measures of appropriate (to the intervention) user information. Researchers and clinicians have been able to assess study participants' self-reported behavior and experiences since the introduction of ESM and the invention of early mobile technologies such as PDAs [1]. However, data on key obesity-related behaviors, including sedentary behavior, physical activity, and dietary behavior, are susceptible to biases that stem from self-reporting, including memory lapses and purposeful omission [58]. The objective, accurate, contextualized, and real- or near-time measurement of obesity-related behavior is one of the central promises of mHealth solutions. The incorporation of validated wearable devices will help to realize these promises by providing insight into participants' behavior with an improved ecological, as well as measurement, validity, and decreased user burden. Measuring complicated behaviors, such as physical activity and dietary behavior, however, is challenging even with wearable sensors. This section will provide an overview of the current use of wearable sensors in measuring key obesity-related behaviors, including physical activity, sedentary behavior, and dietary behavior, in pediatric obesity studies.

A recent review published by Bort-Roig et al. [5] used evidence published through 2013 to systematically examine the current use of technology in measuring and influencing physical activity. Among the 26 unique studies examined, Bort-Roig et al. found that external measurement devices (e.g., pedometers), external (waist- or wrist-worn) acceleration-based motion sensors, and accelerometers inside smartphones are the most commonly used equipment to obtain objective physical activity measurements [5]. Accelerometers, or microelectromechanical systems (MEMS-based accelerometers), are considered the current gold standard for objectively measuring physical activity and sedentary behavior. Accelerometers measure physical activity by converting acceleration captured by built-in transducers into a quantifiable signal [59]. Because many new accelerometers are providing raw data rather than preprocessed data such as "counts," advanced algorithms, using signals captured by accelerometers, can now be processed to yield excellent measurement accuracy when the accelerometers are worn on the waist or hip areas [5]. Besides triaxial accelerometers, more complex approaches such as on-body sensing with a combination of multiple devices (e.g., an accelerometer with a heart rate monitor, gyroscope, and magnetic sensors) [5,32] and smart watches [5] are available to capture physical activity and sedentary behavior. Wearable technologies such as gyroscopes and magnetic sensors have also shown high accuracy in capturing key physical activity and sedentary behaviors such as sitting, standing, walking, and jogging [5]. However, evidence on using real-time data captured by wearable sensors to prevent and treat obesity in natural settings is limited [5], especially among pediatric populations [1,16]. Although Bluetooth and other wireless data transmission technology is available, to date, there is only one pilot study that has incorporated real-time physical activity data in promoting physical activity in a youth sample [16].

Accurate assessment of dietary intake is one of the greatest challenges in obesity research, and depends on the accurate estimation of portion sizes, the identification of ingredients, and the accurate identification of eating occasions. Accurate measurement, inference, and estimation of dietary intake using wearable and deployable sensors remains challenging [9,60]. Although a majority of efforts have been focusing on using mobile technology to enhance recall-based collection methodologies (e.g., providing visualized examples of portion sizes and fully automated self-administered dietary assessment [1,60]), there is a rapidly growing body of literature focusing on memory-independent collection methodologies using wearable sensors [9]. A recent work by Steele provided an overview of technologies that are currently being used for the automated capture of dietary intake information. Among the current technologies, portion-size estimation has largely relied on pattern recognition and image-analysis approaches [9,61]. Besides portion-size estimation, image analysis has also shown some promise in identifying types of food consumed and nutrient-intake estimation [61]. These data have also been accrued using bar code or quick response (QR) code scanners [9,60]. Nonetheless, as image-analysis approaches mainly rely on food appearance features (e.g., color, texture, and shape) and largely ignore the structural features of food (e.g., density of the food in the image) [61], there are inaccuracies inherent in intake estimation using this approach. Another drawback of image-analysis approaches is that they require participant compliance; participants must provide a picture of food before and after consumption, and often need to include in the picture a reference card or fiduciary marker [61] as a reference in order to determine absolute size. Other wearable sensors are currently being developed that require less user effort and compliance including the wrist-worn bite counter (although this must be actively turned on by the participant at each eating event) [62], acoustic-based sensing [63], neck-worn, multisensor lanyards, and "smart" kitchen equipment [9]. Among these devices, wrist-worn bite counters and acoustic-based sensors have been able to fairly accurately measure the amount [62,64] or type [63,64] of food consumed. Nonetheless, each approach still faces some technical limitations. For instance, for pattern recognition, identification of the wide variety of food that participants consume in "free-living" situations remains a tremendous challenge. Although evidence on the usability and acceptability of wearable and deployable technologies in estimating dietary intake in youth is limited [1], the use of mobile health solutions do exhibit preliminary efficacy in the objective measurement of key dimensions of dietary intake [9,61,64].

mHEALTH CHALLENGES: MOVING THE FIELD FORWARD

This chapter provides an overview of the current use of mHealth solutions to prevent and treat pediatric obesity. Several mHealth strategies, including the use of personalized feedback and interactive data visualization, have shown preliminary efficacy in changing key obesity-related behaviors and some of their antecedents in pediatric populations. These strategies capitalize on expanding mobile device ownership and the acceptability of using mobile devices as a means of communication. However, to date most mHealth interventions do not yet capitalize on the full capacities of mHealth technology to develop true JITAIs, providing personalized, adaptive interventions at the moment and in the dose and format that is appropriate for each individual. The true potential of mHealth resides in harnessing rich user information that is constantly streaming from and ubiquitously captured by wearable devices, as suggested in studies that incorporate real-time user information into interventions [16]. However, there are a number of challenges associated with capitalizing on mHealth solutions that need to be considered. These challenges include the need for improved transdisciplinary collaborations, a reconsideration of our measurement and modeling paradigms, and the need for agile and adaptive intervention strategies and evaluation methodologies.

Technology, Transdisciplinarity, and Measurement

mHealth is an inherently transdisciplinary endeavor, and continuing efforts to develop communications among researchers, clinicians, and engineers are essential for designing effective mHealth systems [4,15,65]. Particularly when working with children and minorities, a user-centered approach in designing mHealth systems can be critical in improving both the quality and the effectiveness of the study. Intended participants and patients with "experiential knowledge" can be considered as another one of the "disciplines" that need to be at the table [1]. Another major challenge associated with mHealth technologies is ensuring the security and privacy of data captured by and transmitted from wearable sensors or personal mobile devices [66]. Although ethical issues in mHealth are beyond the scope of this chapter, disciplines that cover data safety and security, as well as medical and research ethics, should be consulted where appropriate [67].

Ensuring the validity and reliability of data collected via wearable sensors and personal mobile devices is essential in attaining quality of the collected data [4,66]. However, using wearable devices and personal mobile devices for data collection in the free-living conditions of natural environments presents different challenges that cannot be simulated in controlled laboratory settings [4,68]. New data streams also bring new issues in measurement and modeling [15]. Although these new areas of research are beyond the scope of this chapter, one example is that, while ascertaining reliability at the group level has been a major concern in measurement methodology, data from new technologies are providing unprecedented opportunities to understand the reliability at the individual level that will, in turn, eventually impact on what are considered "good" measures [69].

Need for New Evaluation Methodologies

Currently, technology development outpaces the evaluation of mHealth intervention across disciplines [1,4,15,16,26]. RCTs have long been the gold standard for evaluating interventions; however, these typically take years. Technology evolves so quickly that a study technology may be outdated or obsolete prior to the completion of a full RCT [4,70]. Agile research designs and agile evaluation frameworks are needed that can accommodate studies that use the full potential of mHealth solutions. An earlier report by an interdisciplinary group of mHealth researchers outlines various innovative research designs and evaluation frameworks that accommodate these needs [4]. This report presents some of the leading new evaluation frameworks, including multiphase optimization strategies (MOST) [18] and sequential multiple assignment randomized trials (SMART) [71]. These frameworks capitalize on the rapid personalization opportunities offered by new technologies to adapt interventions on the fly according to participants' incoming data and to improve intervention efficiency by sequentially randomizing participants within the study.

SUMMARY AND CONCLUSIONS

This chapter discussed the current state of evidence and current challenges for mHealth pediatric obesity prevention and intervention studies. Innovative technologies have been repeatedly demonstrated to be acceptable and feasible tools for collecting objective, contextualized, and real-time data in youth populations [1]. Emerging evidence from recent pediatric obesity prevention and intervention studies has further suggested that personalizing interventions based on these temporally and contextually relevant participant data, whether it is acquired from self-report or ubiquitously captured by wearable sensors, offers promising strategies to change and maintain obesity-related behaviors [16]. To date, both SMS and mobile apps are commonly used platforms for participants to self-report data in a timely fashion through time-based prompting schemes (e.g., random time or stratified time-block prompting schedules) [1]. Nonetheless, pediatric obesity interventions and behavioral assessment studies based on the use of context-sensitive or "event-based" [6] data, whether via self-report or sensed events and contexts, have progressed at a slower pace [1]. The bulk of prevention and intervention science was necessarily built to seek the one best possible solution for the largest number of people [72]. New technologies can now support interventions that provide the best possible solution for each individual in time and context (JITAIs). Intervention dose, timing, content, and modality can be increasingly tailored according to individual needs and adapted over time as the individual changes [13]. These highly individualized and precise interventions are the very near future of personalized behavioral medicine.

REFERENCES

1. Turner T, Spruijt-Metz D, Wen CK, Hingle MD. Prevention and treatment of pediatric obesity using mobile and wireless technologies: A systematic review. *Pediatric Obesity.* 2015;10(6):403–9.
2. The World in 2015: ICT Facts and Figures [Internet]. 2015. Available from: http://www.itu.int/en/ITU-D/Statistics/Documents/facts/ICTFactsFigures2015.pdf.
3. Lenhart A, Duggan M, Perrin A, Stepler R, Rainie L, Parker K. Teens, social media, and technology overview 2015. PEW Research Center: 2015 April 9, 2015.
4. Kumar S, Nilsen WJ, Abernethy A, Atienza A, Patrick K, Pavel M, et al. Mobile health technology evaluation: The mHealth evidence workshop. *American Journal of Preventive Medicine.* 2013;45(2):228–36.
5. Bort-Roig J, Gilson ND, Puig-Ribera A, Contreras RS, Trost SG. Measuring and influencing physical activity with smartphone technology: A systematic review. *Sports Medicine.* 2014;44(5):671–86.

6. Kaplan RM, Stone AA. Bringing the laboratory and clinic to the community: Mobile technologies for health promotion and disease prevention. *Annual Review of Psychology.* 2013;64:471–98.

7. Jimison HB, McKanna J, Ambert K, Hagler S, Hatt WJ, Pavel M. Models of cognitive performance based on home monitoring data. *Conference Proceedings: IEEE Engineering in Medicine and Biology Society.* 2010;2010:5234–7.

8. Wen CKF, Weigensberg M, Schneider S, Weerman B, Spruijt-Metz D. Validity of ZEMI on ambulatory salivary cortisol assessment in an adolescent population. Wireless Health Conference 2015, Bethesda, MD, 2015.

9. Steele R. An overview of the state of the art of automated capture of dietary intake information. *Critical Reviews in Food Science and Nutrition.* 2015;55(13):1929–38.

10. Turner-McGrievy GM, Helander EE, Kaipainen K, Perez-Macias JM, Korhonen I. The use of crowdsourcing for dietary self-monitoring: Crowdsourced ratings of food pictures are comparable to ratings by trained observers. *Journal of the American Medical Informatics Association.* 2015;22(e1):e112–9.

11. Stumbo PJ. New technology in dietary assessment: A review of digital methods in improving food record accuracy. *Proceedings of the Nutrition Society.* 2013;72(1):70–6.

12. Scisco JL, Muth ER, Hoover AW. Examining the utility of a bite-count–based measure of eating activity in free-living human beings. *Journal of the Academy of Nutrition and Dietetics.* 2014;114(3):464–9.

13. Nahum-Shani I, Hekler E, Spruijt-Metz D. Building health behavior models to guide the development of just-in-time adaptive interventions: A pragmatic framework. *Health Psychology.* 2015;34 Suppl:1209–19.

14. Tomlinson M, Rotheram-Borus MJ, Swartz L, Tsai AC. Scaling up mHealth: Where is the evidence? *PLoS Med.* 2013;10(2):e1001382.

15. Spruijt-Metz D, Hekler E, Saranummi N, Intille S, Korhonen I, Nilsen W, et al. Building new computational models to support health behavior change and maintenance: New opportunities in behavioral research. *Translational Behavioral Medicine.* 2015;5(3):335–46.

16. Spruijt-Metz D, Wen CK, O'Reilly G, Li M, Lee S, Emken BA, et al. Innovations in the use of interactive technology to support weight management. *Current Obesity Reports.* 2015;4(4):510–9.

17. Collins LM, Murphy SA, Strecher V. The multiphase optimization strategy (MOST) and the sequential multiple assignment randomized trial (SMART): New methods for more potent eHealth interventions. *American Journal of Preventive Medicine.* 2007;32(5 Suppl):S112–8.

18. Rivera DE, Pew MD, Collins LM. Using engineering control principles to inform the design of adaptive interventions: A conceptual introduction. *Drug and Alcohol Dependence.* 2007;88 Suppl 2:S31–40.

19. Lenhart A. Teens, smartphones & texting. *Pew Internet & American Life Project.* 2012.

20. Woolford SJ, Khan S, Barr KL, Clark SJ, Strecher VJ, Resnicow K. A picture may be worth a thousand texts: Obese adolescents' perspectives on a modified photovoice activity to aid weight loss. *Childhood Obesity.* 2012;8(3):230–6.

21. Hingle M, Nichter M, Medeiros M, Grace S. Texting for health: The use of participatory methods to develop healthy lifestyle messages for teens. *Journal of Nutrition Education and Behavior.* 2013;45(1):12–9.

22. Woolford SJ, Clark SJ, Strecher VJ, Resnicow K. Tailored mobile phone text messages as an adjunct to obesity treatment for adolescents. *Journal of Telemedicine and Telecare.* 2010;16(8):458–61.

23. Woolford SJ, Barr KL, Derry HA, Jepson CM, Clark SJ, Strecher VJ, et al. OMG do not say LOL: Obese adolescents' perspectives on the content of text messages to enhance weight loss efforts. *Obesity (Silver Spring).* 2011;19(12):2382–7.

24. Sharifi M, Dryden EM, Horan CM, Price S, Marshall R, Hacker K, et al. Leveraging text messaging and mobile technology to support pediatric obesity-related behavior change: A qualitative study using parent focus groups and interviews. *Journal of Medical Internet Research.* 2013;15(12):e272.

25. Shapiro JR, Bauer S, Hamer RM, Kordy H, Ward D, Bulik CM. Use of text messaging for monitoring sugar-sweetened beverages, physical activity, and screen time in children: A pilot study. *Journal of Nutrition Education and Behavior.* 2008;40(6):385–91.

26. Cole-Lewis H, Kershaw T. Text messaging as a tool for behavior change in disease prevention and management. *Epidemiologic Reviews.* 2010;32:56–69.

27. de Niet J, Timman R, Bauer S, van den Akker E, Buijks H, de Klerk C, et al. The effect of a short message service maintenance treatment on body mass index and psychological well-being in overweight and obese children: A randomized controlled trial. *Pediatric Obesity.* 2012;7(3):205–19.

28. Nguyen B, Shrewsbury VA, O'Connor J, Steinbeck KS, Hill AJ, Shah S, et al. Two-year outcomes of an adjunctive telephone coaching and electronic contact intervention for adolescent weight-loss maintenance: The Loozit randomized controlled trial. *International Journal of Obesity (London).* 2013;37(3):468–72.

29. Patrick K, Norman GJ, Davila EP, Calfas KJ, Raab F, Gottschalk M, et al. Outcomes of a 12-month technology-based intervention to promote weight loss in adolescents at risk for type 2 diabetes. *Journal of Diabetes Science & Technology*. 2013;7(3):759–70.

30. Sirriyeh R, Lawton R, Ward J. Physical activity and adolescents: An exploratory randomized controlled trial investigating the influence of affective and instrumental text messages. *British Journal of Health Psychology*. 2010;15(Pt 4):825–40.

31. Silva C, Fassnacht DB, Ali K, Gonçalves S, Conceição E, Vaz A, et al. Promoting health behaviour in Portuguese children via Short Message Service: The efficacy of a text-messaging programme. *Journal of Health Psychology*. 2015;20(6):806–15.

32. Emken BA, Li M, Thatte G, Lee S, Annavaram M, Mitra U, et al. Recognition of physical activities in overweight Hispanic youth using KNOWME Networks. *Journal of Physical Activity & Health*. 2012;9(3):432.

33. Byrne S, Gay G, Pollack J, Gonzales A, Retelny D, Lee T, et al. Caring for mobile phone-based virtual pets can influence youth eating behaviors. *Journal of Children and Media*. 2012;6(1):83–99.

34. Lister C, West JH, Cannon B, Sax T, Brodegard D. Just a fad? Gamification in health and fitness apps. *JMIR Serious Games*. 2014;2(2):e9.

35. Schoffman DE, Turner-McGrievy G, Jones SJ, Wilcox S. Mobile apps for pediatric obesity prevention and treatment, healthy eating, and physical activity promotion: Just fun and games? *Translational Behavioral Medicine*. 2013;3(3):320–5.

36. Edwards HM, McDonald S, Zhao T, Humphries L. Design requirements for persuasive technologies to motivate physical activity in adolescents: A field study. *Behaviour & Information Technology*. 2014;33(9):968–86.

37. Guixeres J, Cantero L, Lurbe E, Saiz J, Raya MA, Cebolla A, et al. Effects of virtual reality during exercise in children. *Journal of Universal Computer Science*. 2013;19(9):1199–218.

38. Lu F, Turner K, eds. Improving adolescent fitness attitudes with a mobile fitness game to combat obesity in youth. In *Games Innovation Conference (IGIC), 2013 IEEE International*, Vancouver, BC: IEEE, pp. 148–51, 2013.

39. Nollen NL, Hutcheson T, Carlson S, Rapoff M, Goggin K, Mayfield C, et al. Development and functionality of a handheld computer program to improve fruit and vegetable intake among low-income youth. *Health Education Research*. 2013;28(2):249–64.

40. Toscos T, Faber A, Connelly K, Upoma AM, eds. Encouraging physical activity in teens: Can technology help reduce barriers to physical activity in adolescent girls? In *Pervasive Computing Technologies for Healthcare, 2008 PervasiveHealth 2008 Second International Conference*, Tampere, Finland: IEEE, pp. 218–221, 2008.

41. Valentín G, Howard AM, eds. Dealing with childhood obesity: Passive versus active activity monitoring approaches for engaging individuals in exercise. In *Biosignals and Biorobotics Conference (BRC), 2013 ISSNIP*, Rio de Janerio: IEEE, pp. 1–5, 2013.

42. Arteaga SM, González VM, Kurniawan S, Benavides RA. Mobile games and design requirements to increase teenagers' physical activity. *Pervasive and Mobile Computing*. 2012;8(6):900–8.

43. Schiel R, Kaps A, Bieber G. Electronic health technology for the assessment of physical activity and eating habits in children and adolescents with overweight and obesity IDA. *Appetite*. 2012;58(2):432–7.

44. Clawson J, Patel N, Starner T, eds. Dancing in the streets: The design and evaluation of a wearable health game. In *Wearable Computers (ISWC), 2010 International Symposium on*, Seoul: IEEE, pp. 1–4, 2010.

45. Dunton GF, Liao Y, Intille SS, Spruijt-Metz D, Pentz M. Investigating children's physical activity and sedentary behavior using ecological momentary assessment with mobile phones. *Obesity (Silver Spring)*. 2011;19(6):1205–12.

46. Daugherty BL, Schap TE, Ettienne-Gittens R, Zhu FM, Bosch M, Delp EJ, et al. Novel technologies for assessing dietary intake: Evaluating the usability of a mobile telephone food record among adults and adolescents. *Journal of Medical Internet Research*. 2012;14(2):e58.

47. Vazquez-Briseno M, Navarro-Cota C, Nieto-Hipolito JI, Jimenez-Garcia E, Sanchez-Lopez J, eds. A proposal for using the internet of things concept to increase children's health awareness. In *Electrical Communications and Computers (CONIELECOMP), 2012 22nd International Conference on*, Cholula, Puebla: IEEE, pp. 168–72, 2012.

48. Cushing CC, Jensen CD, Steele RG. An evaluation of a personal electronic device to enhance self-monitoring adherence in a pediatric weight management program using a multiple baseline design. *Journal of Pediatric Psychology*. 2011;36(3):301–7.

49. Rofey DL, Hull EE, Phillips J, Vogt K, Silk JS, Dahl RE. Utilizing Ecological Momentary Assessment in pediatric obesity to quantify behavior, emotion, and sleep. *Obesity (Silver Spring)*. 2010;18(6):1270–2.

50. Bielik P, Tomlein M, Krátky P, Mitrík Š, Barla M, Bieliková M, eds. Move2Play: An innovative approach to encouraging people to be more physically active. In *Proceedings of the 2nd ACM SIGHIT International Health Informatics Symposium,* New York: ACM, pp. 61–70, 2012.

51. Boushey CJ, Kerr DA, Wright J, Lutes KD, Ebert DS, Delp EJ. Use of technology in children's dietary assessment. *Eur J Clin Nutr.* 2009;63 Suppl 1:S50–7.

52. Nollen NL, Mayo MS, Carlson SE, Rapoff MA, Goggin KJ, Ellerbeck EF. Mobile technology for obesity prevention: A randomized pilot study in racial-and ethnic-minority girls. *American Journal of Preventive Medicine.* 2014;46(4):404–8.

53. Smith JJ, Morgan PJ, Plotnikoff RC, Dally KA, Salmon J, Okely AD, et al. Smart-phone obesity prevention trial for adolescent boys in low-income communities: The ATLAS RCT. *Pediatrics.* 2014;134(3):e723–31.

54. Arteaga SM, Kudeki M, Woodworth A, Kurniawan S, eds. Mobile system to motivate teenagers' physical activity. In *Proceedings of the 9th International Conference on Interaction Design and Children,* New York: ACM, pp. 1–10, 2010.

55. Mariappan A, Bosch M, Zhu F, Boushey CJ, Kerr DA, Ebert DS, et al., eds. Personal dietary assessment using mobile devices. In *IS&T/SPIE Electronic Imaging; 2009: International Society for Optics and Photonics,* 2009. http://proceedings.spiedigitallibrary.org/volume.aspx?conference id=1193&volumeid=1872.

56. Lu F, Turner K, Murphy B, eds. Reducing adolescent obesity with a mobile fitness application: Study results of youth age 15 to 17. In *e-Health Networking, Applications & Services (Healthcom), 2013 IEEE 15th International Conference on,* Libson: IEEE, pp. 554–8, 2013.

57. Krebs P, Duncan DT. Health app use among US mobile phone owners: A national survey. *Journal of Medical Internet Research.* 2015;3(4):e101.

58. Spruijt-Metz D, Belcher BR, Hsu YW, McClain AD, Chou CP, Nguyen-Rodriguez S, et al. Temporal relationship between insulin sensitivity and the pubertal decline in physical activity in peripubertal Hispanic and African American females. *Diabetes Care.* 2013;36(11):3739–45.

59. Miller J, ed. Accelerometer technologies, specifications, and limitations. *International Conference on Ambulatory Monitoring and Physical Activity Measurement.* Amherst, MA, 2013.

60. Illner AK, Freisling H, Boeing H, Huybrechts I, Crispim SP, Slimani N. Review and evaluation of innovative technologies for measuring diet in nutritional epidemiology. *International Journal of Epidemiology.* 2012;41(4):1187–203.

61. Probst Y, Nguyen DT, Rollo M, Li W. mHealth diet and nutrition guidance. In S. Adibi (ed.), *mHealth Multidisciplinary Verticals,* p. 65, Boca Raton, FL, CRC Press, 2014.

62. Scisco JL, Muth ER, Dong Y, Hoover AW. Slowing bite-rate reduces energy intake: An application of the bite counter device. *Journal of the American Dietetic Association.* 2011;111(8):1231–5.

63. Amft O, ed. A wearable earpad sensor for chewing monitoring. In *Sensors, 2010 IEEE,* Kona, HI: IEEE, pp. 222–27, 2010.

64. Liu J, Johns E, Atallah L, Pettitt C, Lo B, Frost G, et al., eds. An intelligent food-intake monitoring system using wearable sensors. In *Wearable and Implantable Body Sensor Networks (BSN), 2012 Ninth International Conference on,* London: IEEE, pp. 154–60, 2012.

65. Estrin D, Sim I. Health care delivery. Open mHealth architecture: An engine for health care innovation. *Science.* 2010;330(6005):759–60.

66. Kumar S, Nilsen W, Pavel M, Srivastava M. Mobile health: Revolutionizing healthcare through transdisciplinary research. *Computer.* 2013;(1):28–35.

67. Capron AM, Spruijt-Metz D. Behavioral economics in the physician-patient relationship: A possible role for mobile devices and small data. In Cohen IG, Lynch HF, Robertson CT, eds. *Nudging Health: Health Law and Behavioral Economics,* Baltimore, MD: Johns Hopkins University Press, 233–243.

68. Barnett A, Cerin E, Vandelanotte C, Matsumoto A, Jenkins D. Validity of treadmill-and track-based individual calibration methods for estimating free-living walking speed and VO_2 using the Actigraph accelerometer. *BMC Sports Science, Medicine and Rehabilitation.* 2015;7(1):29.

69. Schneider S, Stone AA. Ambulatory and diary methods can facilitate the measurement of patient-reported outcomes. *Quality of Life Research.* 2015:1–10.

70. Ioannidis JP. Effect of the statistical significance of results on the time to completion and publication of randomized efficacy trials. *JAMA.* 1998;279(4):281–6.

71. Lizotte DJ, Bowling MH, Murphy SA, eds. Efficient reinforcement learning with multiple reward functions for randomized controlled trial analysis. In *Proceedings of the 27th International Conference on Machine Learning (ICML-10)*, 2010.
72. Hekler E, Michie S, Rivera DE, Collins LM, Pavel M, Jimison HB, et al. Advancing models and theories for digital behavior change interventions. *American Journal of Preventive Medicine*. In press.

40 Complementary and Integrative Health Strategies for Addressing Childhood Obesity

Marc J. Weigensberg

CONTENTS

INTRODUCTION AND DEFINITIONS

This chapter introduces a broad range of complementary integrative health approaches to childhood and adolescent obesity. This is a relatively new field, and one with which many in the world of conventional medicine remain unfamiliar. Therefore, before delving directly into the specific modalities, the chapter will first deal with some of the basic concepts and definitions relating to *alternative*, *complementary*, and *integrative* health and medicine.

Multiple terms have been used over the last 20 years to describe the growing use of therapies that have been generally considered nonconventional in the context of Western, allopathic medicine practice. The term *alternative medicine* generally refers to those therapies and practices that are used *in place of* conventional medicine, while *complementary medicine* generally indicates those practices that are used as complements or adjuncts to conventional allopathic therapy. In recent years, the term *integrative medicine* has generally replaced these older terminologies, as a growing research evidence base has demonstrated the effectiveness of some of these therapies once considered alternative by the conventional medical field [1]. Integrative medicine therefore implies and promotes an integration of all health practices and therapies, whether Western based or complementary, using an integrated approach to the treatment of disease and/or the promotion of health and wellness in human beings. Integrative medicine also represents an approach to the whole human being—body, mind, emotion, and spirit—recognizing and encompassing emotional, spiritual, social, cultural, and environmental influences on the overall health of the human organism. The term *integrative health*, in contrast to *integrative medicine*, may be used to designate those practices that promote health, wellness, and well-being, rather than emphasizing those therapies or medicines that treat specific pathological conditions within the Western medicine paradigm. Finally, integrative medicine/health is generally practiced as a collaborative relationship between the patient and a clinician who understands the benefits of both complementary and Western medicine and can guide the patient toward optimal health by integrating the benefits of both.

Given this general overview, the most widely used definitions today to describe these concepts can be taken from national and international institutions that are leading the field of integrative medicine and health. The National Center for Complementary and Integrative Health, part of the National Institutes of Health, uses the terms *complementary health approaches* to discuss non-mainstream therapies and *integrative health* when discussing the incorporation of complementary approaches into mainstream health care [2]. The Academic Consortium for Integrative Medicine and Health views integrative health care as that which promotes dignity and respect, includes a caring therapeutic relationship, honors the whole person—mind, body, and spirit—recognizes the innate capacity to heal, and offers choices for complementary and conventional therapies [3].

Taking all this into account, this chapter will consider integrative approaches to childhood obesity as those patient-centered or relationship-centered therapies that encompass the whole child—mind, body, and spirit—in the promotion of healthy body weight insofar as that is a part of the child's overall health and well-being. This stands in philosophical distinction to the Western, allopathic model, which identifies obesity as a disease requiring a therapeutic intervention to eliminate it. The chapter will focus on those complementary, integrative modalities and approaches that have been demonstrated to be effective through evidence-based research. Due to the relative paucity of research evidence in children, evidence of effectiveness of some integrative modalities in adults will be discussed, and the chapter will conclude with a discussion of the new directions for research needed to build the evidence base necessary to confidently recommend modalities for obese and overweight children.

PREVALENCE OF COMPLEMENTARY INTEGRATIVE MEDICINE USE IN PEDIATRICS

The use of complementary alternative medicine (CAM) or complementary integrative medicine (CIM) in general for all medical conditions has been building steadily over the last 20 years in the United States. The prevalence of CAM use in children has generally been lower than that for adults. For example, in 2007, adult use of CAM therapies averaged close to 40%, with the highest use among Native Americans and Alaskan Natives, and the lowest among black adults [4]. In contrast, about 12% of children had used CAM therapy for any medical condition in the past 12 months, with natural product supplements and mind–body therapies being the most commonly used. Much higher prevalence of CAM use (above 30%) has been reported among children with chronic health problems and in those whose parents use CAM therapies [4–6]. There are no data for the prevalence of CAM use among children specifically for obesity or obesity-related disorders, but it is likely to be relatively low, since the use of CAM modalities in obese adults is known to be similar or lower than in the general population [7].

INTEGRATIVE ASSESSMENT OF THE OBESE CHILD

A proper integrative assessment of an obese child should include not only an assessment of dietary intake and physical activity, but should also pay attention to such other lifestyle factors as degree of life stress and other psychological issues, adequacy and quality of sleep, and social factors such as food insecurity and access to safe places to play or exercise. Family history, maternal history of obesity or diabetes during pregnancy, and exposure to environmental toxins such as bisphenol are further likely to impact childhood obesity status through genetic and epigenetic mechanisms, though a history of exposure to specific environmental toxins may be difficult to obtain [8].

It has become clear that chronic life stress is another potential factor in the development of obesity and its related complications. It is therefore important that the integrative assessment of the obese child evaluates stressors in the child's life and the means by which the child manages such stress. Stress results in a preference for and the ingestion of higher calories, more fat, and calorically dense snack foods, as well as in cortisol secretion [9,10]. Studies in primates [11] and human adults [12,13] suggest that chronic stress, via neuroendocrine mechanisms producing hypothalamic–pituitary–adrenal axis activation and subtle hypercortisolism, can result in a *pseudo-Cushingoid* obesity phenotype characterized by visceral adiposity, insulin resistance, and metabolic syndrome [14]. These factors appear to be present in children as well. Thus, among overweight/obese Latino adolescents, those with metabolic syndrome have higher morning serum cortisol levels [15], and higher serum cortisol predicts future deterioration of insulin sensitivity [16]. Additionally, a blunted diurnal salivary cortisol pattern is linked to increased carotid intima-media thickness—that is, preclinical peripheral vascular pathology—independent of age, height, systolic blood pressure, and ethnicity [17]. Finally, higher morning cortisol levels and dietary sugar intake may interact to promote increased visceral adipose tissue stores [18].

Other psychosocial factors need to be part of the evaluation of the obese child. Decreased sleep duration has been linked to increased body mass index (BMI) in children [19,20]. Depression, history of physical or sexual abuse, disrupted family structure, lower socioeconomic status, food insecurity, neighborhood crime, and gang activity all promote obesity in children and will not easily respond to routine dietary or physical activity recommendations [21]. These factors will generally require attention from other health professionals (e.g., social workers, psychologists) in order to successfully address the psychosocial issue that is physically manifesting as obesity.

SPECIFIC COMPLEMENTARY INTEGRATIVE MEDICINE MODALITIES FOR OBESITY

MIND–BODY APPROACHES TO OBESITY IN YOUTH

Mind–body therapies encompass a diverse array of methods that all utilize the connection of mind, imagery, and attention in ways that affect physiological processes. These therapies include guided imagery (GI), mindfulness-based approaches, meditation, hypnotherapy, biofeedback, relaxation training, and others. GI and mindfulness-based approaches, in particular, have been reported on in recent years in the context of childhood and adolescent obesity.

Guided Imagery

GI is a complementary/alternative, mind–body healing modality that typically involves a series of relaxation techniques followed by the generation of mental images to evoke a state of relaxation (i.e., reduced stress) or achieve a specific health outcome (e.g., reduce pain, lower blood pressure, enhance immune function) [22]. GI is also a proven stress management technique in a wide array of clinical circumstances [23]. In adults, GI has been shown to improve unhealthy eating behaviors, including binge–purge activity in bulimia [24].

The potential to change eating behaviors as well as reduce stress makes GI an attractive target therapy for obese children. Stress reduction–GI was found to be an acceptable and well-liked modality in obese Latino adolescents who were previously quite naïve to any mind–body modalities, as well as leading to acute reduction in salivary cortisol levels [25]. A follow-up study in obese Latino adolescents utilized a 12-week guided-imagery intervention in order to reduce stress, as well as to motivate improved obesity-related lifestyle behaviors. Findings replicated the ability to acutely reduce salivary cortisol levels by approximately 40%, as well as demonstrating significant reductions in sedentary behaviors and increases in moderate physical activity across the 12-week intervention [26]. Larger follow-up studies of this population are currently underway to determine the effects of GI on objective measures of physical activity and eating behaviors, longer-term stress management, adiposity, and insulin resistance.

INTEGRATIVE LIFESTYLE APPROACHES: NUTRITION, PHYSICAL ACTIVITY, STRESS, AND SLEEP

The mainstay of conventional management of the obese child remains attention to lifestyle behaviors to improve eating and physical habits. This is true as well in the integrative approach to the obese child. As conventional nutrition and exercise approaches are covered extensively in other chapters of this book, this section will focus on those integrative approaches that move beyond standard "eat less, exercise more" physical activity prescriptions.

Integrative Nutritional Approaches: Intuitive Eating and Mindful Eating

It is clear that the first approach to childhood obesity must be to ensure adequate nutritional education for both parents and children. However, it is also clear that nutritional education alone, while absolutely necessary, is unlikely to have a sustainable benefit in terms of weight reduction in most cases. True health behavior change—that is, making healthier eating choices and increasing physical activity and movement—takes motivating internal factors that actually change one's relationship to the behavior in question.

Intuitive eating and *mindful eating* (also referred to as *mindfulness-based eating*) represent two very similar *nondieting* approaches to eating that seek to radically change the relationship of an individual to his or her eating behaviors and choices. Intuitive eating is a nondieting philosophy whose major principles include (1) rejecting the *diet mentality* to give oneself unconditional permission to eat when hungry, and to eat whatever food is desired; (2) using internal hunger and satiety cues, rather than external rules on portion size, to determine when and how much to eat; (3) eating for physical rather than emotional reasons; and (4) seeking satisfaction in the eating experience [27,28]. By supporting autonomy in eating and physical activity decision making, intuitive eating is developmentally ideal for adolescents, for whom the pursuit of autonomy is a critical developmental milestone [29]. Multiple studies in young adults, both cross-sectional and longitudinal, have shown positive associations between intuitive eating practices and lower BMI, improved psychological outcomes, and other physical health indicators [30,31]. When intuitive eating was used as one component of an integrative mind–body intervention in obese adolescents, intuitive eating attitudes and practices were increased, and there were no increases in intake of calories, sugars, or fats despite the nondieting intuitive-eating curriculum [26]. Combined with the findings in adults showing positive relationships between intuitive eating practices and BMI and other health markers, these findings suggest that intuitive eating can be used in obese adolescents without fear of sustained consumption of unhealthy foods or worsening obesity status. Further studies are clearly needed to directly test the intuitive-eating approach against conventional dietary approaches.

Mindfulness, a meditation-based mind–body CAM modality, has been defined as paying attention, on purpose, in the present moment, nonjudgmentally, to the unfolding of experience moment by moment [32,33]. One of the key concepts in mindfulness is the lowering of reactivity to stress triggers. Mindful eating, also known as mindfulness-based eating, extends general mindfulness approaches directly to the field of obesity and eating disorders. Mindfulness-based interventions in adults have been found to be effective for obesity and for altering obesity-related eating behaviors such as emotional eating, binge eating, and dietary intake [34,35]. Such approaches have specifically been useful for treating binge-eating disorder [36,37] and obesity in adults [34,38]. A recent report showed that among obese women, a mindfulness intervention for stress-related eating led to a reduction in morning cortisol responses, which was associated with a reduction in abdominal fat [39].

With respect to children and adolescents, recent years have seen increases in mindfulness training programs for a variety of clinical conditions [40]. A recent review exploring theoretical considerations for mindfulness training for obesity and obesity-related eating behaviors in youth suggested that improved executive function, increased attentional control, emotional and cognitive flexibility, and acknowledgment of impulses without reaction might all be mental capacities developed through mindfulness that could result in improved eating behaviors and benefits for obese youth [41]. To date, however, there have been no published reports on the effects of mindfulness-based eating interventions in obese children.

Integrative Physical Activity Approaches: Yoga, Tai Chi, and Qigong

Conventional approaches to physical activity are covered elsewhere in this volume. This section covers complementary approaches to movement and physical activity, including yoga, tai chi, and qigong. It must be noted, however, that these practices each involve a major component of mindfulness, and thus, rather than representing a strictly *physical activity* approach, they each represent an integrative mind–body therapy in and of themselves.

Yoga, though primarily viewed as a movement practice in the Western world, typically involves significant mindfulness, stress reduction, and breathwork, linking all components of mind, body, emotion, spirit, and meaning together, and thus is a fully integrative practice. Early studies suggest that the benefits of yoga in obese adults may include the reduction of BMI and waist circumference and improvements in metabolic outcomes [42–44]. In children, yoga has been reported to reduce stress, improve classroom behavior, prevent eating disorders, foster self-esteem, and have multiple beneficial health effects [45,46]. The minimal information from small intervention studies in obese youth has demonstrated reductions in body fat, BMI, and some lipid parameters [47,48].

Tai chi and qigong represent low-impact movement meditations from the Chinese medicine tradition that each contain both physical activity and mindfulness components. Tai chi has shown reductions in BMI in older adults [49], and adolescents taught tai chi as a "control" exercise intervention showed similar stabilization of body fat during growth to an active kung fu martial arts intervention group [50]. In obese adults with type 2 diabetes, qigong led to reduced weight, waist circumference, insulin resistance, and hemoglobin A1C [51,52]. Studies are absent regarding the use of qigong in obese children or adolescents.

Stress Management

Because of the links between chronic life stress, obesity, and obesity-related morbidities, the assessment and management of stress represents an important part of the integrative approach to the obese child. As discussed in previous sections, most mind–body modalities utilize stress reduction techniques as a major component. These can be as simple as focused breathing, which has been used successfully to reduce stress and stress biomarkers such as cortisol in children for a variety of clinical conditions, including obesity [26]. Other *integrative* stress management activities, such as music, exercise, gardening, or hobbies can be recommended as determined in collaboration with the individual child or adolescent. These need to be determined collaboratively in the integrative assessment of the child, listening closely to the child's narrative of what he or she has previously found useful in managing stress, and then tying that activity into the overall *obesity prescription*.

Sleep

As reviewed in Chapter 28, sleep is another critical piece of lifestyle behavior that is often overlooked in the assessment of the obese child, despite clear evidence that decreased sleep duration is associated with both increased BMI and insulin resistance [19,53,54]. Recommendations to improve sleep quality and duration should thus be given as part of obesity treatment.

HERBS/BOTANICALS AND DIETARY SUPPLEMENTS

Dietary supplements are the most common CAM approach used by obese adults [55]. However, the majority of weight loss supplements advertised and sold have not been demonstrated to be effective and safe in adults, much less in children [56,57]. In adults, some data for modest effects on weight reduction exist for fiber supplements and green tea catechins [58]. Glucomannin and other soluble fiber supplements have been found to be of benefit in weight management in adults [59]. The data are inconclusive or negative for other common supplements such as chromium picolinate, chitosan, conjugated linoleic acid, or *Garcinia cambogia* (hydroxycitric acid) [60].

There is evidence to support a number of herbal therapies in adults with obesity-related complications such as metabolic syndrome and type 2 diabetes. Thus, ginseng (*Panax ginseng*), green tea (*Camellia sinensis*), milk thistle (*Slybum marianum*), and nopales (prickly pear) cactus have all shown glucose-lowering effects in type 2 diabetes or other benefits in obesity-related conditions [61]. Cinnamon has been shown in animals to increase insulin sensitivity, and a recent meta-analysis concluded it has a significant, though modest (~9 mg/dL), effect on reducing fasting glucose values in adults with type 2 diabetes or prediabetes [62]. Finally, preliminary evidence suggests a possible role for other supplements in treating obesity-related insulin resistance and/or type 2 diabetes, including vitamin D, folate, B12, B6, and zinc [1].

Few of these herbal products have been investigated in children with obesity, prediabetes, or diabetes. Zinc has been found to reduce fasting insulin and glucose levels in obese prepubertal children [1]. Fiber supplements have been considered for weight loss in children. The rationale for the use of fiber is supported by the long-known weight loss effects of diets high in fruits and vegetables in children [63]. In general, the current state of knowledge would suggest that fiber is beneficial to children as part of a good healthy diet, and that the major beneficial source of fiber remains natural food sources. The role of additional fiber supplementation beyond dietary fiber in children remains to be determined.

In summary, it is important to state that the evidence to date is not strong enough to clearly establish herbal and dietary supplements as effective therapies in obese children, and there is an absence of good data on the safety profiles of most dietary supplements in children.

BODY-BASED INTEGRATIVE THERAPIES: ACUPUNCTURE, CHIROPRACTIC, OSTEOPATHY, AND MASSAGE

Among these body-based integrative therapeutic approaches to obesity, an evidence base exists only for acupuncture. Acupuncture, though grouped here in the category of body-based approaches, is often instead categorized as a mind–body integrative intervention. Recent meta-analyses and systematic reviews have shown that acupuncture results in significant weight loss (approximately 1.7–4 kg) compared with either sham-treated or lifestyle controls [64,65]. However, most previous trials suffer from suboptimal design and small numbers. There are few data on the use of acupuncture in children, though one uncontrolled, longitudinal study showed significant reductions of 3.5% in BMI (29.03–28.08 kg/m^2) and 16% in visceral adipose fat volume (measured by magnetic resonance imaging [MRI]) in children undergoing acupuncture for obesity [66].

NARRATIVE MEDICINE AND INTEGRATIVE BEHAVIORAL APPROACHES

These approaches are difficult to categorize in the usual framework of what are considered integrative modalities. Nonetheless, these represent approaches that may hold future promise for obesity treatment in children and teens. Narrative medicine encompasses the field of personal story and how it may relate to healing [67]. Having patients tell their story to the clinician, to peers, to family members, often in writing, helps the person feel heard, promotes self-understanding and insight, helps the clinician understand the individual nuances involved, and promotes a much deeper rapport and relationship from which to engage the salient issues. Integrative behavioral approaches include such modalities as motivational interviewing, integrative health coaching, support groups, and other group approaches. Motivational interviewing represents a behavior modification approach that has been used with success in obese adults, and has also been incorporated into pediatric obesity interventions [68,69]. Self-help support groups have been utilized in obesity treatment programs and are highly valued by participants [70]. Finally, the facilitated group process of *council*, based primarily on Native American processes and preliminarily shown to improve well-being and psychosocial outcomes in young adults with diabetes [71], could readily be applied to the treatment of obese adolescents. All of these behavioral approaches rely on the building and nurturing of relationships between patients and intervening professionals, and the use of the integrative model of collaboration and promotion of whole health rather than the disease-based allopathic approach to the individual child with obesity. Much more future research is needed to determine the ultimate benefit of these integrative behavioral approaches.

CONCLUSIONS

It is clear from the discussion in this chapter that while complementary integrative therapies present a promising and hopeful philosophical approach to the obese child or adolescent, for most of the integrative modalities there remains too little evidence base at this time to strongly substantiate the benefits of their use. Despite this, many of these therapies offer promising potential benefit with very little risk in terms of adverse side effects, particularly among the mind–body and integrative-lifestyle modalities. Such therapies can be used in individual children as part of an integrative approach to their obese condition, as long as reasonable discussion is undertaken between the health-care provider and the child/parent in terms of what is known and what remains unknown with respect to any given integrative therapy. Thus, using the integrative health model of assessment and treatment, a collaborative approach can be utilized that takes into account the whole child, addressing obesity as one physical aspect of the child's whole being— mind, body, emotion, and spirit. Such an approach can help minimize the stigma of obesity in the mind of the child, deflect attention from any failure to lose weight immediately, and launch the child on a personal journey to health and wellness, which over the long term can improve the obese child's well-being and potentially his or her overall health, whether or not the obesity itself is reduced. Clearly, much more research is needed in the area of integrative obesity management of children and adolescents in order to substantiate the potential benefits offered by the various forms of integrative therapies. This represents a wide-open area of investigation for those physicians and scientists interested in pursuing an integrative approach to childhood obesity.

REFERENCES

1. Rakel D. *Integrative Medicine* (3rd edn). Philadelphia, PA: Elsevier Saunders, 2012.
2. NIH National Center for Complementary and Integrative Health. Complementary, alternative, or integrative health: What's in a name? Available from: https://nccih.nih.gov/health/integrative-health.
3. Academic Consortium for Integrative Medicine and Health. Mission. https://www.imconsortium.org/about/mission.cfm.
4. Barnes PM, Bloom B, Nahin RL, Statistics NCfH. Complementary and alternative medicine use among adults and children: United States, 2007. US Department of Health and Human Services, Centers for Disease Control and Prevention, National Center for Health Statistics, Hyattsville, MD, 2008.
5. Kemper KJ, Vohra S, Walls R. The use of complementary and alternative medicine in pediatrics. *Pediatrics*. 2008;122(6):1374–86.
6. Birdee GS, Phillips RS, Davis RB, Gardiner P. Factors associated with pediatric use of complementary and alternative medicine. *Pediatrics*. 2010;125(2):249–56.

7. Bertisch SM, Wee CC, McCarthy EP. Use of complementary and alternative therapies by overweight and obese adults. *Obesity*. 2008;16(7):1610–5.

8. Trasande L, Attina TM, Blustein J. Association between urinary bisphenol A concentration and obesity prevalence in children and adolescents. *JAMA*. 2012;308(11):1113–21.

9. Wardle J, Steptoe A, Oliver G, Lipsey Z. Stress, dietary restraint and food intake. *Journal of Psychosomatic Research*. 2000;48(2):195.

10. Epel E, Lapidus R, McEwen B, Brownell K. Stress may add bite to appetite in women: A laboratory study of stress-induced cortisol and eating behavior. *Psychoneuroendocrinology*. 2001;26(1):37.

11. Shively C, Register T, Clarkson T. Social stress, visceral obesity, and coronary artery atherosclerosis in female primates. *Obesity*. 2009;17(8):1513–20.

12. Rosmond R, Dallman MF, Bjorntorp P. Stress-related cortisol secretion in men: Relationships with abdominal obesity and endocrine, metabolic and hemodynamic abnormalities. *Journal of Clinical Endocrinology & Metabolism*. 1998;83(6):1853–9.

13. Epel ES, McEwen B, Seeman T, Matthews K, Castellazzo G, Brownell KD, et al. Stress and body shape: Stress-induced cortisol secretion is consistently greater among women with central fat. *Psychosomatic Medicine*. 2000;62(5):623.

14. Bjorntorp P, Rosmond R. Neuroendocrine abnormalities in visceral obesity. *International Journal of Obesity and Related Metabolic Disorders*. 2000;24(Suppl. 2):S80.

15. Weigensberg MJ, Toledo-Corral CM, Goran MI. Association between the metabolic syndrome and serum cortisol in overweight Latino youth. *Journal of Clinical Endocrinology & Metabolism*. 2008;93(4):1372–8.

16. Adam TC HR, Ventura EE, Toledo-Corral C, Le KA, Mahurkar S, Lane CJ, Weigensberg MJ, Goran MI. Cortisol is negatively associated with insulin sensitivity in overweight Latino youth. *Journal of Clinical Endocrinology & Metabolism*. 2010;95(10):4729–35.

17. Toledo-Corral CM, Myers SJ, Li Y, Hodis HN, Goran MI, Weigensberg MJ. Blunted nocturnal cortisol rise is associated with higher carotid artery intima-media thickness (CIMT) in overweight African American and Latino youth. *Psychoneuroendocrinology*. 2013;38(9):1658–67.

18. Gyllenhammer LE, Weigensberg MJ, Spruijt-Metz D, Allayee H, Goran MI, Davis JN. Modifying influence of dietary sugar in the relationship between cortisol and visceral adipose tissue in minority youth. *Obesity*. 2014;22(2):474–81.

19. Ruan H, Xun P, Cai W, He K, Tang Q. Habitual sleep duration and risk of childhood obesity: Systematic review and dose-response meta-analysis of prospective cohort studies. *Scientific Reports*. 2015;5:16160. doi:10.1038/srep16160.

20. Guidolin M, Gradisar M. Is shortened sleep duration a risk factor for overweight and obesity during adolescence? A review of the empirical literature. *Sleep Medicine*. 2012;13(7):779–86.

21. Campbell MK. Biological, environmental and social influences on childhood obesity. *Pediatric Research*. 2016;79(1–2):131–47.

22. Astin JA, Shapiro SL, Eisenberg DM, Forys KL. Mind–body medicine: State of the science, implications for practice. *The Journal of the American Board of Family Practice*. 2003;16(2):131.

23. Gruzelier JH. A review of the impact of hypnosis, relaxation, guided imagery and individual differences on aspects of immunity and health. *Stress*. 2002;5(2):147.

24. Esplen MJ, Garfinkel PE, Olmsted M, Gallop RM, Kennedy S. A randomized controlled trial of guided imagery in bulimia nervosa. *Psychological Medical*. 1998;28(6):1347.

25. Weigensberg MJ, Lane CJ, Winners O, Wright T, Nguyen-Rodriguez S, Goran MI, et al. Acute effects of stress-reduction Interactive Guided Imagery^SM on salivary cortisol in overweight Latino adolescents. *The Journal of Alternative and Complementary Medicine*. 2009;15(3):297–303.

26. Weigensberg MJ, Lane CJ, Ávila Q, Konersman K, Ventura E, Adam T, et al. Imagine HEALTH: Results from a randomized pilot lifestyle intervention for obese Latino adolescents using Interactive Guided Imagery^SM. *BMC Complementary and Alternative Medicine*. 2014;14(1):28.

27. Tribole E, Resch, E. *Intuitive Eating* (3rd edn; 1st edn, 1995). New York: St Martins Press, 2012.

28. Tylka TL. Development and psychometric evaluation of a measure of intuitive eating. *Journal of Counseling Psychology*. 2006;53(2):226–40.

29. Spruijt-Metz D. *Adolescence, Affect and Health*. Hove, UK: Psychology Press, 1999.

30. Hawks S, Madanat H, Hawks J, Harris A. The relationship between intuitive eating and health indicators among college women. *American Journal of Health Education*. 2005;36(6):331.

31. Van Dyke N, Drinkwater EJ. Relationships between intuitive eating and health indicators: Literature review. *Public Health Nutrition*. 2014;17(08):1757–66.

32. Brown K, Ryan R. The benefits of being present: Mindfulness and its role in psychological well-being. *Journal of Personality and Social Psychology*. 2003;84(4):822–48.

33. Ludwig DS, Kabat-Zinn J. Mindfulness in medicine. *JAMA.* 2008;300(11):1350–2.
34. Godsey J. The role of mindfulness based interventions in the treatment of obesity and eating disorders: An integrative review. *Complementary Therapies in Medicine.* 2013;21(4):430–9.
35. O'Reilly G, Cook L, Spruijt-Metz D, Black D. Mindfulness-based interventions for obesity and related eating behaviours: A literature review. *Obesity Reviews.* 2014;15(6):453–61.
36. Kristeller JL, Hallett C. An exploratory study of a meditation-based intervention for binge eating disorder. *Journal of Health Psychology.* 1999;4:357.
37. Kristeller J, Wolever RQ, Sheets V. Mindfulness-based eating awareness training (MB-EAT) for binge eating: A randomized clinical trial. *Mindfulness.* 2013;5(3):282–97.
38. Dalen J, Smith BW, Shelley BM, Sloan AL, Leahigh L, Begay D. Pilot study: Mindful Eating and Living (MEAL); Weight, eating behavior, and psychological outcomes associated with a mindfulness-based intervention for people with obesity. *Complementary Therapies in Medicine.* 2010;18(6):260–4.
39. Daubenmier J, Kristeller J, Hecht FM, Maninger N, Kuwata M, Jhaveri K, et al. Mindfulness intervention for stress eating to reduce cortisol and abdominal fat among overweight and obese women: An exploratory randomized controlled study. *Journal of Obesity.* 2011;2011:651936.
40. Black DS. *Handbook of Mindfulness: Theory, Research, and Practice*, pp. 283–310. New York: The Guilford Press, 2015.
41. O'Reilly GA, Black DS. Considering mindfulness for obesity-related eating behaviors in children and adolescents. *Journal of Child & Adolescent Behavior.* 2015;3(3):207. doi:10.4172/2375-4494.1000207.
42. Field T. Yoga clinical research review. *Complementary Therapies in Clinical Practice.* 2011;17(1):1–8.
43. McDermott KA, Rao MR, Nagarathna R, Murphy EJ, Burke A, Nagendra RH, et al. A yoga intervention for type 2 diabetes risk reduction: A pilot randomized controlled trial. *BMC Complementary and Alternative Medicine.* 2014;14(1):212.
44. Telles S, Sharma SK, Yadav A, Singh N, Balkrishna A. A comparative controlled trial comparing the effects of yoga and walking for overweight and obese adults. *Medical Science Monitor: International Medical Journal of Experimental and Clinical Research.* 2014;20:894.
45. Birdee GS, Yeh GY, Wayne PM, Phillips RS, Davis RB, Gardiner P. Clinical applications of yoga for the pediatric population: A systematic review. *Academic Pediatrics.* 2009;9(4):212–20.e1–9.
46. Case-Smith J, Shupe Sines J, Klatt M. Perceptions of children who participated in a school-based yoga program. *Journal of Occupational Therapy, Schools, & Early Intervention.* 2010;3(3):226–38.
47. Seo DY, Lee S, Figueroa A, Kim HK, Baek YH, Kwak YS, et al. Yoga training improves metabolic parameters in obese boys. *The Korean Journal of Physiology & Pharmacology.* 2012;16(3):175–80.
48. Benavides S, Caballero J. Ashtanga yoga for children and adolescents for weight management and psychological well being: An uncontrolled open pilot study. *Complementary Therapies in Clinical Practice.* 2009;15(2):110–4.
49. Chen S-C, Ueng K-C, Lee S-H, Sun K-T, Lee M-C. Effect of t'ai chi exercise on biochemical profiles and oxidative stress indicators in obese patients with type 2 diabetes. *The Journal of Alternative and Complementary Medicine.* 2015;16(11):1153–9.
50. Tsang TW, Kohn M, Chow CM, Fiatarone Singh M. A randomized controlled trial of kung fu training for metabolic health in overweight/obese adolescents: The "martial fitness" study. *Journal of Pediatric Endocrinology and Metabolism.* 2009;22(7):595–608.
51. Sun G-C, Lovejoy JC, Gillham S, Putiri A, Sasagawa M, Bradley R. Effects of qigong on glucose control in type 2 diabetes: A randomized controlled pilot study. *Diabetes Care.* 2010;33(1):e8.
52. Liu X, Miller YD, Burton NW, Chang J-H, Brown WJ. Qi-gong mind–body therapy and diabetes control: A randomized controlled trial. *American Journal of Preventive Medicine.* 2011;41(2):152–8.
53. Fatima Y, Mamun A. Longitudinal impact of sleep on overweight and obesity in children and adolescents: A systematic review and bias-adjusted meta-analysis. *Obesity Reviews.* 2015;16(2):137–49.
54. Javaheri S, Storfer-Isser A, Rosen CL, Redline S. Association of short and long sleep durations with insulin sensitivity in adolescents. *The Journal of Pediatrics.* 2011;158(4):617–23.
55. Pillitteri JL, Shiffman S, Rohay JM, Harkins AM, Burton SL, Wadden TA. Use of dietary supplements for weight loss in the United States: Results of a national survey. *Obesity.* 2008;16(4):790–6.
56. Pittler MH, Ernst E. Dietary supplements for body-weight reduction: A systematic review. *The American Journal of Clinical Nutrition.* 2004;79(4):529–36.
57. Rogovik AL, Goldman RD. Should weight-loss supplements be used for pediatric obesity? *Canadian Family Physician.* 2009;55(3):257–9.
58. Thavanesan N. The putative effects of green tea on body fat: An evaluation of the evidence and a review of the potential mechanisms. *British Journal of Nutrition.* 2011;106(09):1297–309.

59. Keithley J, Swanson B. Glucomannan and obesity: A critical review. *Alternative Therapies in Health and Medicine*. 2005;11(6):30.

60. Lovejoy JC. Integrative approaches to obesity treatment. *Integrative Medicine*. 2013;12:30–6.

61. Yeh GY, Eisenberg DM, Kaptchuk TJ, Phillips RS. Systematic review of herbs and dietary supplements for glycemic control in diabetes. *Diabetes Care*. 2003;26(4):1277.

62. Davis PA, Yokoyama W. Cinnamon intake lowers fasting blood glucose: Meta-analysis. *Journal of Medicinal Food*. 2011;14(9):884–9.

63. Epstein LH, Myers MD, Raynor HA, Saelens BE. Treatment of pediatric obesity. *Pediatrics*. 1998;101(3 Pt 2):554.

64. Cho S, Lee J, Thabane L, Lee J. Acupuncture for obesity: A systematic review and meta-analysis. *International Journal of Obesity*. 2009;33(2):183–96.

65. Sui Y, Zhao H, Wong V, Brown N, Li X, Kwan A, et al. A systematic review on use of Chinese medicine and acupuncture for treatment of obesity. *Obesity Reviews*. 2012;13(5):409–30.

66. Zhang H, Peng Y, Liu Z, Li S, Lv Z, Tian L, et al. Effects of acupuncture therapy on abdominal fat and hepatic fat content in obese children: A magnetic resonance imaging and proton magnetic resonance spectroscopy study. *The Journal of Alternative and Complementary Medicine*. 2011;17(5):413–20.

67. Charon R. *Narrative Medicine: Honoring the Stories of Illness*. New York: Oxford University Press, 2006.

68. Resnicow K, Davis R, Rollnick S. Motivational interviewing for pediatric obesity: Conceptual issues and evidence review. *Journal of the American Dietetic Association*. 2006;106(12):2024–33.

69. Davis J, Kelly L, Lane C, Ventura E, Byrd-Williams C, Alexandar K, et al. Randomized control trial to improve adiposity and insulin resistance in overweight Latino adolescents. *Obesity*. 2009;17:1542–8.

70. Kirschenbaum DS, Gierut KJ. Five recent expert recommendations on the treatment of childhood and adolescent obesity: Toward an emerging consensus; A stepped care approach. *Childhood Obesity*. 2013;9(5):376–85.

71. Weigensberg M, Pyatak E, Florindez D, Sequeira P, Spruijt-Metz D, Juarez M, et al. Diabetes empowerment council (DEC): Development and pilot testing of an innovative mind–body group intervention for young adults with type 1 diabetes. *The Journal of Alternative and Complementary Medicine*. 2014;20(5):A69.

Section VI

Public Health and Policy Based Interventions

41 Food Advertising and Marketing Issues Relevant to Childhood Obesity

Tim Lobstein

CONTENTS

> The marketing of foods and non-alcoholic beverages with a high content of fat, sugar or salt reaches children throughout the world. Efforts must be made to ensure that children everywhere are protected against the impact of such marketing and given the opportunity to grow and develop in an enabling food environment—one that fosters and encourages healthy dietary choices and promotes the maintenance of healthy weight.
>
> **Dr. Ala Alwan**
> *Assistant Director-General, World Health Organization, 2010 [1]*

INTRODUCTION

The prevention of child overweight includes moves to encourage children to eat a healthy diet, and in most countries of the world the national food-based dietary guidelines recommend plentiful consumption of fruit, vegetables, pulses, and wholegrain foods, while recommending limiting the consumption of energy-dense, micronutrient-poor processed foods. Yet, in most countries, the mass media shows high levels of commercial promotion of energy-dense foods and relatively little promotion of more healthful foods. In this chapter, we consider current moves to limit children's exposure to such commercial messaging and to rebalance commercial rights in favor of the reduction of risks to children.

POLICY CONTEXT

For more than two decades, concern has been expressed about the commercial promotion of food and beverage products, especially when those products have a nutritional profile that may undermine the healthfulness of diets, and which are not recommended for increased consumption in national dietary guidelines. Campaigns by civil society organizations to restrict the promotion of such unhealthy foods and beverages date back at least to the 1970s and have gained increasing support as the rise in diet-related chronic disease has an impact on health service costs and economic output, in developed and developing economies alike.

"Marketing approaches matter for public health," stated the then director-general of the World Health Organization, Dr. Gro Harlem Bruntland, addressing the World Health Assembly in 2002. "They influence our own—and in particular our children's—patterns of behavior. Given that they are designed to succeed, they have serious consequences for those at whom they are targeted" [2]. This statement triggered official recognition in WHO member states that the promotion of foods that undermine healthy choices represented a major threat to population nutrition security. It was followed a few months later by the WHO's Technical Report 916 [3], which considered the evidence on the nature and strength of the links between diet and chronic diseases, and which classified as "probable" or "convincing":

- The adverse effect of high intake of energy-dense, micronutrient-poor foods
- The adverse effect of high intake of sugar-sweetened beverages
- The adverse effect of heavy marketing of energy-dense foods and fast-food outlets

The technical report was followed by a "Global Strategy on Diet, Physical Activity and Health," endorsed by the World Health Assembly in 2004 [4], which explicitly stated that food advertising influences dietary habits, and that "messages that encourage unhealthy dietary practices or physical inactivity should be discouraged, and positive, healthy messages encouraged." It urges governments to work with stakeholders to develop "multisectoral approaches to deal with the marketing of food to children and to deal with such issues as sponsorship, promotion and advertising."

While policy development was being urged by health advocates and by international health organizations, national governments faced resistance from commercial operators, and in order to take action, needed more concrete evidence to show that market interventions could be justified. For example, one of the counterarguments suggested that advertising of products served only to encourage an exchange from one brand to another, and did not increase overall consumption. The evidence, however, showed that marketing served to increase product sales not only through competition with similar products but also through increased sales of the entire category. A systematic review conducted in 2003 for the UK Food Standards Agency (FSA), concluded:

> Overall, there is evidence that food promotion causes both brand switching and category effects, with stronger support for the latter effect. Although no study provides a thorough comparison of the strength of both types of effect, both types of effect have been examined independently, and there is reasonably strong evidence that both occur. In other words, the effects of food promotion are not limited to brand switching [5].

A second evidence review undertaken by the US Institute of Medicine in 2005 [6] found evidence that television advertising had an impact on overall diet in the short term for children aged 2–11 years, with insufficient evidence for older children. There was also moderate evidence of long-term effects on children aged 6–11, with weak evidence of long-term effects on younger children and weak evidence of no effect for older children. The review also noted strong statistical associations between higher exposure to television advertising and obesity in children aged 2–11 and in youth aged 12–18 years.

Subsequent reviews have largely confirmed and strengthened these associations. A systematic review published by the World Health Organization in 2009 [7] supported the findings of the UK and US reports, and a further review of reviews published in 2013 concluded:

> Food promotions have a direct effect on children's nutrition knowledge, preferences, purchase behaviour, consumption patterns and diet-related health. Current marketing practice predominantly promotes low nutrition foods and beverages. Rebalancing the food marketing landscape' is a recurring policy aim of interventions aimed at constraining food and beverage promotions to children. [8]

Several countries have responded with varying degrees of regulatory action. In the United Kingdom, the communications-regulating agency Ofcom introduced a set of measures implemented over the period 2007–2009 [9] that restricted television advertising for specified foods during children's programing: the age of a child was specified as 16 years, and the definition of the food products that could be advertised was the first example of a nutrient-profiling system defined by a government agency to distinguish acceptable and unacceptable products, based on diet-related public health criteria. In Spain, the government initiative Codigo PAOS (Código de Corregulación de la Publicidad de Alimentos y Bebidas Dirigida a Menores, Prevención de la Obesidad y Salud) [10] consisted of a coregulatory action in which the industry operated a set of definitions and monitored compliance, with government oversight. A similar procedure was developed in Denmark [11]. Several such statutory actions by governments and coregulatory actions (government-agreed, industry-run initiatives) have been developed in several countries in the last decade (see Table 41.1).

Across the globe, sections of the food industry have recognized the need to respond, and some of the largest food-producing companies have offered voluntary pledges to limit their marketing activities in several regions around the world, from 2006 onward [14]. These moves have been welcomed for showing willingness to act and as a method for addressing cross-border advertising concerns. The details have, however, been criticized by civil society organizations on several counts, including the lack of an enforcement structure, the nonbinding nature of the pledges, the lack of application of the pledges to nonsignatory companies, the low threshold for allowing advertising, the limited number of food products that are excluded by the nutritional criteria, the narrow

TABLE 41.1
Examples of Regulatory and Coregulatory Action

Country, Year of Implementation	Regulatory Controls
Iran, 2004, 2014	Statutory prohibition on broadcast advertising of soft drinks; proposals to prohibit 24 food products.
Spain, 2005	Coregulation operated by food industry with government oversight; restricts marketing specified foods and beverages.
United Kingdom, 2007, 2008	Statutory prohibition of the advertising and product placement of specified foods during TV and radio programs with 20% more viewers under 16 years old relative to the general viewing population.
Denmark, 2008	Coregulation operated by food industry under government approval; restricts promotion of specified food and beverages to children aged 13 and under via media including TV, radio, Internet, SMS, newspapers, and comic books.
South Korea, 2010	Statutory prohibition of TV advertising of certain categories of food 5:00–7:00 p.m.; further restrictions on advertising on radio and Internet.
Ireland, 2013	Statutory prohibition of the advertising, sponsorship, teleshopping, and product placement of certain foods during TV and radio programs where over 50% of the audience are under 18 years old, and at any time a restriction of such advertising to no more than 25% of total advertising.
Norway, 2013	General statutory prohibition on advertising to children, with additional coregulatory agreement on the promotion of specified foods and beverages in a wide range of media.
Mexico, 2014, 2015	Statutory prohibition on advertising certain foods and beverages 2:30–7:30 p.m. on weekdays and 7:00 a.m.–7:30 p.m. on weekends, if over 35% of the audience is under age 13.

Sources: World Obesity Federation [Internet resource provided by the World Obesity Federation. Available at: http://www.worldobesity.org/what-we-do/policy-prevention/projects/marketing-children/policy-map/, accessed January 14, 2016; World Cancer Research Fund. Internet resource provided by the World Cancer Research Fund. Available at: http://www.wcrf.org/int/policy/nourishing-framework/restrict-food-marketing, accessed January 14, 2016].

definition of advertising, and the restricted set of media (primarily TV and some Internet activities) included in the pledges [15].

PROMOTIONAL METHODS

The promotion of food products toward children occurs in a variety of forms and in many different settings. Parental food messages are among the first and continue to be significant throughout childhood. Messages from schools are also important and carry cultural significance, as they are in effect authorized by a school's staff, the governing body, and the educational authority. Messages from peers become increasingly influential as children mix socially and develop friendship networks and group loyalties.

Messages from commercial interests are also important, and recent scientific research has strengthened the evidence base demonstrating links between the exposure of children to marketing messages and consequential changes in their dietary behavior, thus reinforcing the case for intervention. At the same time, the technology for advertising has changed, with new and rapidly expanding forms of media (digital TV, online marketing, cellphones and smartphones, and social networking) becoming available to larger numbers of children and offering low-cost, effective means of reaching them directly for marketing purposes.

Food purchase choices and food consumption behavior depend on a range of external factors, including price, availability, and adequate information about the products, as well as the individual's personal preferences and cultural values. For both adults and children, food marketing can influence all these factors: prices (e.g., through promotional "special offers" and discounts), availability (e.g., through positioning at the checkout), information (generally through food advertising and specifically through, e.g., health claims), presentation (e.g., the packaging, labeling, and formulation of the product), personal taste (e.g., through the use of coloring or flavoring additives in the foods), and cultural values (e.g., through the use of celebrities and sports personalities in product promotions).

Messages are delivered by food producers and food service operators as part of their general marketing strategy. Promotional marketing is an economic activity in which organizations promote demand for their goods or services, using paid-for advertising in third-party media or internal activities such as company-owned websites and product and packaging design. Examples of the various ways in which commercial messages about food and beverage products may be delivered are shown in Table 41.2.

EXTENT OF ADVERTISING

Food and beverage advertising during both children's and family TV schedules and during peak and nonpeak viewing hours is largely for unhealthy foods [17–19]. An international survey [17] examined TV food advertising to children in 11 different countries—Australia, Brazil, Canada, China, Germany, Greece, Italy, Spain, Sweden, the United Kingdom, and the United States—and found that, during peak children's viewing time on the three commercial channels most watched by children, food advertising comprised 11%–29% of total exposure to advertising. The proportion of advertisements for unhealthy foods varied between countries but was always the dominant form of food advertising, with little airtime devoted to the promotion of healthy products. Items such as fast food, sugar-sweetened beverages, high-sugar breakfast cereals, cookies, salted snacks, sweet desserts, and confectionery dominate advertising during children's peak viewing times. While advertisements directed at children and at adults differ in theme, they differ little in nutritional value [20], with food products and restaurant experiences being marketed to children on themes of fun and taste, often featuring promotional characters and cartoon animals of particular appeal to children and adolescents [21].

A high level of advertising for unhealthy food has been seen during children's viewing in the United States [22] during a period when voluntary pledges by the food and beverage industry were supposed to reduce children's exposure to such marketing. In the United Kingdom, between 2008 (a period of partial regulation) and 2010 (when full regulation was effective) there was a clear fall in

TABLE 41.2

Examples of Media through Which Children Are Exposed to Product and Brand Promotion

Broadcast
TV and radio advertising
TV and radio program sponsorship
TV program product placement

Nonbroadcast
Cinema advertising
Film product placement
Posters and advertising boards
Print media: e.g., magazines and comic books
Branded books: e.g., counting books for preschoolers
Internet: e.g., email clubs, chat rooms, free ringtones
Websites: e.g., puzzles, interactive games
Promotional sales by telephone
Text messaging to mobile phone
Direct marketing: e.g., home catalogs, mail shots, leafleting
Sponsorship of events and venues
Sponsorship of teams and sports "heroes"
Cross-branding of logos on household goods
Branded toys: e.g., a fast-food store as a playhouse
Branded computer games, product placement in computer games

In Store
On-shelf displays
Displays at checkout till
Special offers and pricing incentives
Purchase-linked gifts, toys, and collectibles
Free samples and tastings

On Or in the Product
Product formulation: colors and shapes
Product portions: e.g., "king size"
In-pack promotions: e.g., gifts, vouchers
On-pack promotions: e.g., games, puzzles, vouchers
Packaging design: Imagery, colors, play shapes

In School
Sponsorship of educational materials and equipment
Vending machines in schools and youth clubs
School participation in promotion and sampling schemes

Source: World Health Organization [World Health Organization, *The Challenge of Obesity in the WHO European Region and the Strategies for Response*, World Health Organization Regional Office for Europe, Copenhagen, Denmark, 2007].

food advertising during children's TV programing but no reduction in food and beverage advertising during family scheduling, which is when most children are watching television.

Analyses of trends in expenditure on food and beverage advertising to children in the United States indicates that TV expenditure is falling, but children and teens still see 12–16 TV advertisements per day for products generally high in saturated fat, sugar, or sodium [22,23]. In addition, marketing using newer digital media is increasing, as is expenditure on advertising using product placement, movies/videos, cross-promotion licenses, athletic sponsorship, celebrity fees, events, and philanthropy [23]. Content analysis of food and beverage advertising on popular children's websites found 84% of products were high in fat, sugar, and/or sodium [24], while food companies' own websites can be highly attractive to children but promote nutritionally poor choices [25].

In a study conducted in Canada [26], 24 websites sponsored by 10 food and beverage companies (all of which were members of the Canadian Children's Food and Beverage Advertising Initiative [27]) were examined, and most (83%) were found to target children below the age of 12 years. Half of the websites had a mechanism for children to recommend them to a friend. Brand and product imagery permeated all these sites, with *spokescharacters* (brand equity characters) being by far the most common device used. Brand logos appeared and were used to link to games, as game pieces, scenery, and as game "buttons." This is of some concern, as this age group may lack the ability to recognize advertising content on the Internet compared with broadcast media.

A systematic review published in 2013 of children's exposure to the marketing of foods and beverages found that high levels of advertising of less healthy foods continue to be found in many different countries worldwide, despite the evidence provided in industry-sponsored reports that indicates a remarkably high adherence to voluntary codes [28]. The authors concluded "adherence to voluntary codes may not sufficiently reduce the advertising of foods that undermine healthy diets, or reduce children's exposure to this advertising." A second review reached similar conclusions: "Statutory regulation could reduce the volume of and children's exposure to advertising for foods HFSS, and had potential to impact more widely. Self-regulatory approaches showed varied results in reducing children's exposure" [29].

EFFECTS OF ADVERTISING

The 2003 systematic review of the impact of advertising on children's food preferences, choices, and diets, undertaken for the UK FSA noted earlier [5], identified over 29,000 potentially relevant papers, from which it selected 55 of sufficient relevance and quality. The Institute of Medicine, in its 2006 report, based its conclusions on 155 relevant papers [6]. The subsequent decade has seen a substantial increase in scientific research specifically examining the extent of food advertising and brand promotion, children's recognition and understanding of advertising messages, and the effect of advertising on children's preferences, eating patterns, and dietary behavior. We give a brief narrative summary here.

The recognition of commercial brands and logos starts early in childhood and by the age of 4 years is associated with different expressions of eating behavior and weight status. Robinson et al. [30] showed that brand imagery on food packaging affects children's perceptions of the taste of food they are eating. Forman et al. [31] showed that overweight children in particular react to branded food packaging by increasing their food consumption. The inclusion of licensed characters (such as those from children's films) on food product packaging improves children's ratings of the product's taste [32,33].

There is a strong link between TV viewing and obesity in children. Using data collected in a survey of TV advertising to children, Lobstein and Dibb [34] compared the prevalence of overweight among children in nine participating countries with the extent of advertising of energy-dense foods, and the extent of advertising of healthier foods and nonfood products. They found a significant positive correlation between overweight prevalence and the promotion of energy-dense foods but a weak negative correlation with the promotion of healthier foods and nonfood products, indicating a specific association with the types of products being advertised. More direct evidence of a link is shown in one study [35] in which viewing of advertisements was a predictor of subsequent excess body weight, even when physical activity and eating in front of the TV were taken into account. These data indicate the powerful influence of the commercial content of TV on children's health.

The quantity of TV viewed may be an indicator of susceptibility to advertising. A study in the United Kingdom found that the food preferences of children and young adolescents who habitually viewed a large amount of commercial TV were more affected by experimental exposure to food advertisements than those of children who watched less commercial TV [36]. This was particularly apparent in their selection of branded food items following the viewing of food advertisements. Parental concern may not help and could make matters worse: a study in the United States [37] found parental input to have little impact on food choices following exposure to advertisements, and a Dutch study [38] found that children reporting the highest maternal encouragement to be thin ate the most food when exposed to advertisements for energy-dense products in the absence of their caregivers.

The effectiveness of advertising may lie outside direct cognitive control, especially for those most susceptible. A study by Bruce et al. [39] of neural responses to images of food brand logos showed greater motivational responses from children who were obese and greater cognitive control responses from children of normal weight. There is evidence that children at least as old as 12 years may not recognize online advertising for what it is [40]. A Swedish study using eye tracking showed that while adolescents (14–16 years) were surfing the Internet, food and beverage advertising had a relatively greater impact on their attention than other forms of promotion [41]. The adolescents were unaware of much of the advertising to which they had been exposed.

RIGHTS AND RISKS

The protection of children from exploitation has a long legislative history. Marketing to children has been described as inherently exploitative because children may be incapable of discerning its commercial intent and yet are susceptible to its influence [42]. A rights-based approach builds on the United Nations Convention on the Rights of the Child [43], the right to adequate food [44], and the right to freedom from obesity [45]. The rights-based approach is based on the concept of a civilized society's responsibility to protect its citizens, especially the more vulnerable.

An alternative is the risk-based (or risk/benefit-based) approach, where an attempt is made to weigh up the multiple likelihoods of harm and benefit in terms of outcomes, to minimize the risk of harm and maximize the benefit. It recognizes conflicting interests and the costs to different stakeholders, and the need for proportionate action to balance commercial and economic costs against health gains.

In the World Health Organization's 2010 recommendations on marketing to children [46], the approach is primarily one of reducing health risks while not constraining responsible marketing. Specifically, the document calls on member states to adopt policies that reduce the extent of exposure to, and the power of, marketing messages that promote the consumption of "foods high in saturated fats, trans-fatty acids, free sugars, or salt" in order to reduce the risk of noncommunicable diseases.

Risk-based policies have been enacted in France, the United Kingdom, and several other countries (see Table 41.1). A rights-based approach is more comprehensive in nature and can be more easily formulated. A risk-based approach has to define which marketing messages are and are not allowable, based on an evaluation of the likelihood of harm, and it has to specify the products permitted to be advertised, the age group whose exposure is being protected, and the methods, media, and messages being used. Such a risk-based set of specifications may also need to be set against costs and an evaluation of the proportionality of the market restriction in order to justify the measures taken; an example of this is provided by the UK communications regulator, Ofcom [47].

A rights-based approach usually puts human health and well-being ahead of economic interests and so is likely to be intrinsically more favorable to the protection of children, whereas a risk-based approach offers some protection to the free working of markets and commerce. In practice, rights-based policies have already been enacted in several countries to protect children from commercial marketing messages generally, including Canada (the province of Quebec) and Sweden. A broadening of the rights-based approach to justify restrictions of the commercial promotion of unhealthful food products has been recommended by several international civil society organizations and supported by leading international lawyers, including UN special rapporteurs on cultural rights [48], rights to health [49], and rights to food [50].

REFERENCES

1. Alwan A. Foreword to: Set of recommendations on the marketing of foods and non-alcoholic beverages to children. Geneva, Switzerland: World Health Organization, 2010.
2. Brundtland GH. Address by Dr. Gro Harlem Brundtland, director-general to the Fifty-Fifth World Health Assembly. Document A55/3. Geneva, Switzerland: World Health Organization, May 13, 2002.
3. World Health Organization. Report of a joint WHO/FAO expert consultation: Diet, nutrition and the prevention of chronic diseases. WHO Technical Report Series no. 916. Geneva, Switzerland: World Health Organization, 2002.
4. World Health Organization. Global strategy on diet, physical activity and health. Geneva, Switzerland: World Health Organization, 2004.
5. Hastings G, Stead M, McDermott L, et al. Review of research on the effects of food promotion to children: Final report. Stirling: University of Stirling, UK, 2003.
6. Institute of Medicine, Committee on Food Marketing and the Diets of Children and Youth, McGinnis JM, Gootman JA, Kraak VI, eds. *Food Marketing to Children and Youth: Threat or Opportunity?* Washington, DC: National Academies Press, 2006.
7. Cairns G, Angus K, Hastings G. The extent, nature and effects of food promotion to children: A review of the evidence to December 2008. Geneva, Switzerland: World Health Organization, 2009.
8. Cairns G, Angus K, Hastings G, Caraher M. Systematic reviews of the evidence on the nature, extent and effects of food marketing to children: A retrospective summary. *Appetite*. 2013;62:209–15.
9. Ofcom. Television advertising of food and drink products to children: Final statement. London: Office of Communications, 2007. Available at: http://stakeholders.ofcom.org.uk/consultations/foodads_new/statement/ [accessed January 14, 2016].
10. Ministerio de sanidad, servicios sociales e igualdad. Publicity and marketing PAOS code. Madrid: Government of Spain, 2016. Available at: http://www.naos.aesan.msps.es/en/naos/publicidad/ [accessed January 14, 2016].
11. Forum of Responsible Food Marketing Communication. Code of responsible food marketing communication to children. Copenhagen: Forum for Fødevarereklamer, 2014. Available at: http://kodeksforfoedevarereklamer.di.dk/english/Pages/english.aspx [accessed January 14, 2016].
12. Internet resource provided by the World Obesity Federation. Available at: http://www.worldobesity.org/what-we-do/policy-prevention/projects/marketing-children/policy-map/ [accessed January 14, 2016].
13. Internet resource provided by the World Cancer Research Fund. Available at: http://www.wcrf.org/int/policy/nourishing-framework/restrict-food-marketing [accessed January 14, 2016].
14. International Food and Beverage Alliance. Responsible marketing & advertising to children. Available at: https://ifballiance.org/our-commitments/responsible-marketing-advertising-to-children/ [accessed January 14, 2016].
15. Lobstein T, Parn T, Aikenhead A. A junk free childhood: Responsible standards for marketing foods and beverages to children. London, UK: International Association for the Study of Obesity, 2011.
16. World Health Organization, Branca F, Nikogosian H, Lobstein T, eds. The challenge of obesity in the WHO European region and the strategies for response. Copenhagen, Denmark: World Health Organization Regional Office for Europe, 2007.
17. Kelly B, Halford JC, Boyland EJ, et al. Television food advertising to children: A global perspective. *Am J Public Health*. 2010;100:1730–6.
18. Kunkel DL, Castonguay JS, Filer CR. Evaluating industry self-regulation of food marketing to children. *Am J Prev Med*. 2015;49:181–7.

19. Boyland EJ, Harrold JA, Kirkham TC, Halford JC. The extent of food advertising to children on UK television in 2008. *Int J Pediatr Obes.* 2011;6:455–61.
20. Boyland EJ, Harrold JA, Kirkham TC, Halford JC. Persuasive techniques used in television advertisements to market foods to UK children. *Appetite.* 2012;58:658–64.
21. Kraak VI, Story M. Influence of food companies' brand mascots and entertainment companies' cartoon media characters on children's diet and health: A systematic review and research needs. *Obes Rev.* 2015;16:107–26.
22. Powell LM, Szczypka G, Chaloupka FJ. Trends in exposure to television food advertisements among children and adolescents in the United States. *Arch Pediatr Adolesc Med.* 2010;164:794–802.
23. Powell LM, Harris JL, Fox T. Food marketing expenditures aimed at youth: Putting the numbers in context. *Am J Prev Med.* 2013;45:453–61.
24. Ustjanauskas AE, Harris JL, Schwartz MB. Food and beverage advertising on children's web sites. *Pediatr Obes.* 2014;9:362–72.
25. Cheyne AD, Dorfman L, Bukofzer E, Harris JL. Marketing sugary cereals to children in the digital age: A content analysis of 17 child-targeted websites. *J Health Commun.* 2013;18:563–82.
26. Brady J, Mendelson R, Farrell A, Wong S. Online marketing of food beverages to children: A content analysis. *Can J Diet Prac Res.* 2010;71:166–71.
27. Canadian Children's Food & Beverage Advertising Initiative. Core principles. Toronto: Advertising Standards Canada, 2016. Available at: http://www.adstandards.com/en/childrensinitiative/CCFBAI_EN.pdf [accessed January 14, 2016].
28. Galbraith-Emami S, Lobstein T. The impact of initiatives to limit the advertising of food and beverage products to children: A systematic review. *Obes Rev.* 2013;14:960–74.
29. Chambers SA, Freeman R, Anderson AS, MacGillivray S. Reducing the volume, exposure and negative impacts of advertising for foods high in fat, sugar and salt to children: A systematic review of the evidence from statutory and self-regulatory actions and educational measures. *Prev Med.* 2015;75:32–43.
30. Robinson TN, Borzekowski DL, Matheson DM, Kraemer HC. Effects of fast food branding on young children's taste preferences. *Arch Pediatr Adolesc Med.* 2007;161:792–7.
31. Forman J, Halford JC, Summe H, MacDougall M, Keller KL. Food branding influences ad libitum intake differently in children depending on weight status: Results of a pilot study. *Appetite.* 2009;53:76–83.
32. Roberto CA, Baik J, Harris JL, Brownell KD. Influence of licensed characters on children's taste and snack preferences. *Pediatrics.* 2010;126:88–93.
33. Lapierre MA, Vaala SE, Linebarger DL. Influence of licensed spokescharacters and health cues on children's ratings of cereal taste. *Arch Pediatr Adolesc Med.* 2011;165:229–34.
34. Lobstein T, Dibb S. Evidence of a possible link between obesogenic food advertising and child overweight. *Obes Rev.* 2005;6:203–8.
35. Zimmerman FJ, Bell JF. Associations of television content type and obesity in children. *Am J Public Health.* 2010;100:334–40.
36. Boyland EJ, Harrold JA, Kirkham TC, et al. Food commercials increase preference for energy-dense foods, particularly in children who watch more television. *Pediatrics.* 2011;128:e93–100.
37. Ferguson CJ, Muñoz ME, Medrano MR. Advertising influences on young children's food choices and parental influence. *J Pediatr.* 2012;160:452–5.
38. Anschutz DJ, Engels RC, Van Strien T. Maternal encouragement to be thin moderates the effect of commercials on children's snack food intake. *Appetite.* 2010;55:117–23.
39. Bruce AS, Lepping RJ, Bruce JM, et al. Brain responses to food logos in obese and healthy weight children. *J Pediatr.* 2013;162:759–64.
40. Blades M, Oates C, Li S. Children's recognition of advertisements on television and on web pages. *Appetite.* 2013;62:190–3.
41. Sandberg H, Gidlof K, Holmberg N. Children's exposure to and perceptions of online advertising. *Int J Comm.* 2011;5:21–50.
42. Swinburn B, Sacks G, Lobstein T, et al. The "Sydney Principles" for reducing the commercial promotion of foods and beverages to children. *Public Health Nutr.* 2008;11:881–6.
43. UN General Assembly. Convention on the rights of the child. Geneva, Switzerland: Office of the United Nations High Commissioner for Human Rights, 1989.
44. UN Committee on Economic, Social and Cultural Rights. General comment 12: The right to adequate food. Document E/C.12/1999/5. New York, United Nations, 1999.
45. UN Standing Committee on Nutrition. The human right of children and adolescents to adequate food and to be free from obesity and related diseases: The responsibilities of food and beverage corporations and related media and marketing industries. Rome, Italy: 34th session of the SCN, February 26–March 1, 2007.

46. World Health Organization. Set of recommendations on the marketing of foods and non-alcoholic beverages to children. Geneva, Switzerland: World Health Organization, 2010.

47. Ofcom. HFSS advertising restrictions: Final review. London, UK: Ofcom, 2010. Available at: http://stakeholders.ofcom.org.uk/market-data-research/other/tv-research/hfss-final-review/ [accessed January 14, 2016].

48. Shaheed F. Statement made by the special rapporteur on cultural rights at the 69th session of the General Assembly. New York: United Nations, October 28, 2014. Available at: http://www.ohchr.org/EN/NewsEvents/Pages/DisplayNews.aspx?NewsID=15864&LangID=E [accessed January 16, 2016].

49. Grover A. Statement: Special rapporteur on the right of everyone to the enjoyment of the highest attainable standard of physical and mental health. High-Level Meeting of the UN General Assembly to undertake a comprehensive review and assessment on the prevention and control of NCDs. New York: United Nations, July 10–11, 2014. Available at: http://www.unscn.org/files/Announcements/Other_announcements/Statement_UNGA_comments_final.pdf [accessed January 14, 2016].

50. De Schutter O. Unhealthy diets greater threat to health than tobacco: UN expert calls for global regulation. May 19, 2014. Available at: http://www.srfood.org/en/unhealthy-diets-greater-threat-to-health-than-tobacco-un-expert-calls-for-global-regulation [accessed 16 January 2016].

42 Connecting the Dots
Translating Systems Thinking into Innovative Solutions for Childhood Obesity

Terry T.-K. Huang and Emily B. Ferris

CONTENTS

INTRODUCTION

The opening article of the second *Lancet* "Obesity" series describes the false dichotomies behind conventional approaches to obesity prevention [1]. These false dichotomies include either/or arguments around the significance of individual responsibility or government policies, prevention or treatment interventions, and public- or private-sector actions, for example. However, as this and other papers [2–6] in the *Lancet* "Obesity" series point out, the reality is that solutions to the obesity problem require the integration and coordination of all these approaches. Nevertheless, how these diverse approaches can and should be integrated remains a daunting challenge. This dilemma lies at the heart of the complexity of obesity. Systems approaches provide a way to address this dilemma.

In the last decade, there has been increasing interest in the concept of systems approaches to obesity prevention and control. The term *systems science* in the context of obesity and chronic disease was first coined and solidified by the Office of Behavioral and Social Sciences Research at the National Institutes of Health (NIH) [7]. Although the science of systems approaches to complex problems has been in development since at least the mid-twentieth century, its introduction to the chronic disease prevention field has been fairly recent. Many competing schools of thought and methodologies exist within the broader field of complexity science. In an effort to bridge these differences and adopt a more applied approach to solving modern-day public health problems that seem so intractable, the NIH proposed a relatively neutral term—*systems science*—to embody the overarching principles and methods of complex systems as a whole.

Around the same time as systems science was introduced to the biomedical and public health research community, the Eunice Kennedy Shriver National Institute of Child Health and Human

Development at the NIH hosted an international conference entitled "Beyond Individual Behavior: Multidimensional Research in Obesity Linking Biology to Society." This was the first attempt at the NIH to bring together basic, clinical, population, and policy scientists, along with representatives from government and industry, to discuss how interconnections across these diverse silos could be cultivated and how a new roadmap for childhood obesity prevention and control could be developed through a systems lens. The conference yielded insights into new cross-disciplinary research questions, the need to integrate individual and policy research, the capacity required to undertake such a systems approach, and the importance of learning from a global mindset [8,9]. A subsequent series of papers stemming from this discussion focused in greater detail on how biology–society interactions [10], developmental trajectories [11], and multistakeholder partnerships [12] could all cohere around a common systems framework [9].

Much progress has occurred since the 2000s on the field's thinking around systems approaches to obesity prevention and control. The goal of this chapter is to review and summarize the complex dimensions of childhood obesity, how systems thinking and systems insights can inform innovative solutions, and how to implement a systems framework in real-world settings.

CHILDHOOD OBESITY AS A COMPLEX PROBLEM

The UK Foresight Programme first published the complexity map of obesity in 2007 (Figure 42.1) [13]. This map illustrates several features that are inherent in a complex problem. First, there is a great deal of *heterogeneity* in the actors, factors, and sectors that contribute to energy balance. The map shows how energy intake and output are connected to, for example, the food and the built environment; diverse social, economic, and political forces; and multiple institutions and sectors that have greater control over these environmental dimensions than individuals alone. Many publications on obesity in the last decade have focused on dissecting this heterogeneity; fewer, however, have focused on how the heterogeneous components are linked [9]. This leads to the second obvious attribute in the map—that is, the multiplicity of *feedback* loops that connect these actors, factors, and sectors. These feedbacks give rise to system behaviors that are not simply the addition of all the system's parts—also known as *emergence*. The phenomenon of emergence makes it difficult to use traditional reductionist methods to isolate cause and effect. In addition, feedbacks in a complex system create delays in system behaviors. Much as how there is a delay in getting hot water when we turn on the faucet, delays are everywhere in a social and public health system. Consideration of delays is critical for intervention design so that undesirable delays in effects can be managed and appropriate outcomes to capture intervention effects within a specific time horizon can be selected.

The heterogeneity and feedbacks in the complex system of childhood obesity contribute to the formation of highly interactive and dynamic networks of actors and actions. Recent research has shown how obesity in the population "spreads"—or emerges—through such a network effect [14]. The complexity of this effect is that individuals are usually embedded in multiple networks that may all influence individual energy intake and output. For example, a recent paper showed the simultaneous effect of peer and parental influence on children's unhealthy behaviors and how this in turn affects prevention and treatment intervention outcomes [15]. Another aspect of network complexity is the fact that they are dynamic, meaning they change, learn, and adapt over time. Just as the body adjusts its energy metabolism, where diet- or physical activity–induced weight loss occurs in a downward exponential fashion and eventually plateaus after 3–4 years [16], a social system also adapts to changes in the actors, factors, and sectors involved over time. This has important implications—such as how obesity intervention strategies should be combined and sequenced—that need to be considered *a priori*. The obesity field is quite far yet from taking obesity intervention research to this next level, but there are emerging methodological advances in adaptive interventions—albeit limited to experimental models thus far—that can be of utility [17].

Predicting system behaviors is challenging. As such, public health researchers and practitioners often cannot anticipate the unintended consequences of obesity interventions. Yet,

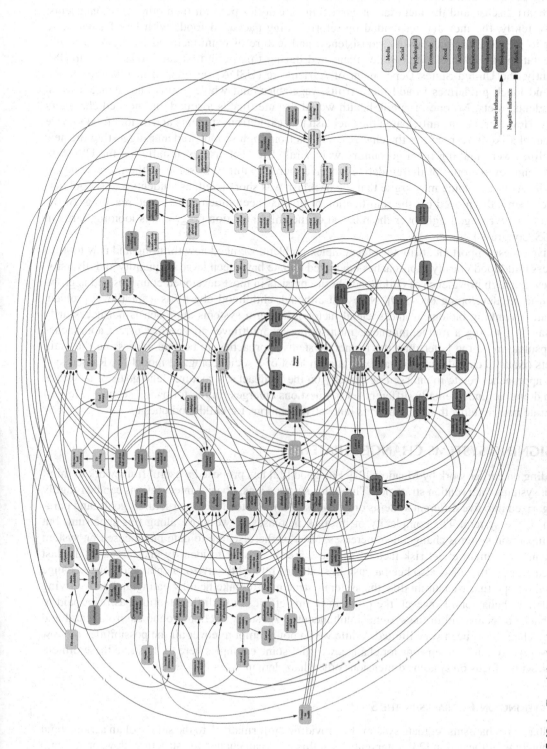

FIGURE 42.1 Foresight obesity system map. The UK Foresight Programme first published the complexity map of obesity in 2007. The map illustrates several features that are inherent in a complex problem. [From: Vandenbroeck IP, Goossens J, Clemens M. *Tackling Obesities: Future Choices; Obesity System Atlas.* London, UK: Foresight (Government Office for Science), 2007.]

unintended consequences occur more frequently than we think. In the 1980s and 1990s, there was a strong public health emphasis on reducing fat intake because of research showing its association with heart disease and the fact that fat carried more calories per unit than other macronutrients. Inadvertently, the industry responded by reformulating packaged foods with less fat but more sugar to preserve the palatability, consistency, and texture of manufactured foods. As a result, while fat intake in the United States plateaued during this period, sugar intake went up [18]. Recently, the United States Department of Agriculture (USDA) introduced new school breakfast and lunch guidelines to add more fruits, vegetables, and whole grains and reduce sodium in students' diets. No one in public health would dispute this as a sound and needed change in policy. However, no one anticipated the backlash that came from students and school food service personnel alike in response to the changes. Videos from high school students suggesting the new guidelines were making them go hungry went viral. The backlash eventually led the USDA to revisit and revise some of the guidelines to give more flexibility to some of the more stringent criteria. Although some may argue that the backlash was short-lived, as students and school personnel eventually moved on, the ramification of this has been much more broad reaching. At the time of this writing, a fight over the renewal of the child nutrition programs is looming large in the US Congress [19].

Given these important attributes of a complex problem, we need new thinking and new tools to address childhood obesity. Approaches attempted to date have been large in quantity and diversity. However, a high prevalence of childhood obesity persists in most developed countries and is growing in many developing ones [20]. Note that although childhood obesity is a multilevel problem by nature (linking biological and societal factors), taking a systems approach is not necessarily the same as taking a multicomponent, multisetting, or multilevel approach. Current approaches encapsulate more the latter than the former. Systems approaches go beyond addressing the main effects (isolated causal factors) that exist at each level of a socioecological model [9]. Rather, systems approaches relate to intervening directly on the feedbacks, structures, and goals of a system. In so doing, a fundamentally different set of questions emerges. In the following sections, we will illustrate how systems thinking informs innovative solutions for childhood obesity.

DESIGNING SYSTEMS CHANGE STRATEGIES

Building on earlier work by Meadow [21], Finegood [22] has proposed a useful framework to think about systems intervention strategies. Through a systems lens, obesity interventions can be roughly categorized into five different systems dimensions: elements, feedbacks, structures, goals, and paradigm of the system. The complexity of the task increases as we move along this spectrum, but the impact on systems change also increases. Most of the research to date has focused on system elements (i.e., main-effect risk factors), as these are the easiest to identify and target. In the last 10 years or so, there has also been a push in strategies related to environmental and policy change with the hope that we can modify the system's structure to make healthy eating and active living the default behaviors. However, the problem in this effort is that little attention has been paid to feedbacks or goals within the system simultaneously. As such, traction around environmental and policy change has been very limited. While we do not attempt to cover all the possibilities on how to leverage systems dimensions for change, we offer some examples here to illustrate these dimensions, with a focus on systems dimensions other than elements.

INTERVENING ON FEEDBACKS IN THE SYSTEM

Feedback mechanisms regulate systems by providing "information" to the source of an action about the outcome of the action [23]. Interventions at this level can change the structure, flow, or strength of information channels within a system. Feedback interventions can enhance positive feedback mechanisms, disrupt negative feedback mechanisms, or create new feedback loops.

Intervening on feedback mechanisms is not necessarily a new approach to childhood obesity prevention and reduction. However, most of the attempts to date have focused on individual-level information feedback, with the assumption that information alone, along with rational mental processing, would lead to behavior change. For example, interventions based on cognitive behavioral therapy (CBT) help participants better understand and change the thoughts, attitudes, or expectations that influence their actions and well-being, thereby altering the psychosocial feedback mechanisms related to health behaviors [24–28]. Other intervention strategies with modest success have focused on stimulus control (i.e., disrupting an obesogenic feedback) or self-monitoring (i.e., establishing a new information feedback loop) of weight, eating, and physical activity [29–34]. Mindfulness-based interventions have gained popularity in recent years, and preliminary findings appear to be positive [35,36]. Biofeedback therapies provide another example of existing interventions at the individual level that may help mitigate the stress-coping mechanisms associated with obesity. Visual biofeedback (e.g., electrodermal activity) paired with food stimuli has shown positive effects on food-related self-efficacy and perceived stress in obese adults by desensitizing the reward value of food or redirecting coping strategies among participants [37]. A similar approach has shown potential benefits in girls with anorexia [38], but the impact on children with obesity is unknown.

The impact of interventions targeting feedbacks can be enhanced if such feedbacks are reinforced by additional social or environmental strategies. For example, it has been shown that the facilitation of social support further increases the effectiveness of CBT-based interventions on reducing child adiposity and obesogenic behaviors [26,39–41]. Other novel, promising strategies include Pushcart, an app being developed by the Small Data Lab at Cornell Tech, which harnesses consumer information through online grocery purchases (popular in many large US cities) and maps this information to users' health goals (e.g., fruit and vegetable servings per week) to guide future food purchases [42]. Presumably, such a system can incorporate *nudging* or *choice architecture* principles in a virtual environment to prompt consumers with specific purchase options that are more likely to help them meet their dietary goals, thus reinforcing the positive information feedback loop toward greater behavior change. Recently, the Children's Use of the Built Environment (CUBE) study showed that adolescents increased their physical activity when GPS- and accelerometer-captured activity patterns were fed back to participants along with strategies for increasing physical activity within the context of each participant's built environment (e.g., taking a different transit path) [43]. The same researchers are exploring scaling this up and adding social networking and environmental change opportunities to such a feedback platform [44].

Sometimes, when we intervene on system feedbacks, especially feedbacks at an institutional or community level, such interventions over time alter the structure of the system. For example, farm-to-school initiatives create a new demand–supply feedback loop at the local level in hopes of improving student awareness of where foods come from and increasing access to fresh ingredients in school meals [45,46]. Though currently still experimental on a small scale, there is a broader local foods movement that can shift the structure of the food value chain [47]. Calorie menu-labeling initiatives add transparency to foods at the point of purchase; however, the greatest impact of such initiatives may not be at the level of individual purchase behavior but rather at the level of food reformulation by restaurants [48–51].

INTERVENING ON STRUCTURES IN THE SYSTEM

Interventions on the system's structures alter the interactions or interconnections between components or actors within the system or between subsystems [23]. Interventions can introduce new elements into the system, such as enhanced built-environment infrastructure, to increase opportunities for healthy foods or physical activity [52,53] or to alter individuals' interaction with the environment, such as through choice architecture [54–57]. For example, active design interventions in schools can alter students' interactions with the built environment and impact physical activity behaviors [58,59]. Switching to more healthful default side options for children's meals can impact eating behaviors [60–62]. One study in San Francisco found a significant decrease over time in the total fat and sodium content in children's orders after a chain restaurant switched to a more healthful default side dish and replaced the accompanying low-fat beverage with a fat-free beverage [60].

Many policy strategies advocated by public health are also designed to alter the system's structure [63]. Policy strategies can create new economic incentives or disincentives for consumer behavior and accelerate environmental changes deemed important to healthy lifestyles. Because of the population reach of policies, such interventions, when effective, can tip the system toward a large-scale shift in system behavior. However, policy interventions are also likely to create unintended consequences (i.e., compensatory responses elsewhere in the system) that need to be anticipated and managed.

Interventions on the system's structures can also shift existing structural dynamics by fostering collaboration and/or competition among actors to increase productivity or innovation. It is possible to leverage collaboration and competition simultaneously if they work on different levels to create a virtuous cycle [64]. Competition between teams leads to the selection of players that are more collaborative within teams, and in turn, this leads teams to become more competitive. This has important implications for how we structure different community organizations or government agencies, for example, to create both synergy and innovative solutions to obesity. One example of this at work relates to the Access to Nutrition Index (ATNI), which rates and ranks food and beverage companies in terms of their contribution to global nutrition [65]. While ATNI creates a new public information feedback loop to hold companies accountable, where ATNI may exert its most powerful impact lies in its adoption by value investors who are increasingly looking to put their money in companies that contribute to social good. Indices on environmental sustainability, access to medicine, and corporate social responsibility are used in a similar fashion [66–69]. ATNI also fosters collaboration across divergent voices (e.g., sales vs. public affairs) within companies in order for each company to be more competitive against others in ATNI rankings.

Last but not least, interventions on structure can include efforts to align the capacity of actors with the complexity of the tasks by either scaling up actor capacity, reducing the complexity through distributed actions, or both. Healthy Together Victoria, a statewide initiative in Victoria, Australia, created a new prevention infrastructure that embedded defined programmatic, evaluation, communication, and outreach functionalities both horizontally across communities and vertically between the local and state levels (i.e., distributed actions with coordination). In addition, the scaling up of systems-thinking capacity among its prevention workforce was central to the initiative, so that the individual actors were equipped to cope with the complexity of the system [70]. Elsewhere, the Missouri Foundation's Social Innovation for Missouri initiative seeks to alter the existing infrastructure by integrating health strategies into a holistic paradigm (e.g., tackling tobacco cessation and obesity prevention together) and investing in multisectoral partnerships to increase the system's capacity [71,72].

Intervening on Goals of the System

The goals of a system inform all of the interactions and feedback mechanisms within the system. Interventions on system goals can alter the aim of the system with the potential for considerable impact. In order for the overall paradigm to shift, new targets must be set and met [23]. The true goals of the system are not always the goals identified by actors within the system [21], so it is critical to examine the system's actual goals and set new goals if the existing goals contradict the desired paradigm shift. As mentioned at the start of this chapter, the obesity prevention field has grappled with various dichotomous goals—for example, prevention versus treatment, obesity versus hunger, food regulation versus individual preference, multisectoral approaches versus no collaboration with industry, and so on. However, these are false dichotomies that are incompatible with the complexity of the system in which obesity arises. Top-down goals cannot be at the exclusion of creating the demand for healthy products, policies, and places [2]. There has been relatively little attention paid to the demand-side strategies. Huang et al. [2] describe several examples showing how public demand can be mobilized through political strategies including streamlined messaging, media advocacy, the harnessing of citizen engagement and protest, and investment in a favorable political environment. As Hawkes et al. [3] point out in their paper on food policies and food preferences, the goal of the system is not to make the healthy choices the default choices; rather, the goal ought to be making the healthy choices the preferred choices. Reemphasizing the system goal around demand-side issues necessarily introduces a whole new set of system elements thus far not considered. The paper by Huang et al. [2] illustrates how the fundamental questions for each sector shift as a result. For example, rather than focusing on obesity specifically, a recent study focused on enhancing the readiness of a Latino community to embrace health as an issue in general through the use of youth activism and social media [73,74]. In the burgeoning field of school design, there have been efforts to dovetail school goals around learning and sustainability to incorporate design-based strategies for healthy eating and physical activity [58,59,75–77]. Thus, shifting system goals opens up new opportunities for both research and practice as we move toward systems solutions for childhood obesity.

SHIFTING THE PARADIGM OF THE SYSTEM

Shifting the system's paradigm is the most difficult place to intervene in a complex system but also has the potential to create the most substantial impact. Shifting the system's paradigm requires changing the deep beliefs and values that inform the goals and the many interactions, interconnections, and structures within the system [23]. An important paradigm shift in the obesity context relates to moving from a problem-oriented to a solution-oriented frame. Recognizing the "causes" of obesity does not necessarily lead to ideas about how to solve it [78]. For childhood obesity specifically, we need a shift from a cost/savings perspective to a moralistic or human rights perspective. In the United States, we also need to go from a system created to generate health care to one that values and generates health. These paradigm shifts happen gradually but require systematic planning and effort. We recently published a commentary illustrating how lessons from the gay marriage movement in the United States can be adapted to create a movement that leads us to healthier lifestyles and communities [79].

MODELING AS A TOOL TO MANAGE COMPLEXITY

Systems modeling (SM), with a strong tradition in engineering, business, ecology, and some corners of the social sciences, is an emerging methodology in the field of chronic disease. Researchers increasingly recognize its potential to frame and analyze the complex systems involved in obesity and related chronic diseases. SM can be qualitative or quantitative. It allows researchers to better understand complex interactions, identify potential intervention levers, predict system behaviors, test or generate new hypotheses, model intervention effects, and anticipate unintended consequences. SM is particularly powerful because it can accommodate nonlinear dynamics, feedback mechanisms, time delays, multiple interactions, and diverse sources of data, all of which are challenging using conventional research tools [22,80,81]. A review of SM in the obesity prevention field demonstrates the versatility of SM to explore different facets of the complex systems dynamics related to obesity and to generate compelling, actionable new knowledge.

In the context of childhood obesity, one particularly useful function of SM is its ability to model the potential impact of policies or interventions. The knowledge generated from SM can be an invaluable tool for informing researchers' and policymakers' work. The Baltimore Low Income Food Environment (BLIFE) model is an agent-based model of the Baltimore City food environment [82]. Researchers have used it to simulate the potential impact of different types and combinations of small food store interventions to reduce obesity in adolescents [83]. They found that while healthy food availability interventions in corner stores were more effective than in takeout restaurants, a combined approach to address healthy food availability in both settings was the most effective and had the potential to reduce adolescents' BMI by an average of 3.9 centile points over a 5-year period [83]. This new knowledge can help policymakers leverage the ideal combinations of interventions to create the most impact or prioritize the best use of limited resources.

SM can also help inform how interventions may impact different subpopulations or how environmental or socioeconomic characteristics may influence interventions' effectiveness. An agent-based model of walking behaviors explored the interactions between different intervention approaches, walking behaviors, income differentials of walking behaviors, and aspects of the built environment [84,85]. One simulation found that while interventions to increase positive attitudes around walking may initially improve walking behaviors, they are unsustainable if the built environment is not conducive to walking [85]. Another simulation from this model focused on travel costs, such as parking tickets and gas prices, and found that changes in travel costs may impact the walking behavior of individuals in lower socioeconomic groups, but that high-income groups are relatively insensitive to changes in travel costs [84].

A third example by Hammond et al. [86] illustrates how individual neurological and physiological development can be integrated with different environmental contexts in a virtual, agent-based environment to help anticipate how environmental exposures might influence future behaviors. In this study, researchers showed that early-life exposure to a highly palatable and highly rewarding food environment strongly shapes the individual reward valuation system over time and that such early exposure may be more important than current exposure.

SM can be a helpful tool in better understanding the complexity of childhood obesity and its potential interventions. However, SM is only a tool to manage complexity. Systems thinking is a much broader philosophy to master and can be pursued by modelers and nonmodelers alike.

IMPLEMENTING SYSTEMS CHANGE

Though systems change provides a powerful approach to conceptualizing and addressing childhood obesity, the complexity of the task can be daunting. Once systems change has been identified as an important course of action, where does one start? Just as SM provides a way to better understand the complexity of the childhood obesity system, implementing and operationalizing systems change may greatly benefit from the lessons of frameworks and approaches in other fields.

Though not explicitly developed as a systems thinking tool, the philosophy and aims of the collective impact (CI) model dovetail in a compelling and mutually beneficial way with the systems-thinking approach. The CI model identifies the components necessary to create change at a systems level and scaffolds the design, implementation, and evaluation of each component [87]. The CI model comprises five main ingredients: a common agenda, a shared measurement system, mutually reinforcing activities, continuous communication, and a strong backbone organization [87]. Stakeholders can use these five elements to identify common goals, align their expertise and resources, and create change by synergistically working across the systems levels.

Stakeholders can leverage each component of the CI model to manage the complex task of systems change interventions to address childhood obesity. By defining a common agenda, stakeholders establish a shared understanding of the problem, agree to a course of action, and identify the goals needed to resolve the problem. The process can help participants better understand the existing paradigm, scrutinize whether the actual goals of the system match the desired goals, and, if not, articulate the new goals necessary to shift the paradigm.

By establishing a backbone organization and aligning activities so that they are mutually reinforcing, multisector stakeholders can coordinate and leverage their combined efforts. This synergistic approach has the potential to shift the systems' structure and alter the existing interactions and feedback loops between different actors and sectors. Mutually reinforcing activities help harness the power of the complex system dynamics in support of the desired goals. A shared measurement platform and continuous communication develop new feedback mechanisms to further shift interactions between systems actors and subsystems and ensure alignment among collaborators. A shared measurement system helps track progress toward goals and can alert actors if interventions are causing unexpected or negative consequences. Continuous communication between actors builds capacity, trust, and motivation, and helps actors better understand the system dynamics.

The CI model offers a structured, action-oriented framework with specific tools to help design, align, and launch multisectoral systems change interventions to impact childhood obesity. CI case studies demonstrate the possibilities of collective action and the model can be both an inspiration and a foundation for systems change [88].

INNOVATING THROUGH DESIGN THINKING

To optimize the potential of systems change in childhood obesity, creativity and innovation are key. Creativity and innovation come only when we operate in an environment where it is safe to fail—and fail frequently—so that lessons learned about what leads to failure can be rapidly parlayed into new solution ideas. Implementing a systems approach to childhood obesity must therefore be iterative and adaptable. Design thinking is a useful framework to facilitate this process [89]. The design-thinking approach embraces complexity and provides a way of thinking and a set of tools to help public health researchers and practitioners experience the needs of people and communities, empathize with the everyday challenges in weight prevention or management, and rapidly ideate, prototype, and test potential solutions [90]. Design thinking is nonlinear, provides a systematized way of engaging in community-based participatory research and practice [91], and can be embedded within a broader CI implementation framework. Though design thinking is a relatively new approach in public health, its concepts have been successfully applied to complex systems in other fields including business [90,92], engineering [93,94], and social services [95].

CONCLUSIONS

There is no debate that childhood obesity is a complex problem. The question is how to solve it. In this chapter, we summarized our thinking around what we call *translational systems science*—the idea that systems science is not only used to unravel complexity but to inform real-world solutions. In the traditional reductionist approach, the goal is to isolate "causes" that lead to obesity. In so doing, we lose sight of the bigger picture, including all the interconnections and dynamics across the elements, feedbacks, structures, and goals in the complex system in which childhood obesity occurs. A systems approach seeks to understand and manage such complexity with the hope that we can find sets of solutions that work in synergistic ways to ultimately shift the behavior of the system to favor healthy environments and healthy behaviors. Thinking in systems compels us to ask different questions and leads us to consider solutions that target system feedbacks, structures, and goals directly. Altering these systems dimensions is key to shifting the system paradigm. Tools exist outside the traditional public health field to facilitate systems change. CI and design thinking are two such tools that can help us put together a plan for implementation and evaluation in the real-world setting. Attempts at systems changes will inevitably lead to many failed starts, but not taking a systems approach is unlikely to lead to new solutions to effectively solve the childhood obesity epidemic.

REFERENCES

1. Roberto CA, Swinburn B, Hawkes C, Huang TT, Costa SA, Ashe M, et al. Patchy progress on obesity prevention: Emerging examples, entrenched barriers, and new thinking. *Lancet (London, England)*. 2015;385(9985):2400–9.
2. Huang TT, Cawley JH, Ashe M, Costa SA, Frerichs LM, Zwicker L, et al. Mobilisation of public support for policy actions to prevent obesity. *Lancet (London, England)*. 2015;385(9985):2422–31.

3. Hawkes C, Smith TG, Jewell J, Wardle J, Hammond RA, Friel S, et al. Smart food policies for obesity prevention. *Lancet (London, England)*. 2015;385(9985):2410–21.

4. Dietz WH, Baur LA, Hall K, Puhl RM, Taveras EM, Uauy R, et al. Management of obesity: Improvement of health-care training and systems for prevention and care. *Lancet (London, England)*. 2015;385(9986):2521–33.

5. Lobstein T, Jackson-Leach R, Moodie ML, Hall KD, Gortmaker SL, Swinburn BA, et al. Child and adolescent obesity: Part of a bigger picture. *Lancet (London, England)*. 2015;385(9986):2510–20.

6. Swinburn B, Kraak V, Rutter H, Vandevijvere S, Lobstein T, Sacks G, et al. Strengthening of accountability systems to create healthy food environments and reduce global obesity. *Lancet (London, England)*. 2015;385(9986):2534–45.

7. Mabry PL, Olster DH, Morgan GD, Abrams DB. Interdisciplinarity and systems science to improve population health: A view from the NIH Office of Behavioral and Social Sciences Research. *American Journal of Preventive Medicine*. 2008;35(2 Suppl.):S211–24.

8. Huang TT, Glass TA. Transforming research strategies for understanding and preventing obesity. *JAMA*. 2008;300(15):1811–3.

9. Huang TT, Drewnoski A, Kumanyika S, Glass TA. A systems-oriented multilevel framework for addressing obesity in the 21st century. *Preventing Chronic Disease*. 2009;6(3):A82.

10. Haemer MA, Huang TT, Daniels SR. The effect of neurohormonal factors, epigenetic factors, and gut microbiota on risk of obesity. *Preventing Chronic Disease*. 2009;6(3):A96.

11. Esposito L, Fisher JO, Mennella JA, Hoelscher DM, Huang TT. Developmental perspectives on nutrition and obesity from gestation to adolescence. *Preventing Chronic Disease*. 2009;6(3):A94.

12. Huang TT, Yaroch AL. A public-private partnership model for obesity prevention. *Preventing Chronic Disease*. 2009;6(3):A110.

13. Vandenbroeck IP, Goossens J, Clemens M. *Tackling Obesities: Future Choices; Obesity System Atlas*. London, UK: Foresight (Government Office for Science), 2007.

14. Christakis NA, Fowler JH. The spread of obesity in a large social network over 32 years. *The New England Journal of Medicine*. 2007;357(4):370–9.

15. Frerichs LM, Araz OM, Huang TTK. Modeling social transmission dynamics of unhealthy behaviors for evaluating prevention and treatment interventions on childhood obesity. *PLoS ONE*. 2013;8(12):e82887.

16. Hall KD, Sacks G, Chandramohan D, Chow CC, Wang YC, Gortmaker SL, et al. Quantification of the effect of energy imbalance on bodyweight. *Lancet (London, England)*. 2011;378(9793):826–37.

17. The Methodology Center, Pennsylvania State University. Why use a SMART design to build an adaptive intervention? 2015 [September 2015]. Available from: https://methodology.psu.edu/ra/adap-inter/research.

18. Organisation for Economic Co-operation and Development. Non-medical determinants of health: Food consumption, 2015 [cited October 1, 2015]. Available from: http://stats.oecd.org/index.aspx?DataSetCode=HEALTH_STAT#.

19. Rushton C. School lunch programs will suffer if Congress fails to act. *USA Today* [Internet]. September 28, 2015. Available from: http://www.usatoday.com/story/news/health/2015/09/08/school-lunch-programs-suffer-if-congress-fails-act-tom-vilsack-usda-healthy-hunger-free-kids-act/71893222/%29.

20. World Health Organization. Facts and figures on childhood obesity, 2014 [updated October 29; cited September 28, 2015]. Available from: http://www.who.int/end-childhood-obesity/facts/en/.

21. Meadows DH. *Thinking in Systems: A Primer*. River Junction, VT: Chelsea Green Publishing, 2008.

22. Finegood DT. The complex systems science of obesity. In Cawley JH, ed. *The Oxford Handbook of the Social Science of Obesity*, pp. 208–36. New York: Oxford University Press, 2011.

23. Johnston LM, Matteson CL, Finegood DT. Systems science and obesity policy: A novel framework for analyzing and rethinking population-level planning. *American Journal of Public Health*. 2014;104(7):1270–8.

24. Vanderlinden J, Adriaensen A, Vancampfort D, Pieters G, Probst M, Vansteelandt K. A cognitive-behavioral therapeutic program for patients with obesity and binge eating disorder: Short- and long-term follow-up data of a prospective study. *Behavior Modification*. 2012;36(5):670–86.

25. Annesi JJ, Smith AE, Tennant GA. Effects of a cognitive-behaviorally based physical activity treatment for 4- and 5-year-old children attending US preschools. *International Journal of Behavioral Medicine*. 2013;20(4):562–6.

26. Tsiros MD, Sinn N, Brennan L, Coates AM, Walkley JW, Petkov J, et al. Cognitive behavioral therapy improves diet and body composition in overweight and obese adolescents. *The American Journal of Clinical Nutrition*. 2008;87(5):1134–40.

27. Brennan L, Walkley J, Wilks R, Fraser SF, Greenway K. Physiological and behavioural outcomes of a randomised controlled trial of a cognitive behavioural lifestyle intervention for overweight and obese adolescents. *Obesity Research & Clinical Practice.* 2013;7(1):e23–41.

28. Institute for Quality and Efficiency in Health Care. Cognitive behavioral therapy, 2013 [cited October 1, 2015]. Available from: http://www.ncbi.nlm.nih.gov/pubmedhealth/PMH0072481/.

29. Faith M, Saelens B, Wilfley D, Allison D. Behavioral treatment of childhood and adolescent obesity: Current status, challenges, and future directions. In Thompson JK, Smolak L, eds. *Body Image, Eating Disorders, and Obesity in Youth: Assessment, Prevention, and Treatment*, pp. 313–9. Washington, DC: American Psychological Association, 2001.

30. Graves T, Meyers AW, Clark L. An evaluation of parental problem-solving training in the behavioral treatment of childhood obesity. *Journal of Consulting and Clinical Psychology.* 1988;56(2):246–50.

31. Young KM, Northern JJ, Lister KM, Drummond JA, O'Brien WH. A meta-analysis of family-behavioral weight-loss treatments for children. *Clinical Psychology Review.* 2007;27(2):240–9.

32. Epstein LH, Myers MD, Raynor HA, Saelens BE. Treatment of pediatric obesity. *Pediatrics.* 1998;101(3 Pt 2):554–70.

33. Wilfley DE, Welch RR, Stein RI, Spurrell EB, Cohen LR, Saelens BE, et al. A randomized comparison of group cognitive-behavioral therapy and group interpersonal psychotherapy for the treatment of overweight individuals with binge-eating disorder. *Archives of General Psychiatry.* 2002;59(8):713–21.

34. Wilfley DE, Kolko RP, Kass AE. Cognitive-behavioral therapy for weight management and eating disorders in children and adolescents. *Child and Adolescent Psychiatric Clinics of North America.* 2011;20(2):271–85.

35. O'Reilly GA, Cook L, Spruijt-Metz D, Black DS. Mindfulness-based interventions for obesity-related eating behaviours: A literature review. *Obesity Reviews: An Official Journal of the International Association for the Study of Obesity.* 2014;15(6):453–61.

36. Katterman SN, Kleinman BM, Hood MM, Nackers LM, Corsica JA. Mindfulness meditation as an intervention for binge eating, emotional eating, and weight loss: A systematic review. *Eating Behaviors.* 2014;15(2):197–204.

37. Teufel M, Stephan K, Kowalski A, Kasberger S, Enck P, Zipfel S, et al. Impact of biofeedback on self-efficacy and stress reduction in obesity: A randomized controlled pilot study. *Applied Psychophysiology and Biofeedback.* 2013;38(3):177–84.

38. Pop-Jordanova N. Psychological characteristics and biofeedback mitigation in preadolescents with eating disorders. *Pediatrics International: Official Journal of the Japan Pediatric Society.* 2000;42(1):76–81.

39. Wilfley DE, Tibbs TL, Van Buren DJ, Reach KP, Walker MS, Epstein LH. Lifestyle interventions in the treatment of childhood overweight: A meta-analytic review of randomized controlled trials. *Health Psychology: Official Journal of the Division of Health Psychology, American Psychological Association.* 2007;26(5):521–32.

40. Epstein LH, Wing RR, Woodall K, Penner BC, Kress MJ, Koeske R. Effects of family-based behavioral treatment on obese 5-to-8-year-old children. *Behavior Therapy.* 1985;16(2):205–12.

41. Epstein LH, Paluch RA, Roemmich JN, Beecher MD. Family-based obesity treatment, then and now: Twenty-five years of pediatric obesity treatment. *Health Psychology: Official Journal of the Division of Health Psychology, American Psychological Association.* 2007;26(4):381–91.

42. Cornell Tech Small Data Lab. Pushcart [cited September 28, 2015]. Available from: http://gopushcart.com/.

43. Oreskovic NM, Goodman E, Park ER, Robinson AI, Winickoff JP. Design and implementation of a physical activity intervention to enhance children's use of the built environment (the CUBE study). *Contemporary Clinical Trials.* 2015;40:172–9.

44. Oreskovic NM, Huang TT, Moon J. Integrating mHealth and systems science: A combination approach to prevent and treat chronic health conditions. *JMIR mHealth and uHealth.* 2015;3(2):e62.

45. Joshi A, Ratcliffe MM. Causal pathways linking farm to school to childhood obesity prevention. *Childhood Obesity (Print).* 2012;8(4):305–14.

46. Marshall C, Feenstra G, Zajfen V. Increasing access to fresh, local produce: Building values-based supply chains in San Diego Unified School District. *Childhood Obesity (Print).* 2012;8(4):388–91.

47. Pirog R, Miller C, Way L, Hazekamp C, Kim E. *The Local Food Movement: Setting the Stage for Good Food*. MSU Center for Regional Food Systems, 2014.

48. Oh A, Nguyen AB, Patrick H. Correlates of reported use and perceived helpfulness of calorie information in restaurants among U.S. adults. *American Journal of Health Promotion: AJHP.* 2015.

49. Bleich SN, Wolfson JA, Jarlenski MP. Calorie changes in chain restaurant menu items: Implications for obesity and evaluations of menu labeling. *American Journal of Preventive Medicine.* 2015;48(1):70–5.

50. Cioffi CE, Levitsky DA, Pacanowski CR, Bertz F. A nudge in a healthy direction: The effect of nutrition labels on food purchasing behaviors in university dining facilities. *Appetite*. 2015;92:7–14.

51. Chen R, Smyser M, Chan N, Ta M, Saelens BE, Krieger J. Changes in awareness and use of calorie information after mandatory menu labeling in restaurants in King County, Washington. *American Journal of Public Health*. 2015;105(3):546–53.

52. Dobbins M, Tirilis D. Built environment: A synthesis of review of evidence. *Population Health Improvement Research Network*. 2011:S1(3).

53. Chawla N, Thamarangsi T. Effectiveness of school built environment on physical activity in children: A systematic review. *Journal of Health Science*. 2014;23(4).

54. Thorndike AN, Sonnenberg L, Riis J, Barraclough S, Levy DE. A 2-phase labeling and choice architecture intervention to improve healthy food and beverage choices. *American Journal of Public Health*. 2012;102(3):527–33.

55. Skov LR, Lourenco S, Hansen GL, Mikkelsen BE, Schofield C. Choice architecture as a means to change eating behaviour in self-service settings: A systematic review. *Obesity Reviews: An Official Journal of the International Association for the Study of Obesity*. 2013;14(3):187–96.

56. Wansink B, Just DR, Hanks AS, Smith LE. Pre-sliced fruit in school cafeterias: Children's selection and intake. *American Journal of Preventive Medicine*. 2013;44(5):477–80.

57. Wansink B, Just DR, Payne CR, Klinger MZ. Attractive names sustain increased vegetable intake in schools. *Preventive Medicine*. 2012;55(4):330–2.

58. Huang TT, Sorensen D, Davis S, Frerichs L, Brittin J, Celentano J, et al. Healthy eating design guidelines for school architecture. *Preventing Chronic Disease*. 2013;10:E27.

59. Brittin J, Sorensen D, Trowbridge M, Lee KK, Breithecker D, Frerichs L, et al. Physical activity design guidelines for school architecture. *PLoS ONE*. 2015;10(7):e0132597.

60. Otten JJ, Saelens BE, Kapphahn KI, Hekler EB, Buman MP, Goldstein BA, et al. Impact of San Francisco's toy ordinance on restaurants and children's food purchases, 2011–2012. *Preventing Chronic Disease*. 2014;11:E122.

61. Henry HK, Borzekowski DL. Well, that's what came with it: A qualitative study of U.S. mothers' perceptions of healthier default options for children's meals at fast-food restaurants. *Appetite*. 2015;87:108–15.

62. Anzman-Frasca S, Dawes F, Sliwa S, Dolan PR, Nelson ME, Washburn K, et al. Healthier side dishes at restaurants: An analysis of children's perspectives, menu content, and energy impacts. *The International Journal of Behavioral Nutrition and Physical Activity*. 2014;11:81.

63. Glickman D, Parker L, Sim LJ, Del Valle Cook H, Miller EA, eds. *Accelerating Progress in Obesity Prevention: Solving the Weight of the Nation*. Washington, DC: Institute of Medicine of the The National Academies, 2012.

64. Bar-Yam Y. *Making Things Work: Solving Complex Problems in a Complex World*. Cambridge, MA: NECSI Knowledge Press, 2004.

65. Access to Nutrition Index. Access to Nutrition Foundation [cited September 28, 2015]. Available from: https://www.accesstonutrition.org/.

66. S & P Dow Jones Indices. Dow Jones Sustainability Indices [cited October 1, 2015]. Available from: http://www.djindexes.com/sustainability/.

67. Yale University. Environmental Performance Index, 2015 [cited October 1, 2015]. Available from: http://epi.yale.edu/.

68. Access to Medicine Index, 2012 [cited October 1, 2015]. Available from: http://www.accesstomedicineindex.org/.

69. Business in the Community. The Corporate Responsibility Index, 2015 [cited October 1, 2015]. Available from: http://www.bitc.org.uk/services/benchmarking/cr-index.

70. Healthy Together Victoria [cited September 28, 2015]. Available from: http://healthytogether.vic.gov.au/.

71. Missouri Foundation for Health. Social Innovation for Missouri (SIM), 2015 [cited September 28, 2015]. Available from: https://www.mffh.org/content/485/social-innovation-for-missouri-sim.aspx.

72. Schoen MW, Moreland-Russell S, Prewitt K, Carothers BJ. Social network analysis of public health programs to measure partnership. *Social Science & Medicine*. 2014;123:90–5.

73. Frerichs L, Brittin J, Stewart C, Robbins R, Riggs C, Mayberger S, et al. SaludableOmaha: Development of a youth advocacy initiative to increase community readiness for obesity prevention, 2011–2012. *Preventing Chronic Disease*. 2012;9:E173.

74. Frerichs L, Brittin J, Robbins R, Steenson S, Stewart C, Fisher C, et al. SaludABLEOmaha: Improving readiness to address obesity through healthy lifestyle in a Midwestern Latino community, 2011–2013. *Preventing Chronic Disease*. 2015;12:E20.

75. Brittin J, Frerichs L, Sirard J, Wells N, Myers B, Garcia J, et al. Impact of active school design on school-time sedentary behavior: A longitudinal study. Obesity Week, Los Angeles, CA, 2015.

76. Frerichs L, Brittin J, Intolubbe-Chmil L, Trowbridge M, Sorenson D, Huang TT. Influence of design and architecture on elementary school staff and student healthy eating outcomes. *Journal of School Health*. In press.

77. Sorensen D, Brittin J, Frerichs L, Trowbridge MJ, Huang TT. *Moving Schools Forward: A Design Recipe for Health; Buckingham County Primary & Elementary School, Dillwyn, Virginia*. Dillwyn, VA: AIA Design & Health, 2014.

78. Robinson TN, Sirard JR. Preventing childhood obesity: A solution-oriented research paradigm. *American Journal of Preventive Medicine*. 2005;28(2 Suppl. 2):194–201.

79. Costa SA, Ferris E, Huang TT. What the obesity prevention field can learn from the gay marriage movement. *Obesity (Silver Spring, Md)*. 2015;23(10):1939–40.

80. Levy DT, Mabry PL, Wang YC, Gortmaker S, Huang TTK, Marsh T, et al. Simulation models of obesity: A review of the literature and implications for research and policy. *Obesity Reviews*. 2011;12(5):378–94.

81. Ip EH, Rahmandad H, Shoham DA, Hammond R, Huang TT-K, Wang Y, et al. Reconciling statistical and systems science approaches to public health. *Health Education & Behavior*. 2013;40(1 Suppl.):123S–31S.

82. Gittelsohn J, Mui Y, Adam A, Lin S, Kharmats A, Igusa T, et al. Incorporating systems science principles into the development of obesity prevention interventions: Principles, benefits, and challenges. *Current Obesity Reports*. 2015;4(2):174–81.

83. Mui Y, Oke J, Igusa T, Lee B, Anderson Steeves E, Gittelshon J, eds. An agent-based model simulates interventions in small food sources to improve the urban food environment and curb obesity. International Congress on Obesity, Kuala Lumpur, Malaysia, 2014.

84. Yang Y, Auchincloss AH, Rodriguez DA, Brown DG, Riolo R, Diez-Roux AV. Modeling spatial segregation and travel cost influences on utilitarian walking: Towards policy intervention. *Computers, Environment and Urban Systems*. 2015;51:59–69.

85. Yang Y, Diez Roux AV, Auchincloss AH, Rodriguez DA, Brown DG. Exploring walking differences by socioeconomic status using a spatial agent-based model. *Health & Place*. 2012;18(1):96–9.

86. Hammond RA, Ornstein JT, Fellows LK, Dubé L, Levitan R, Dagher A. A model of food reward learning with dynamic reward exposure. *Frontiers in Computational Neuroscience*. 2012;6:82.

87. Collective Impact Forum, 2014 [cited October 21, 2015]. Available from: http://collectiveimpactforum. org/.

88. Collective Impact Forum. Featured initiative stories, 2014 [cited October 5, 2015]. Available from: http://collectiveimpactforum.org/initiative-stories.

89. Stempfle J, Badke-Schaub P. Thinking in design teams: An analysis of team communication. *Design Studies*. 2002;23:473–96.

90. Brown T. *Change by Design: How Design Thinking Transforms Organizations and Inspires Innovation*. New York: HarperCollins, 2009.

91. Vechakul J, Shrimali BP, Sandhu JS. Human-centered design as an approach for place-based innovation in public health: A case study from Oakland, California. *Maternal and Child Health Journal*. 2015;19:2552–9.

92. Lockwood T, Walton T, eds. *Building Design Strategy: Using Design to Achieve Key Business Objectives*. New York: Allworth Press, 2008.

93. Renger M KG, de Vreede GJ. Challenges in collaborative modelling: A literature review and research agenda. *International Journal of Simulation and Process Modelling*. 2008;4(3/4):248–63.

94. Kolfschoten G, de Vreede G. A design approach for collaboration processes: A multimethod design science study in collaboration engineering. *Journal of Management Information Systems*. 2009;26(1):225–56.

95. Participle [cited September 28, 2015]. Available from: http://www.participle.net/.

43 Food Policy for Childhood Obesity Prevention
A Global Perspective

Alanna Soupen, Stefanie Vandevijvere,
Hillary Tolley, and Boyd Swinburn

CONTENTS

INTRODUCTION

Reversing the global obesity epidemic is one of the most serious public health challenges of the twenty-first century [1]. It is now widely accepted that obesity is a complex problem that needs to be addressed through comprehensive multisectoral action [2]. Over the last 15 years, the World Health Organization (WHO) and member states have collaborated to develop global strategies for the prevention and control of obesity and noncommunicable diseases (NCDs) [2–6] and to improve maternal and child health [7]. Reducing childhood obesity has been an important part of these comprehensive strategies. This is motivated by the need to protect children from harm, ensure their right to healthy food, and to reduce the global burden of diet-related NCDs, for which obesity is a major risk factor [2]. Most recently, in 2014, to better inform the development and implementation of comprehensive policy approaches, the WHO established the Commission on Ending Childhood Obesity [2]. As a result of these global efforts, there are now agreed high-level policies, strategies, and targets for addressing childhood obesity. However, translating these global recommendations into specific policy actions at the national level remains challenging [8]. No country has comprehensively adopted the recommended strategies [8]. Policy adoption is often characterized by the implementation of a few isolated interventions. These have mostly focused on the *soft policy* options of social marketing and education, rather than on comprehensive policy programs, including policies to create healthy food environments [8].

Given the complex nature of the obesity epidemic, the implementation of isolated policies is unlikely to be successful [8]. But moving toward comprehensive approaches will involve tackling several corporate, political, and societal barriers. While there are multiple macro challenges in reversing the obesity epidemic, this chapter focuses mainly on food policies and their implementation. Challenges in implementing policies aimed at increasing physical activity, such as active transport policies and urban design solutions, have been discussed in detail in the *Lancet* "Physical Activity" series.* The aims of this chapter are to

- Highlight the importance of reducing childhood obesity
- Provide a brief overview of the key global policy developments relating to the prevention of childhood obesity
- Discuss some of the main challenges related to the implementation of food policies to reduce childhood obesity: developing a shared narrative, rebalancing the power, and strengthening accountability of the main actors
- Identify priority strategies in moving from patchy progress to comprehensive policy approaches

REDUCING CHILDHOOD OBESITY

The simultaneous increases in obesity observed worldwide appear to be primarily driven by changes in the global food system [9]. These changes have led to mass production of increasingly processed, affordable, and effectively marketed food [9,10]. It is now widely recognized that children are growing up in increasingly obesogenic food environments, and unlike adult populations, bear little or no responsibility for their obesity and its health complications [2]. For this reason, efforts to prevent childhood obesity are often viewed as efforts to protect vulnerable children from social harm [2]. In addition, the prevention of unhealthy weight gain among children is a more achievable prospect than reducing the body weight of the large proportions of adults who are already overweight or obese. To tackle other NCD risk factors, such as smoking, high blood pressure, and high blood cholesterol, effective evidence-based interventions have been established and widely applied in adult populations to achieve reductions in the prevalence of those risk factors [9]. This is not the case, however, for obesity, where sustained weight loss is a challenge even for motivated individuals, let alone across a population [9]. This has major implications for the time scale for reducing the prevalence of obesity-driven diseases, especially type 2 diabetes [9]. While the upswing of the obesity epidemic occurred at roughly the same rate in all age groups (the hallmark of an environmentally induced epidemic affecting the whole population), the scenario of the downswing of the obesity epidemic is unlikely to be the mirror image of the upswing, simply because the large proportion of people who are overweight or obese are unlikely to lose large amounts of weight en masse. A more likely scenario will be major cohort effects as childhood obesity reduces over time and those leaner childhood populations become leaner adult populations. Preventing and treating childhood obesity is thus likely to play a major role in reducing the global burden of NCDs, particularly type 2 diabetes.

KEY POLICY DEVELOPMENTS

Initially, the focus of global recommendations to address risk factors for obesity and diet-related NCDs was on adult populations. The first WHO document to focus entirely on obesity was the 2000 Technical Report 894, entitled "Obesity: Preventing and Managing the Global Epidemic" [3]. The release of this report put the prevention and control of obesity squarely on the global public health agenda. In the 15 years that have followed, significant other global policy milestones have been

---

* See http://www.thelancet.com/series/physical-activity.

reached. While the recommended policies and strategies have grown in sophistication over time, global policy documents have consistently recommended a government-led, comprehensive, preventive approach that integrates prevention with policies aimed at helping populations lose weight and maintain healthy weights. They have also consistently specified that, while government is to take the lead, the success of prevention efforts depends equally on input from the private sector and civil society. The key global policy documents have been summarized in chronological order in Table 43.1. The table specifies whether policy recommendations have been aimed at children specifically or the general population. It also specifies whether the focus of each document is explicitly on obesity or on the prevention and control of NCDs.

The first WHO report to include specific recommendations for preventing and controlling obesity in children was Technical Report 916: "Diet, Nutrition and the Prevention of Chronic Diseases," published in 2003 [12]. It was also the first report to include an analysis of environmental factors as determinants of the obesity epidemic and global dietary and physical activity recommendations. The implementation of these recommendations was outlined in the 2004 "Global Strategy on Diet,

TABLE 43.1
Key Global Policy Documents

Year	Document	Target Population	Focus
2000	Obesity: Preventing and managing the global epidemic [3].	General	Obesity
2000	Global strategy for the prevention and control of NCDs [11].	General	NCDs
2003	Diet, nutrition and the prevention of chronic diseases [12].	General	NCDs
2004	Global strategy on diet, physical activity and health [13].	General	Nutrition and physical activity
2008	2008–2013 Action plan for the global strategy for the prevention and control of NCDs [14].	General	NCDs
2008	School policy framework: Implementation of the WHO global strategy on diet, physical activity and health [15].	Children	Diet and physical activity
2010	Set of recommendations on the marketing of food and nonalcoholic beverages to children [16].	Children	Marketing of unhealthy food
2011	Political declaration of the High-Level Meeting of the General Assembly on the Prevention and Control of Non-communicable Diseases [17].	General	NCDs
2011	Global recommendations on physical activity for health: 5–17 years old [18].	Children	Physical activity
2012	Population-based approaches to childhood obesity prevention [1].	Children	Obesity
2012	Prioritizing areas for action in the field of population-based prevention of childhood obesity [19].	Children	Obesity
2013	Noncommunicable diseases global monitoring framework (*includes target of 0% increase in adolescent obesity*) [20].	General	NCDs
2013	Global action plan for the prevention and control of noncommunicable diseases 2013–2020 [21].	General	NCDs
2014	UN Food and Agriculture Organization, Second International Conference on Nutrition [22].	General	Nutrition and agricultural policy
2014	Comprehensive implementation plan on maternal, infant and young child nutrition (*includes target of 0% increase in childhood obesity*) [7].	Mothers and children	Maternal and child nutrition
2015	Report of the Commission on Ending Childhood Obesity [2].	Children	Obesity

Physical Activity and Health"; no strategies were aimed specifically at child populations [13]. The focus on childhood obesity sharpened between 2010 and 2015. In 2010, the 63rd World Health Assembly adopted resolution WHA63.23 on infant and young child nutrition [23], followed by the release of a comprehensive implementation plan on maternal, infant, and young child nutrition by the WHO in 2014 [7]. For the first time, the prevention of over- and undernutrition were explicitly linked [23]. The assembly also adopted WHA63.14, which outlined a set of recommendations on restricting junk food marketing to children [15]. The following year, the 2011 UN Declaration on the Prevention and Control of NCDs was adopted, representing a major political effort to seriously address the global NCD burden [17]. Following the declaration, "halting the rise in adult and adolescent obesity" was set as a target in the WHO NCD global monitoring framework [20].

Between 2011 and 2015, significant work was done by the WHO to develop specific tools and frameworks to translate global strategies into specific policy recommendations for childhood obesity. The comprehensive implementation plan on maternal, infant, and young child nutrition was the first document to set an obesity reduction target for children (no increase in childhood obesity) [7]. During this period, global recommendations for adolescent physical activity, recommendations for population-based approaches to childhood obesity prevention, guidelines for priority setting in childhood obesity prevention, and a framework for implementing the "Global Strategy on Diet, Physical Activity, and Health" in schools were also published by the WHO [1,15–18]. Furthermore, in 2014, the WHO established a high-level Commission on Ending Childhood Obesity (ECHO). The final report of the commission reaffirmed the message of earlier documents: that governments have the essential role in providing leadership in addressing childhood obesity [2]. The report identified the need for constructive relationships between government, the private sector, and civil society to move forward. Furthermore, it emphasized that policy implementation requires consideration of contextual differences and inequalities between and within countries. The report also highlighted the need for a monitoring and accountability framework at a national level to ensure effective policy implementation and action.

FEATURES OF A COMPREHENSIVE APPROACH TO PREVENT CHILDHOOD OBESITY

In "Population-Based Approaches to Childhood Obesity Prevention," the WHO identified six key features that a comprehensive approach to preventing childhood obesity should include [1]

1. A mixture of government-driven, "top-down," and community-based actions
2. A mixture of policy instruments, including legislative and fiscal tools, to ensure the availability and affordability of healthy foods and physical activity opportunities (see Box 43.2 for some examples of specific policies)
3. The integration of policies for childhood obesity prevention into existing structures to ensure sustainability of action
4. Interventions across a range of settings, including early child-care settings, schools, and community organizations
5. The establishment of cross-sectoral platforms and a multisectoral approach to childhood obesity
6. Strengthening structural components within government to support action on childhood obesity

In this document, the WHO further categorizes these policy instruments into three "components" of a comprehensive strategy: (1) supportive structures within government, (2) population-wide policies and initiatives, and (3) community-based interventions.

INFRASTRUCTURE SUPPORT

While supportive structures within government are often critical to intervention success, they are also frequently overlooked [1]. Strengthening these components is essential to support the implementation of more "direct" population-wide and community-based interventions [1,24]. The International Network for Food and Obesity/Non-communicable Diseases Research, Monitoring and Action Support (INFORMAS) framework for benchmarking and monitoring food environments identifies six key domains of infrastructure support that are derived from the WHO system's building blocks [25]:

1. Leadership
2. Governance
3. Monitoring and intelligence
4. Funding and resources
5. Platforms for interaction
6. Health-in-all policies

Two examples of best-practice infrastructure support systems are described in Box 43.1.

POPULATION-WIDE PREVENTION STRATEGIES

There are a range of population-wide policy options recommended by the WHO and other organizations. Building on the work of these organizations, options have been categorized by the World Cancer Research Fund's NOURISHING framework [4]. This framework classifies different food

---

BOX 43.1   INFRASTRUCTURE SYSTEMS WITHIN GOVERNMENT TO SUPPORT CHILDHOOD OBESITY PREVENTION POLICIES AND INTERVENTIONS

MONITORING AND INTELLIGENCE: ENGLAND'S NATIONAL CHILD MEASUREMENT PROGRAMME

The National Child Measurement Programme was established in 2006 and aims to measure all children in England in the first (4–5) and last (10–11) years of primary school. In 2011–2012, 565,662 children were measured on beginning primary school and 491,118 children were measured in the last year of primary school. The large sample size allows for detailed data on prevalence and trends at a very local level and in particular subgroups of the population. [26]

HEALTH-IN-ALL POLICIES: FINLAND'S HEALTH CARE ACT REFORM

One recent example of positive change has been the Finnish city of Seinäjoki, where 6 years ago one in five 5-year-olds was obese. Through collaboration between the municipality's health department and childcare, education, nutrition, recreation, and urban planning departments to ensure all day-care centers and schools provide the same quality of services, *this proportion has now halved*. This collaboration was facilitated by a reform of the Health Care Act in 2011 to mandate health promotion services and require municipalities to involve all sectors in their plans. Reform enabled many municipalities, including Seinäjoki, to provide free health-care counseling and health examinations of equal quality to all children and their families. Without reform, it is likely that many municipalities would have lacked the resources to hire additional public health staff to support their programs to improve child health. [27]

policies implemented around the world, providing a policy development tool for governments. The framework divides actions into the following 10 categories:

1. Nutrition label standards and regulations on the use of claims and implied claims on foods
2. Offer healthy foods and set standards in public institutions and other specific settings
3. Use economic tools to address food affordability and purchase incentives (such as taxes on unhealthy food)
4. Restrict food advertising and other forms of commercial promotion
5. Improve the quality of the whole food supply
6. Set incentives and rules to create a healthy retail and food service environment
7. Harness supply chain and actions across sectors to ensure coherence with health
8. Inform people about food and nutrition through public awareness
9. Nutrition advice and counseling in health-care settings
10. Give nutrition education and skills

Of these strategies, educational approaches and information campaigns have most frequently been used by governments. To date, over 20 jurisdictions have implemented some form of tax on unhealthy foods and beverages [28]. The implementation of a sugar-sweetened beverage (SSB) tax in Mexico provides an example of successful population-wide policy adoption and implementation. This is described further in Box 43.2.

COMMUNITY-BASED APPROACHES

Community-based approaches are those involving strong community engagement or participation [1]. Those that adopt a systems-based approach, addressing multiple components concurrently, are more likely to be achievable and sustainable at scale [1]. Other key factors that are likely to determine success include adapting the intervention to the local context, ensuring cultural and environmental appropriateness, using existing social and organizational structures of a community, and incorporating the ongoing involvement of all key community stakeholders [1]. One example of a large-scale systems-based approach is described in Box 43.3.

The Ensemble Prevenons l'besité des Enfants (EPODE; Together let's prevent childhood obesity) program is a coordinated, capacity-building approach for communities to implement effective and

---

BOX 43.2   POPULATION-WIDE STRATEGIES AND INITIATIVES

INTRODUCTION OF A SUGAR-SWEETENED BEVERAGE TAX IN MEXICO

In December 2013, Mexico passed two new taxes as part of their "National Strategy for the Prevention and Control of Overweight, Obesity and Diabetes," which came into force in January 2014. One of these was a tax on SSBs, which applied an excise duty of 1 peso ($0.07) per liter to sugary drinks (defined as all drinks with added sugar, excluding milk or yoghurt). The revenue from the tax was to be invested in providing safe drinking water in schools. Initial price monitoring indicated that this increased the price of sugary drinks by around 10%, and all revenue was allocated to the general budget. A recent study conducted by the Mexican Institute of Public Health and the University of North Carolina suggests that, on average, the tax cut SSB sales by 6% in 2014, and by as much as 12% in the latter part of the year. While reductions occurred across all socioeconomic groups, they were higher among lower socioeconomic households, averaging a 9% decline over 2014 and up to a 17% decline by December 2014. There was also an increase of roughly 4% in purchases of untaxed beverages over 2014, mainly driven by an increase in purchased bottled plain water. [28,29]

BOX 43.3 SYSTEMS-BASED COMMUNITY APPROACHES

HEALTHY TOGETHER VICTORIA (AUSTRALIA)

Healthy Together Victoria was established in 2011 as part of a national effort to strengthen prevention [30]. It was led by the Victoria state government and worked through local government. It involved multiple players at the community level, including child-care centers, schools, workplaces, food outlets, sporting clubs, businesses, local governments, health professionals, and other stakeholders to create healthier environments. Taking a complex *whole of systems* approach to prevention, it used multiple strategies, policies, and initiatives at both state and local levels. Some strategies were aimed at the entire Victorian population, but most resources were concentrated at the community level in 12 Healthy Together Communities. These communities covered 1.3 million Victorians (25% of the Victorian population) through 520 schools, 938 early childhood services, and 4409 medium-to-large workplaces. The core driver creating system change was a dynamic and innovative workforce, both within the 12 Healthy Together Communities and more broadly across the state. Unfortunately, as the initiative was starting to achieve significant changes in community systems, the incoming federal and state governments defunded prevention, including Healthy Together Victoria.

sustainable strategies to promote healthier lifestyles and prevent childhood obesity [1]. Although it has not incorporated a full systems approach, EPODE appears to be having some success in reducing childhood obesity [31].

CONSIDERATION OF NUTRITION IN AGRICULTURE AND TRADE

At a global level, there is a pressing need to make population nutrition goals a central consideration in the development of food and agricultural policies and international food and agricultural trade agreements, including food security initiatives. Policy work on "nutrition-sensitive agricultural policies" was progressed at the joint WHO/Food and Agricultural Organization's Second International Conference on Nutrition in 2014 [22]. While this meeting recognized that many low- and middle-income countries are struggling with a double burden of under- and overnutrition, the final set of commitments from member states fell well short of what would be needed to truly reorient agricultural policies toward reducing the very high global burden of diet-related diseases [22].

Trade and foreign direct investment (FDI) agreements, such as the Trans-Pacific Partnership [10] and the Transatlantic Trade and Investment Partnership, present a threat to the nutritional health of populations, especially through the FDI clauses that allow transnational corporations to sue governments for loss of investment due to government policies that adversely affect their profits. Such suits are heard offshore in secret settlement tribunals (investor–state dispute settlements) [10]. The threats to population nutrition from trade and FDI agreements have been outlined by Friel et al. [10,32]. Some of the major threats identified by Friel et al. have been summarized as follows [10]:

- **Imports: Access to nutritious foods:** The reduction of tariff and nontariff barriers to trade through trade liberalization policies has resulted in disproportionately large increases in the import and domestic production of processed foods, creating an oversupply of highly processed foods that are calorie rich and nutrient poor.
- **Tax revenues and government spending:** Tariff reduction could affect nutrition through its potential to reduce the size of tax revenue available to fund health programs.
- **Increasing foreign direct investment and integrated food supply chains:** Many trade liberalization policies have facilitated greater foreign direct investment, which enables

transnational corporations to extend their supply chains. This has allowed for greater penetration of transnational food corporations into many developing countries, which has led to the global diffusion of highly processed, nutrient-poor food.

The annual "Global Nutrition Report," which was launched in 2014, reports on progress toward nutrition goals, including reducing childhood underweight and overweight, globally and by country [33].

REASONS FOR PATCHY PROGRESS ON REDUCING CHILDHOOD OBESITY

Although there is global consensus on high-level strategies needed to comprehensively address childhood obesity, policy uptake has been low [8]. In the 2015 *Lancet* "Obesity" series, Roberto and colleagues described the implementation of the recommended strategies as being "patchy" at best, being limited to the implementation of isolated interventions [8]. However, there were some positive examples of policy implementation emerging globally, suggesting that there is reason to be optimistic about the future of obesity prevention. The series identified several reasons for the poor translation of global recommendations into national policies, including the power imbalance between the private sector and government/civil society, ineffective accountability mechanisms, and the need to improve the transfer of policy knowledge [8]. These are discussed further in the following sections.

REBALANCING POWER AND DEVELOPING SHARED NARRATIVES

Power to influence health-related policy decisions often rests disproportionately with commercial interests, an imbalance facilitated by the spread of neoliberal politics [34,35]. The idea that government intervention in health should be kept to a bare minimum has been a core narrative in the many countries that have adopted the economic and governance philosophies of neoliberalism [35]. The spread of these philosophies with their prioritization of free-market ideals has made deregulated markets the norm in many countries and privileged commercial interests in influencing policymaking [35]. The corporate political activity of *Big Food* and *Big Soda* in halting or slowing down efforts to introduce public health regulation of the food and beverage industry is clear [36]. Even in regions where pressure from civil society on government is strong, political lobbying by the food and beverage industry is stronger [37]. In some low- and middle-income countries, where civil society has successfully lobbied government to regulate the food and beverage industry, Big Food and Big Soda have still managed to intervene [37]. In Brazil, Chile, and Thailand, interference by Big Food and Big Soda has slowed or halted progress in industry regulation, even in the final stages of policymaking [37]. Thailand, for example, initiated a program to ban unhealthy beverages from schools [37]. However, the impact of the program has been slowed by the food industry's financially remunerative contracts with schools to provide SSBs and junk food [37].

The power of commercial interests to influence public health grants them considerable sway over core narratives about obesity, its drivers, and its solutions [34–36]. In most countries, the obesity epidemic is viewed through two broad and distinct frames: for some, obesity is driven by environmental factors and can only be addressed through government-led action; for others, obesity is primarily caused by individual behavior and, therefore, is the responsibility of the individual not the government [35]. Roberto and colleagues identify the existence of such dichotomous narratives as a major obstacle for collaboration in preventing and reducing obesity [8]. Table 43.2 illustrates some of the dichotomies and their intersections in obesity narratives.

In most countries, the narratives in column A are predominant. However, as the second *Lancet* series on obesity highlighted, oversimplifying the issue into a series of dichotomies does not do justice to the understanding of the problems or solutions [8]. While the evidence suggests that both frames have some merit, it is often at the intersection of the dichotomy where key insights lie, as

TABLE 43.2

Dichotomies and Intersections in Obesity Narratives

Issue	Narrative Dichotomies A	B	Intersection
Drivers of obesity	Individual choices	Environmental pressures	Commercial interests shape environments to exploit individual vulnerabilities, thus creating unhealthy preferences [8].
Consumption of unhealthy food	Demand driven	Supply driven	The supply of unhealthy foods in early years creates preference for unhealthy foods, thus fueling the demand for unhealthy foods over the life course, sustaining a vicious cycle [2,8].
Nutrition	Undernutrition	Overnutrition	Under- and overnutrition have some common drivers and solutions. Linking prevention of all forms of malnutrition could bring greater benefit [8,33].
Solutions	Treatment	Prevention	Prevention and treatment reinforce each other. Healthier food environments support people trying to lose weight; medical advocacy for prevention strategies and people trying to lose weight advocate for healthier food environments [8,12,21].
Regulation	Industry self-regulation	Government statutory regulation	In reality, it may be that a combination (coregulation) and/or something in the middle (quasi-regulation) will be more feasible and effective [8,35].
Pressure for change	Bottom-up (consumer demand)	Top-down (regulation)	Both approaches reinforce each other and combined approaches will be effective [8,38].

shown in the table. To work together effectively, government, the private sector, and civil society will need to come to a more integrated understanding of childhood obesity [2,8].

ENHANCING ACCOUNTABILITY FOR ACTION ON CHILDHOOD OBESITY

For multisectoral partnerships to be effective, they have to be supportive of population nutrition goals rather than corporate interests [38]. Governments need to ensure that power and accountability structures are aligned so that the influence of governments and civil society, acting on behalf of public interest, are not dominated by the commercial interests of the private sector [38]. At present, however, accountability mechanisms in most countries are weak and do not provide the necessary infrastructure to support effective partnerships [35]. In the second *Lancet* series on obesity, Swinburn and colleagues described effective accountability frameworks as those where (1) the principles of all parties are aligned, (2) a clear understanding of lines of accountability exists, and (3) sanctions are in place for noncompliance or poor performance [35]. They propose a four-step cycle of taking, sharing, holding, and ensuring a response to the account as follows [35] (Figure 43.1).

For obesity, *taking the account* must include regular monitoring of adult and childhood body mass index (BMI) as well as regular monitoring of food and physical activity policies and environments. Monitoring systems for food policies and environments have been developed and data are currently being collected by INFORMAS. INFORMAS data on food environments will complement the WHO NCD global monitoring framework, and the group will provide independent assessments of the policy efforts of government and the corporate activity of the food and beverage industry [35]. There is a need for an equivalent set of monitoring systems for physical activity environments.

Sharing the account will involve the wide dissemination of information collected through monitoring efforts. *Holding [actors] to account* will involve stakeholders acknowledging achievements and sanctioning poor performance of each other. This is currently the weakest step in the

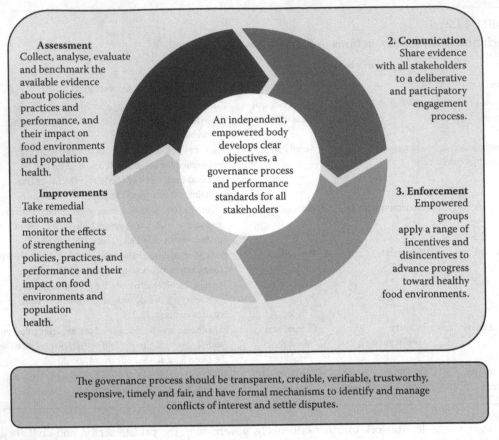

Assessment
Collect, analyse, evaluate and benchmark the available evidence about policies. practices and performance, and their impact on food environments and population health.

Improvements
Take remedial actions and monitor the effects of strengthening policies, practices, and performance and their impact on food environments and population health.

An independent, empowered body develops clear objectives, a governance process and performance standards for all stakeholders

2. Comunication
Share evidence with all stakeholders to a deliberative and participatory engagement process.

3. Enforcement
Empowered groups apply a range of incentives and disincentives to advance progress toward healthy food environments.

The governance process should be transparent, credible, verifiable, trustworthy, responsive, timely and fair, and have formal mechanisms to identify and manage conflicts of interest and settle disputes.

FIGURE 43.1 An accountability framework to promote healthy food environments. (Adapted from Kraak and colleagues, Cambridge University Press [license number 3695590621337]. With permission.)

accountability framework, especially when governments do not provide strong leadership of the accountability processes. The fourth step aims to ensure an active *response to the account* and will entail changes in policies and practices of governments, as well as in the food and beverage industry.

In this framework, government is responsible for holding the private sector to account, and civil society is responsible for holding both the private sector and government to account. It identifies six categories of accountability mechanisms that government and civil society actors have at their disposal—that is, legal, quasi-regulatory, political, market-based mechanisms, and the use of public and private communications. The strongest accountability lever available to governments is the use of legal mechanisms. However, while several countries now have regulatory accountability measures in place, enforcing sanctions remains the weakest component of the cycle [35]. In today's globalized environment, national governance has become more and more complex as governments face the disjunction between soft obligations to implement WHO recommendations approved at the World Health Assembly and hard obligations to adhere to multinational trade and investment agreements [35]. In addition, global trade agreements can impose demanding evidentiary hurdles that must be crossed before public health regulations that may affect trade and foreign investment can be implemented [35].

In today's political environment, where many countries have adopted neoliberal economic outlooks, it comes as no surprise that trade obligations are generally privileged over health obligations. However, while governments probably need to implement regulatory measures, the adoption of quasi-regulatory approaches is generally underutilized and could provide useful alternative pathways [35]. Although voluntary food industry commitments often lack transparency and are weakly enforced, governments can play a role in strengthening these frameworks [35]. Through establishing a clear policy framework and identifying measurable contributions that private stakeholders are expected to make, transparency and enforcement can be improved [35]. Furthermore, governments can take a *legislative scaffolding* approach, where they create a credible expectation that more direct forms of regulation will follow if the industry underperforms on its goals [35].

STRENGTHENING CIVIL SOCIETY

Civil society can also use a range of mechanisms to hold government and the private sector to account [35]. In most countries, however, civil society levers are relatively weak—even in countries with democratic political systems, independent media and judicial systems, and a low tolerance for corruption [35]. Government can strengthen civil society through improving participatory governance structures so that policymaking is weighted toward population nutrition goals rather than commercial interests [35]. In Brazil, for example, the Brazilian Food and Nutrition Council, which is responsible for translating nutrition conference recommendations into policy proposals, has two-thirds representation from civil society [35]. Private sector actors are included in the remaining third of its members, but only if they do not have substantial conflicts of interest with population nutrition goals.

Public health researchers and organizations can also play a role in strengthening the influence of civil society by mobilizing public support for action on obesity. "Bottom-up" or "grassroots" pressure for public health change has played a crucial role in the success of many public health campaigns [33]. Huang and colleagues identify several strategies that can be used to increase public support for action on obesity [38]. These include the refinement and streamlining of public information, the identification of obesity frames most effective for each population, improving media advocacy, the building of citizen protest and engagement, and developing a receptive political environment where change agents work across multiple organizations and sectors.

IMPROVING THE IMPACT OF RESEARCH

Learning from countries that have successfully implemented comprehensive approaches can help catalyze and improve policy implementation at the national level. The World Cancer Research Fund's NOURISHING framework and corresponding policy database represents a major international effort in this area. Collecting data on international policy efforts will also help provide benchmarks from which to identify best-practice policies. However, in addition to improving data collection and monitoring, there is also a pressing need to improve the translation of research into policy and practice [39]. The concept of *strategic science* provides a conceptual framework for collaborations between researchers and change agents—those who can convert the knowledge into action [39]. The starting point is the cocreation of the research question by researchers and change agents. They may or may not collaborate in the actual data collection and analyses but certainly do so in the interpretation and communication of the findings. Research results should be communicated not only in academic publications, as with traditional science, but also in forms more relevant to policymakers. This collaboration creates a two-way policy "bridge" that ensures issues relevant to policy are addressed, and that research findings are communicated in real time to policymakers, who must often make decisions quickly.

CONCLUSION

It is clear that over the last 15 years, significant progress has been made in developing global strategies for the prevention and control of obesity and diet-related NCDs, including reducing childhood obesity. However, the translation of higher-level recommendations to the national level remains difficult. The disproportionate sway over public policymaking held by commercial interests, and their influence over obesity narratives, have contributed significantly to the patchy progress observed at national levels. In this chapter, improving accountability mechanisms, mobilizing public support, and improving the collection and transfer of policy knowledge have been identified as key strategies in improving policy uptake and implementation of comprehensive policy approaches to prevent childhood obesity.

REFERENCES

1. World Health Organization. Population-based approaches to childhood obesity prevention. Geneva, Switzerland: World Health Organization, 2012.
2. World Health Organization. Report of the Commission on Ending Childhood Obesity. Geneva, Switzerland: World Health Organization, 2015.
3. World Health Organization. Obesity: Preventing and managing the global epidemic. Report of a WHO consultation. WHO Technical Report Series, no. 894. Geneva, Switzerland: World Health Organization, 2000.
4. Hawkes C, Jewell J, Allen K. A food policy package for healthy diets and the prevention of obesity and diet-related non-communicable diseases: The NOURISHING framework. *Obesity Reviews.* 2013;14:159–68.
5. Committee on Accelerating Progress in Obesity Prevention, Glickman D, Institute of Medicine. *Accelerating Progress in Obesity Prevention: Solving the Weight of the Nation.* Washington, DC: National Academies Press, 2012.
6. Birch LL, Parker L, Burns A, Institute of Medicine. *Early Childhood Obesity Prevention Policies.* Washington, DC: National Academies Press, 2011.
7. World Health Organization. Comprehensive implementation plan on maternal, infant and young child nutrition. Geneva: World Health Organization, 2014.
8. Roberto CA, Swinburn B, Hawkes C, Huang TTK, Costa SA, Ashe M, et al. Patchy progress on obesity prevention: Emerging examples, entrenched barriers, and new thinking. *The Lancet.* 2015;385(9985):2400–9.
9. Swinburn BA, Sacks G, Hall KD, McPherson K, Finegood DT, Moodie ML, et al. The global obesity pandemic: Shaped by global drivers and local environments. *The Lancet.* 2011;378(9793):804–14.
10. Friel S, Gleeson D, Thow A-M, Labonte R, Stuckler D, Kay A, et al. A new generation of trade policy: Potential risks to diet-related health from the trans pacific partnership agreement. *Globalization and Health.* 2013;9(1):46.
11. World Health Organization. Global strategy for the prevention and control of NCDs. Geneva, Switzerland: World Health Organization, 2000.
12. World Health Organization. Diet, nutrition and the prevention of chronic diseases. WHO Technical Report Series, no. 916. Geneva, Switzerland: World Health Organization, 2003.
13. World Health Organization. Global strategy on diet, physical activity and health. Geneva, Switzerland: World Health Organization, 2004.
15. World Health Organization. School policy framework: Implementation of the WHO Global Strategy on Diet, Physical Activity and Health. Geneva, Switzerland: World Health Organization, 2008.
14. World Health Organization. 2008–2013 Action plan for the global strategy for the prevention and control of noncommunicable diseases. Geneva, Switzerland: World Health Organization, 2008.
16. World Health Organization. Set of recommendations on the marketing of foods and non-alcoholic beverages to children. Geneva, Switzerland: World Health Organization, 2010.
17. UN General Assembly. Political declaration of the High-Level Meeting of the General Assembly on the Prevention and Control of Non-communicable Diseases. New York: United Nations, 2011.
18. World Health Organization. Non-communicable diseases global monitoring framework. Geneva, Switzerland: World Health Organization, 2013.
19. World Health Organization. Global recommendations on physical activity for health: 5–17 years old. Geneva, Switzerland: World Health Organization, 2011.
20. Sacks G, Shill J, Snowdon W, Swinburn B, Armstrong T, Irwin R, et al. Prioritizing areas for action in the field of population-based prevention of childhood obesity. Geneva, Switzerland: World Health Organization, 2012.
21. World Health Organization. Global action plan for the prevention and control of noncommunicable diseases 2013–2020. Geneva, Switzerland: World Health Organization, 2013.

22. Food and Agricultural Organization of the United Nations, World Health Organization. Conference outcome document: Framework for action. Second International Conference on Nutrition. Rome, Italy, 2014.

23. World Health Organization. Resolution WHA63.23. Infant and young child nutrition. Geneva, Switzerland: World Health Organization, 2010.

24. Bell C, Simmons A, Sanigorski A, Kremer P, Swinburn B. Preventing childhood obesity: The sentinel site for obesity prevention in Victoria, Australia. *Health Promotion International*. 2008;23(4):328–6.

25. Swinburn B, Vandevijvere S, Kraak V, Sacks G, Snowdon W, Hawkes C, et al. Monitoring and benchmarking government policies and actions to improve the healthiness of food environments: A proposed Government Healthy Food Environment Policy Index. *Obesity Reviews*. 2013;14(S1):24–37.

26. Dinsdale H, Rutter H. National Child Measurement Programme: Detailed analysis of the 2006/07 national dataset. London: Department of Health, 2008.

27. World Health Organization. Finland curbs childhood obesity by integrating health in all policies. Geneva, Switzerland: World Health Organization, 2015.

28. Colchero MA, Popkin BM, Rivera JA, Ng SW. Beverage purchases from stores in Mexico under the excise tax on sugar sweetened beverages: Observational study. *BMJ*. 2016;352:h6704. http://dx.doi.org/10.1136/bmj.h6704.

29. Instituto nacional de salud publica. Reduction in the consumption of taxed beverages after the implementation of a tax in Mexico. 2015. Available from: http://www.insp.mx/epppo/blog/3666-reduccion-consumo-bebidas.html.

30. Healthy Together Victoria. About Healthy Together Victoria, 2015. http://www.healthytogether.vic.gov.au/.

31. Romon M, Lommez A, Tafflet M, Basdevant A, Oppert JM, Bresson JL, et al. Downward trends in the prevalence of childhood overweight in the setting of 12-year school-and community-based programmes. *Public Health Nutrition*. 2009;12(10):1735–42.

32. Friel S, Hattersley L, Snowdon W, Thow AM, Lobstein T, Sanders D, et al. Monitoring the impacts of trade agreements on food environments. *Obesity Reviews*. 2013;14(S1):120–34.

33. Haddad LJ, Achadi E, Ag Bendech M, Ahuja A, Bhatia K, Bhutta Z, et al. Global nutrition report 2014: Actions and accountability to accelerate the world's progress on nutrition. Washington, DC: International Food Policy Research Institute, 2014.

34. Moodie R, Stuckler D, Monteiro C, Sheron N, Neal B, Thamarangsi T, et al. Profits and pandemics: Prevention of harmful effects of tobacco, alcohol, and ultra-processed food and drink industries. *The Lancet*. 2013;381(9867):670–9.

35. Swinburn B, Kraak V, Rutter H, Vandevijvere S, Lobstein T, Sacks G, et al. Strengthening of accountability systems to create healthy food environments and reduce global obesity. *The Lancet*. 2015;385(9986):2534–45.

36. Stuckler D, Nestle M. Big food, food systems, and global health. *PLoS Medicine*. 2012;9(6):e1001242.

37. Popkin B, Monteiro C, Swinburn B. Overview: Bellagio conference on program and policy options for preventing obesity in the low- and middle-income countries. *Obesity Reviews*. 2013;14:1–8.

38. Huang TT-K, Cawley JH, Ashe M, Costa SA, Frerichs LM, Lindsey Z, et al. Mobilisation of public support for policy actions to prevent obesity. *The Lancet*. 2015;385(9985):2422–31.

39. Brownell KD, Roberto CA. Strategic science with policy impact. *The Lancet*. 2015;385(9986):2445–6.

Index

Printed in the United States
by Baker & Taylor Publisher Services